Disorders of the Central Nervous System: Cognitive Deficits

Disorders of the Central Nervous System: Cognitive Deficits

Editor: Fred Cole

AMERICAN
MEDICAL PUBLISHERS
www.americanmedicalpublishers.com

AMERICAN
MEDICAL PUBLISHERS
www.americanmedicalpublishers.com

Cataloging-in-Publication Data

Disorders of the central nervous system : cognitive deficits / edited by Fred Cole.
p. cm.
Includes bibliographical references and index.
ISBN 978-1-63927-293-8
1. Central nervous system--Diseases. 2. Central nervous system--Abnormalities.
3. Central nervous system--Wounds and injuries. 4. Cognitive neuroscience. I. Cole, Fred.
RC360 .D57 2022
616.8--dc23

American Medical Publishers,
41 Flatbush Avenue,
1st Floor, New York,
NY 11217, USA

ISBN 978-1-63927-293-8 (Hardback)

Contents

Preface IX

Chapter 1 **Simulating real world functioning in schizophrenia using a naturalistic city environment and single-trial, goal-directed navigation** 1
John A. Zawadzki, Todd A. Girard, George Foussias, Alicia Rodrigues, Ishraq Siddiqui, Jason P. Lerch, Cheryl Grady, Gary Remington and Albert H. C. Wong

Chapter 2 **A virtual reality task based on animal research – spatial learning and memory in patients after the first episode of schizophrenia** 11
Iveta Fajnerová, Mabel Rodriguez, David Levčík, Lucie Konrádová, Pavol Mikoláš, Cyril Brom, Aleš Stuchlík, Kamil Vlček and Jiří Horáček

Chapter 3 **Structural hippocampal anomalies in a schizophrenia population correlate with navigation performance on a wayfinding task** 26
Andrée-Anne Ledoux, Patrice Boyer, Jennifer L. Phillips, Alain Labelle, Andra Smith and Véronique D. Bohbot

Chapter 4 **Bridging disparate symptoms of schizophrenia: a triple network dysfunction theory** 36
Tereza Nekovarova, Iveta Fajnerova, Jiri Horacek and Filip Spaniel

Chapter 5 **Tandospirone, a 5-HT_{1A} partial agonist, ameliorates aberrant lactate production in the prefrontal cortex of rats exposed to blockade of N-methy-D-aspartate receptors; toward the therapeutics of cognitive impairment of schizophrenia** 46
Takashi Uehara, Tadasu Matsuoka and Tomiki Sumiyoshi

Chapter 6 **Mismatch negativity and P3a/reorienting complex in subjects with schizophrenia or at-risk mental state** 54
Yuko Higuchi, Tomonori Seo, Tomohiro Miyanishi, Yasuhiro Kawasaki, Michio Suzuki and Tomiki Sumiyoshi

Chapter 7 **Distinct phenotypes of new transmembrane-domain neuregulin 1 mutant mice and the rescue effects of valproate on the observed schizophrenia-related cognitive deficits** 64
Ju-Chun Pei, Chih-Min Liu and Wen-Sung Lai

Chapter 8 **The effect of psilocin on memory acquisition, retrieval, and consolidation in the rat** 84
Lukas Rambousek, Tomas Palenicek, Karel Vales and Ales Stuchlik

Chapter 9 **MK-801 impairs cognitive coordination on a rotating arena (Carousel) and contextual specificity of hippocampal immediate-early gene expression in a rat model of psychosis** 91
Štěpán Kubík, Helena Buchtová, Karel Valeš and Aleš Stuchlík

Chapter 10 **Reduced expression of Nogo-A leads to motivational deficits in rats** **106**
Thomas Enkel, Stefan M. Berger, Kai Schönig, Björn Tews and Dusan Bartsch

Chapter 11 **Nogo-A-deficient transgenic rats show deficits in higher cognitive functions, decreased anxiety, and altered circadian activity patterns** **113**
Tomas Petrasek, Iva Prokopova, Martin Sladek, Kamila Weissova, Iveta Vojtechova, Stepan Bahnik, Anna Zemanova, Kai Schönig, Stefan Berger, Björn Tews, Dusan Bartsch, Martin E. Schwab, Alena Sumova and Ales Stuchlik

Chapter 12 **Low-dose memantine-induced working memory improvement in the allothetic place avoidance alternation task (APAAT) in young adult male rats** **128**
Malgorzata J. Wesierska, Weronika Duda and Colleen A. Dockery

Chapter 13 **Neurosonological examination: a non-invasive approach for the detection of cerebrovascular impairment in AD** **140**
Barbora Urbanova, Ales Tomek, Robert Mikulik, Hana Magerova, Daniel Horinek and Jakub Hort

Chapter 14 **Neural correlates of spatial navigation changes in mild cognitive impairment and Alzheimer's disease** **152**
Kamil Vlček and Jan Laczó

Chapter 15 **Effect of meditation on cognitive functions in context of aging and neurodegenerative diseases** **158**
Rafał Marciniak, Katerina Sheardova, Pavla Čermáková, Daniel Hudeček, Rastislav Šumec and Jakub Hort

Chapter 16 **Pregnanolone glutamate, a novel use-dependent NMDA receptor inhibitor, exerts antidepressant-like properties in animal models** **166**
Kristina Holubova, Tereza Nekovarova, Jana Pistovcakova, Alexandra Sulcova, Ales Stuchlík and Karel Vales

Chapter 17 **Common mechanisms of pain and depression: are antidepressants also analgesics?** **176**
Tereza Nekovarova, Anna Yamamotova, Karel Vales, Ales Stuchlik, Jitka Fricova and Richard Rokyta

Chapter 18 **Spatial reversal learning in chronically sensitized rats and in undrugged sensitized rats with dopamine D2-like receptor agonist quinpirole** **188**
Hana Hatalova, Dominika Radostova, Adela Pistikova, Karel Vales and Ales Stuchlik

Chapter 19 **Consequences of early postnatal benzodiazepines exposure in rats. I. Cognitive-like behavior** **200**
Anna Mikulecká, Martin Šubrt, Aleš Stuchlík and Hana Kubová

Chapter 20 **Dynamic learning and memory, synaptic plasticity and neurogenesis: an update** **209**
Ales Stuchlik

Chapter 21 **Consequences of early postnatal benzodiazepines exposure in rats. II. Social behavior** **215**
Anna Mikulecká, Martin Šubrt, Martina Pařízková, Pavel Mareš and Hana Kubová

Chapter 22 **Links between circadian rhythms and psychiatric disease** ... **226**
Ilia N. Karatsoreos

Chapter 23 **Does sleep improve memory organization?** ... **231**
Masashi Takeuchi, Hisakazu Furuta, Tomiki Sumiyoshi, Michio Suzuki, Yoko Ochiai, Munehito Hosokawa, Mie Matsui and Masayoshi Kurachi

Permissions

List of Contributors

Index

Preface

This book has been an outcome of determined endeavour from a group of educationists in the field. The primary objective was to involve a broad spectrum of professionals from diverse cultural background involved in the field for developing new researches. The book not only targets students but also scholars pursuing higher research for further enhancement of the theoretical and practical applications of the subject.

The portion of the nervous system which is composed of the spinal cord and the brain is termed as central nervous system. It assembles the received information and coordinates the actions of all the parts of the body in most of the multicellular animals. The disorders of the central nervous system encompass early-onset neurological disorders, infections, late-onset neurodegenerative diseases, tumors, genetic disorders, etc. A few of them are addiction, attention deficit/hyperactivity disorder (ADHD), brain tumors, encephalitis, Alzheimer's and Parkinson's. The treatment of the disorders of the central nervous system can consist of medications, neural rehabilitation and surgery. This book aims to shed light on some of the unexplored aspects of the disorders of the nervous system. It will also provide interesting topics for research which interested readers can take up. Researchers and students in this field will be assisted by this book.

It was an honour to edit such a profound book and also a challenging task to compile and examine all the relevant data for accuracy and originality. I wish to acknowledge the efforts of the contributors for submitting such brilliant and diverse chapters in the field and for endlessly working for the completion of the book. Last, but not the least; I thank my family for being a constant source of support in all my research endeavours.

Editor

1

Simulating real world functioning in schizophrenia using a naturalistic city environment and single-trial, goal-directed navigation

John A. Zawadzki[1,2], Todd A. Girard[3], George Foussias[1,2,4], Alicia Rodrigues[2,5], Ishraq Siddiqui[1,2], Jason P. Lerch[6,7], Cheryl Grady[8,9], Gary Remington[1,2,4] and Albert H. C. Wong[1,2,4]*

[1] *Institute of Medical Science, University of Toronto, ON, Canada*
[2] *Centre for Addiction and Mental Health, Campbell Family Mental Health Research Institute, Toronto, ON, Canada*
[3] *Department of Psychology, Ryerson University, Toronto, ON, Canada*
[4] *Department of Psychiatry, University of Toronto, ON, Canada*
[5] *Collaborative Program in Neuroscience, University of Toronto, ON, Canada*
[6] *Department of Medical Biophysics, University of Toronto, ON, Canada*
[7] *Program in Neuroscience and Mental Health, The Hospital for Sick Children, Toronto, ON, Canada*
[8] *Departments of Psychology and Psychiatry, University of Toronto, ON, Canada*
[9] *Rotman Research Institute at Baycrest, Toronto, ON, Canada*

Edited by:
Ales Stuchlik, Academy of Sciences of the Czech Republic, Czech Republic

***Correspondence:**
Albert H. C. Wong, Centre for Addiction and Mental Health, Campbell Family Mental Health Research Institute, 250 College St., Room 323, Toronto, ON M5T 1R8, Canada
e-mail: albert.wong@utoronto.ca

Objective: To develop a virtual reality platform that would serve as a functionally meaningful measure of cognition in schizophrenia and that would also complement standard batteries of cognitive tests during clinical trials for cognitive treatments in schizophrenia, be amenable to human neuroimaging research, yet lend itself to neurobiological comparison with rodent analogs.

Method: Thirty-three patients with schizophrenia and 33 healthy controls matched for age, sex, video gaming experience, and education completed eight rapid, single-trial virtual navigation tasks within a naturalistic virtual city. Four trials tested their ability to find different targets seen during the passive viewing of a closed path that led them around different city blocks. Four subsequent trials tested their ability to return to four different starting points after viewing a path that took them several blocks away from the starting position.

Results: Individuals with schizophrenia had difficulties in way-finding, measured as distance travelled to find targets previously encountered within the virtual city. They were also more likely not to notice the target during passive viewing, less likely to find novel shortcuts to targets, and more likely to become lost and fail completely in finding the target. Total travel distances across all eight trials strongly correlated (negatively) with neurocognitive measures and, for 49 participants who completed the Quality of Life Scale, psychosocial functioning.

Conclusion: Single-trial, goal-directed navigation in a naturalistic virtual environment is a functionally meaningful measure of cognitive functioning in schizophrenia.

Keywords: schizophrenia, cognition, psychosocial functioning, virtual reality, navigation

INTRODUCTION

Schizophrenia is a chronic mental illness presenting with psychotic symptoms of delusions and hallucinations against a background of neurocognitive impairment, poor motivation, and poor psychosocial functioning (Heinrichs and Zakzanis, 1998; Wong et al., 2003). Cognitive deficits are a significant predictor of functional outcome (Green, 1996; Harvey et al., 1998; Green et al., 2000, 2004), and are current targets for psychopharmacological treatment (Hyman and Fenton, 2003).

A number of neuropsychological tests assess cognitive domains that are particularly impaired in schizophrenia (Nuechterlein et al., 2004). These have been incorporated into a standard battery of cognitive tests for use in clinical trials by the Measurement and Treatment Research to Improve Cognition in Schizophrenia (MATRICS) initiative (Nuechterlein et al., 2008). In order to provide tools for clinical trial evaluation, the Cognitive Neuroscience Treatment Research to Improve Cognition in Schizophrenia (CNTRICS) initiative identified additional tests from cognitive neuroscience literature that are sensitive to schizophrenia (Barch et al., 2009). However, the US Food and Drug Administration stipulates a requirement for a functionally meaningful measure of overall outcome in addition to an accepted battery of cognitive tests for clinical trials for cognitive treatments in schizophrenia (Green et al., 2011).

Goal-directed navigation offers a powerful paradigm for studying neural system interactions during complex human behaviors (Spiers and Maguire, 2006). Rodent models have detailed the neurobiology of various cognitive processes including perception, motivation, planning, and decision making at molecular, cellular, and systems level analysis (Burgess, 2008; Moser et al., 2008; Penner and Mizumori, 2012). The neurotransmitter dopamine, an important target in schizophrenia research (Laruelle and Abi-Dargham, 1999), plays a dominant role in the modulation of the neuroanatomical structures and networks engaged in rodent navigation (Penner and Mizumori, 2012).

Several core brain regions involved in successful goal-directed navigation in humans (Aguirre et al., 1996; Wolbers et al., 2004; Wolbers and Hegarty, 2010) including the hippocampus, prefrontal cortex and striatum (Maguire et al., 1998; Astur et al., 2002; Driscoll et al., 2003; Ekstrom et al., 2003; Hartley et al., 2003; Iaria et al., 2003; Bohbot et al., 2004; Voermans et al., 2004; Spiers and Maguire, 2006; Doeller et al., 2008; Brown et al., 2012), are also strongly implicated in the pathophysiology of schizophrenia (Weinberger et al., 1986; Goldberg et al., 1987; Weinberger, 1987; Bogerts et al., 1990; Csernansky et al., 1999; Laruelle and Abi-Dargham, 1999). Optimum navigation is associated with the ability to flexibly switch between hippocampal and striatal networks (Hartley et al., 2003; Iaria et al., 2003; Etchamendy and Bohbot, 2007) and to integrate wayfinding networks with prefrontal cortex working memory (Wolbers et al., 2007; Hanlon et al., 2012) and executive functions (Maguire et al., 1998; Hartley et al., 2003). The virtual reality (VR) navigation paradigms used for schizophrenia research, by focusing on specific neural structures or cognitive domains, have tended to be based on rodent models or necessarily circumscribed environments within a paradigm of trial and error learning or extensive exploratory activity prior to testing to ensure familiarity with landmark locations (Astur et al., 2004; Hanlon et al., 2006, 2012; Weniger and Irle, 2008; Folley et al., 2010; Spieker et al., 2012).

Table 1 | Patients with schizophrenia were individually matched with healthy controls for age (within 4 years), sex, and video gaming experience (within 1 level of difference).

	Age		Gaming experience		Education		WAIS-III pro-rated FSIQ	
	SZ	HC	SZ	HC	SZ	HC	SZ	HC
Mean	40	39	0.8	0.7	4.1	4.2	107	116
Median	43	43	0	1	4	4	108	116
Standard deviation	10.9	11.3	1.3	0.9	0.9	1.0	17.8	14.0
Range	21–54	21–55	0–4	0–4	2–5	2–5	78–137	91–145

As a group they were also matched for education. HC, healthy controls; SZ, patients with schizophrenia; FSIQ, pro-rated full scale IQ. Gaming experience: 0 = never, 1 = a few times per year, 2 = a few times per month, 3 = a few times per week; 4 = daily; Education: 1 = less than high school, 2 = some high school, 3 = completed high school, 4 = some post-secondary, 5 = completed post-secondary.

We sought to extend this work by designing a more realistic human VR task that would assess goal-directed navigation in a naturalistic city environment. In addition, rather than using a multiple-trial incremental learning paradigm, we developed a single-trial paradigm more analogous to daily events such as going to a shopping mall and trying to find the shop you spotted on your way to the drug store or trying to find your way back to your parked car. Here we report on the results of the behavioral testing of performance by patients with schizophrenia using a single-trial navigation paradigm in a naturalistic virtual city.

MATERIALS AND METHODS

PARTICIPANTS

All experiments were conducted with the approval of our institutional research ethics board. Informed consent was obtained from all participants. Diagnosis was based on the Mini International Neuropsychiatric Inventory (MINI) (Sheehan et al., 1998) which enables diagnosis based on DSM-IV. Thirty-three outpatients diagnosed with schizophrenia ($n = 22$) or schizoaffective disorder ($n = 11$) and on stable doses of antipsychotics for the preceding 4 weeks took part in this study. All patients were chronically ill with durations of illness ranging from 2 to 39 years ($M = 15$, median $= 11.5$). Thirty-three healthy controls were individually matched with patients for age, sex (total 42 male, 24 female), and experience with first person action computer games. As a group, patients, and controls were also matched in education (**Table 1**).

Patients were recruited from the Center for Addiction and Mental Health, Toronto, Canada. Healthy controls were recruited by advertisements within the local community. Exclusion criteria for healthy controls were—no personal or family history of psychiatric dysfunction; for patients—no other DSM-IV Axis I disorder. Inclusion/exclusion criteria for both groups were: (1) 18–55 years of age; (2) no history of substance abuse in the past 3 months; (3) no history of neurological disease or loss of consciousness longer than 15 min; (4) a Wechsler Adult Intelligence Scale-III (WAIS-III) (Wechsler, 1997) prorated full scale IQ score greater than 75; and, (5) fluency in English.

CLINICAL AND NEUROPSYCHOLOGICAL ASSESSMENT

Current positive and negative symptoms were assessed by using the Scales for the Assessment of Positive Symptoms (SAPS) and Negative Symptoms (SANS) (Andreasen, 1983, 1984). General intellectual ability was assessed using four subscales (vocabulary, similarities, block design, and matrix reasoning) of the WAIS-III (Wechsler, 1997), prorated to obtain estimated full scale IQ scores (Schrimsher et al., 2008). Participants also completed the Repeatable Battery for the Assessment of Neuropsychological Status (RBANS; Randolph, 1998). Education level was classified along five categories: "less-than-high-school," "some high school," "completed high school," "some post-secondary," and, "completed-post- secondary." Forty-nine of the participants in this study (twenty-five with schizophrenia and twenty-four healthy controls) participated in a concurrent study that used the Quality of Life Scale (Heinrichs et al., 1984) to evaluate current psychosocial status. Those results were incorporated into this study. Clinical evaluations were completed during one session, typically 1–2 weeks prior to a single session of cognitive, and navigation trials.

VIRTUAL REALITY ENVIRONMENT

The VR environment consisted of a 6 x 6 block cityscape with a central park and over 80 residential, commercial, institutional, and office buildings. Embedded within the city were various "targets" such as a playground and hospital (**Figures 1**, **2**). The environment included distal cues to aid in orienting such as a mountain range along one boundary, a hot air balloon, and a tall radio tower. Participants used a video game controller with simple forward/reverse and left/right levers to navigate. A 5 min practice session of free navigation before the beginning of trials, restricted to an area of the virtual city not used during subsequent trials, ensured familiarity with controller operations.

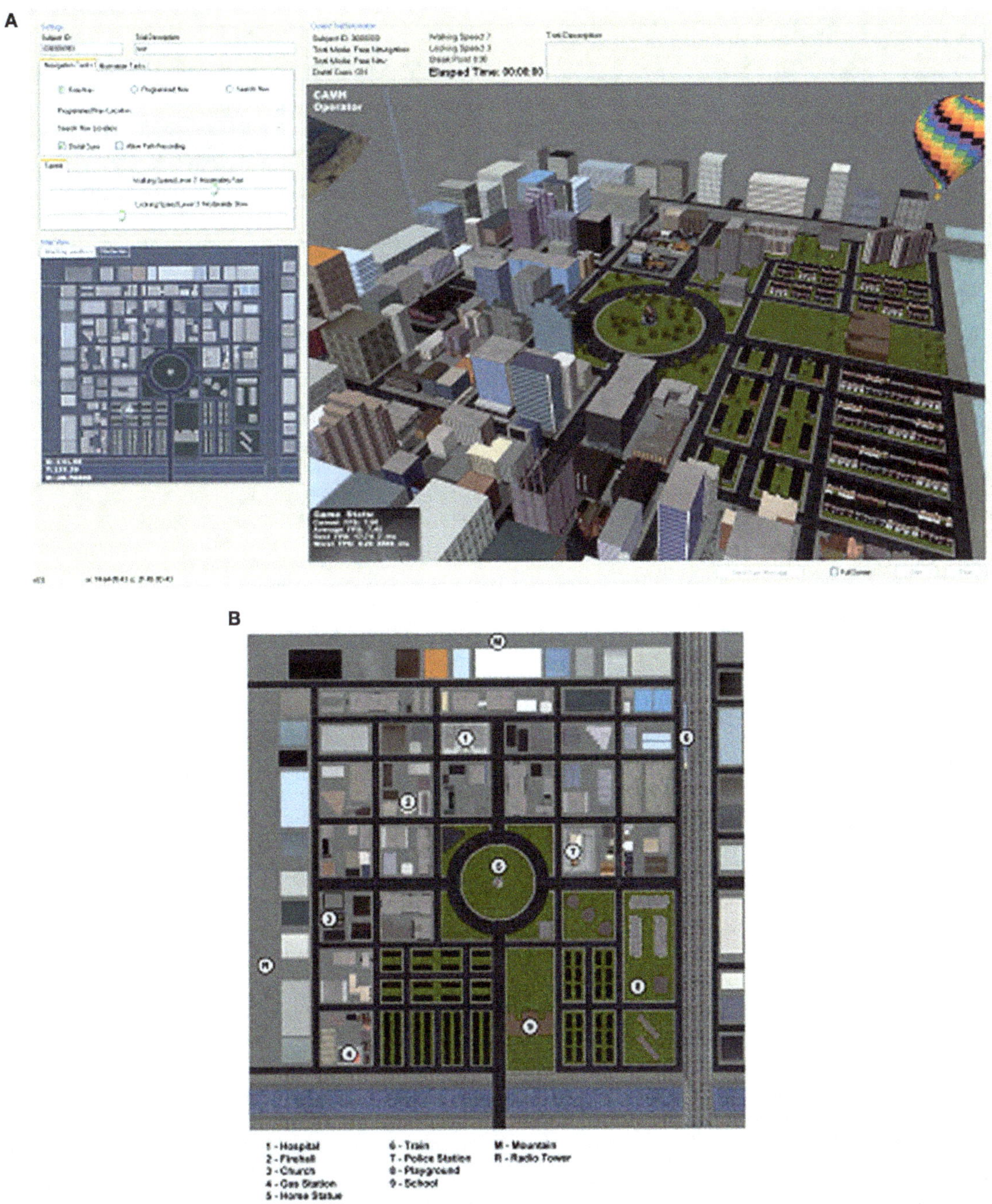

FIGURE 1 | Virtual city. (A) Screen shot of the VR software operator showing an aerial map view of the virtual city and a 3-D isometric projection of the 6 × 6 block city. **(B)** Detailed aerial view showing the location of a few landmarks. These views were not seen by the participants.

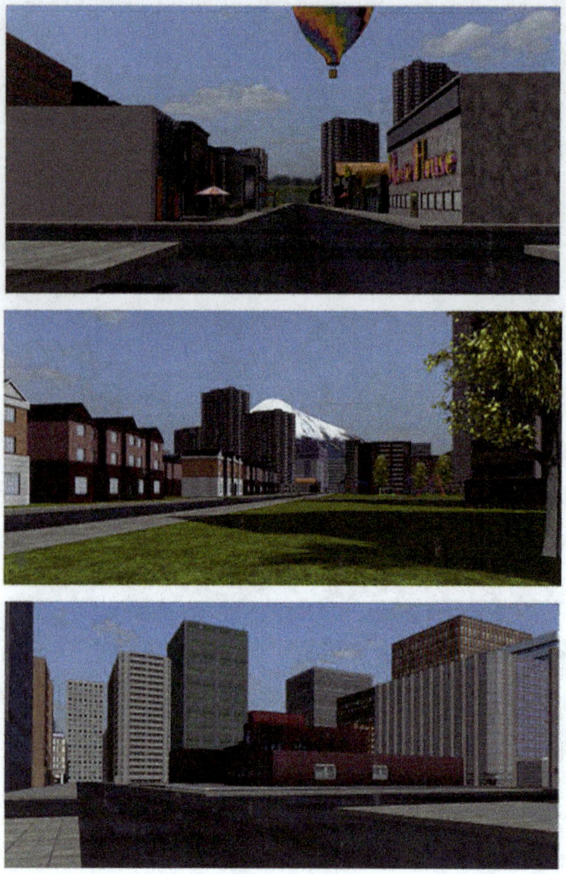

FIGURE 2 | Virtual city. Examples of subject views of the environment are shown.

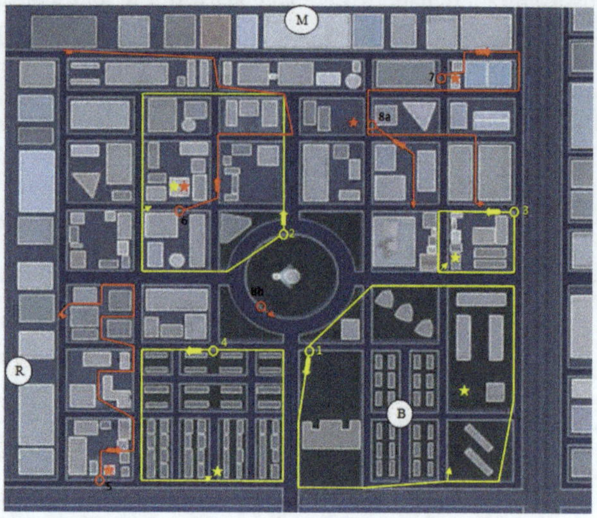

FIGURE 3 | Prerecorded paths viewed by participants during the passive viewing of each trial. Shown is the aerial view of each path. During eye-level passive viewing the paths shown in yellow (four closed loop paths numbered according to order of presentation) and red (four return paths, similarly ordered) were followed by the participant starting at the open circle. For the closed loop trials the star represents the target and the small arrow pointing to the target indicates the position along the path where path movement temporarily halted and attention was directed toward the target for 2–3 s before proceeding to the end of the path. For the return path trials the star represents the target focused on at the start of the trial and the small arrow at the end of the path the direction of view at the end of the prerecorded path. At the end of the passive viewing portion of each trial the participant was asked to locate the target using the shortest route they could think of, beginning where the passive viewing portion ended. 8a represents the passive viewing portion of trial 8, ending at a position affording a view of the overhead balloon (B) and radio tower (R); 8b represents the starting position, facing the overhead balloon, for the subsequent attempt, during trial 8, by the participant to return to the starting position at 8a. M, mountain range.

NAVIGATION TRIALS

A total of eight different navigation trials were carried out, each within different areas of the VR city. Each trial commenced with passive viewing of a pre-recorded path taken along several blocks of the virtual city, followed by a single attempt by the participant to locate a target shown during the passive viewing portion of the trial. The first four trials assessed participant ability to find a target seen during the passive viewing of a closed path that led them in a loop around one or more city blocks ("closed-loop" trials, **Figure 3**). The second four trials assessed participant ability to return to a starting point after viewing a path that took them a few blocks away from the starting position ("return-path" trials, **Figure 3**). All trials were presented in the same fixed random order to all participants.

For all trials, participants were instructed to take the shortest route possible to find the targets. Participants were asked to confirm that they had noticed the target immediately after passive viewing in each of the trials. Targets were typically focused on for 2–3 s during path viewing. Those who failed to see the target were allowed to view the pre-recorded path a second time. For those who failed to find the target, distances travelled were measured as total distances travelled until the participant admitted being lost and gave up further searching.

Each of the navigation trials took approximately 2–5 min to complete. Completion of all 8 trials ranged from a low of 15 min to a high of 60 min with an overall average of 30 min for patients and 22 min for controls.

HARDWARE AND SOFTWARE

The VR environment was rendered and presented on the testing computer to participants using an advanced graphics workstation and a 30′ widescreen LCD display. A separate computer, connected via a local area network to the testing computer, controlled task settings for each trial. The scene assets for the 3D virtual city were created in Maya and Adobe Photoshop. The simulation was rendered using Ogre, an open source 3D graphics engine. Data on distance travelled, time on task, and path directions travelled were stored automatically throughout the trials, and a video recording of the path followed by participants was made during each trial.

STATISTICAL ANALYSES

Success at finding targets or returning to original starting positions was measured as the distance travelled to find the target or return to origin. Non-parametric statistics were used because all trials showed non-normal distributions in total distances travelled, with Shapiro-Wilk statistics typically significant at $p < 0.01$. The two matched samples were compared using the Wilcoxon Signed-ranks test (SRT) which yields a Z-statistic. Corresponding effect sizes were calculated as the SRT Z-value divided by the square root of sample size. Correlation analysis (Spearman's rho) was used to assess the relationships between distances travelled across all eight trials and scores on clinical (SAPS/SANS), cognitive (WAIS-III and RBANS), and psychosocial functioning (Quality of Life) measures. A logistic regression was undertaken to determine the role played by VR performance (distance travelled) in predicting group membership as compared to cognitive testing (RBANS total score, prorated WAIS-III full scale IQ), and psychosocial functioning (total score on the Quality of Life Scale). Pearson's r was used to assess relationships between normally distributed cognitive and clinical symptom scores. Correlations between task performance (distance travelled) and cognitive tests (RBANS, pro-rated WAIS-III full scale IQ) as well as the Quality of Life Scale scores were conducted on all subjects. Regression analysis of task performance with cognitive and psychosocial tests similarly represents all subjects. Correlations with clinical tests (SAPS/SANS) were conducted only on patients. Results were evaluated at an alpha-level of 0.05. SPSS v13.0 was used for the statistical analysis.

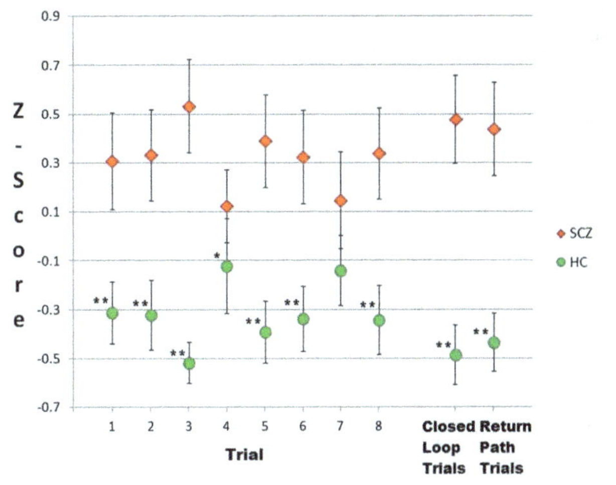

FIGURE 4 | Individuals with schizophrenia travelled further to find targets in a virtual city than healthy controls. Shown are the standardized distances (z-scores) travelled across each of eight trials. Group means and standard errors are illustrated. Trials 1–4 = closed loop trials; trials 5–8 = return path trials. Asterisks represent between-group comparisons; $^*p \leq 0.05$; $^{**}p < 0.01$.

RESULTS

In order to compare performances across trials, distances travelled were standardized by conversion to z-scores (**Figure 4**). A Friedman test of the four closed-loop trials indicated that there were no significant differences in difficulty between the trials for either schizophrenia [$\chi^2_{(3)} = 0.82$, $p = 0.85$] or control subjects [$\chi^2_{(3)} = 3.22$, $p = 0.37$]. Similarly, a Friedman test of the four return-path trials showed no significant differences in difficulty for either schizophrenia [$\chi^2_{(3)} = 2.56$, $p = 0.47$] or healthy participants [$\chi^2_{(3)} = 7.01$, $p = 0.07$]. Distances across each of the four trials were therefore added together for a composite distance travelled score for the closed-loop and return-path trials. Across the four closed-loop trials, patients travelled significantly further (median = 9564) than their matched healthy controls (median = 5467), $Z = -4.05$, $p < 0.001$, $r = 0.50$ (**Table 2**). Across the four return-path trials the patient group again travelled significantly further (median = 19,214) than controls (median = 12,579), $Z = -3.58$, $p < 0.001$, $r = 0.44$ (**Table 2**). **Figure 5** illustrates, using one of the closed loop trials, differences between the two groups' path trajectories based on the representative median for each group.

The time parameter had similar results. Across the four closed-loop trials, patients took significantly longer in their attempts to find their targets (median = 8.3 min., range = 2.6–20.4 min.) than their matched healthy controls (median = 4.4 min., range = 1.9–14.5 min.), $Z = -3.92$, $p < 0.001$, $r = 0.48$. Across the four return-path trials the patient group again took significantly longer (median = 13.2 min, range = 5.0–38.0 min.) than controls (median = 8.5 min., range = 4.0–22.0 min.), $Z = -3.23$, $p < 0.001$, $r = 0.40$.

Twenty-three of the pre-recorded portions of the trials were repeated a second time because thirteen individuals with schizophrenia and three healthy controls reported failure to notice targets during passive viewing—a statistically significant difference between groups, $\chi^2_{(1, n=66)} = 8.25$, $p = 0.004$, phi = − 0.35. Twenty-nine individuals with schizophrenia were unable to find at least one of the eight targets (median = 2, range = 0–6) compared to twenty healthy controls (median = 1, range = 0–4); a statistically significant difference as measured by a Wilcoxon SRT, $Z = -4.21$, $p < 0.001$, $r = -0.52$. Healthy controls were more likely to use shortcuts during wayfinding to locate targets than individuals with schizophrenia. Thirty healthy controls were able to find the shortcut for at least one of the trials (median = 3 trials) compared to twenty-two individuals with schizophrenia (median = 1 trial), a statistically significant difference as measured by a Wilcoxon SRT, $Z = -3.82$, $p < 0.001$, $r = -0.47$.

Although patients diagnosed with schizoaffective disorder travelled numerically shorter distances to find targets (median = 15,875, range = 8,490–27,409) than patients diagnosed with schizophrenia (median = 21,492, range = 13,523–51,901) the differences, measured by Mann Whitney U, were not statistically significant, $Z = -1.53$, $p = 0.13$. Similarly, there were no significant differences in the number of targets not found, the number of shortcuts used and the number of prerecorded portions of trials that had to be repeated because of failure to notice targets during passive viewing.

Total target-finding distances across all eight trials were significantly and negatively correlated with RBANS total score (rho = − 0.48, $p < 0.001$) and the WAIS III pro-rated full scale IQ (rho = − 0.40, $p < 0.001$). Moreover, the differences in standardized z-scores between individuals with schizophrenia and controls in our goal-directed navigation task were as robust as RBANS total scores and almost double that of estimated full scale IQ (**Table 2**). However, as shown in **Table 2**, there was

Table 2 | A comparison of mean differences between patient and control groups illustrates the ability of goal-directed navigation to obtain results similar to that of standard neurocognitive measures.

	SCZ		HC		Difference in group means(a)
	Mean	*SD*	Mean	*SD*	
NAVIGATION TRIALS					
1–4 total	10,328	4611	6029	3128	– 0.96
5–8 total	20,856	8606	14,115	5350	– 0.86
1–8 total	31,185	11,045	20,143	7065	– 1.03
RBANS					
Immediate memory	92	20	105	14	– 0.71
Visuospatial/Constructional	86	17	104	15	– 0.95
Language	94	13	101	14	– 0.53
Attention	89	18	104	14	– 0.88
Delayed memory	88	17	101	8	– 0.91
Total	86	15	105	14	– 1.08
WAIS-III					
Pro-rated verbal IQ	109	21	113	14	– 0.27
Pro-rated performance IQ	105	18	116	16	– 0.63
Pro-rated full scale IQ	107	18	116	14	– 0.54

Distances are expressed in virtual units wherein 500 units = approximately 1 virtual block; N = 66; (a) = scores were standardized prior to group comparisons; HC, healthy controls; SCZ, individuals with schizophrenia. For consistency, all variables were scored such that (–) differences represent a schizophrenia-related deficit.

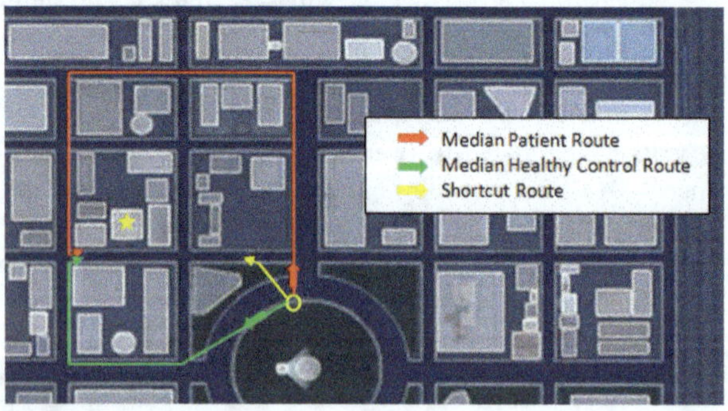

FIGURE 5 | Individuals with schizophrenia used longer routes to find targets than healthy controls. Shown are the median distances travelled and their respective routes by patients and healthy controls for closed loop trial #2. The target, identified by the yellow star, is a fire hall. The yellow circle marks the trial start position. Participants unable to recognize a shortcut route typically attempted to retrace the forward path seen during passive viewing or attempted a reverse path to the target. Errors typically occurred when individuals failed to turn at the proper intersection.

some variation across individual indices, with RBANS z-scores for group differences ranging from 0.53 (language) to 0.95 (visualspatial/construction) and WAIS-III performance deficits more than double the effect-size for verbal. These results highlight the importance of assessing visual-spatial abilities in schizophrenia and that our task is at least as sensitive to detecting cognitive deficits as the standardized batteries.

Spearman correlations of distances travelled by individuals with schizophrenia to find targets and clinical symptoms, as measured by SAPS/SANS were non-significant: SAPS (rho = −0.17); SANS (rho = −0.01). Correlations between clinical symptoms and cognitive scores were weak for SAPS (RBANS, $r = 0.10$; WAIS FSIQ, $r = 0.004$) to moderate for SANS (RBANS, $r = -0.26$; WAIS FSIQ, $r = -0.31$). Spearman correlations of distances travelled by individuals with schizophrenia to find targets and antipsychotic medications, computed as chlorpromazine equivalents, were non-significant, rho = −0.06. For the 49 individuals in this study that also completed the Quality of Life scale (25 with schizophrenia, 24 healthy controls), distances travelled across all eight trials correlated negatively with total score results (rho = −0.37, $p = 0.009$); i.e., longer travel distances correlated with lower psychosocial functioning. The correlation between distances travelled and psychosocial function was largely, but not completely, reflective of group differences.

A logistic regression analysis was conducted to predict group membership (schizophrenia or healthy control) using distance travelled, RBANS total score, pro-rated WAIS full scale IQ, and Quality of Life total score as predictors. A test of the full model against a constant only model was statistically significant, indicating that the predictors as a set reliably distinguished between individuals with schizophrenia and healthy controls (chi square = 40.49, $p < 0.001$). Nagelkerke's R^2 of 0.750 indicated a moderately strong relationship between prediction and grouping. Prediction success overall was 83.7% (84% for schizophrenia, 83.3% for healthy controls). The Wald criterion demonstrated that only Quality of Life (Wald = 8.45) and distance travelled (Wald = 6.67) made significant contribution to prediction ($p = 0.004$, $p = 0.01$, respectively). Neither pro-rated WAIS full scale IQ (Wald = 1.24) nor RBANS (Wald = 2.72) made significant contributions ($p = 0.23$, $p = 0.1$., respectively). Running the model using only Quality of Life and distance travelled as predictors provided an overall prediction success rate of 81.6% (80% for schizophrenia and 83.3% for healthy controls).

DISCUSSION

The present study investigated the ability of people with schizophrenia to return to a starting position or accurately find a target within a naturalistic virtual cityscape after a single exposure to the target while passively viewing a path taken within the virtual environment. Individuals with schizophrenia had significantly more difficulty than healthy controls matched for age, sex, gaming experience, and education during these rapid, single-trial navigation tasks. Patients travelled significantly further than controls, were less likely to find novel shortcuts to targets, and were more likely to fail in finding the target. Although patients were also more likely to fail to notice the target during passive viewing, the above difficulties persisted even after the passive viewing segments of the trials were repeated to ensure participants saw the relevant target.

Both types of trials posed equal levels of difficulty for individuals with schizophrenia compared to healthy controls and were as effective as RBANS and WAIS III prorated full scale IQ in separating patient from control performance (**Table 2**). Navigation distance on our task also significantly correlated (negatively) with RBANS total score and the WAIS III pro-rated full scale IQ. We also found that navigation performance across trials was significantly inversely correlated with psychosocial functioning. Logistic regression demonstrated that of the three cognitive variables—distance travelled, RBANS and pro-rated WAIS full scale IQ, only distance travelled made a significant contribution to predicting group membership in a model that included Quality of Life self reports. The combination of Quality of Life self reports and distances travelled demonstrated an overall prediction of group membership success rate of 81.6%. Green and colleagues, in their study of meaningful measures of functioning for use in clinical trials (Green et al., 2011) considered both performance-based and interview-based measures as potential coprimary measures. These results would suggest that a combination of the two might be the more effective strategy.

With respect to clinical symptoms, SANS scores were moderately and SAPS scores weakly correlated with cognitive performance, while correlations between distance travelled and clinical symptoms were non-significant. Schizophrenia symptom correlations with cognitive performance have tended to be inconsistent, but generally minimal for positive symptoms and modest for negative or disorganized symptoms (Gold, 2004; Keefe et al., 2006). The relative independence of cognitive impairment from psychotic symptoms, combined with the presence of cognitive problems before symptom onset (David et al., 1997; Cornblatt et al., 1999; Reichenberg et al., 2002; Niendam et al., 2003; Khandaker et al., 2011; Dickson et al., 2012) and strong relationship to functional outcome (Green, 1996; Harvey et al., 1998; Green et al., 2000, 2004), support the recent focus on cognitive impairment as a unique target for treatment (Hyman and Fenton, 2003).

However, cognitive deficits in schizophrenia are broad and display significant heterogeneity (Joyce and Roiser, 2007). Various factor analytic studies have demonstrated a high level of interrelatedness for domains found to be impaired in schizophrenia (Gladsjo et al., 2004; Dickinson et al., 2006; Keefe et al., 2006; Dickinson and Harvey, 2009). These observations are consistent with the argument that schizophrenia may be a neurodevelopmental disorder (Weinberger, 1987; Seidman, 1990; Lewis and Levitt, 2002) characterized by disturbed functional connectivity (Weinberger et al., 1992; Friston and Frith, 1995; Bullmore et al., 1997; Friston, 1999; Meyer-Lindenberg et al., 2001; Stephan et al., 2006, 2009; Garrity et al., 2007; Liu et al., 2008; Ellison-Wright and Bullmore, 2009; Rotarska-Jagiela et al., 2010). While separate tests for different cognitive domains have shown to be effective for identifying localized dysfunctional areas in the brain, they may not be adequate for understanding functional coordination difficulties. Indeed, the growing use of neuroimaging methodologies such as functional magnetic resonance imaging has led to an increased awareness and emphasis on neural circuits or systems implicated in schizophrenia rather than traditional neuropsychological taxonomies (Minzenberg and Carter, 2012; Gold and Dickinson, 2013).

To the best of our knowledge, all the virtual navigation studies in schizophrenia have used a necessarily constrained paradigm of place learning using rodent models such as the Morris water maze (Morris et al., 1982; Astur et al., 2004; Hanlon et al., 2006, 2012; Folley et al., 2010) and radial arm maze (Olton and Samuelson, 1976; Spieker et al., 2012) or circumscribed environments such as a virtual park (Weniger and Irle, 2008) and virtual town (Ledoux et al., 2013). These were designed to test specific neural structures, principally the hippocampus, and/or specific cognitive domains, such as allocentric memory (Weniger and Irle, 2008; Folley et al., 2010), working and reference memory (Spieker et al., 2012), working and relational memory (Hanlon et al., 2012), and episodic memory (Ledoux et al., 2013). These studies were typically based on a multiple-trial learning paradigm where performance is measured across repetitive trial and error attempts to find one or more game-like rewards, or required extensive exploratory navigation prior to testing to ensure familiarity with all the landmarks subsequently used as targets.

When combined with brain imaging these simplified navigation environments are capable of uncovering dysfunctional circuitry associated with other neural structures and networks in schizophrenia. For example, Astur et al. (2004), in addition to finding reduced hippocampal activation in schizophrenia, also found altered cingulate, insular, and prefrontal cortex activations during virtual navigation. Folley et al. (2010) found anomalous patterns in four widely distributed neural circuits. Hanlon et al. (2012) found lower frontotemporal anatomical connectivity using diffusion tensor imaging. Hanlon et al. (2012) also found that longer path lengths to find the submerged platform in the Morris water maze predicted lower everyday functioning as measured by the UCSD Performance-Based Skills Assessment (UPSA; Patterson et al., 2001). However, the Morris water maze or radial arm maze might not be considered functionally meaningful tests of overall outcome for human clinical trial testing. In addition, Folley et al. (2010), using the virtual Morris water maze, found that impaired performance for both the hidden and exposed platforms was associated with negative symptom severity, suggesting possible motivation difficulties by patients using their paradigm based on a rodent task.

Although not a study of schizophrenia, Spiers and Maguire (2006), using a very realistic model of downtown London (UK) and a single-trial challenge, were able to demonstrate that human goal-directed navigation is not simply a hippocampal place learning phenomenon but rather, a "complex choreography of neural dynamics." Their model, however, required extensive previous driving experience within this particular city environment.

Our study builds upon these prior findings in presenting a paradigm based on a single-trial attempt at finding typical urban facilities previously seen and located within different areas of a novel realistic virtual city. Each of the four closed-loop trials could be viewed as somewhat similar to trying to find the shortcut to the recreational facility spotted while a passenger during a round trip shopping excursion. Each of the return-path trials were somewhat similar to finding the shortest way back home after being driven to a doctor's appointment. The trial designs of this study have been shown to be as effective as the navigation paradigms used to-date in schizophrenia research in identifying poor functional performance by individuals with schizophrenia and have demonstrated significant correlations with neuropsychological testing and functional outcome. In addition they represent a meaningful test of every day functioning and were judged by most participants as engaging and challenging. The lack of correlation between distance travelled and SANS scores are consistent with these self-reports, and that, unlike the Folley et al. (2010) results based on the virtual Morris water maze, decreased motivation to perform was not apparent during our more naturalistic virtual environment. It should be noted, however, that Hanlon et al. (2012), also using the virtual Morris water maze, found no evidence of amotivation in their results.

The results of these trials support the use of single-trial goal-directed navigation in a naturalistic virtual environment as a measure of cognitive functioning with specific, real life consequences (e.g., getting lost). Future applications will verify successful replication of the task findings, including among subsamples other than the high-functioning patients used here, and more directly explore both specific and global neurocognitive mechanisms accounting for impaired performance among patients. For clinical trial use, the four closed loop trials would appear to be adequate in assessing cognitive functioning, thereby reducing overall trial durations to an average of 15 min plus 5 min for practice and explanation of procedure. In addition, the amenability of this tool in neuroimaging studies in humans and cross referencing results with those of rodent studies will aid in uncovering the aetiology and pathophysiology of schizophrenia.

AUTHOR CONTRIBUTIONS

Albert H. C. Wong and Todd A. Girard designed the study and wrote the original protocol. John A. Zawadzki and Jason P. Lerch refined the protocol. John A. Zawadzki and Alicia Rodrigues recruited the participants, obtained the informed consents, performed the behavioral testing and collected the data. Ishraq Siddiqui completed various VR software refinements. John A. Zawadzki processed the data and undertook the statistical analysis. Todd A. Girard, George Foussias and Cheryl Grady contributed to data interpretation. John A. Zawadzki wrote the first draft of the manuscript. Albert H. C. Wong supervised the study. All authors discussed the results and contributed to the final version of the paper and have approved its final version.

ACKNOWLEDGMENTS

The authors would like to thank the two reviewers whose helpful comments served to improve the quality of the final manuscript. We would also like to thank Sathasan Thavabalasingam, Nasteho Hasan, and Krysta McDonald for their assistance with data collection on this study and Ed Sykes, Bob Jones, Song Ahn, Ian Howatson, Jonathan Eger, and Damian Domagala of the Visualization Design Institute (VDI) of the Sheridan Institute of Technology and Advanced Learning and Darian Segura for their work in developing the VR application. John A. Zawadzki was supported by an Ontario Graduate Scholarship, Ontario Ministry of Training, Colleges and Universities and a Fellowship from the Institute of Medical Sciences, University of Toronto. Albert H. C. Wong was supported by a CIHR Clinician-Scientist Fellowship, a NARSAD Independent Investigator award and an OMHF Mid-career Investigator Fellowship. We would like to thank the Ministry of Health and Long-Term Care (MOHLTC) for supporting this research through the Academic Health Science Center AFP Innovation Fund. This research was also supported by the Canadian Foundation for Innovation (#16014 and #20289), the Ontario Ministry of Research and Innovation, the CAMH Foundation, the Schizophrenia Society of Ontario (Gary Remington and George Foussias) and a CIHR Clinician-Scientist Training Award (George Foussias).

REFERENCES

Aguirre, G. K., Detre, J. A., Alsop, D. C., and Desposito, M. (1996). The parahippocampus subserves topographical learning in man. *Cereb. Cortex* 6, 823–829. doi: 10.1093/cercor/6.6.823

Andreasen, N. C. (1983). *Scale for the Assessment of Negative Symptoms (SANS)*. Iowa City, University of Iowa.

Andreasen, N. C. (1984). *Scale for the Assessment of Positive Symptoms (SAPS)*. Iowa City, University of Iowa.

Astur, R. S., St Germain, S., Mathalon, D. H., D'Souza, D. C., Krystal, J. K., Constable, R. T., et al. (2004). Using virtual reality to investigate functioning of the hippocampus in schizophrenia. *Cyberpsychol. Behav.* 7, 269–269.

Astur, R. S., Taylor, L. B., Mamelak, A. N., Philpott, L., and Sutherland, R. J. (2002). Humans with hippocampus damage display severe spatial memory impairments in a virtual Morris water task. *Behav. Brain Res.* 132, 77–84. doi: 10.1016/S0166-4328(01)00399-0

Barch, D. M., Carter, C. S., Arnsten, A., Buchanan, R. W., Cohen, J. D., Geyer, M., et al. (2009). Selecting paradigms from cognitive neuroscience for translation into use in clinical trials: proceedings of the third CNTRICS meeting. *Schizophr. Bull.* 35, 109–114. doi: 10.1093/schbul/sbn163

Bogerts, B., Ashtari, M., Degreef, G., Alvir, J. M. J., Bilder, R. M., and Lieberman, J. A. (1990). Reduced temporal limbic structure volumes on magnetic-resonance images in 1st episode schizophrenia. *Psychiatry Res.* 35, 1–13. doi: 10.1016/0925-4927(90)90004-P

Bohbot, V. D., Iaria, G., and Petrides, M. (2004). Hippocampal function and spatial memory: evidence from functional neuroimaging in healthy participants and performance of patients with medial temporal lobe resections. *Neuropsychology* 18, 418–425. doi: 10.1037/0894-4105.18.3.418

Brown, T. I., Ross, R. S., Tobyne, S. M., and Stern, C. E. (2012). Cooperative interactions between hippocampal and striatal systems support flexible navigation. *Neuroimage* 60, 1316–1330. doi: 10.1016/j.neuroimage.2012.01.046

Bullmore, E. T., Frangou, S., and Murray, R. M. (1997). The dysplastic net hypothesis: an integration of developmental and dysconnectivity theories of schizophrenia. *Schizophr. Res.* 28, 143–156. doi: 10.1016/S0920-9964(97)00114-X

Burgess, N. (2008). "Spatial cognition and the brain," in *Year in Cognitive Neuroscience 2008*. (Malden, MA: Wiley-Blackwell), 77–97.

Cornblatt, B., Obuchowski, M., Roberts, S., Pollack, S., and Erlenmeyer-Kimling, L. (1999). Cognitive and behavioral precursors of schizophrenia. *Dev. Psychopathol.* 11, 487–508. doi: 10.1017/S0954579499002175

Csernansky, J. G., Wang, L., Joshi, S., Gado, M., Kido, D., Morris, J. C., et al. (1999). Hippocampal shape deformities specific to schizophrenia suggest a disturbance of hippocampal-prefrontal connections. *Schizophr. Res.* 36, 193–194.

David, A. S., Malmberg, A., Brandt, L., Allebeck, P., and Lewis, G. (1997). IQ and risk for schizophrenia: a population-based cohort study. *Psychol. Med.* 27, 1311–1323. doi: 10.1017/S0033291797005680

Dickinson, D., and Harvey, P. D. (2009). Systemic hypotheses for generalized cognitive deficits in schizophrenia: a new take on an old problem. *Schizophr. Bull.* 35, 403–414. doi: 10.1093/schbul/sbn097

Dickinson, D., Ragland, J. D., Calkins, M. E., Gold, J. M., and Gur, R. C. (2006). A comparison of cognitive structure in schizophrenia patients and healthy controls using confirmatory factor analysis. *Schizophr. Res.* 85, 20–29. doi: 10.1016/j.schres.2006.03.003

Dickson, H., Laurens, K. R., Cullen, A. E., and Hodgins, S. (2012). Meta-analyses of cognitive and motor function in youth aged 16 years and younger who subsequently develop schizophrenia. *Psychol. Med.* 42, 743–755. doi: 10.1017/S0033291711001693

Doeller, C. F., King, J. A., and Burgess, N. (2008). Parallel striatal and hippocampal systems for landmarks and boundaries in spatial memory. *Proc. Natl. Acad. Sci. U.S.A.* 105, 5915–5920. doi: 10.1073/pnas.0801489105

Driscoll, I., Hamilton, D. A., Petropoulos, H., Yeo, R. A., Brooks, W. M., Baumgartner, R. N., et al. (2003). The aging hippocampus: cognitive, biochemical and structural findings. *Cereb. Cortex* 13, 1344–1351. doi: 10.1093/cercor/bhg081

Ekstrom, A. D., Kahana, M. J., Caplan, J. B., Fields, T. A., Isham, E. A., Newman, E. L., et al. (2003). Cellular networks underlying human spatial navigation. *Nature* 425, 184–187. doi: 10.1038/nature01964

Ellison-Wright, I., and Bullmore, E. (2009). Meta-analysis of diffusion tensor imaging studies in schizophrenia. *Schizophr. Res.* 108, 3–10. doi: 10.1016/j.schres.2008.11.021

Etchamendy, N., and Bohbot, V. D. (2007). Spontaneous navigational strategies and performance in the virtual town. *Hippocampus* 17, 595–599. doi: 10.1002/hipo.20303

Folley, B. S., Astur, R., Jagannathan, K., Calhoun, V. D., and Pearlson, G. D. (2010). Anomalous neural circuit function in schizophrenia during a virtual Morris water task. *Neuroimage* 49, 3373–3384. doi: 10.1016/j.neuroimage.2009.11.034

Friston, K. J. (1999). Schizophrenia and the disconnection hypothesis. *Acta Psychiatr. Scand. Suppl.* 395, 68–79. doi: 10.1111/j.1600-0447.1999.tb05985.x

Friston, K. J., and Frith, C. D. (1995). Schizophrenia—a disconnection syndrome. *Clin. Neurosci.* 3, 89–97.

Garrity, A. G., Pearlson, G. D., McKiernan, K., Lloyd, D., Kiehl, K. A., and Calhoun, V. D. (2007). Aberrant "default mode" functional connectivity in schizophrenia. *Am. J. Psychiatry* 164, 450–457. doi: 10.1176/appi.ajp.164.3.450

Gladsjo, J. A., McAdams, L. A., Palmer, B. W., Moore, D. J., Jeste, D. V., and Heaton, R. K. (2004). A six-factor model of cognition in schizophrenia and related psychotic disorders: relationships with clinical symptoms and functional capacity. *Schizophr. Bull.* 30, 739–754. doi: 10.1093/oxfordjournals.schbul.a007127

Gold, J. M. (2004). Cognitive deficits as treatment targets in schizophrenia. *Schizophr. Res.* 72, 21–28. doi: 10.1016/j.schres.2004.09.008

Gold, J. M., and Dickinson, D. (2013). "Generalized cognitive deficit" in schizophrenia: overused or underappreciated? *Schizophr. Bull.* 39, 263–265. doi: 10.1093/schbul/sbs143

Goldberg, T. E., Weinberger, D. R., Berman, K. F., Pliskin, N. H., and Podd, M. H. (1987). Further evidence for dementia of the prefrontal type in schizophrenia—A controlled-study of teaching the Wisconsin Card Sorting Test. *Arch. Gen. Psychiatry* 44, 1008–1014. doi: 10.1001/archpsyc.1987.01800230088014

Green, M. F. (1996). What are the functional consequences of neurocognitive deficits in schizophrenia? *Am. J. Psychiatry* 153, 321–330.

Green, M. F., Kern, R. S., Braff, D. L., and Mintz, J. (2000). Neurocognitive deficits and functional outcome in schizophrenia: are we measuring the "right stuff"? *Schizophr. Bull.* 26, 119–136. doi: 10.1093/oxfordjournals.schbul.a033430

Green, M. F., Kern, R. S., and Heaton, R. K. (2004). Longitudinal studies of cognition and functional outcome in schizophrenia: implications for MATRICS. *Schizophr. Res.* 72, 41–51. doi: 10.1016/j.schres.2004.09.009

Green, M. F., Schooler, N. R., Kern, R. S., Frese, F. J., Granberry, W., Harvey, P. D., et al. (2011). Evaluation of functionally meaningful measures for clinical trials of cognition enhancement in schizophrenia. *Am. J. Psychiatry* 168, 400–407. doi: 10.1176/appi.ajp.2010.10030414

Hanlon, F. M., Houck, J. M., Klimaj, S. D., Caprihan, A., Mayer, A. R., Weisend, M. P., et al. (2012). Frontotemporal anatomical connectivity and working-relational memory performance predict everyday functioning in schizophrenia. *Psychophysiology* 49, 1340–1352. doi: 10.1111/j.1469-8986.2012.01448.x

Hanlon, F. M., Weisend, M. P., Hamilton, D. A., Jones, A. P., Thoma, R. J., Huang, M. X., et al. (2006). Impairment on the hippocampal-dependent virtual Morris water task in schizophrenia. *Schizophr. Res.* 87, 67–80. doi: 10.1016/j.schres.2006.05.021

Hartley, T., Maguire, E. A., Spiers, H. J., and Burgess, N. (2003). The well-worn route and the path less traveled: distinct neural bases of route following and wayfinding in humans. *Neuron* 37, 877–888. doi: 10.1016/S0896-6273(03)00095-3

Harvey, P. D., Howanitz, E., Parrella, M., White, L., Davidson, M., Mohs, R. C., et al. (1998). Symptoms, cognitive functioning, and adaptive skills in geriatric patients with lifelong schizophrenia: a comparison across treatment sites. *Am. J. Psychiatry* 155, 1080–1086.

Heinrichs, D. W., Hanlon, T. E., and Carpenter, W. T. (1984). The quality of life scale—an instrument for rating the schizophrenic deficit syndrome. *Schizophr. Bull.* 10, 388–398. doi: 10.1093/schbul/10.3.388

Heinrichs, R. W., and Zakzanis, K. K. (1998). Neurocognitive deficit in schizophrenia: a quantitative review of the evidence. *Neuropsychology* 12, 426–445. doi: 10.1037/0894-4105.12.3.426

Hyman, S. E., and Fenton, W. S. (2003). Medicine: what are the right targets for psychopharmacology? *Science* 299, 350–351. doi: 10.1126/science.1077141

Iaria, G., Petrides, M., Dagher, A., Pike, B., and Bohbot, V. D. (2003). Cognitive strategies dependent on the hippocampus and caudate nucleus in human navigation: variability and change with practice. *J. Neurosci.* 23, 5945–5952.

Joyce, E. M., and Roiser, J. P. (2007). Cognitive heterogeneity in schizophrenia. *Curr. Opin. Psychiatry* 20, 268–272. doi: 10.1097/YCO.0b013e3280ba4975

Keefe, R. S., Bilder, R. M., Harvey, P. D., Davis, S. M., Palmer, B. W., Gold, J. M., et al. (2006). Baseline neurocognitive deficits in the CATIE schizophrenia trial. *Neuropsychopharmacology* 31, 2033–2046. doi: 10.1038/sj.npp.1301072

Khandaker, G. M., Barnett, J. H., White, I. R., and Jones, P. B. (2011). A quantitative meta-analysis of population-based studies of premorbid intelligence and schizophrenia. *Schizophr. Res.* 132, 220–227. doi: 10.1016/j.schres.2011.06.017

Laruelle, M., and Abi-Dargham, P. (1999). Dopamine as the wind of the psychotic fire: new evidence from brain imaging studies. *J. Psychopharmacol.* 13, 358–371. doi: 10.1177/026988119901300405

Ledoux, A.-A., Lynne Phillips, J., Labelle, A., Smith, A., Deborah Bohbot, V., and Boyer, P. (2013). Decreased fMRI activity in the hippocampus of patients with schizophrenia compared to healthy control participants, tested on a wayfinding task in a virtual town. *Psychiatry Res.* 211, 47–56. doi: 10.1016/j.pscychresns.2012.10.005

Lewis, D. A., and Levitt, P. (2002). Schizophrenia as a disorder of neurodevelopment. *Annu. Rev. Neurosci.* 25, 409–432. doi: 10.1146/annurev.neuro.25.112701.142754

Liu, Y., Liang, M., Zhou, Y., He, Y., Hao, Y. H., Song, M., et al. (2008). Disrupted small-world networks in schizophrenia. *Brain* 131, 945–961. doi: 10.1093/brain/awn018

Maguire, E. A., Burgess, N., Donnett, J. G., Frackowiak, R. S., Frith, C. D., and O'Keefe, J. (1998). Knowing where and getting there: a human navigation network. *Science* 280, 921–924. doi: 10.1126/science.280.5365.921

Meyer-Lindenberg, A., Poline, J. B., Kohn, P. D., Holt, J. L., Egan, M. F., Weinberger, D. R., et al. (2001). Evidence for abnormal cortical functional connectivity during working memory in schizophrenia. *Am. J. Psychiatry* 158, 1809–1817. doi: 10.1176/appi.ajp.158.11.1809

Minzenberg, M. J., and Carter, C. S. (2012). Developing treatments for impaired cognition in schizophrenia. *Trends Cogn. Sci.* 16, 35–42. doi: 10.1016/j.tics.2011.11.017

Morris, R. G. M., Garrud, P., Rawlins, J. N. P., and Okeefe, J. (1982). Place navigation impaired in rats with hippocampal-lesions. *Nature* 297, 681–683. doi: 10.1038/297681a0

Moser, E. I., Kropff, E., and Moser, M. B. (2008). Place cells, grid cells, and the brain's spatial representation system. *Annu. Rev. Neurosci.* 31, 69–89. doi: 10.1146/annurev.neuro.31.061307.090723

Niendam, T. A., Bearden, C. E., Rosso, I. M., Sanchez, L. E., Hadley, T., Nuechterlein, K. H., et al. (2003). A prospective study of childhood neurocognitive functioning in schizophrenic patients and their siblings. *Am. J. Psychiatry* 160, 2060–2062. doi: 10.1176/appi.ajp.160.11.2060

Nuechterlein, K. H., Barch, D. M., Gold, J. M., Goldberg, T. E., Green, M. F., and Heaton, R. K. (2004). Identification of separable cognitive factors in schizophrenia. *Schizophr. Res.* 72, 29–39. doi: 10.1016/j.schres.2004.09.007

Nuechterlein, K. H., Green, M. F., Kern, R. S., Baade, L. E., Barch, D. M., Cohen, J. D., et al. (2008). The MATRICS consensus cognitive battery, part 1: test selection, reliability, and validity. *Am. J. Psychiatry* 165, 203–213. doi: 10.1176/appi.ajp.2007.07010042

Olton, D. S., and Samuelson, R. J. (1976). Remembrance of places passed—spatial memory in rats. *J. Exp. Psychol.Anim. Behav. Process.* 2, 97–116. doi: 10.1037/0097-7403.2.2.97

Patterson, T. L., Goldman, S., McKibbin, C. L., Hughs, T., and Jeste, D. V. (2001). UCSD performance-based skills assessment: development of a new measure of everyday functioning for severely mentally ill adults. *Schizophr. Bull.* 27, 235–245. doi: 10.1093/oxfordjournals.schbul.a006870

Penner, M. R., and Mizumori, S. J. Y. (2012). Neural systems analysis of decision making during goal-directed navigation. *Prog. Neurobiol.* 96, 96–135. doi: 10.1016/j.pneurobio.2011.08.010

Randolph, C. (1998). *Repeatable Battery for the Assessment of Neuropsychological Status (RBANS).* San Antonio, Tx: Harcourt Brace and Company.

Reichenberg, A., Weiser, M., Rabinowitz, J., Caspi, A., Schmeidler, J., Mark, M., et al. (2002). A population-based cohort study of premorbid intellectual, language, and behavioral functioning in patients with schizophrenia, schizoaffective disorder, and nonpsychotic bipolar disorder. *Am. J. Psychiatry* 159, 2027–2035. doi: 10.1176/appi.ajp.159.12.2027

Rotarska-Jagiela, A., van de Ven, V., Oertel-Knochel, V., Uhlhaas, P. J., Vogeley, K., and Linden, D. E. J. (2010). Resting-state functional network correlates of psychotic symptoms in schizophrenia. *Schizophr. Res.* 117, 21–30. doi: 10.1016/j.schres.2010.01.001

Schrimsher, G. W., O'bryant, S. E., O'Jile, J. R., and Sutker, P. B. (2008). Comparison of tetradic WAIS-III short forms in predicting full scale IQ scores in neuropsychiatric clinic settings. *J. Psychopathol. Behav. Assess.* 30, 235–240. doi: 10.1007/s10862-007-9066-9

Seidman, L. J. (1990). The neuropsychology of schizophrenia: a neurodevelopmental and case study approach. *J. Neuropsychiatry Clin. Neurosci.* 2, 301–312.

Sheehan, D. V., Janavs, J., Baker, R., Harnett-Sheehan, K., Knapp, E., Sheehan, M., et al. (1998). MINI—Mini International Neuropsychiatric Interview—English Version 5.0.0—DSM-IV. *J. Clin. Psychiatry* 59, 34–57.

Spiers, H. J., and Maguire, E. A. (2006). Thoughts, behaviour, and brain dynamics during navigation in the real world. *Neuroimage* 31, 1826–1840. doi: 10.1016/j.neuroimage.2006.01.037

Stephan, K. E., Baldeweg, T., and Friston, K. J. (2006). Synaptic plasticity and dysconnection in schizophrenia. *Biol. Psychiatry* 59, 929–939. doi: 10.1016/j.biopsych.2005.10.005

Stephan, K. E., Friston, K. J., and Frith, C. D. (2009). Dysconnection in schizophrenia: from abnormal synaptic plasticity to failures of self-monitoring. *Schizophr. Bull.* 35, 509–527. doi: 10.1093/schbul/sbn176

Voermans, N. C., Petersson, K. M., Daudey, L., Weber, B., Van Spaendonck, K. P., Kremer, H. P. H., et al. (2004). Interaction between the human hippocampus and the caudate nucleus during route recognition. *Neuron* 43, 427–435. doi: 10.1016/j.neuron.2004.07.009

Wechsler, D. (1997). *Wechsler Adult Intelligence Scale-III.* San Antonio, TX: The Psychological Corporation.

Weinberger, D. R. (1987). Implications of normal brain-development for the pathogenesis of schizophrenia. *Arch. Gen. Psychiatry* 44, 660–669. doi: 10.1001/archpsyc.1987.01800190080012

Weinberger, D. R., Berman, K. F., Suddath, R., and Torrey, E. F. (1992). Evidence of dysfunction of a prefrontal-limbic network in schizophrenia—a magnetic-resonance-imaging and regional cerebral blood-flow study of discordant monozygotic twins. *Am. J. Psychiatry* 149, 890–897.

Weinberger, D. R., Berman, K. F., and Zec, R. F. (1986). Physiological dysfunction of dorsolateral prefrontal cortex in schizophrenia.1. regional cerebral blood-flow evidence. *Arch. Gen. Psychiatry* 43, 114–124. doi: 10.1001/archpsyc.1986.01800020020004

Weniger, G., and Irle, E. (2008). Allocentric memory impaired and egocentric memory intact as assessed by virtual reality in recent-onset schizophrenia. *Schizophr. Res.* 101, 201–209. doi: 10.1016/j.schres.2008.01.011

Wolbers, T., and Hegarty, M. (2010). What determines our navigational abilities? *Trends Cogn. Sci.* 14, 138–146. doi: 10.1016/j.tics.2010.01.001

Wolbers, T., Weiller, C., and Buchel, C. (2004). Neural foundations of emerging route knowledge in complex spatial environments. *Cogn. Brain Res.* 21, 401–411. doi: 10.1016/j.cogbrainres.2004.06.013

Wolbers, T., Wiener, J. M., Mallot, H. A., and Buchel, C. (2007). Differential recruitment of the hippocampus, medial prefrontal cortex, and the human motion complex during path integration in humans. *J. Neurosci.* 27, 9408–9416. doi: 10.1523/JNEUROSCI.2146-07.2007

Wong, A. H. C., Macciardi, F., Klempan, T., Kawczynski, W., Barr, C. L., Lakatoo, S., et al. (2003). Identification of candidate genes for psychosis in rat models, and possible association between schizophrenia and the 14-13-3 gene. *Mol. Psychiatry* 8, 156–166. doi: 10.1038/sj.mp.4001237

2

A virtual reality task based on animal research – spatial learning and memory in patients after the first episode of schizophrenia

Iveta Fajnerová[1,2,3]*, Mabel Rodriguez[1], David Levčík[2], Lucie Konrádová[1], Pavol Mikoláš[1,3], Cyril Brom[4], Aleš Stuchlík[2], Kamil Vlček[2] and Jiří Horáček[1,3]

[1] Prague Psychiatric Center, Prague, Czech Republic
[2] Department of Neurophysiology of Memory, Institute of Physiology, Academy of Sciences of the Czech Republic v.v.i., Prague, Czech Republic
[3] Department of Psychiatry and Medical Psychology, 3rd Faculty of Medicine, Charles University in Prague, Prague, Czech Republic
[4] Department of Software and Computer Science Education, Faculty of Mathematics and Physics, Charles University in Prague, Prague, Czech Republic

Edited by:
Tomiki Sumiyoshi, National Center of Neurology and Psychiatry, Japan

****Correspondence:***
Iveta Fajnerová, Prague Psychiatric Center, Ústavní 91, 181 03 Prague 8 – Bohnice, Czech Republic
e-mail: fajnerova@pcp.lf3.cuni.cz

Objectives: Cognitive deficit is considered to be a characteristic feature of schizophrenia disorder. A similar cognitive dysfunction was demonstrated in animal models of schizophrenia. However, the poor comparability of methods used to assess cognition in animals and humans could be responsible for low predictive validity of current animal models. In order to assess spatial abilities in schizophrenia and compare our results with the data obtained in animal models, we designed a virtual analog of the Morris water maze (MWM), the *virtual Four Goals Navigation (vFGN) task.*

Methods: Twenty-nine patients after the first psychotic episode with schizophrenia symptoms and a matched group of healthy volunteers performed the *vFGN* task. They were required to find and remember four hidden goal positions in an enclosed virtual arena. The task consisted of two parts. The Reference memory (RM) session with a stable goal position was designed to test spatial learning. The Delayed-matching-to-place (DMP) session presented a modified working memory protocol designed to test the ability to remember a sequence of three hidden goal positions.

Results: Data obtained in the RM session show impaired spatial learning in schizophrenia patients compared to the healthy controls in pointing and navigation accuracy. The DMP session showed impaired spatial memory in schizophrenia during the recall of spatial sequence and a similar deficit in spatial bias in the probe trials. The pointing accuracy and the quadrant preference showed higher sensitivity toward the cognitive deficit than the navigation accuracy. Direct navigation to the goal was affected by sex and age of the tested subjects. The age affected spatial performance only in healthy controls.

Conclusions: Despite some limitations of the study, our results correspond well with the previous studies in animal models of schizophrenia and support the decline of spatial cognition in schizophrenia, indicating the usefulness of the vFGN task in comparative research.

Keywords: schizophrenia, spatial navigation, learning and memory, virtual reality environment, cognitive deficit, Morris Water Maze (MWM), psychotic disorders, spatial behavior

INTRODUCTION

The impairment of cognitive functions is considered to be a characteristic and permanent manifestation in patients with schizophrenia disorder (Andreasen, 1999; Elvevag and Goldberg, 2000). The MATRICS (Measurement and Treatment Research to Improve Cognition in Schizophrenia) initiative identified seven crucial cognitive areas typically influenced in schizophrenia: attention, psychomotor speed, working memory, logical thinking, problem solving, social cognition, and verbal and visuo-spatial learning (Green et al., 2004). Although the extent of cognitive decline in schizophrenia has considerable inter-individual variability, it has been shown that the overall performance in neuropsychological tests is more than 1 SD lower in schizophrenia when compared to the healthy population (Keefe et al., 2005). This deficit is demonstrated in 82–84% of the patients (Reichenberg et al., 2009).

Various "paper-and-pencil" or simple computer tests are traditionally used to assess cognitive deficit in schizophrenia. However, these methods are not comparable with the behavioral tasks used in animal research and such limitation can be shown in a low predictive validity of the animal models of schizophrenia (Pratt et al., 2012). Considerable attention is therefore devoted to the assessment of visuo-spatial abilities in schizophrenia and in animal models of this disorder, since spatial behavior and spatial memory can be measured using similar methods in various species. It was demonstrated that schizophrenia patients exhibit

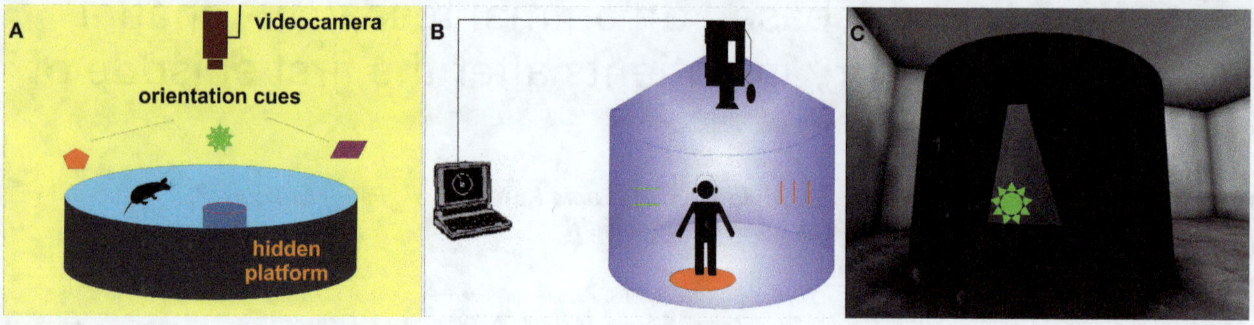

FIGURE 1 | Morris water maze—the hidden platform paradigm - and its human analogs. (A) Scheme of the original MWM apparatus for rats. **(B)** Schematic view of the real human analog called Blue Velvet Arena (BVA). **(C)** Virtual analog of BVA (view of the virtual tent from the outside).

impaired performance on all levels of spatial cognition, from the most basic level of mental rotations of letters and objects (de Vignemont et al., 2006) to more complex spatial navigation abilities (Weniger and Irle, 2008; Landgraf et al., 2010). Numerous studies demonstrated the deficit of the visuo-spatial working memory in schizophrenia (see review; Piskulic et al., 2007) using various tasks. These findings motivate the development of human analogs of animal spatial tasks for application in comparative clinical research.

One of the most often used spatial tasks in animal research is the *Morris water maze* (MWM; Morris, 1981). This goal-directed task was originally developed for rats and requires them to learn and remember the position of a hidden platform located in a circular swimming pool in relation to distal visual cues (**Figure 1A**). The MWM apparatus is used in several basic versions (shortly described in Morris, 2008) or protocols (for further information see section Materials and Methods): (1) the *reference memory protocol*, with the hidden platform placed in a stable position; (2) the *reversal protocol*, with a changing platform position; (3) the *delayed-matching-to-place (DMP) protocol* often referred to as the "working memory protocol" which uses variable inter-trial intervals and 4) the *probe trial* with the platform removed. Measurable impairment of visuo-spatial abilities in MWM has already been demonstrated in several animal models of schizophrenia (see review; Bubenikova-Valesova et al., 2008). Several animal studies including the work of our group confirmed that the rodent model of schizophrenia based on administration of MK-801 (dizocilpine, a non-competitive NMDA glutamate receptor antagonist) leads to decreased cognitive functioning in rats, resulting in compromised performance in all variants (reference, reversal, and working memory protocol) of the MWM task (Stuchlik et al., 2004; Vales et al., 2006; van der Staay et al., 2011; Lobellova et al., 2013).

Several real space human MWM analogs have been developed to test the human spatial navigation, mostly in dry circular arenas (Overman et al., 1996; Skolimowska et al., 2011). A real analog of the MWM has also been developed in our laboratory as an apparatus named the "Blue Velvet Arena (BVA)" (Stepankova et al., 1999; Laczo et al., 2010; see **Figure 1B**). The development of virtual environments (VE) provided a significant methodological advance, allowing the detailed recording of the subject's behavior, along with easy handling and presentation of stimuli. Several virtual reality versions of the MWM have been designed using the reference memory protocol with a stable goal position (Bohbot et al., 1998; Jacobs et al., 1998; Moffat and Resnick, 2002; Astur et al., 2004; Mueller et al., 2008; Goodrich-Hunsaker et al., 2009) or working memory paradigm (Rodriguez, 2010). However, only the reference memory protocol has been applied to schizophrenia patients (Hanlon et al., 2006; Folley et al., 2010).

Thus, our aim was to extend the current comparative research by attempting to incorporate several MWM variants into a small test battery named the "*virtual Four Goals Navigation*" *(vFGN) task*. The vFGN task is completed in a virtual analog of the real BVA apparatus designed previously by our group (Stepankova et al., 1999; depicted in the **Figure 1C**). The presented study describes the newly-developed vFGN task and presents first data obtained in a group of patients after the first episode of schizophrenia psychosis in comparison to a group of healthy volunteers, in order to express its sensitivity toward the present cognitive deficit. To minimize possible effects of sex, age and education level, both groups were carefully matched according to these variables. In order to assess the usefulness of the vFGN task in preclinical studies, we compare the data obtained in the vFGN task with the previously published animal studies.

On the basis of animal and human literature, we hypothesized that the schizophrenia patients would perform worse compared to the healthy controls in the vFGN task in terms of: (1) impaired spatial learning during the Reference memory (RM) session; and (2) decreased working memory performance in the Delayed-matching-to-place (DMP) session. Since several studies described sex differences in spatial abilities of rodents (see meta-analysis by Jonasson, 2005) and humans (e.g., Astur et al., 1998, 2004), we hypothesized to find similar differences in our subjects as well. In addition, the effect of age variable was analyzed in order to understand how the age affects performance in the vFGN task and if this effect is the same in both groups. Moreover, the effect of several clinical parameters, such as the duration of untreated psychosis (DUP), general functioning (GAF score), clinical symptoms (PANSS scores) and antipsychotic medication [dose calculated in chlorpromazine (CPZ) equivalents], was evaluated in the group of patients.

MATERIALS AND METHODS

EXPERIMENTAL SUBJECTS

Twenty-nine patients (17 males and 12 females) after the first psychotic episode with schizophrenia symptoms were recruited for the study. All patients have been diagnosed with schizophrenia or related psychotic disorders according to ICD-10 criteria (Paranoid Schizophrenia F20.0: $n = 3$; Undifferentiated Schizophrenia F20.3: $n = 1$; Simplex Schizophrenia F20.6: $n = 1$; Acute psychotic disorder: F23.0: $n = 4$; F23.1: $n = 18$; F23.2: $n = 2$). They were recruited in the early remission phase during their first psychiatric hospitalization (therefore considered to be first-episode psychotic patients with schizophrenia symptoms, FEP) with a variable duration of untreated psychosis (DUP, 6.4 ± 13 months). DUP defined as the duration of untreated but clearly presented psychotic symptoms, was obtained from the detailed interview with the patients and family members. All of the patients were tested prior to the end of their hospitalization. In order to cover the whole spectrum of the first episodes of schizophrenia, both early and late onset patients were recruited for the study (in the age between 18 and 35 years).

The patients were individually matched to healthy volunteers ($n = 29$; see **Table 1**) in terms of sex, age (within 2 years difference), education level and gaming experiences (both within 1 level of difference). Healthy subjects were recruited from the same socio-demographic background via a local advertisement. To provide sufficient homogeneity of the examined group, most of the recruited participants were regular users of computer devices with none or mild gaming experience. The inclusion criteria for both groups were: (1) no history of neurological disease or loss of consciousness longer than 10 min; and (2) native in Czech/Slovak

Table 1 | Patients with schizophrenia were individually matched with healthy controls for sex, age (within 2 years), education level and gaming experience (both within one level of difference).

	Group mean (*SD*)		Group differences	
Demographic variable	**Schizophrenia patients (SZ)**	**Healthy Controls (HC)**	**Mann-Whitney U**	***p*-value**
N	29	29		
Sex (M: F)	17: 12	17: 12		
Age	25.8 ± 6.2	25.7 ± 5.4	419.5	0.994
Education level (1–6)	3.1 ± 1.6	3.7 ± 1.2	323	0.131
Gaming experience (0–2)	1.1 ± 0.7	0.6 ± 0.5	258	0.012
Clinical assessment	**SZ**	**HC**		
PANSS score	56 ± 16	–		
PANSS-positive	13.6 ± 6	–		
PANSS-negative	15 ± 6	–		
PANS-general	27 ± 7.7	–		
GAF	64 ± 20.5	–		
Duration of illness	12 ± 20.8	–		
DUP	6.4 ± 13	–		
Hospitalization duration	30 ± 12	–		
Medication (CPZ equivalents)	426 ± 145	–		
Neurocognitive assessment	**Raw test scores—Mean (*SD*)**			
	SZ	**HC**	**Mann-Whitney U**	***p*-value**
TMT—*A*	38 ± 12.1	26.5 ± 8	131.5	0.0001
TMT—*B*	98 ± 44	50 ± 11.5	82	0.0001
RCFT—copy	31.6 ± 5	35.7 ± 0.9	98.5	0.0001
RCFT—3 min recall	17.2 ± 8	26.2 ± 5.5	108.510	0.0001
RCFT—30 min recall	17.7 ± 7	26 ± 4.9	4.5	0.0001
Digit Span (WAIS-III)—*forward*	9.3 ± 3.7	10 ± 2.3	254.5	0.09
Digit Span (WAIS-III)—backward	5.3 ± 2.1	7.4 ± 2.1	137.5	0.0001
Spatial Span (WMS-III)—*forward*	8.5 ± 1.8	9 ± 1.4	281.5	0.42
Spatial Span (WMS-III)—*backward*	7.5 ± 2.5	9 ± 1.4	218.5	0.046

SZ, first episodes schizophrenia patients; HC, healthy controls; Education level: 1 = less than high school, 2 = started high school, 3 = completed high school, 4 = started university, 5 = completed university, 6 = started postgraduate studies; Gaming experience: 0 = none, 1 = mild, 2 = good; PANSS, Positive and Negative Symptoms Scale; GAF, Global of Assessment of Functioning; DUP, duration of untreated psychosis; TMT, Trial Making Test; RCFT, Rey-Osterrieth Complex Figure. WMS-III, Wechsler Memory Scale III edition; WAIS-III, Wechsler adult intelligence scale III edition.

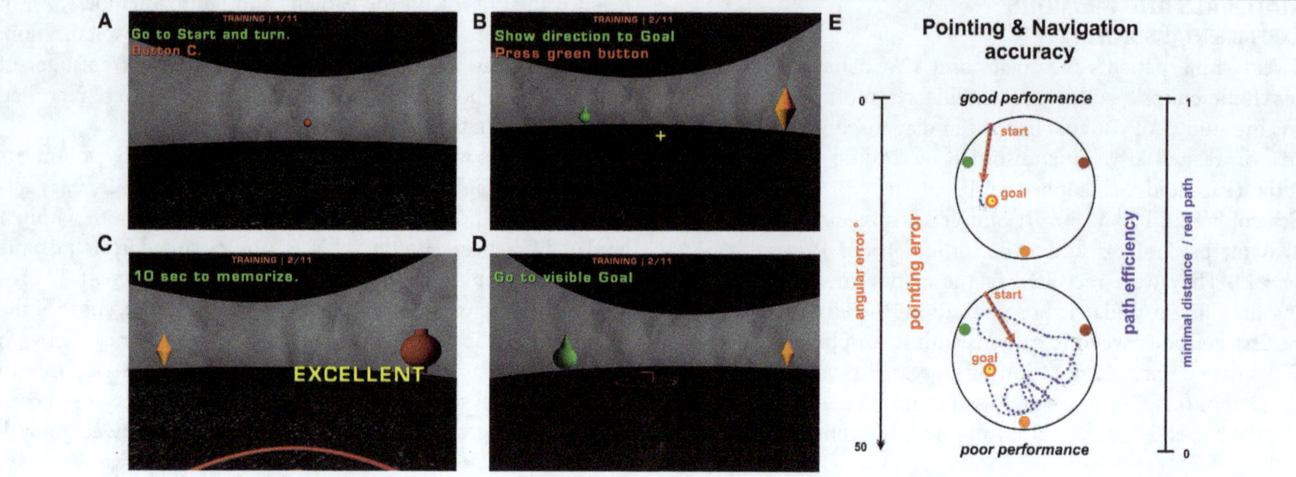

FIGURE 2 | Virtual version of the BVA apparatus from the inside—one trial procedure. (A–D) demonstrate individual phases of one trial using the first-person previews from the vFGN task. The short instructions used as a reminder for the participants were translated to English. **(A)** The starting position is presented as a red sphere. **(B)** Two visible orientation cues (from a set of three cues with various shapes and colors) and yellow cross in the middle of the screen used to point toward the hidden goal direction. **(C)** Goal position visualized after 60 s trial time limit. **(D)** Movement blocked after the entrance to the goal position enabling only rotational movement in 10 s memorizing. **(E)** Illustration of the two parameters measured in all trials (except the probe trial). Lateral axis present the interval of values gained in both parameters. The central pictures illustrate good and poor performance in the vFGN task. Trajectories (line of blue points) from the both tested groups are presented as an overview scheme of the spatial configuration in one hidden-goal trial. The red arrow illustrates the pointing error parameter. The trajectory length is transformed to the path efficiency parameter.

language. The main exclusion criterion for the control subjects was personal history of any psychiatric disorder. All tested subjects signed a written informed consent approved by the Ethics Committee.

APPARATUS AND SOFTWARE

The virtual scene was displayed on a 24″ LCD monitor using the Unreal Tournament game engine (UT2004; Epic Games, 2004). A Java software toolkit called *"SpaNav"* (Šupalová, 2009) was programmed to configure an experimental setup and to record detailed experimental data for further analysis. A three-dimensional circular arena was designed as a virtual model of the *BVA* apparatus, an arena enclosed by a white curtain wall and with floor covered with a gray carpet (Stepankova et al., 2003), with the utmost realism. Because the virtual environment enabled us to enlarge the size of the virtual arena, an arena 20 times larger than the original BVA apparatus (2.8 m in diameter) was used. Three orientation cues were located in the arena near the circular wall. These objects were fully colored and had various rotational shapes. The goal location had a circular shape with a red border and occupied about 10% of the arena diameter (see **Figure 2C**). The tested subject moved through the virtual maze in a first person view. In order to facilitate movement in VE for participants without gaming experience, only one stick of the gamepad device (Logitech F310) was used, enabling only forward/backward movement and left/right rotation.

CLINICAL AND NEUROPSYCHOLOGICAL ASSESSMENT

All of the patients completed a psychiatric interview prior to the experiment in order to obtain information about their current symptoms using the Positive and Negative Symptoms Scale (PANSS; Kay et al., 1987) and the GAF (Global Assessment of Functioning) scale (Jones et al., 1995). Only stabilized patients who mainly scored 3 points or lower in their individual scores were recruited for the experiment. All of the patients were treated by second generation antipsychotics (olanzapin, risperidon, and amisulpirid). The dose of antipsychotic medication was CPZ equivalents (according to Woods, 2003; Andreasen et al., 2010). For details on the clinical parameters see **Table 1**.

Overall cognitive performance was measured in both patients and healthy controls with several neuropsychological tests compatible with the MATRICS battery to assess psychomotor speed, mental flexibility, learning, and memory (see **Table 1**): *Trial Making Test* (A and B; Reitan and Wolfson, 1993 modified by Preiss, 1997); *Rey-Osterrieth Complex Figure* (Meyers and Meyers, 1995); *Digit span* of the WAIS-III (Wechsler, 1997a); *Spatial span* (computer version adapted from the Corsi block test in the PEBL battery (PEBL, 2012) and modified according to Spatial span of the WMS-III (Wechsler, 1997b).

PRE-TRAINING OF MOTOR CONTROL

Prior to the task, all of the participants underwent a short (5 min long) pre-training of movement control using the gamepad apparatus (see time schedule in **Figure 3**). Afterwards, the participants performed a simple task in a complex virtual labyrinth maze with instructions to "follow the route highlighted by six objects (stars) on each crossroad and get to the end of the route as fast as possible." After completing the pre-training, all of the tested subjects performed the vFGN task.

THE VIRTUAL FOUR GOALS NAVIGATION (vFGN) TASK

In each trial of the vFGN task the subjects were required to find a hidden circular goal placed on the arena floor using the direct trajectory to the goal. Each trial started by moving toward a pseudorandom starting position displayed as a red sphere near the arena wall (see **Figure 2A**). Then, three orientation cues were

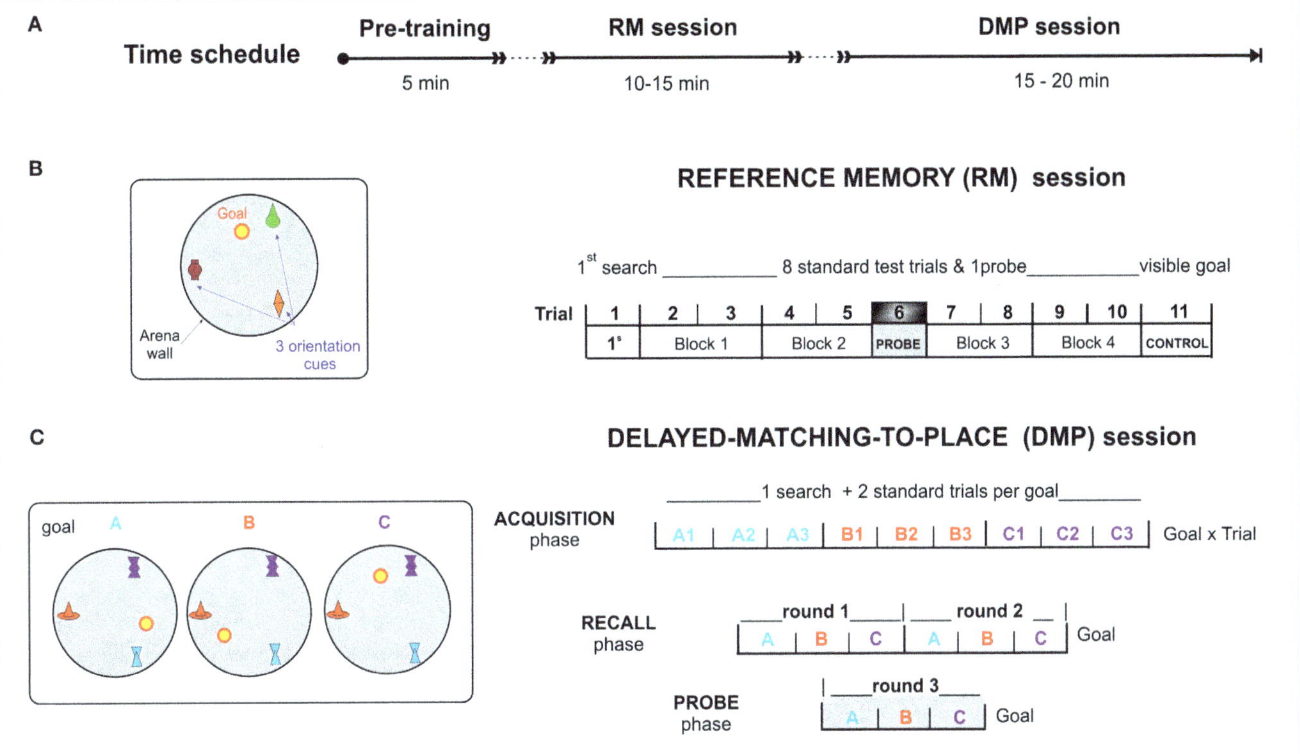

FIGURE 3 | The virtual Four Goals Navigation (vFGN) task. (A) upper panel presents the time schedule of the experiment. Spatial configurations with the goal positions used in individual sessions are presented on the left and the procedure of individual parts of the task on the right. **(B)** REFERENCE MEMORY session with a stable goal position over 11 trials. T1, 1st search trial; Block 1-Block 4, pairs of standard trials with repeated search for hidden goal; T6, probe trial with inactivated goal position; T11, control trial testing navigation toward a visible goal. **(C)** DELAYED-MATCHING-TO-PLACE session with goal in three possible positions ordered in a spatial sequence (A,B,C). ACQUISITION phase, each goal position is repeated in 3 consecutive trials (9 trials in total); RECALL phase, two rounds of the spatial sequence ABC (6 trials in total); PROBE phase, one spatial sequence ABC with inactivated goal positions (3 trials).

visualized in the arena. At this moment, the subject's movement was blocked at the starting position and only rotational movements were enabled. Apart from the first trial when the goal position was unknown, the subject was instructed to point toward the hidden goal position using the yellow cross in the middle of the screen (see **Figure 2B**) and then press the green button on the gamepad (in all standard, probe, and control trials) to activate his or her movement. Thereafter, the 60 s time limit for locating the hidden goal began. After entering the correct area, the goal became visible and a short beeping sound was played. If the goal was not found within the 60 s time limit, it became visible (see **Figure 2C**) and a short warning beep was played. The subject was then instructed to enter the visible goal position. Upon entering the goal area, the movement was blocked in the middle of the goal position and the participant had 10 s to remember the goal position for consecutive trials using only rotational movements (see **Figure 2D**). This "learning time" represented the analogy of an animal standing on a platform for several seconds after each trial.

The vFGN task consisted of two parts: the RM and the DMP sessions; both administered successively in 1 day protocol (Time schedule in **Figure 3**).

Part I—Reference memory (RM) session

In the session completed at the beginning of the vFGN task, was designed according to the original reference memory protocol (Morris, 1981, 1984; Morris et al., 1982). Similar to other human MWM analogs (Jacobs et al., 1998; Astur et al., 2002) the task was shortened into 1 day protocol to test spatial learning and memory by monitoring the performance improvement in 11 consecutive trials (see **Figure 3B**). In the "first search" trial (T1) the participants were instructed to find the hidden goal location on the arena floor by free exploration of the arena and to remember it for the following trials using the three orientation cues. In the following standard trials T2-T5 and T7-T10, displayed as four blocks of 2 trials in **Figures 3**, **4**, the subjects were required to look for the hidden goal repeatedly while starting from pseudo-randomized starting positions. One probe trial (T6) was inserted in the middle of the RM session in order to test the effect of extinction process as a sort of interference in the course of learning (inspired by the human learning tasks). This probe trial was aimed at memory precision and confidence (by evaluating the time spent in the goal proximity) while the goal was inactivated. The final CONTROL trial (T11) used the navigation toward the visible goal and served as a test of secondary effects generated by impairment of vision and motor abilities.

Part II—Delayed-matching-to-place (DMP) session

In order to prevent any transfer from the RM session, the color and the shape of the orientation cues were changed for the following DMP session. The DMP session was designed as a working

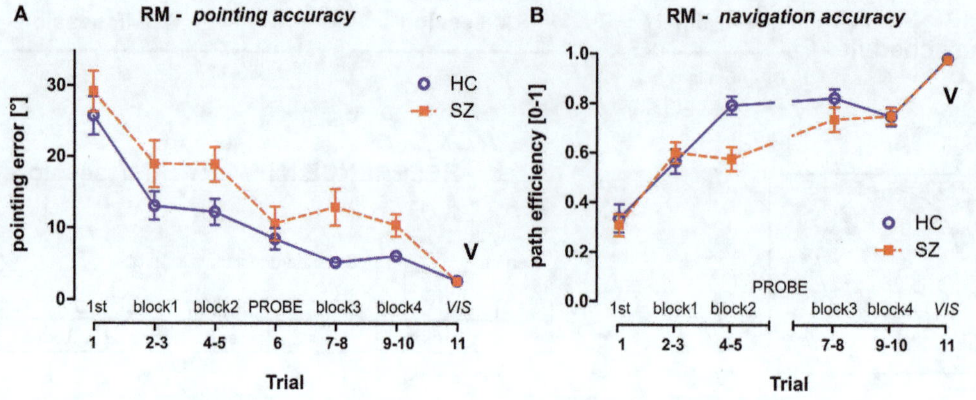

FIGURE 4 | Reference Memory (RM) session group performance. (A) The pointing error (mean ± s.e.m) and **(B)** the path efficiency (mean ± s.e.m) measured in individual trials and/or blocks of trials. The probe trial T6 is not depicted in the path efficiency parameter, the control trial T11 is marked by letter V (as displayed). HC—Healthy controls; SZ—first-episode schizophrenia patients.

memory protocol constructed by combining two different animal protocols for assessment of working memory adapted for humans. The DMP session consists of three consecutive phases (graphically depicted on **Figure 3C**):

(1) The **ACQUISITION** phase involved 9 trials with the goal placed successively in three various positions (A, B, or C) in relation to three distal orientation cues. The goal was moved after each 3 trials (see **Figure 3B**). It was based on a modified *reversal protocol* of the MWM, in which the goal position is changed over the days used to test mental flexibility (Lipp et al., 1998; Vorhees and Williams, 2006; Garthe et al., 2009; Lobellova et al., 2013) and/or working memory (Morris et al., 1986). Unlike in rats, the change in goal position was separated not by days of testing but by an announcement to the subjects, in order to test their memory for spatial sequence (ABC) in the subsequent phases.
(2) The **RECALL** phase together with the Acquisition phase represents a modified version of the DMP paradigm (for review see Dudchenko, 2004; also in Morris et al., 1986; Steele and Morris, 1999; O'Carroll et al., 2006) designed for assessment of the working memory functions in rodents using delayed recall. Our task was designed to test spatial memory processes by evaluating the performance decline measured between the Acquisition and the Recall phase. To increase the difficulty and adapt the task for human participants, the task combined the DMP protocol applied in rats with the spatial sequence encoding in the Corsi Block Test (developed by Corsi in 1972) used in many variants to test spatial working memory in humans (Fischer, 2001). This modified protocol required them to retrieve the correct sequence of three goal positions (ABC) previously learned in the Acquisition trials and identify them successively (according to instructions) in two consecutive rounds (see **Figure 3B**).
(3) The **PROBE** phase, involving 3 trials with inactivated goal position, was conducted directly after the Recall phase as a final third round of the spatial sequenced recall (see **Figure 3B**). The probe trials, with a removed hidden platform adopted from the animal studies, provide an important demonstration of memory processes in terms of spatial bias (Morris et al., 1982, 1990; Sutherland et al., 1983; Whishaw, 1991). In rats probe trials are usually conducted in the reference memory protocols, but sometimes after reversal condition as well (Lobellova et al., 2013).

MEASURED PARAMETERS AND DATA ANALYSIS

Latency to find the goal and distance traveled to reach it are usually measured in standard trials in animals (for review see D'Hooge and De Deyn, 2001) and in human studies (Hanlon et al., 2006; Moffat, 2009; Folley et al., 2010). In our study the latency parameter was not evaluated, since the decision about the correct goal position was already done while pointing to it. Therefore, we address the spatial performance in all trials except probes using the *pointing accuracy* later referred to as the **pointing error**. This parameter was recorded at the moment when the subject stands on the starting position and points toward the hidden goal by pressing one of the gamepad keys. It was calculated as the absolute angular difference between the pointed and linear direction toward the goal position and its value decreases with growing precision in pointing performance (see **Figure 2E**). The distance parameter expresses the *navigation accuracy* and it is referred to as **path efficiency** (abbr. **path eff**) with the range of 0–1. It was calculated as a ratio between the minimal possible path length (the actual distance between the start and the goal position) and the real distance traveled by the subject, using the following formula: path eff $= \text{path}_{\text{min}}/\text{path}_{\text{real}}$ (see **Figure 2E**). Contrary to the standard *distance* parameter its value increases with the precision of navigation and enables us a direct comparison between individual trials by considering the possible minimal distance. In addition, we measured two common parameters in all of the probe trials: **goal quadrant preference** calculated as a proportion of the overall trial time spent in the goal quadrant (arena quadrant containing the hidden goal in its center); and **number of entrances** calculated as number of crossings through the inactivated goal position.

To analyze the data recorded in SpaNav, a custom-made PHP program called drf2track was used to produce primary data tables and trajectory pictures. Further statistical analysis was performed using the Statistica software (Statistica v.9, StatSoft, Czech

Republic). The group differences in the demographic variables (age, education level and gaming experience) are calculated using non-parametric Mann-Whitney U Test. Identical method was used to analyze the raw scores obtained in neuropsychological tests. The group and sex differences in individual parts of the vFGN task were calculated using the GLM repeated measure analysis of variance with two categorical predictors (group × sex). Significant interactions were analyzed using a Newman-Keuls *post-hoc* test. A correlation analysis was performed separately for both groups between the age variable and the spatial performance of individual subjects averaged for individual parts of the vFGN task. The *t*-test for independent groups was used to compare the groups in a single visible goal trial and in a single probe trial in the RM session. The *t*-test for single means against a reference constant was used in order to show that the quadrant preference measured in probe trials is different from the chance level (0.25). The effect of clinical characteristics (age of illness onset, DUP, PANSS, and GAF scores and antipsychotic medication calculated in CPZ equivalents) on averaged performance in the vFGN task was calculated using forward stepwise multiple linear regression analysis (with F to enter set to 1.00 and F to remove to 0). The overall level of significance was set to 0.05.

RESULTS

The groups did not differ significantly in any of the demographic parameters, except the gaming experience, where patients showed to be more experienced than the healthy controls (see **Table 1**). As expected, group of patients showed significantly lower cognitive performance on all neuropsychological tests, except the forward Digital and Spatial Span task performance (see **Table 1**). The modification from 3D to 2D version of the Spatial Span could cause lower sensitivity of the test in comparison to other standard methods. Group differences measured in individual parts of the vFGN task are graphically depicted as performance curves for all of the evaluated parameters (see **Figures 4–8**).

GROUP DIFFERENCES IN THE vFGN TASK

RM session

To analyze the group differences in the RM session a GLM analysis was performed with the group as one of the main factors (group × sex) and block (pairs of standard trials, see **Figure 3A**) as a repeated measure factor. This analysis showed impaired learning performance of the schizophrenia group in both measured parameters (see **Figure 4**). While a robust effect of the group factor was identified in the pointing error parameter [$F_{(1,54)} = 9.5$; $p < 0.01$], a significant interaction (block × group) was found in path efficiency parameter [$F_{(3,162)} = 6.2$; $p < 0.001$]. A *post-hoc* test on this interaction revealed that the groups differed in path eff (on level $p < 0.01$) in the second block of trials (T4 and T5). Interestingly, the navigation performance in healthy controls improved significantly in the beginning of training between the first two blocks of trials ($p < 0.001$), while in the group of patients similar improvement occurred later on after the completion of probe trial in the middle of the training (only blocks completed before the probe trial showed lower performance than blocks completed after the probe trial; $p < 0.05$). Block as repetition factor was significant in both tested parameters ($p < 0.001$).

To compare the first search trial (T1) of the RM session with the remaining standard trials, another GLM analysis was performed on individual trials. The interaction identified between the group and repetition trials was tested by the *post-hoc* test and revealed that T1 differed significantly from all of the following standard trials in the RM session ($p < 0.05$) in both of the measured parameters. This demonstrates fast learning of the goal position after one learning episode.

One probe trial (T6) was inserted in the middle of the RM session (see **Figure 5**) to assess spatial memory by evaluating the goal quadrant preference. While the control subjects spent 75 ± 11% of the trial time in the correct arena quadrant, the mean value in the patients was only 57 ± 23%. The goal quadrant preference of both groups differed from the chance level (25%). The *t*-test revealed a main group effect in the goal quadrant preference [$t_{(56)} = 3.9$, $p < 0.001$] but not in the number of entrances to the inactivated goal [$t_{(56)} = 1.4$, $p = 0.16$].

The visible goal trial (T11, marked as V in **Figure 4**) used as a control of visuo-motor functioning at the end of the RM session showed minimal interpersonal variability. No group effect was revealed by the *t*-test for two independent samples in either of the parameters; in pointing error [$t_{(56)} = 0.57$; $p = 0.57$] or in path eff parameter [$t_{(56)} = 0.09$; $p = 0.93$].

DMP—ACQUISITION phase

The main effect of the trial as repeated measures factor was found in the Acquisition phase of the DMP session ($p < 0.001$)

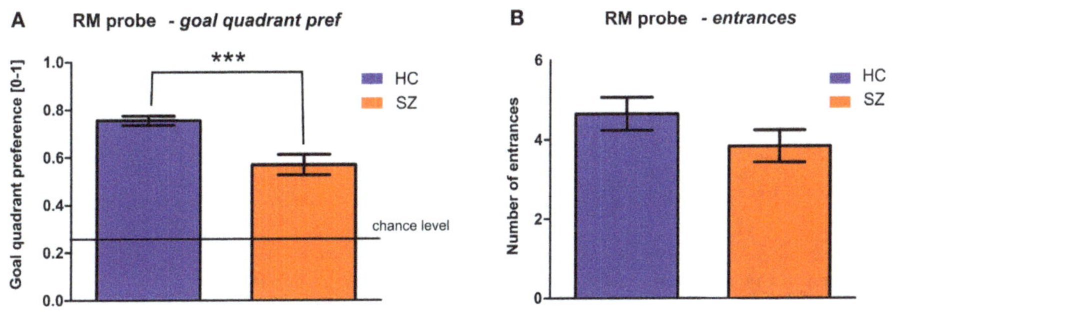

FIGURE 5 | Probe trial (trial T6) performance in the middle of RM session. (A) The goal quadrant preference (mean ± s.e.m) and **(B)** the number of entrances (mean ± s.e.m) into the inactivated goal position. Annotation: ***$p < 0.001$ group difference. HC, Healthy controls; SZ, first-episode schizophrenia patients.

tested using GLM analysis (group × sex) with repeated measures (goal × trial) (see **Figure 6**). The main group effect was found in the pointing accuracy for trials 2 and 3 [$F_{(1,\ 54)} = 7.8$; $p < 0.01$]. The 1st search trials—A1, B1, C1—representing the free exploration trials were excluded from the analysis as they represent random performance. However, no group differences were identified in the path efficiency parameter, even the interaction effect (trial × group) only approached the significance level [$F_{(2,108)} = 2.8$, $p = 0.068$]. No other significant interactions were obtained from the analysis.

DMP—RECALL phase

The GLM analysis with repeated measures (round × goal) was used to analyze the performance in the two Recall rounds in comparison to the performance observed in the last Acquisition trials—A3, B3, and C3 (see **Figure 7**). The analysis performed on both Recall rounds showed significant group differences in both measured parameters, as a main effect in pointing error [$F_{(1,\ 54)} = 20.4$; $p < 0.001$] and in path eff [$F_{(1,\ 54)} = 9.9$; $p < 0.01$]. Interestingly, while the path efficiency parameter showed only main effect of round as repetition factor ($p < 0.001$), we identified an interaction effect (group × round) in the pointing error [$F_{(2,\ 108)} = 4.4$; $p < 0.05$]. The *post-hoc* test on this interaction revealed that healthy controls showed stable performance over the DMP session (individual rounds did not differ in the group of healthy controls), but the schizophrenia group showed significant drop of performance after the time delay between the last trials of the Acquisition phase (trials 3) and the first Recall round ($p < 0.001$). No differences have been identified between the two Recall rounds. Interestingly, no main effects or interactions of the goal position were identified.

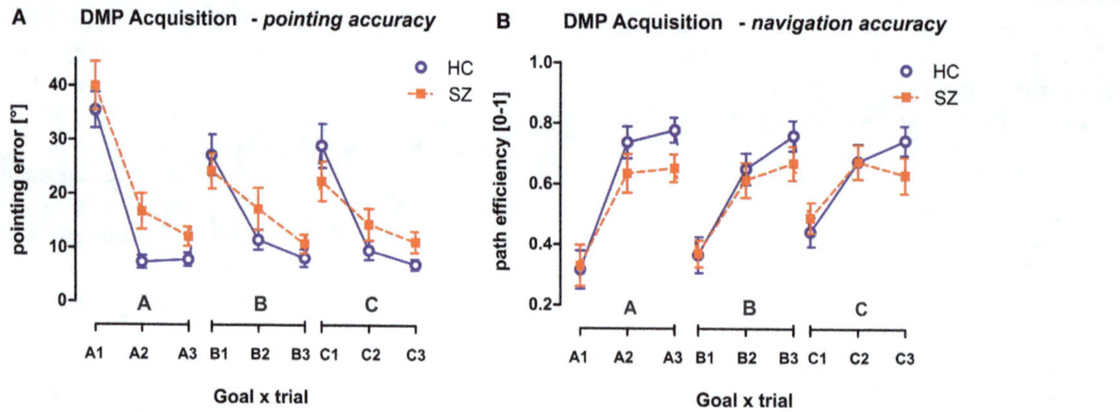

FIGURE 6 | The performance of both groups in the Acquisition phase of the DMP session. The behavior is measured after three consecutive spatial changes, the hidden goal is placed in three possible goal positions (A, B, C), in different relationships to the orientation cues. Trials marked as A1, B1, and C1 required the subject to search for the hidden goal after announcement of the positional change. The next 2 trials required repeated search for the hidden goal. The behavior is shown in all 9 trials presented in the order applied during the Acquisition phase using the two following parameters: **(A)** The pointing error (mean ± s.e.m) and **(B)** the path efficiency (mean ± s.e.m). HC, Healthy controls; SZ, first-episode schizophrenia patients.

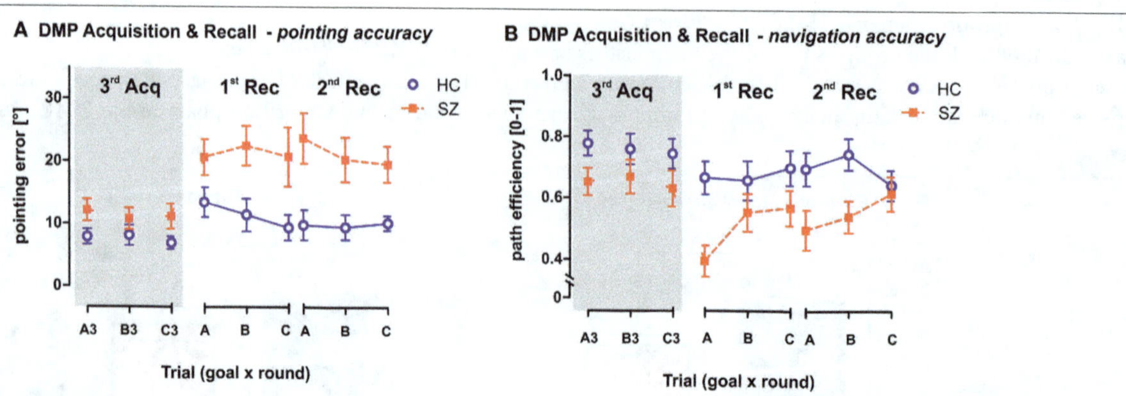

FIGURE 7 | Pointing and Navigation accuracy in the Recall phase of the DMP session in comparison to the performance in the 3rd trial of the Acquisition phase. (A) The pointing error (mean ± s.e.m) and **(B)** the path efficiency (mean ± s.e.m) measured in individual trials. Panels 1st Rec and 2nd Rec show the group performance in the two rounds of the Recall phase. Each round requires recalling the previously learned goal positions in the correct sequence (ABC). Gray area on the left (marked as 3rd Acq) represents the performance achieved in the last (3rd) repetitions of each goal position (A3, B3, and C3) in the Acquisition phase. It illustrates the drop in behavioral performance due to time delay between the last Acquisition trial and the Recall phase. HC, Healthy controls; SZ, first-episode schizophrenia patients.

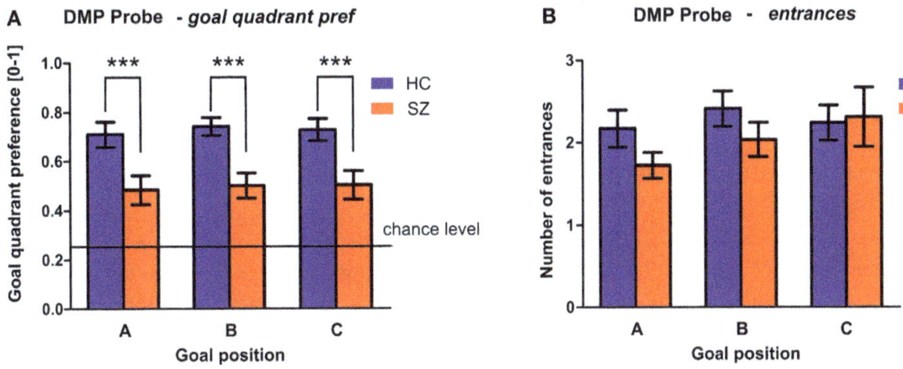

FIGURE 8 | PROBE phase of the DMP session. (A) The goal quadrant preference (mean ± s.e.m) and **(B)** the number of entrances (mean ± s.e.m) into the inactivated goal position presented separately for individual goal positions. Annotation: ***$p < 0.01$ group difference. HC, Healthy controls; SZ, first-episode schizophrenia patients.

Table 2 | Correlation analysis between the age variable and the performances averaged for individual parts of the vFGN task, analyzed separately for group of schizophrenia patients and healthy volunteers.

Correlation analysis	Age correlations					
	Schizophrenia patients $N = 29$			Healthy Controls $N = 29$		
Averaged performance	$r(X,Y)$	t	p	$r(X,Y)$	t	p
avgPath-RM1	−0.48	−2.83	0.009	0.10	0.50	0.62
avgPoint-RM1	0.14	0.77	0.456	−0.20	−1.04	0.31
avgPath-AcqDMP	−0.38	−2.12	0.043	−0.06	−0.31	0.76
avgPoint-AcqDMP	0.33	1.82	0.079	0.10	0.55	0.59
avgPath-RecDMP	−0.49	−2.95	0.006	0.01	0.06	0.95
avgPoint-RecDMP	0.42	2.43	0.022	0.14	0.76	0.45
avgQuadrant- ProbeDMP	−0.36	−2.01	0.054	0.01	0.07	0.95
avgEntrances-ProbeDMP	−0.49	−2.92	0.007	−0.18	−0.96	0.35

avgPath, averaged path efficiency performance; avgPoint, averaged pointing error; avgQuadrant, averaged goal quadrant preference; avgEntrances, averaged number of entrances to the goal; RM1, first half of the RM session; AcqDMP, Acquisition phase of the DMP session; RecDMP, Recall phase of the DMP session; ProbeDMP, Probe phase of the DMP session; r (X,Y), correlation coefficient.

DMP—PROBE phase

The performance of both groups in the PROBE phase (conducted as the last repetition of the spatial sequence after the Recall session) is shown in **Figure 8**. Despite the fact that the performance of both groups differed from the chance level (0.25), the GLM analysis with goal as repetition factor identified significant group differences in the goal quadrant preference [$F_{(1,54)} = 16.9$; $p < 0.001$]. However, we found no differences between the individual goal positions. The performance in healthy controls shows that well-trained subjects search for all three goal positions most of the time in the correct quadrant of the arena, as can be seen in their goal quadrant preference of around 73 ± 18%. The averaged performance in the schizophrenia group is lower for all three goals (50 ± 23%). No significant group differences were identified in the number of entrances to the goal position.

SEX AND AGE DIFFERENCES

In order to show the possible effects of sex on spatial performance in the vFGN task, sex has been used as additional main factor in the GLM analysis (group × sex) with repeated measures performed on individual phases of the task. Interestingly, some sex differences have been observed in almost all parts of the task but exclusively only for the parameter of path efficiency. The main effect of sex was found significant only in the path efficiency in the RM session [$F_{(1, 54)} = 4.2$, $p < 0.05$]. Sex differences approached the significance level in the path efficiency measured in the Acquisition [$F_{(1, 54)} = 3.6$, $p = 0.064$] and the Recall phase [$F_{(1, 54)} = 3.7$, $p = 0.06$] of the DMP session. In all cases males showed superior performance in comparison to females. No differences have been observed either in the pointing accuracy or in the quadrant preference measured in the probe trials. Importantly, no interaction of sex and group factor was observed.

In order to analyze how the age of our participants had affected their performance in the vFGN task, we performed a correlation analysis. The spatial performance of individual participants was averaged for all trials in individual parts of the vFGN task and correlated with the age variable, separately for group of patients and for healthy volunteers (see **Table 2**). The averaged path efficiency in the group of healthy volunteers negatively correlated with the age of individual subjects in all parts of the task. Similarly, the averaged pointing error in the Recall phase and the number of entrances in the Probe phase was significantly affected by the age variable. Importantly, no such correlation was identified for the group of schizophrenia patients.

REGRESSION MODEL OF CLINICAL VARIABLES EFFECT ON PERFORMANCE IN THE vFGN TASK

From the set of the potential clinical and demographic factors that could contribute to the cognitive decline observed in the group of patients, the following predictors were added to the regression model (age, DUP, PANSS-P, PANSS-N, PANSS-G, GAF, and CPZ level) analyzing their effect on performance measured in the vFGN task (averaged separately for individual vFGN parts—RM session and three parts of the DMP session). A stepwise forward multiple regression analysis employed using these predictors only identified the following significant effects—positive effect of GAF score on spatial learning ability expressed as the averaged pointing accuracy ($b_{GAF} = -0.52$; $p < 0.05$) and the navigation accuracy ($b_{GAF} = 0.49$; $p < 0.05$) in the RM session. The full model was significant only for pointing accuracy ($R = 0.57$; $R^2 = 32\%$; $p = 0.045$), but not for the path efficiency ($R = 0.54$; $R^2 = 30\%$; $p = 0.06$), both with GAF and DUP predictors added in 2 steps (all other predictors were removed). In the Recall DMP phase measured by the path efficiency, a significant effect of PANSS-G ($b_{PANSS-G} = 0.68$; $p < 0.05$) and CPZ level ($b_{GAF} = 0.7$; $p < 0.05$) was identified. The whole model, with non-significant DUP and PANSS-N as additional predictors added in the succeeding steps, was not significant ($R = 0.67$; $R^2 = 44\%$; $p = 0.066$). No other significant effects were found by applying this regression model.

DISCUSSION

Both parts of the newly developed virtual vFGN task demonstrated sufficient sensitivity toward the impairment of visuospatial functions identified in our schizophrenia patients using standard neuropsychological methods. First, it is important to discuss the sensitivity of the parameters measured in our study. The pointing error parameter has yet not been applied in similar studies, with the exception of the bearing error used to address spatial abilities in a virtual maze (Waller et al., 2001). This pointing error parameter showed higher sensitivity toward behavioral impairment in schizophrenia than the path efficiency parameter. This finding indicates that the simple pointing paradigm could be used to assess spatial abilities separately. Possible explanation of different sensitivity of measured parameters is that the navigation accuracy (expressed in path eff) could be more affected by sex and age differences, connected to skill learning abilities. The common spatial bias parameter (Morris, 1984, 2008) calculated as percentage of time in the correct arena quadrant was more sensitive toward the impairment in schizophrenia than the other applied parameter, the number of entrances to the goal.

SPATIAL LEARNING PERFORMANCE IN THE RM SESSION

The spatial performance measured during the RM session in our participants strengthen the idea of spatial learning impairment in schizophrenia demonstrated in other human studies (Hanlon et al., 2006; Folley et al., 2010) and animal models of schizophrenia (Gorter and de Bruin, 1992; Latysheva and Rayevsky, 2003; Sircar, 2003; Stuchlik et al., 2004). We found decreased performance in the schizophrenia patients in both pointing and navigation accuracy to the goal. However, the navigation accuracy was decreased only in the first half of the RM session.

We were able to demonstrate the continual improvement of performance in healthy controls during the whole RM session, expressed by the decreasing pointing error and path shortening (growing path efficiency). This is in agreement with the evidence that the latency is shortened in animals during consecutive RM sessions (D'Hooge and De Deyn, 2001; Mulder and Pritchett, 2003; Vorhees and Williams, 2006) and in RM blocks tested in human virtual analogs (Nadel et al., 1998; Leplow et al., 2003). Similar continual improvement was present in our group of schizophrenia patients, but interestingly only in the pointing accuracy. In agreement with another human study (Hanlon et al., 2006) the path efficiency of the schizophrenia group did not improve in the first half of the RM session (trial T2-T5). The discrepancy between these two measured parameters supports the idea that navigation performance could be divided into two distinct parts (directional vs. place navigation in Hamilton et al., 2008): (1) selection of direction to the goal at the beginning of the navigation process represented here by the pointing accuracy and (2) precise determination of goal position represented by the path efficiency. We assume that while the patients do improve in directional navigation by remembering the approximate position of the goal (near a particular cue), they do not improve in direct navigation to the goal due to imprecise perception and memorizing of spatial information.

This assumption is supported by the fact that the navigation accuracy improved after the insertion of a single probe trial (in the middle of the RM session) that could facilitate their motivation to focus on important spatial information due to the previous unsuccessful search. This finding supports our assumption that the measured spatial performance is affected by attention deficit measured using standard neuropsychological tests (TMT and Digit span, see **Table 1**).

In addition, results obtained in the probe trial showed impairment of spatial bias in schizophrenia, in accordance to animal studies (Norris and Foster, 1999; Stuchlik et al., 2004). In rats, the probe test is known to start extinction process; we expected human subjects to respond similarly. The probe trial was therefore applied in the middle of the RM session as a form of interference (often used in learning tasks). Interestingly in animal studies only first half of the probe trial (first 30 s) shows group differences in rodent model of schizophrenia (e.g., Entlerova et al., 2013), as afterwards even the intact animals tend to leave the unrewarded position. However, due to the verbal instruction, our subjects tend to look for the goal during the whole trial. Despite these differences, the human analog of probe trial shows the same pattern as observed in the rodent model of the MWM; lower occupancy of the goal quadrant in the group of schizophrenia patients in comparison to the healthy controls. On the other hand, the number of entrances parameter failed to show significant group differences. This discrepancy indicates that most of the subjects (from both groups) identified the correct goal position, but only the healthy controls tend to stay in the goal area.

Importantly, the final *visible goal trial* showed that the impaired performance observed in the group of schizophrenia patients was not produced by locomotor or sensory deficits. This one-trial finding is in accordance with other human (Hanlon et al., 2006) and animal studies (e.g., Gorter and de Bruin, 1992; Vales et al., 2006), suggesting that the usual block (of several trials) procedure is not essential for demonstrating the control performance of navigation toward a visible goal. Taken together, our findings confirm the designed RM session as a useful tool for assessing visuo-spatial learning in schizophrenia.

MENTAL FLEXIBILITY AND WORKING MEMORY PERFORMANCE IN THE DMP SESSION

The ACQUISITION phase

A major performance improvement in the Acquisition phase of the DMP session appeared immediately after the 1st search trial. Similar behavior was also observed in animal studies where only an improvement between the first and the second trial is present in well-trained animals in the DMP or reversal protocol (Garthe et al., 2009; Saab et al., 2011). Despite the observed group differences in the pointing accuracy, the announcement of positional change to our participants was probably responsible for the low group differences in this part of vFGN task. In addition, in order to be able to compare the group performance in later recall of the spatial sequence regardless of individual goal positions, the goals were placed in identical positions (in the meaning of spatial relationship between the goal position and the orientation cues). Such settings could be a source of skill learning effect that could explain the lack of between-group differences observed in the navigation accuracy. Nevertheless, the low sensitivity of the reversal protocol toward the cognitive deficit in schizophrenia is in accordance with the animal studies that failed to find group differences after application of lower doses of MK-801 (Watson and Stanton, 2009; Lobellova et al., 2013). Interestingly, similar reversal protocol applied in the avoidance task on the rotating arena showed that the pre-training of animals in the task (as in our RM session) can lead to lack of group differences after application of MK-801 (Zemanova et al., 2013).

Importantly, the performance of individual groups achieved in the Acquisition phase (in the last repetition of the goal positions A3, B3, and C3) did not differ between the three goal positions, enabling us to test the consecutive recall of this sequence after a time delay.

The RECALL phase

Our study was the first to demonstrate impairment in schizophrenia patients using the analog of the DMP MWM protocol. Our results showed impaired recall of spatial sequence in schizophrenia patients in both pointing and navigation accuracy. The working memory performance was here expressed in the performance decrease observed after the time delay between the Acquisition phase and the first round of the Recall phase. The strong performance decline in the group of patients (but not in healthy controls) demonstrates the working and/or long-term memory deficit in schizophrenia. These findings are in agreement with the data obtained in animal models of schizophrenia using the DMP protocol (van der Staay et al., 2011).

The PROBE phase

We demonstrated the schizophrenia specific disturbance of spatial bias expressed as decreased *goal quadrant preference* in the PROBE trials completed in the end of the task. The observed behavioral impairment is similar to the observations of rats injected with dizocilpine or scopolamine in pharmacological screening models of schizophrenia and dementia, respectively (Entlerova et al., 2013; Lobellova et al., 2013), which exhibit disturbed performance in probe trials. Nevertheless, in most of the schizophrenia patients the observed probe trial performance was better than in rats after lesion of the hippocampus (Morris et al., 1982; Sutherland et al., 1983) performing by random search patterns.

EFFECT OF DEMOGRAPHIC VARIABLES

Based on the studies describing sex differences in spatial abilities of both rodents (e.g., Roof and Stein, 1999; Cimadevilla et al., 2000) and humans (e.g., Astur et al., 1998, 2004), we expected to find similar effects in spatial abilities measured by the vFGN task. However, we identified significant sex differences only in learning abilities assessed in the RM session. In addition, sex differences have been observed exclusively for the navigation accuracy (path eff) parameter. This fact and the lack of significant sex differences in other parts of the task suggest the following: (1) the simple circular environment prevents the usage of abilities found to be affected by sex (environmental geometry); (2) the directional information was gained similarly in males and females, yet females tend to use less precise trajectories when navigating toward the goal. This could be due to sex differences in motor skill learning; (3) the animal experiments done with pre-training in MWM protocol showed to exhibit smaller sex differences (Jonasson, 2005), as all the three goal positions have been placed in geometrically identical positions. The lack of interaction between sex and group factor in the measured parameters shows that the presented group effects are independent of the sex differences.

According to the current literature describing negative effect of aging on spatial learning and memory processes (e.g., (Moffat and Resnick, 2002; Moffat, 2009)), we expected to find significant correlation between the age and spatial performance in the vFGN task, both during learning and recall of the spatial information. We confirmed this hypothesis as we observed age effects in all parts of the vFGN task in our healthy volunteers. Interestingly, such effect was fully suppressed in schizophrenia patients. This finding supports the idea that the observed cognitive decline is a characteristic pattern in schizophrenia disorder. This result is in contrary to the current meta-analysis (Rajji et al., 2009), which assumed a better prognosis and less expressed cognitive deficit in patients with a lower age of illness onset. However, our study describes the visuo-spatial deficit only in the early remission phase after the first psychotic episode; repeated assessment in the full remission could reveal a different pattern.

EFFECT OF PSYCHIATRIC SYMPTOMS AND ANTIPSYCHOTIC MEDICATION

One of the currently monitored clinical parameter is the *DUP* defined as the time from appearance of the first psychotic symptom to the initiation of suitable antipsychotic treatment (for review see; Marshall et al., 2005). In accordance to a recently published follow-up study (Barnes et al., 2008), we found no significant effect of DUP.

Current literature describes a strong association of cognitive functions and negative symptoms, but the absence of a positive symptom effect on cognitive deficit in schizophrenia (e.g., Addington et al., 1991; Rossi et al., 1997). Interestingly, we found no significant effect of negative or positive symptoms on the performance in the vFGN task. However, we observed a strong connection between the GAF score and spatial learning performance in the RM session and effect of generalized symptoms in the Recall phase of the DMP session. These results demonstrate that high-functioning patients perform better in the cognitive tasks than the low-functioning individuals in the group of schizophrenia patients (Green et al., 2004).

Older studies described negative effects of the first-generation antipsychotic treatment on the cognitive functioning in schizophrenia (Spohn and Strauss, 1989). On the contrary, the current studies addressing atypical antipsychotics reported slightly positive effects of some drugs on the cognitive functioning in schizophrenia patients (e.g., Meltzer and McGurk, 1999) and in an NMDA model of schizophrenia in rats (Bubenikova et al., 2005). Interestingly, only the memory deficit found in the Recall phase of the DMP session was affected by the antipsychotic dosage calculated in CPZ equivalents in the navigation accuracy parameter. We did not find any other effect of the atypical antipsychotic treatment on the overall cognitive performance in the vFGN task. Nevertheless, our study was not aimed at individual antipsychotic compounds and this could distort the analysis.

LIMITATIONS OF THE STUDY

There are some limitations to the current study. Firstly, both animal protocols (RM and DMP) were modified in order to test the human subjects, inducing possible behavioral changes.

The lack of a strong reward motivation present in animal studies (escape from water reaching the platform) could change the motivation to higher performance in the task. However, we assume that our subjects had been motivated as they all voluntarily participated in the study. Moreover, in the group of patients, the vFGN task was performed in the time of neuropsychological assessment aimed to support the diagnostic process. We do believe that during this time period our patients were motivated toward higher performance in general. In addition, both groups judged the level of entertainment during the task similarly as averaged (not reported). Nevertheless, some positive reward could be applied in order to prevent possible lack of motivation in future studies.

In order to enable fast assessment of our participants in only 1 day, the RM protocol could be considered too short to assess long-term memory processes. However, 1-day protocols are common in human studies testing learning abilities and long-term memory in standard tasks (such as verbal or non-verbal learning memory tasks) and in virtual MWMs that have been considered a valid human analogy of spatial RM in rats, and supported by both behavioral data (e.g., Jacobs et al., 1998) and dependence on hippocampal function (e.g., Astur et al., 2002; Goodrich-Hunsaker et al., 2009).

Also the DMP session in our study is not fully comparable to the animal DMP protocol and was modified in the following three details: (1) The inter-trial interval was not controlled directly but was naturally formed by the number of trials included before the recall trial (6 trials for goal A, 4 for B and 2 for C); and (2) Positional changes applied in our study between acquisition and recall of the goal position are not usual in animal studies; (3) The acquisition of the goal position (spatial sequence) was repeated for several (3) trials, as an analog to a reversal protocol, and due to that the spatial information could be retained in the long-term and not the working memory. Despite these modifications we were able to demonstrate that the results obtained in the individual phases of the vFGN task could be compared to the performance patterns obtained in the animal models.

Secondly, despite the smaller number of participants in our study, we were able to demonstrate the deficit in spatial cognition in schizophrenia group. However, matching of the healthy controls to the patients produced an unbalanced distribution in demographic variables, such as the two-peak age distribution in analyzed groups and variable age distribution in males and females caused by the typical age of the early and late onset of schizophrenia.

Thirdly, it is important to note that the navigation performance of schizophrenia patient group observed in the vFGN task was not unitary and showed higher individual variability than the performance in the healthy control group. This variability could be partly produced by the early assessment of patients. Despite these limitations, our findings are supported by the results of studies describing variability of the cognitive deficit level measured in individual first-episode schizophrenia patients (Keefe et al., 2005). In order to understand how the spatial performance was affected by the present attention or memory deficits, further analysis of the spatial performance measured in the vFGN task and its association to standard measures of cognitive deficit is required. A separate paper will be devoted to tracking the possible effects of demographic variables, gaming experiences and cognitive functioning in the group of healthy volunteers, in order to produce normative data for vFGN task performance (in preparation).

CONCLUDING REMARKS

The novel vFGN task covered several MWM protocols in a single task and was sensitive toward the impairment of spatial navigation performance, which was observed in nearly all parts of the designed battery. Our results documented strong parallels between the real animal MWM and the presented virtual analog for humans. Therefore, this novel computer task could serve as a useful method of preclinical trials for assessment of spatial behavior and complex cognitive processes in schizophrenia. According to the animal studies, we propose that the vFGN task could be used to assess spatial learning, attention, mental flexibility and spatial working and/or long-term memory processes in three-dimensional space. Future work should confirm the validity of the individual parts of the designed task using a simultaneous examination of the related cognitive functions by standardized neuropsychological methods.

FUTURE DIRECTIONS

The data presented in this paper demonstrated the sensitivity of the vFGN task toward the cognitive deficit in the first episodes of schizophrenia, confirmed by standard neuropsychological methods. We do believe that the vFGN task assessing complex visuospatial behavior could serve as an ecologically valid screening method more sensitive toward the future course of illness in individual patients than the standard methods measuring single cognitive functions. In order to test this sensitivity, a second assessment session takes place 1 year later in the same patients. This time delay is used to evaluate possible cognitive deficit persisting in our patients after the full remission of symptoms or due to potential relapse of the illness. Longitudinal data revealing the trajectory of vFGN performance during the course of schizophrenia are needed.

AUTHOR CONTRIBUTIONS

Mabel Rodriguez and Iveta Fajnerová designed the study and together with Kamil Vlček wrote the original protocol. Jiří Horáček refined the protocol. Iveta Fajnerová and Kamil Vlček prepared the VR experiment. Iveta Fajnerová, David Levčík and Lucie Konrádová recruited the participants, performed the behavioral and neuropsychological testing and Pavol Mikoláš collected the clinical data. Cyril Brom and his students provided all VR software used in the study. Iveta Fajnerová and Kamil Vlček processed the data and undertook the statistical analysis. Mabel Rodriguez, Kamil Vlček and Jiří Horáček supervised the study. Iveta Fajnerová wrote the first draft of the manuscript. Jiří Horáček, Aleš Stuchlík and Kamil Vlček contributed to data interpretation. All of the authors discussed the results and contributed to the final version of the paper and have approved it.

ACKNOWLEDGMENTS

We are grateful first of all to Prof. Jan Bureš† and Věra Bubeníková-Valešová for their scientific inspiration and valuable advice at the beginning of the project. We would like to thank the reviewers that helped improve the quality of the manuscript. We thank Karolína Dvorská, Martina Ungrmanová, Filip Španiel and his ESO team members for their assistance in the collection of clinical data. We would like to thank Zbyněk Krulich for VE design and Michal Bída for his modifications to the SpaNav software. The study was supported mainly by IGA MZ CR grant No. NT13386 and partially by projects No. NT14291 and NT13843. The institutional support from the Academy of Sciences of the CR (RVO: 67985823) and from the Prague Psychiatric Center by MH CZ - DRO (PCP, 00023752) covered the salaries and other institutional costs.

REFERENCES

Addington, J., Addington, D., and Maticka-Tyndale, E. (1991). Cognitive functioning and positive and negative symptoms in schizophrenia. *Schizophr. Res.* 5, 123–134. doi: 10.1016/0920-9964(91)90039-T

Andreasen, N. C. (1999). A unitary model of schizophrenia: bleuler's fragmented phrene as schizencephaly. *Arch. Gen. Psychiatry* 56, 781–787. doi: 10.1001/archpsyc.56.9.781

Andreasen, N. C., Pressler, M., Nopoulos, P., Miller, D., and Ho, B. C. (2010). Antipsychotic dose equivalents and dose-years: a standardized method for comparing exposure to different drugs. *Biol. Psychiatry* 67, 255–262. doi: 10.1016/j.biopsych.2009.08.040

Astur, R. S., Ortiz, M. L., and Sutherland, R. J. (1998). A characterization of performance by men and women in a virtual Morris water task: a large and reliable sex difference. *Behav. Brain Res.* 93, 185–190. doi: 10.1016/S0166-4328(98)00019-9

Astur, R. S., Taylor, L. B., Mamelak, A. N., Philpott, L., and Sutherland, R. J. (2002). Humans with hippocampus damage display severe spatial memory impairments in a virtual Morris water task. *Behav. Brain Res.* 132, 77–84. doi: 10.1016/S0166-4328(01)00399-0

Astur, R. S., Tropp, J., Sava, S., Constable, R. T., and Markus, E. J. (2004). Sex differences and correlations in a virtual Morris water task, a virtual radial arm maze, and mental rotation. *Behav. Brain Res.* 151, 103–115. doi: 10.1016/j.bbr.2003.08.024

Barnes, T. R., Leeson, V. C., Mutsatsa, S. H., Watt, H. C., Hutton, S. B., and Joyce, E. M. (2008). Duration of untreated psychosis and social function: 1-year follow-up study of first-episode schizophrenia. *Br. J. Psychiatry* 193, 203–209. doi: 10.1192/bjp.bp.108.049718

Bohbot, V. D., Kalina, M., Stepankova, K., Spackova, N., Petrides, M., and Nadel, L. (1998). Spatial memory deficits in patients with lesions to the right hippocampus and to the right parahippocampal cortex. *Neuropsychologia* 36, 1217–1238. doi: 10.1016/S0028-3932(97)00161-9

Bubenikova, V., Votava, M., Horacek, J., Palenicek, T., and Dockery, C. (2005). The effect of zotepine, risperidone, clozapine and olanzapine on MK-801-disrupted sensorimotor gating. *Pharmacol. Biochem. Behav.* 80, 591–596. doi: 10.1016/j.pbb.2005.01.012

Bubenikova-Valesova, V., Horacek, J., Vrajova, M., and Hoschl, C. (2008). Models of schizophrenia in humans and animals based on inhibition of NMDA receptors. *Neurosci. Biobehav. Rev.* 32, 1014–1023. doi: 10.1016/j.neubiorev.2008.03.012

Cimadevilla, J. M., Fenton, A. A., and Bures, J. (2000). Continuous place avoidance task reveals differences in spatial navigation in male and female rats. *Behav. Brain Res.* 107, 161–169. doi: 10.1016/S0166-4328(99)00128-X

de Vignemont, F., Zalla, T., Posada, A., Louvegnez, A., Koenig, O., Georgieff, N., et al. (2006). Mental rotation in schizophrenia. *Conscious. Cogn.* 15, 295–309. doi: 10.1016/j.concog.2005.08.001

D'Hooge, R., and De Deyn, P. P. (2001). Applications of the Morris water maze in the study of learning and memory. *Brain Res. Brain Res. Rev.* 36, 60–90. doi: 10.1016/S0165-0173(01)00067-4

Dudchenko, P. A. (2004). An overview of the tasks used to test working memory in rodents. *Neurosci. Biobehav. Rev.* 28, 699–709. doi: 10.1016/j.neubiorev.2004.09.002

Elvevag, B., and Goldberg, T. E. (2000). Cognitive impairment in schizophrenia is the core of the disorder. *Crit. Rev. Neurobiol.* 14, 1–21. doi: 10.1615/CritRevNeurobiol.v14.i1.10

Entlerova, M., Lobellova, V., Hatalova, H., Zemanova, A., Vales, K., and Stuchlik, A. (2013). Comparison of Long-Evans and Wistar rats in sensitivity to central cholinergic blockade with scopolamine in two spatial tasks: an active place avoidance and the Morris water maze. *Physiol. Behav.* 120, 11–18. doi: 10.1016/j.physbeh.2013.06.024

Fischer, M. H. (2001). Probing spatial working memory with the Corsi Blocks task. *Brain Cogn.* 45, 143–154. doi: 10.1006/brcg.2000.1221

Folley, B. S., Astur, R., Jagannathan, K., Calhoun, V. D., and Pearlson, G. D. (2010). Anomalous neural circuit function in schizophrenia during a virtual Morris water task. *Neuroimage* 49, 3373–3384. doi: 10.1016/j.neuroimage.2009.11.034

Garthe, A., Behr, J., and Kempermann, G. (2009). Adult-generated hippocampal neurons allow the flexible use of spatially precise learning strategies. *PLoS ONE* 4:e5464. doi: 10.1371/journal.pone.0005464

Goodrich-Hunsaker, N. J., Livingstone, S. A., Skelton, R. W., and Hopkins, R. O. (2009). Spatial deficits in a virtual water maze in amnesic participants with hippocampal damage. *Hippocampus* 119, 1307–1315. doi: 10.1002/hipo.20651

Gorter, J. A., and de Bruin, J. P. (1992). Chronic neonatal MK-801 treatment results in an impairment of spatial learning in the adult rat. *Brain Res.* 580, 12–17. doi: 10.1016/0006-8993(92)90921-U

Green, M. F., Kern, R. S., and Heaton, R. K. (2004). Longitudinal studies of cognition and functional outcome in schizophrenia: implications for MATRICS. *Schizophr. Res.* 72, 41–51. doi: 10.1016/j.schres.2004.09.009

Hamilton, D. A., Akers, K. G., Johnson, T. E., Rice, J. P., Candelaria, F. T., Sutherland, R. J., et al. (2008). The relative influence of place and direction in the Morris water task. *J. Exp. Psychol. Anim. Behav. Process.* 34, 31–53. doi: 10.1037/0097-7403.34.1.31

Hanlon, F. M., Weisend, M. P., Hamilton, D. A., Jones, A. P., Thoma, R. J., Huang, M., et al. (2006). Impairment on the hippocampal-dependent virtual Morris water task in schizophrenia. *Schizophr. Res.* 87, 67–80. doi: 10.1016/j.schres.2006.05.021

Jacobs, L. F., Thomas, K. G. F., Laurance, H. E., and Nadel, L. (1998). Place learning in virtual space II: topographical relations as one dimension of stimulus control. *Learn. Motiv.* 29, 288–308. doi: 10.1006/lmot.1998.1008

Jonasson, Z. (2005). Meta-analysis of sex differences in rodent models of learning and memory: a review of behavioral and biological data. *Neurosci. Biobehav. Rev.* 28, 811–825. doi: 10.1016/j.neubiorev.2004.10.006

Jones, S. H., Thornicroft, G., Coffey, M., and Dunn, G. (1995). A brief mental health outcome scale-reliability and validity of the Global Assessment of Functioning (GAF). *Br. J. Psychiatry* 166, 654–659. doi: 10.1192/bjp.166.5.654

Kay, S. R., Fiszbein, A., and Opler, L. A. (1987). The positive and negative syndrome scale (PANSS) for schizophrenia. *Schizophr. Bull.* 13, 261–276. doi: 10.1093/schbul/13.2.261

Keefe, R. S., Eesley, C. E., and Poe, M. P. (2005). Defining a cognitive function decrement in schizophrenia. *Biol. Psychiatry* 57, 688–691. doi: 10.1016/j.biopsych.2005.01.003

Laczo, J., Andel, R., Vyhnalek, M., Vlcek, K., Magerova, H., Varjassyova, A., et al. (2010). Human analogue of the Morris water maze for testing subjects at risk of Alzheimer's disease. *Neurodegener. Dis.* 7, 148–152. doi: 10.1159/000289226

Landgraf, S., Krebs, M. O., Olie, J. P., Committeri, G., van der, M. E., Berthoz, A., et al. (2010). Real world referencing and schizophrenia: are we experiencing the same reality? *Neuropsychologia* 48, 2922–2930. doi: 10.1016/j.neuropsychologia.2010.05.034

Latysheva, N. V., and Rayevsky, K. S. (2003). Chronic neonatal N-methyl-D-aspartate receptor blockade induces learning deficits and transient hypoactivity in young rats. *Prog. Neuropsychopharmacol. Biol. Psychiatry* 27, 787–794. doi: 10.1016/S0278-5846(03)00110-6

Leplow, B., Lehnung, M., Pohl, J., Herzog, A., Ferstl, R., and Mehdorn, M. (2003). Navigational place learning in children and young adults as assessed with a standardized locomotor search task. *Br. J. Psychol.* 94, 299–317. doi: 10.1348/000712603767876244

Lipp, H. P., Stagliar-Bozicevic, M., Fischer, M., and Wolfer, D. P. (1998). A 2-year longitudinal study of swimming navigation in mice devoid of the prion protein: no evidence for neurological anomalies or spatial learning impairments. *Behav. Brain Res.* 95, 47–54. doi: 10.1016/S0166-4328(97)00209-X

Lobellova, V., Entlerova, M., Svojanovska, B., Hatalova, H., Prokopova, I., Petrasek, T., et al. (2013). Two learning tasks provide evidence for disrupted behavioural flexibility in an animal model of schizophrenia-like behaviour induced by acute MK-801: a dose-response study. *Behav. Brain Res.* 246, 55–62. doi: 10.1016/j.bbr.2013.03.006

Marshall, M., Lewis, S., Lockwood, A., Drake, R., Jones, P., and Croudace, T. (2005). Association between duration of untreated psychosis and outcome in cohorts of first-episode patients: a systematic review. *Arch. Gen. Psychiatry* 62, 975–983. doi: 10.1001/archpsyc.62.9.975

Meltzer, H. Y., and McGurk, S. R. (1999). The effects of clozapine, risperidone, and olanzapine on cognitive function in schizophrenia. *Schizophr. Bull.* 25, 233–255. doi: 10.1093/oxfordjournals.schbul.a033376

Meyers, J. E., and Meyers, K. R. (1995). *Rey Complex Figure Test and Recognition Trial.* Lutz, FL: Psychological Assessment Resources.

Moffat, S. D. (2009). Aging and spatial navigation: what do we know and where do we go? *Neuropsychol. Rev.* 19, 478–489. doi: 10.1007/s11065-009-9120-3

Moffat, S. D., and Resnick, S. M. (2002). Effects of age on virtual environment place navigation and allocentric cognitive mapping. *Behav. Neurosci.* 116, 851–859. doi: 10.1037/0735-7044.116.5.851

Morris, R. (1984). Developments of a water-maze procedure for studying spatial learning in the rat. *J. Neurosci. Methods* 11, 47–60. doi: 10.1016/0165-0270(84)90007-4

Morris, R. G., Garrud, P., Rawlins, J. N., and O'Keefe, J. (1982). Place navigation impaired in rats with hippocampal lesions. *Nature* 297, 681–683. doi: 10.1038/297681a0

Morris, R. G., Hagan, J. J., and Rawlins, J. N. (1986). Allocentric spatial learning by hippocampectomised rats: a further test of the spatial mapping and working memory theories of hippocampal function. *Q. J. Exp. Psychol. B* 38, 365–395.

Morris, R. G., Schenk, F., Tweedie, F., and Jarrard, L. E. (1990). Ibotenate lesions of hippocampus and/or subiculum: dissociating components of allocentric spatial learning. *Eur. J. Neurosci.* 2, 1016–1028. doi: 10.1111/j.1460-9568.1990.tb00014.x

Morris, R. G. M. (1981). Spatial localization does not require the presence of local cues. *Learn. Motiv.* 12, 239–261. doi: 10.1016/0023-9690(81)90020-5

Morris, R. G. M. (2008). Morris water maze. *Scholarpedia* 3:6315. doi: 10.4249/scholarpedia.6315

Mueller, S. C., Jackson, C. P., and Skelton, R. W. (2008). Sex differences in a virtual water maze: an eye tracking and pupillometry study. *Behav. Brain Res.* 193, 209–215. doi: 10.1016/j.bbr.2008.05.017

Mulder, G. B., and Pritchett, K. (2003). The Morris water maze. *Contemp. Top. Lab. Anim. Sci.* 42, 49–50.

Nadel, L., Thomas, K. G. F., Laurance, H. E., Skelton, R., Tal, T., and Jacobs, W. J. (1998). Human place learning in a computer generated arena. *Lect. Notes Comput. Sci.* 1404, 399–428. doi: 10.1007/3-540-69342-4_19

Norris, C. M., and Foster, T. C. (1999). MK-801 improves retention in aged rats: implications for altered neural plasticity in age-related memory deficits. *Neurobiol. Learn. Mem.* 71, 194–206. doi: 10.1006/nlme.1998.3864

O'Carroll, C. M., Martin, S. J., Sandin, J., Frenguelli, B., and Morris, R. G. (2006). Dopaminergic modulation of the persistence of one-trial hippocampus-dependent memory. *Learn. Mem.* 13, 760–769. doi: 10.1101/lm.321006

Overman, W. H., Pate, B. J., Moore, K., and Peuster, A. (1996). Ontogeny of place learning in children as measured in the radial arm maze, Morris search task, and open field task. *Behav. Neurosci.* 110, 1205–1228. doi: 10.1037/0735-7044.110.6.1205

PEBL. (2012). *The Psychology Experiment Building Language. (Version 0.12, Test Battery 0.7).* Michigan Technological University. Available online at: http://pebl.sourceforge.net/battery.html

Piskulic, D., Olver, J. S., Norman, T. R., and Maruff, P. (2007). Behavioural studies of spatial working memory dysfunction in schizophrenia: a quantitative literature review. *Psychiatry Res.* 150, 111–121. doi: 10.1016/j.psychres.2006.03.018

Pratt, J., Winchester, C., Dawson, N., and Morris, B. (2012). Advancing schizophrenia drug discovery: optimizing rodent models to bridge the translational gap. *Nat. Rev. Drug Discov.* 11, 560–579. doi: 10.1038/nrd3649

Preiss, M. (1997). *Trail Making test Pro Děti a Dospělé. Manuál.* Bratislava: Psychodiagnostika.

Rajji, T. K., Ismail, Z., and Mulsant, B. H. (2009). Age at onset and cognition in schizophrenia: meta-analysis. *Br. J. Psychiatry* 195, 286–293. doi: 10.1192/bjp.bp.108.060723

Reichenberg, A., Harvey, P. D., Bowie, C. R., Mojtabai, R., Rabinowitz, J., Heaton, R. K., et al. (2009). Neuropsychological function and dysfunction in schizophrenia and psychotic affective disorders. *Schizophr. Bull.* 35, 1022–1029. doi: 10.1093/schbul/sbn044

Reitan, R. M., and Wolfson, D. (1993). *The Halstead-Reitan Neuropsychological Test battery: Theory and Clinical Interpretation.* 2nd edn. Tuscon, AZ: Neuropsychology Press.

Rodriguez, P. F. (2010). Human navigation that requires calculating heading vectors recruits parietal cortex in a virtual and visually sparse water maze task in fMRI. *Behav. Neurosci.* 124, 532–540. doi: 10.1037/a0020231

Roof, R. L., and Stein, D. G. (1999). Gender differences in Morris water maze performance depend on task parameters. *Physiol Behav.* 68, 81–86. doi: 10.1016/S0031-9384(99)00162-6

Rossi, A., Mancini, F., Stratta, P., Mattei, P., Gismondi, R., Pozzi, F., et al. (1997). Risperidone, negative symptoms and cognitive deficit in schizophrenia: an open study. *Acta Psychiatr. Scand.* 95, 40–43. doi: 10.1111/j.1600-0447.1997.tb00371.x

Saab, B. J., Luca, R. M., Yuen, W. B., Saab, A. M., and Roder, J. C. (2011). Memantine affects cognitive flexibility in the Morris water maze. *J. Alzheimers. Dis.* 27, 477–482. doi: 10.3233/JAD-2011-110650

Sircar, R. (2003). Postnatal phencyclidine-induced deficit in adult water maze performance is associated with N-methyl-D-aspartate receptor upregulation. *Int. J. Dev. Neurosci.* 21, 159–167. doi: 10.1016/S0736-5748(03)00026-1

Skolimowska, J., Wesierska, M., Lewandowska, M., Szymaszek, A., and Szelag, E. (2011). Divergent effects of age on performance in spatial associative learning and real idiothetic memory in humans. *Behav. Brain Res.* 218, 87–93. doi: 10.1016/j.bbr.2010.11.035

Spohn, H. E., and Strauss, M. E. (1989). Relation of neuroleptic and anticholinergic medication to cognitive functions in schizophrenia. *J. Abnorm. Psychol.* 98, 367–380. doi: 10.1037/0021-843X.98.4.367

Steele, R. J., and Morris, R. G. (1999). Delay-dependent impairment of a matching-to-place task with chronic and intrahippocampal infusion of the NMDA-antagonist D-AP5. *Hippocampus* 9, 118–136.

Stepankova, K., Pastalkova, E., Kalova, E., Kalina, M., and Bures, J. (2003). A battery of tests for quantitative examination of idiothetic and allothetic place navigation modes in humans. *Behav. Brain Res.* 147, 95–105. doi: 10.1016/S0166-4328(03)00141-4

Stepankova, K., Pastalkova, E., Kaminsky, Y., Fenton, A. A., and Bures, J. (1999). Allothetic and idiothetic navigation in healthy young humans. *Physiol. Res.* 48, 123.

Stuchlik, A., Rezacova, L., Vales, K., Bubenikova, V., and Kubik, S. (2004). Application of a novel Active Allothetic Place Avoidance task (AAPA) in testing a pharmacological model of psychosis in rats: comparison with the Morris Water Maze. *Neurosci. Lett.* 366, 162–166. doi: 10.1016/j.neulet.2004.05.037

Šupalová, I. (2009). *Orientace v Prostoru Zkoumaná ve Virtuální Realitě. (Adaptation Of Spatial Navigation Tests To Virtual Reality).* Charles University in Prague.

Sutherland, R. J., Whishaw, I. Q., and Kolb, B. (1983). A behavioural analysis of spatial localization following electrolytic, kainate- or colchicine-induced damage to the hippocampal formation in the rat. *Behav. Brain Res.* 7, 133–153. doi: 10.1016/0166-4328(83)90188-2

Vales, K., Bubenikova-Valesova, V., Klement, D., and Stuchlik, A. (2006). Analysis of sensitivity to MK-801 treatment in a novel active allothetic place avoidance task and in the working memory version of the Morris water maze reveals differences between Long-Evans and Wistar rats. *Neurosci. Res.* 55, 383–388. doi: 10.1016/j.neures.2006.04.007

Vorhees, C. V., and Williams, M. T. (2006). Morris water maze: procedures for assessing spatial and related forms of learning and memory. *Nat. Protoc.* 1, 848–858. doi: 10.1038/nprot.2006.116

Waller, D., Knapp, D., and Hunt, E. (2001). Spatial representations of virtual mazes: the role of visual fidelity and individual differences. *Hum. Factors.* 43, 147–158. doi: 10.1518/001872001775992561

Watson, D. J., and Stanton, M. E. (2009). Intrahippocampal administration of an NMDA-receptor antagonist impairs spatial discrimination reversal learning in weanling rats. *Neurobiol. Learn. Mem.* 92, 89–98. doi: 10.1016/j.nlm.2009.02.005

Wechsler, D. (1997a). *Wechsler Adult Intelligence Scale-III* San Antonio, TX: The Psychological Corporation. Czech translation by Hogrefe–Testcentrum, Praha 2010.

Wechsler, D. (1997b). *Manual for the Wechsler Memory Scale-III.* San Antonio, TX: Psychological Corporation. Czech translation by Psychodiagnostika, Bratislava 1999.

Weniger, G., and Irle, E. (2008). Allocentric memory impaired and egocentric memory intact as assessed by virtual reality in recent-onset schizophrenia. *Schizophr. Res.* 101, 201–209. doi: 10.1016/j.schres.2008.01.011

Whishaw, I. Q. (1991). Latent learning in a swimming pool place task by rats: evidence for the use of associative and not cognitive mapping processes. *Q. J. Exp. Psychol. B* 43, 83–103.

Woods, S. W. (2003). Chlorpromazine equivalent doses for the newer atypical antipsychotics. *J. Clin. Psychiatry* 64, 663–667. doi: 10.4088/JCP.v64n0607

Zemanova, A., Stankova, A., Lobellova, V., Svoboda, J., Vales, K., Vlcek, K., et al. (2013). Visuospatial working memory is impaired in an animal model of schizophrenia induced by acute MK-801: an effect of pretraining. *Pharmacol. Biochem. Behav.* 106, 117–123. doi: 10.1016/j.pbb.2013.03.014

Structural hippocampal anomalies in a schizophrenia population correlate with navigation performance on a wayfinding task

Andrée-Anne Ledoux[1,2,*], Patrice Boyer[1,3], Jennifer L. Phillips[1], Alain Labelle[1], Andra Smith[2] and Véronique D. Bohbot[4]

[1] University of Ottawa Institute of Mental Health Research, Ottawa, ON, Canada
[2] School of Psychology, University of Ottawa, Ottawa, ON, Canada
[3] Université Paris Diderot – Paris 7, Paris, France
[4] Douglas Mental Health University Institute, McGill University, Montreal, QC, Canada

Edited by:
Tomiki Sumiyoshi, National Center of Neurology and Psychiatry, Japan

***Correspondence:**
Andrée-Anne Ledoux, University of Ottawa School of Psychology, 136 Jean-Jacques Lussier, Ottawa, ON K1N 6N5, Canada
e-mail: aledoux@uottawa.ca

Episodic memory, related to the hippocampus, has been found to be impaired in schizophrenia. Further, hippocampal anomalies have also been observed in schizophrenia. This study investigated whether average hippocampal gray matter (GM) would differentiate performance on a hippocampus-dependent memory task in patients with schizophrenia and healthy controls. Twenty-one patients with schizophrenia and 22 control participants were scanned with an MRI while being tested on a wayfinding task in a virtual town (e.g., find the grocery store from the school). Regressions were performed for both groups individually and together using GM and performance on the wayfinding task. Results indicate that controls successfully completed the task more often than patients, took less time, and made fewer errors. Additionally, controls had significantly more hippocampal GM than patients. Poor performance was associated with a GM decrease in the right hippocampus for both groups. Within group regressions found an association between right hippocampi GM and performance in controls and an association between the left hippocampi GM and performance in patients. A second analysis revealed that different anatomical GM regions, known to be associated with the hippocampus, such as the parahippocampal cortex, amygdala, medial, and orbital prefrontal cortices, covaried with the hippocampus in the control group. Interestingly, the cuneus and cingulate gyrus also covaried with the hippocampus in the patient group but the orbital frontal cortex did not, supporting the hypothesis of impaired connectivity between the hippocampus and the frontal cortex in schizophrenia. These results present important implications for creating intervention programs aimed at measuring functional and structural changes in the hippocampus in schizophrenia.

Keywords: psychiatric population, VBM, allocentric strategy, episodic memory, spatial memory, hippocampus

INTRODUCTION

Cognitive dysfunction is believed to be among the core features of schizophrenia. Despite abundant evidence of a prefrontal impairment in schizophrenia, this type of deficit is not specific to schizophrenia and has been extensively reported in different psychiatric disorders (e.g., mood disorders, OCD spectrum; Clark et al., 2010). Emerging research indicates that other types of deficits are more characteristic of schizophrenia, such as an episodic memory deficit, thought to be related to a dysfunction at the level of the hippocampal formation (Aleman et al., 1999; Boyer et al., 2007).

One of the most robust findings in schizophrenia is the abnormal hippocampal structure (Weiss et al., 2005). Abundant evidence from post-mortem evaluations (Bogerts et al., 1990) and *in vivo* magnetic resonance imaging (MRI) studies has demonstrated a reduced volume of the hippocampal regions (Nelson et al., 1998; Wright et al., 2000). These MRI findings have also been observed in prodromal and first episode subjects (Pantelis et al., 2003). Structural MRI studies have demonstrated that the hippocampal volume deficit is diffused throughout the anterior and posterior portions and not localized to any given parts of the hippocampus (Weiss et al., 2005). Studies have demonstrated shape differences (Shenton et al., 2002) in the hippocampal structure but also morphological differences (size, organization, and shape) in the hippocampal neurons. Post-mortem studies have demonstrated reduced neuronal size (Benes et al., 1991; Arnold et al., 1995; Zaidel et al., 1997) and disorganized pyramidal cell (Luts et al., 1998) in the hippocampus proper subfields CA1 (Arnold et al., 1995), CA2, and CA3 (Zaidel et al., 1997) and subiculum (Kovelman and Scheibel, 1984; Arnold et al., 1995). Further, there have been reports of decreased density of dendritic spines, and less extensive apical dendritic trees in the pyramidal neurons of the subicular complex (Rosoklija et al., 2000) and in the granule cells of the dentate gyrus (Lauer et al., 2003).

It is now commonly accepted that the hippocampus plays a critical role in learning, long-term memory, and spatial memory. When the hippocampus is selectively lesioned, humans present with severe spatial memory deficits (Bohbot et al., 1998). It has also been demonstrated that hippocampal lesions in rats produce difficulties in solving spatial navigation tasks (Morris et al., 1982). Visuospatial navigation has been shown to be critically dependent on the hippocampus. Navigating is a cognitively demanding task, and requires individuals to construct a mental representation of the environment with allocentric and egocentric frameworks. The allocentric representation of the environment is dependant on the cognitive map. In other words to be successful at a task one must learn the relations between landmarks (stimulus–stimulus association; Bohbot et al., 2007). According to the cognitive map theory, the main function of the hippocampus is to construct and maintain spatial maps (learning the relationship between environmental landmarks) of the environment (O'Keefe and Nadel, 1978; Kumaran and Maguire, 2005). Therefore, the cognitive map allows a target to be reached in a direct path from any given direction. In contrast, individuals can use stimulus-response learning (Packard et al., 1989) for example using a single landmark as a reference (e.g., at the coffee shop turn left) or make decisions based on their body movement, independent of landmarks in their environment (Iaria et al., 2003). Patients with lesions at the level of the hippocampus are unable to complete spatial allocentric tasks (Bohbot et al., 1998). Recently, it was found in a behavioral study that individuals with schizophrenia exhibit impairments in allocentric memory while egocentric memory remained intact (Weniger and Irle, 2008). Similarly, patients with brain damage to the medial temporal lobe, which includes the hippocampus, are impaired when they spontaneously use an allocentric spatial memory strategy in a dual-solution task (Bohbot et al., 1998). However, similar patients who spontaneously use the stimulus-response strategy are not impaired (Bohbot et al., 2004). Neuroimaging studies have greatly contributed to the literature by providing confirmatory evidence that the hippocampus, together with the parahippocampal gyrus, posterior parietal cortices, medial prefrontal cortex, and striatum are engaged in visuospatial navigation (Aguirre et al., 1996; Maguire et al., 1998; Burgess et al., 2001).

In a previous fMRI study that included the same research participants (schizophrenia and control groups) as those included in the current study, Ledoux et al. (2013) demonstrated an episodic memory deficit in the schizophrenia group. Further, controls performed significantly better on a virtual visuospatial navigation task called the wayfinding task and had significantly increased fMRI activity in the hippocampus compared to these patients while performing the wayfinding task. The wayfinding task used by Ledoux et al. (2013) and in the current study is identical to the one used by Etchamendy and Bohbot (2007), and is modeled after the task used by Hartley et al. (2003). In this task, participants are required to use allocentric representations in order to be successful at finding their way in the environment taking the shortest path. Therefore, in the current paper, we asked whether the wayfinding deficit found in patients with schizophrenia was associated with gray matter (GM) loss in the hippocampus.

Though it is known that the hippocampus is involved in a more general class of memory, such as episodic memory including memory across temporal delays such as trace conditioning (Gruart et al., 2006), explicit memory (Eichenbaum et al., 2012), or relational memory (Clarke et al., 2010), the current paper focuses on the role of the hippocampus in spatial memory (Burgess et al., 2002). The current study used voxel-based morphometry (VBM) to investigate hippocampal GM in patients with schizophrenia and healthy controls previously studied by Ledoux et al. (2013) and examined the relationship between the region of interest in the hippocampus and behavioral performance on the wayfinding task. In this study, we sought to investigate whether performance on the wayfinding task has a predictive relation with the morphological differences in the hippocampus of patients and control participants. Further, we investigated whether the different regions known to be anatomically connected to the hippocampus in a healthy population were associated with the hippocampal GM in the schizophrenia group. It was hypothesized that the patient group would have hippocampal GM differences compared to the control group and that the GM in the hippocampus would play a significant role in performance on the hippocampus-dependent spatial memory task in patients with schizophrenia and in healthy control participants. Finally, in previous studies it was demonstrated that individuals with more GM in the hippocampus also had more GM in an associated network of neuroanatomically connected regions, which include the orbital prefrontal cortex, the parahippocampal cortex, entorhinal and perirhinal cortices, and amygdala (Bohbot et al., 2007; Konishi and Bohbot, 2013). Taking these previous studies into consideration and the disconnectivity theories suggesting connectivity impairments between the hippocampus and prefrontal cortex (Weinberger et al., 1992), it was hypothesized that the patient group would demonstrate differences in the associated network of neuroanatomically connected regions, notably in the orbital prefrontal cortex.

MATERIALS AND METHODS

PARTICIPANTS

A total of 43 study participants who comprised two groups: (1) 21 schizophrenia patients and (2) 22 control participants were recruited for this study. Participants were male and female between 18 and 40 years old inclusively and right-handed (determined by the Handedness Inventory; Oldfield, 1971) due to documented differences in hippocampal areas linked to navigation skills associated with the non-dominant hemisphere. Patients with a primary diagnosis of schizophrenia were recruited from the Outpatient Schizophrenia Clinic at the Royal Ottawa Mental Health Centre. Controls were recruited via newspaper and poster advertisement. The control group was closely matched to the schizophrenia patients in terms of age, sex, and education level. Ethics for the current study were accepted by the Research Ethics Board of the University of Ottawa, Institute of Mental Health Research in Ottawa. Prior to starting the study, all participants signed an informed consent form authorizing the researcher to conduct research with their information. Participants were paid a sum of $75 to take part in the study.

Inclusion criteria for the patient group

Participants of this group needed to be clinically diagnosed with schizophrenia by a psychiatrist, therefore they had to meet the Diagnostic and Statistical Manual of Mental Disorders – Fourth Edition criteria (DSM-IV-TR; American Psychiatric Association, 2000). Patients meeting the DSM-IV criteria for schizophrenia, disorganized, undifferentiated, or paranoid subtypes, were eligible to participate in the study; catatonia subtypes and schizoaffective patients were excluded from the study. Patients needed to be clinically stabilized. Stabilization is defined as having had no significant change in symptom severity (i.e., level of severity), and no changes in medication type or dosage or therapeutic methods following a 3-month retrospective chart review determined by their psychiatrist.

Exclusion criteria for patient group

Participants with an acute psychotic episode on the total Positive Negative Symptoms Scale (PANSS; Kay et al., 1987) or having a score of 4 on two or more of the following PANSS items (conceptual disorganization, P2; hallucinatory behavior, P3; suspiciousness, P6; unusual thought content, G9) were excluded. Further, participants exhibiting comorbid depressive symptoms [Calgary Depression Scale (CDS) score ≥7; Addington et al., 1990], taking typical antipsychotics, benzodiazepines, or receiving electroconvulsive therapy (ECT) were excluded from this study. Finally, the presence of extrapyramidal symptoms (EPS), or overt signs of tremor or movement disorder could affect the quality of MRI image acquisition. Therefore, patients exhibiting those symptoms were also excluded from this study.

Exclusion criteria for control group

Presentation of a psychiatric condition corresponding to an Axis 1 DSM-IV TR diagnosis (using SCID-NP interview) was considered an exclusion criteria. Also, participants reporting a psychiatric history concerning their siblings or other first-degree relatives did not qualify for the study. Finally, having depressive symptoms [Hamilton Scale for Depression (HAMD) score ≥10; Hamilton, 1960] excluded participants from the study.

Exclusion criteria common for patient and control groups

Current diagnosis of alcohol abuse or other kinds of dependence in the previous 12 months [Alcohol Use Disorders Identification Test (AUDIT) score ≥8 in men or ≥7 in women; Saunders et al., 1993] or current diagnosis or history of drug abuse or dependence in the past 12 months [Drug and Abuse Screening Test (DAST) score ≥6; Skinner, 1982] were exclusion criterion. Participants with neurological disease, history of head injury, cardiovascular disease, or stroke (determined by Medical Questionnaire) were also excluded. The presence of any non-removable magnetic metal on or in the body (such as cardiac pacemakers, metal prostheses), as determined by the Medical Questionnaire, was also reason for exclusion from the study.

MATERIAL AND PROCEDURE

Clinical assessment

The clinical assessment was a 2 h session separated into two parts. The first hour of the assessment was the clinical interview where the SCID, CDS, or HAMD, PANSS (for patients only) were administered. The second part of the assessment consisted of self-report questionnaires answered by participants. Participants were required to assess themselves on the following questionnaires: AUDIT, DAST.

MRI session

The MRI portion of this project occurred in two phases performed on the same day: the pre-scan training phase followed within 1 h by the scan phase. Since familiarity with first-person videogames may have an impact in the virtual reality task performance, before the pre-scan training participants were asked about their video game habits [e.g., what type(s) of video game played]. During the pre-scan training, participants were first familiarized with the keyboard to ensure their ability to maneuver through the environment. This was done in a virtual environment different from the virtual town used for the experiment. They then navigated in the virtual town created with the game editor of a commercially available computer game (Unreal Tournament 2003; Epic Games, Raleigh, NC, USA). The virtual town is a visually complex computer-based environment, which includes several roads, intersections, and buildings, in addition to distinct landmarks (easily recognizable, labeled locations such as a school or a hospital). Participants engaged in a free exploration of the town for 20–30 min. During exploration, participants were required to encounter every landmark twice and to travel along all roads. The path taken and the amount of time participants visited each landmark was recorded. The free exploration provided an opportunity for participants to encode and construct a cognitive map of the environment by building relationships between landmarks in the town. Participants were not permitted sufficient exploration time to form habitual routes between landmarks. Creating the paradigm using a modified video game framework provided participants with a first-person perspective while navigating. Following the training outside the MRI, participants were scanned while performing tasks based on the navigation paradigm. In the MRI, participants underwent a 15 min T1 structural scan. During fMRI scanning which followed, participants were required to complete the Navigation Task. For each eight navigation trials, participants were placed in one location in the city (e.g., school) and were required to navigate from there to another landmark (e.g., movie theater) within the city. Successful completion of this task required taking the shortest route by deriving it from a cognitive map, a task that critically requires the hippocampus. During completion of the navigation trials, participants were timed and their precise paths were recorded on a 2D aerial view of the town.

Magnetic resonance imaging scans were acquired using a 1.5 Tesla Siemens Magnetom Symphony. The protocol generated T1-weighted image volumes with a 1 mm isotropic resolution using a three-dimensional spoiled gradient echo acquisition with sagittal volume excitation (repetition time, 22; echo time, 9.2; flip angle, 30°; field of view, 256 mm; 160 1 mm sagittal slices). An MRI-compatible virtual reality system, Silent Vision™ Model SV-7021 Fiber Optic Visual System with In Control Software (Avotec, Inc.), was acquired for this study, as well as a four button fiber optic touch pad.

DATA ANALYSES

Participants were matched according to their age, sex, and level of education for all analyses in this study. Behavioral data (demographics and navigation performances) were analyzed using SPSS (SPSS, 2008) software. Neuroimaging data was analyzed with

Statistical Parametric Mapping software (SPM8, 2008) and the VBM8 toolbox (http://dbm.neuro.uni-jena.de/vbm/).

Behavioral data

The first hypothesis of a significant difference between patient and control groups within the behavioral navigation performance was analyzed with a multivariate ANOVA. Variables considered for the analysis of navigation performance were Accuracy (i.e., percentage of target locations reached), Percent error (i.e., percentage of extra distance traveled + distance remaining to reach the goal compared to shortest distance needed to reach goal location), and mean time.

$$\text{Percent error}: \left((x+z) - y/(x+z) \times 100\right)$$

(i.e., x = total distance traveled, z = distance remaining to reach the goal, y = shortest distance to goal). The z variable was included to account for incomplete trials where the target landmark was not reached. Since incomplete trials by definition are missing part of the way to the goal location, the z variable was made to include this missing distance. Therefore, the shortest distance from the end point at which the trial was interrupted to the goal location is added to the distance traveled $(x + z)$.

Voxel-based morphometry and statistical analysis

We applied VBM as implemented in the VBM8 toolbox with default parameters. Images were bias-corrected, tissue classified, and registered using linear (12-parameter affine) and non-linear transformations (warping), within a unified model (Ashburner and Friston, 2005). Subsequently, analyses were performed on GM and white matter (WM) segments, which were multiplied by the non-linear components derived from the normalization matrix in order to preserve actual GM and WM values locally (modulated GM and WM average). Finally, the modulated volumes were smoothed with a Gaussian kernel of 12 mm full width at half maximum (FWHM). GM, WM, and Cerebral Spinal Fluid (CSF) maps were combined for total intracranial volume (TIV). Voxel-wise GM and WM differences between schizophrenia patients and controls were examined using independent-sample t-tests. In order to avoid possible edge effects between different tissue types, we excluded all voxels with GM or WM values of less than 0.1 (absolute threshold masking).

A first regression was performed on GM and navigation performance to determine whether GM regressed with the percentage errors made during the task, accuracy, and time.

The purpose of our study was primarily focused on the hippocampal structure, and secondly the prefrontal cortex and caudate nucleus. Region of interests (ROI) analyses were restricted to the hippocampus, parahippocampal gyrus, caudate nucleus, superior medial, and orbital prefrontal cortices. We created a mask for all specified ROI with the Pick Atlas extension (Maldjian et al., 2003) using the automated anatomical labeling atlas (Tzourio-Mazoyer et al., 2002). This mask was then inserted as the explicit mask in the VBM factorial analyses. Within the masks, significance was set at a threshold of uncorrected $p < 0.001$, with a cluster-wise correction at pFWE $= 0.05$ and a set cluster size larger than 10 voxels.

Pearson correlations were performed between subtracted hippocampal GM regions at the peak voxel (MNI space $x = 24$, $y = -21$, $z = -15$ and $x = -24$, $y = -21$, $z = -18$) and the navigation behavioral variables in both groups.

Results of the first VBM regression were used to regress the GM value at the peak voxel (MNI space coordinates, $x = 24$, $y = -21$, $z = -15$) in the hippocampus against the entire MRI volume in the control and patient groups. This second regression tested and compared whether GM in the network of regions known to be anatomically linked to the hippocampus covaried with hippocampal GM in patients. A similar regression was also performed in Bohbot et al. (2007) showing that navigational strategies correlate with GM in the hippocampus or caudate of healthy participants. In turn, GM in the hippocampus correlated with a network of brain regions, known to be anatomically connected (i.e., orbital prefrontal cortex, the parahippocampal, entorhinal and perirhinal cortices, and amygdala).

RESULTS

DEMOGRAPHICS

Twenty-one patients with schizophrenia and 22 healthy controls qualified and completed the study. All together, 20 pairs were matched on age, sex and education. However, one patient (male age 30) and three controls (one female age 22 and two males age 19 and 37) were not matched because their respective matched partner was withdrawn from the study due to miscellaneous difficulties (e.g., WM abnormalities, experiencing excessive anxiety in the scanner). Therefore, matching of our samples was done at a group level. Participant demographics are demonstrated in **Table 1**. No significant differences were found in the main matching criteria variables: age, sex, education, and no significant differences were found in IQ scores, experience with first-person videogames, or mean number of time participants visited the landmarks during the learning phase (visited landmarks), $p > 0.05$ (**Table 1**). Patients' mean PANSS global score of 64 represents a very moderate severity and slightly predominant but not marked negative symptoms (18.4 vs. 15.4), in summary, a moderate and stabilized population.

Table 1 | Participant demographics.

	Controls ($n = 22$; SD)	Patients ($n = 21$; SD)
Sex (F/M)	6/16	5/16
Age (years)	30.45 (1.25)	32.05 (1.08)
Education (years)	16.68 (2.64)	15.10 (2.09)
IQ (NART)	111.32 (1.67)	109.09 (1.47)
Played first-person videogame (yes/no)	13/9	13/8
Visited landmarks	20.64 (4.76)	21.38 (5.36)
Age of onset (years)		20.52 (4.81)
Duration of illness (years)		11.38 (4.93)
PANSS total		64 (13.0)
PANSS positive		15.14 (4.33)
PANSS negative		18.14 (5.68)
PANSS general score		30.71 (6.93)

$p > 0.05$ on all measures.

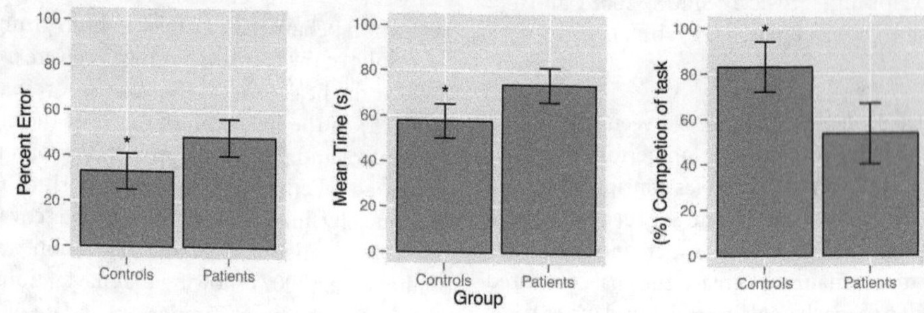

FIGURE 1 | Bar plot demonstrating differences between patient and control groups for the behavioral navigation variables: percent error [*F* (1,41) = 9.64, *p* = 0.003]; mean time [*F* (1,41) = 12.28, *p* = 0.001]; and accuracy [*F* (1,41) = 15.47, *p* = 0.000].

BEHAVIORAL NAVIGATION SCORES

Compared to controls, patients with schizophrenia found fewer target landmarks [$F(1, 41) = 15.47$, $p = 0.000$], traveled longer distances [$F(1, 41) = 9.639$, $p = 0.003$], and took more time [$F(1, 41) = 12.28$, $p = 0.001$] to find target landmarks, **Figure 1**.

REGIONAL GM REDUCTION IN PATIENTS COMPARED TO CONTROL PARTICIPANTS

Groups did not differ in overall TIV ($t_{41} = -0.96$, $p = 0.34$). In order to investigate whether there were whole brain GM and WM differences, independent-sample t-tests were performed. Since there was no significant difference in age or TIV, these variables were not used as covariables. Significant differences in GM (**Table 2** and **Figure 2**) were found between groups (Controls > Patients). WM analysis showed significant differences between controls and patients in the right middle frontal cortex (MNI coordinates: 33, 18, 21; $t = 4.48$) and right frontal inferior triangularis gyrus (MNI coordinates: 30, 39, 21; $t = 4.02$), as well as in the ROI of the posterior left hippocampus (−12, −33, 9; $t = 4.22$).

First regression: association between GM and behavioral variables

Whole group regressions were performed with GM and the behavioral variables. Results (**Table 3**) indicate an inverse association between the behavioral variables (Time and Percent error) and the right hippocampus and right parahippocampal cortex GM. Along the same lines, a positive correlation was found between the right parahippocampal cortex GM and Accuracy. Scatter plots of Percent error against hippocampus GM derived from this analysis shows that the control group forms two separate groups (**Figure 3B**) even if the scores in each axis seem almost normally distributed. A subsequent analysis confirms a significant difference between both subgroups for the variables percent error and right hippocampus GM ($F = 40.88$, $p < 0.01$; $F = 24.24$, $p < 0.01$). In addition, **Figures 3A,B** shows that patients have less hippocampal GM and poorer navigation performance. Regression analyses for the separated groups show a significant negative correlation ($p_{\text{uncorr.}} < 0.001$) between selected brain areas including predominantly the right hippocampus, right parahippocampal cortex, and left caudate GM and Time and Percent error in controls. In addition, we found a significant negative correlation

Table 2 | Reductions of GM volume in patients with schizophrenia compared to healthy controls (controls > patients).

Region	Side	MNI coordinates			*Z* value	*t* value
		x	*y*	*z*		
Insula	L	−28	20	−2	5.98	7.61
Insula	R	34	15	−20	4.60	5.29
Middle frontal gyrus	R	34	36	18	4.50	5.15
Gyrus rectus	L	−2	39	−18	4.49	5.15
Frontal inferior triangular gyrus	R	39	33	3	4.48	5.12
ROI						
Hippocampus	L	−22	−22	−17	3.81	4.21
Hippocampus	L	−36	−12	−17	3.39	3.67
Hippocampus	R	38	−9	−15	3.80	4.18
Hippocampus	R	30	−15	−12	3.23	3.48
Caudate	R	22	24	−2	3.90	4.32
Front inferior orbital	L	−30	27	−5	5.29	6.39
Frontal superior orbital	L	−26	14	−14	5.24	6.30
Frontal superior orbital	R	22	18	−14	4.91	5.78
Frontal inferior orbital	R	34	14	−20	4.51	5.16
Frontal medial orbital	L	−3	39	−15	4.39	5.00
Frontal medial orbital	R	3	68	−2	4.20	4.73

ROI investigation at threshold 0.001 uncorrected, $P_{FWE} = 0.05$ cluster-wise correction.

($p_{\text{uncorr}} = 0.05$) between predominantly the left hippocampus and right parahippocampal cortex GM and time and percent error in patients. A positive correlation was found between the right parahippocampal cortex and accuracy in controls and the right parahippocampal cortex and left hippocampus and accuracy for the patient group ($p_{\text{uncorr.}} < 0.01$). Bivariate Pearson correlations support these results where the right hippocampus seed region correlated significantly with percent error and time in controls ($r = -0.484$, $p = 0.01$; $r = -0.482$, $p = 0.01$) but not in patients ($r = -0.318$, $p = 0.80$; $r = -0.277$, $p = 0.11$) and the left hippocampus seed region correlated significantly with percent error and time in the patient group ($r = -0.401$, $p = 0.036$; $r = -0.429$, $p = 0.026$) but not in the control group ($r = -0.344$, $p = 0.06$; $r = -0.235$, $p = 0.15$).

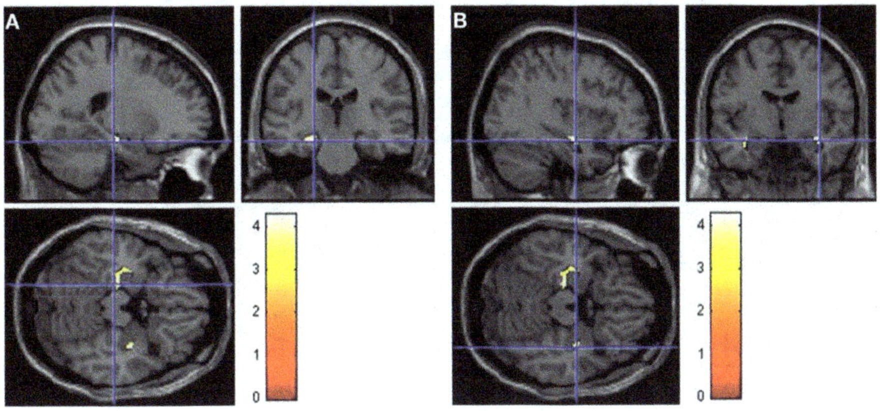

FIGURE 2 | Images demonstrating GM differences of the hippocampus when contrasting controls and patients (controls > patients). The *t* maps are superimposed onto an anatomical brain and displayed in the sagittal, coronal, and horizontal planes. **(A)** GM differences in the left hippocampus when contrasting the control group to the patient group (−22, −22, −17). **(B)** GM differences in the right hippocampus when contrasting the control group to the patient group right (36, −9, −15).

Table 3 | All participants.

Condition	Region	MNI coordinates			K_E	*t* value	*Z* value
		x	*y*	*z*			
Accuracy (+)	R parahippocampal cortex	33	−34	−15	80	3.89	3.57
	R caudate	10	16	−11	80	4.00	3.65
	L caudate	−10	18	−11	104	3.78	3.48
Time (−)	R parahippocampal cortex	33	−34	−15	274	4.62	4.12
	R hippocampus	24	−21	−14	88	3.68	3.40
	R caudate	10	15	−12	74	4.13	3.76
	L caudate	−8	−16	−11	139	3.84	3.53
	L frontal inferior orbital	−34	23	−9	760	4.27	3.86
	L frontal superior orbital	−22	17	−15	760	4.20	3.80
	R frontal superior medial	8	35	60	193	3.80	3.49
Percent error (−)	R parahippocampal cortex	30	−31	−17	222	4.12	3.74
	R hippocampus	24	−21	−15	78	3.82	3.51

ROI investigation at threshold 0.001 uncorrected, $P_{FWE} = 0.05$ cluster-wise correction and k > 10, (R > right, L = Left, (+) = positive, (−) = negative).

Second regression: regression at the seed voxel of the hippocampus

In the control group, the regions covarying significantly with the right hippocampus were the bilateral parahippocampal cortex, left entorhinal cortex, contralateral hippocampus, amygdala, frontal middle orbital cortex, and frontal superior medial gyrus GM (**Figure 4A**). For the patient group, the bilateral parahippocampal cortex, contralateral hippocampus, amygdala, cuneus, frontal superior medial gyrus, and middle cingulate gyrus GM covaried with the right hippocampus (**Figure 4B**). To summarize, in the patient group the right hippocampus did not covary with the entorhinal and middle orbital cortex as within the control group but did covary with the cuneus and middle cingulate gyrus, which was not the case in the control group.

DISCUSSION

The goal of this study was to investigate whether GM in the hippocampus would predict performance on a hippocampus-dependent spatial memory task in patients with schizophrenia and in control participants. Furthermore, this study sought to explore whether regions known to be anatomically connected with the hippocampus covaried with the right hippocampus GM region derived from the VBM regression analysis. To assess spatial memory, a wayfinding task was utilized where participants explored a virtual town and had to remember the location of several landmarks. Spatial memory was tested by asking participants to navigate from one landmark to another by taking the shortest route possible. It was hypothesized that the patient group would have a smaller hippocampal GM average compared to the

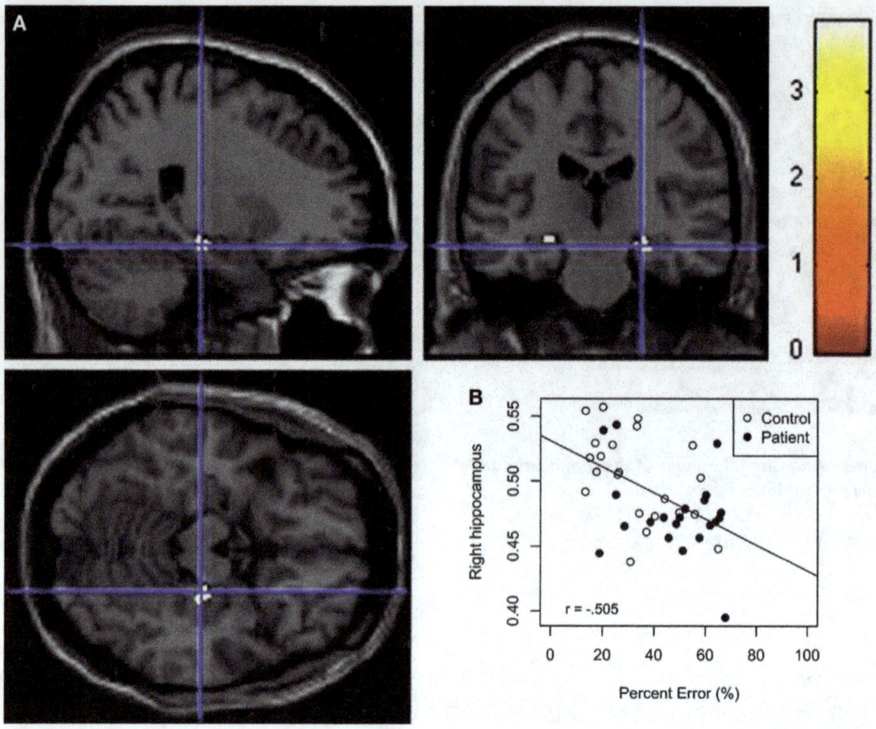

FIGURE 3 | (A) VBM Regression analysis of right hippocampus GM against percent error on the wayfinding task (pFWEcorr. < 0.05). The *t* maps are superimposed onto an anatomical brain and displayed in the sagittal, coronal, and horizontal planes. **(B)** Scatter plot regression of right hippocampal cluster at seed voxel (24, −21, −15; $p < 0.001$) with Percent error on the wayfinding task. Pearson correlation between right hippocampus GM and percept error for the control group ($r = -0.484$, $p = 0.01$) and patient group ($r = -0.318$, $p = 0.08$).

control group and the size of the hippocampus could predict the performance on the navigation task.

During the navigation task, individuals with schizophrenia reached the target goal less often, took more time, and deviated from the shortest route possible significantly more than controls. When comparing controls to patients, GM volumetric analysis revealed significantly lower GM average in the hippocampus of the patient group. This analysis also revealed GM average differences in the insula, middle, and inferior frontal gyrus, gyrus rectus, caudate nucleus, and frontal orbital cortex.

Whole group regression analysis revealed increased latency and deviation from the shortest route were associated with a decrease in the right hippocampus GM, indicating that more GM in the hippocampus is associated with better performance (finding the landmark by making fewer errors and taking less time to complete the task). The anterior right hippocampus has also been associated with performance in navigation in other studies. Bohbot et al. (2007) found that individuals using spontaneous spatial strategies had greater GM in the hippocampus compared to individuals using non-spatial strategies. As seen in the scatter plot (**Figure 3**) there appears to be two clusters in the control group, the good performers with greater right hippocampal GM and poor performers with lower right hippocampal GM. In support of these findings, Etchamendy and Bohbot (2007) found that approximately 50% of their participants used a spontaneous spatial strategy and those who maintained that strategy on the 4-on-8 virtual maze (the task used to dissociate spatial and response strategies) performed significantly better on the wayfinding task than participants who used a response strategy navigating from their starting position. Spatial learners on the 4-on-8 virtual maze also had significantly more GM in the hippocampus than response learners, which would be consistent with the current results. Head and Isom (2010) also demonstrated more GM in individuals who were better at the wayfinding task. Clearly, the current results show an association between hippocampus GM and the ability to learn the relations between the environmental landmarks in order to perform the task successfully.

Compared to controls participants, patients performed significantly worse at the navigation task and had a smaller hippocampus. Low GM volumes have been previously reported in schizophrenia (Wright et al., 2000) and also in first episode groups (Pantelis et al., 2003). Lower GM volumes may be a risk factor for schizophrenia. These anatomical hippocampal anomalies may be the cause of spatial learning impairments and other important cognitive deficits seen in schizophrenia, such as an episodic memory deficit. We previously demonstrated significant differences between both groups, whereby patients made more errors at the immediate and delayed recall of the family picture subtest of the Weschler memory test (Wechsler, 1987) compared to the control group (Ledoux et al., 2013), which is, an assessment that specifically tests the ability to associate together the context and content of an event. The literature postulates that the episodic memory deficit seen in

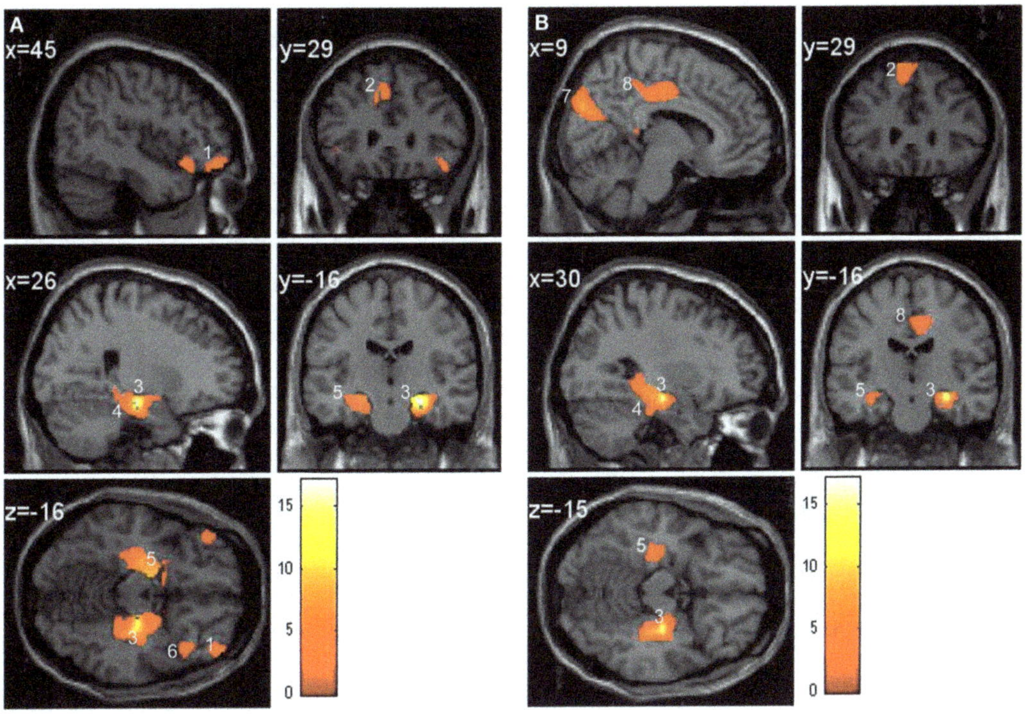

FIGURE 4 | Regression at the seed voxel of the right hippocampus (24, −21, −15) in controls (A) and in patients (B). The *t* maps are superimposed onto an anatomical brain and displayed in the sagittal, coronal, and horizontal planes. **(A)** Right hippocampus (region 3) in controls covaries significantly with the frontal middle orbital cortex (region 1), superior medial gyrus (region 2), right parahippocampal cortex (region 4), and left hippocampus (region 5). Inferior orbital cortex (region 6) does not significantly correlate with the right hippocampus. **(B)** Right hippocampus (region 3) of patients covaries significantly with the cuneus (region 7), middle cingulate gyrus (region 8), superior medial frontal gyrus (region 2), parahippocampal cortex (region 4), and left hippocampus (region 5).

schizophrenia might be mediated by a contextual binding deficit (Boyer et al., 2007), the ability to make associations between the content ("what") and the contextual features (the "where" and "when") of an event. Since the hippocampus is critical for contextual binding in episodic memory (Burgess et al., 2002; Maguire and Frith, 2004), it seems appropriate to use the wayfinding task which assesses similar mechanisms [i.e., in order to reach the target location, participants are required to learn the relations between the environmental landmarks (association of the event with its spatial context)].

Interestingly, the wayfinding-hippocampus GM relation in the patient group (**Figure 3**) shows a cluster, which overlaps with the poor performers in the control group, i.e., with the lower right hippocampus GM group. This indicates that both the patient and the poor performer control groups are in the lower range in terms of GM in the hippocampus and performance on the spatial navigation task. Since, patients in their prodromal and first psychotic episode groups have low hippocampus GM (Pantelis et al., 2003), data in the literature suggest that healthy participants with low hippocampus GM, similar to those in our poor performer control group, may be at risk for neurological and psychiatric disorders such as schizophrenia. The current results suggest that the wayfinding task may be sensitive to abnormalities in the hippocampus for different types of populations.

The prefrontal cortex, striatum, and parahippocampal gyrus are all regions that have been implicated in previous visuospatial navigation studies (Aguirre et al., 1996; Bohbot et al., 1998; Maguire et al., 1998; Burgess et al., 2002; Hartley et al., 2003; Iaria et al., 2003). In this study, it was found that the GM of these regions was also associated with the performance on the wayfinding task.

Regression between the seed region in the right hippocampus and the entire brain demonstrates that the parahippocampal cortex, entorhinal cortex, contralateral hippocampus, amygdala, frontal middle orbital cortex, and frontal superior medial gyrus GM regions correlate with the hippocampus in the control group. In other words, when GM is greater in the hippocampus it will also be greater in the above mentioned regions. These regions are known to be anatomically connected to the hippocampus and were also found to positively covary with the hippocampus in similar navigation studies (Bohbot et al., 2007; Konishi and Bohbot, 2013). Contrary to the control group, in the patient group the cuneus and cingulate gyrus also covaried with the right hippocampus but not the entorhinal and frontal orbital cortices. These regions might be recruited to compensate for the structural and functional deficit seen in schizophrenia while navigating. As previously mentioned the frontal orbital and hippocampal regions were found to have less GM in the patient group. Empirical evidence supports a connection involving neuroanatomical projections from the CA1 and subiculum fields to the medial prefrontal and orbital frontal cortices (Thierry et al., 2000). The hippocampo-prefrontal pathway represents one of the major factors in learning and memory (Laroche et al., 2000). These results provide support to the hippocampal-prefrontal connectivity hypothesis in schizophrenia, which suggests that the prefrontal deficit (such as executive functioning) may in fact be more closely linked to a temporal lobe deficit or associated with connectivity deficits between the temporal lobe and the prefrontal cortex (Weinberger et al., 1992).

Maguire et al. (2000), found that taxi cab drivers, whom have extensive navigation experience, had greater hippocampal volumes than the control group, and a recent study by Lerch et al. (2011), demonstrated in mice that spatial memory training causes neuroanatomical volume changes in the hippocampus. The wayfinding task employed in this study seems to be particularly sensitive to the hippocampus. Training individuals with schizophrenia on hippocampal-dependent tasks, could potentially be used as a form of therapy to help improve the function and structure of the hippocampus, potentially alleviating cognitive deficits seen in this population such as episodic memory problems and executive dysfunction.

Finally, for future research, a study with a larger sample of participants in each group would be a better sample to generalize these results to this population (Steen et al., 2007).

CONCLUSION

In the current study, we investigated whether performance in a wayfinding task could predictably be related to GM in a healthy control group and in a schizophrenia patient group and explore whether the same GM regions in both groups covaried with the hippocampus. Control participants successfully found more target locations in the environment than patients, took less time to complete the task, and made fewer errors compared to patients. Controls had a greater hippocampal GM average than patients. Whole group performance was significantly related to the right hippocampus. Patients' poor performance, contextual binding deficit, and reduced hippocampal activity while performing the wayfinding task, as demonstrated in our previous study, may be attributed to hippocampal anomalies. However, a greater sample size would be necessary to confirm these results. The second VBM regression analysis demonstrated that orbital frontal cortex does not relate with the hippocampal GM in the patient group, a result congruent with the hippocampal-prefrontal connectivity hypothesis of schizophrenia. Results of this study demonstrate that individuals with schizophrenia have a hippocampal disorder and directly targeting the hippocampal structure might be important for improving cognitive impairments.

AUTHORS CONTRIBUTION

Andrée-Anne Ledoux contributed substantially to the conception and design of the experiment design and manuscript; she did the acquisition/collection of the clinical, cognitive, and neuroimaging data, helped in the creation of the neuroimaging paradigm (virtual town), analyzed and interpreted the data, and wrote the paper. Patrice Boyer contributed substantially to the conception or experimental design and hypotheses; he also trained authors on the acquisition of clinical data, revised the work critically for important intellectual content, approved final version of the document, and ensured accuracy and integrity of clinical, navigation, and neuroimaging component of the work and that they are appropriately investigated and resolved. Jennifer L. Phillips contributed at the conception of the experimental design, recruited participants, collected clinical, and neuroimaging data, edited, revised and approved the final version of the manuscript. Andra Smith contributed at the conception of the experimental neuroimaging design, ensured accuracy, and integrity in the neuroimaging data and approved the final version of the paper. Alain Labelle recruited schizophrenia patients, revised the work critically for important intellectual content and approved the final version of the paper. Véronique D. Bohbot contributed substantially to the conception or design of the work and hypotheses; helped with the acquisition parameters of the neuroimaging data, trained the first author on the creation of the neuroimaging paradigm, revised the work critically for important intellectual content, approved the final version to be published and ensured accuracy and integrity of navigation and neuroimaging work and made sure the work was appropriately investigated.

ACKNOWLEDGMENTS

This study was funded by the Canada Foundation for Innovation, the University of Ottawa Medical Research Fund, the Ontario Ministry of Development and Trade, the Royal Ottawa Health Care Foundation and CIHR fund number 64381 to Véronique D. Bohbot. Andrée-Anne Ledoux is supported by the Canadian Institutes of Health Research, and the University of Ottawa. We thank François Rousseau Ph.D., Catherine Smith M.A., and Guylaine Veillette.

REFERENCES

Addington, D., Addington, J., and Schissel, B. (1990). A depression rating scale for schizophrenics. *Schizophr. Res.* 3, 247–251. doi:10.1016/0920-9964(90)90005-R

Aguirre, G. K., Detre, J. A., Alsop, D. C., and D'Esposito, M. (1996). The parahippocampus subserves topographical learning in man. *Cereb. Cortex* 6, 823–829. doi:10.1093/cercor/6.6.823

Aleman, A., Hijman, R., de Haan, E. H., and Kahn, R. S. (1999). Memory impairment in schizophrenia: a meta-analysis. *Am. J. Psychiatry* 156, 1358–1366.

American Psychiatric Association. (2000). *Diagnostic and Statistical Manual of Mental Disorders, 4th Edition, Text Revision (DSM-IV-TR, Text Revision)*. Washington, DC: American Psychiatric Association.

Arnold, S. E., Franz, B. R., Gur, R. C., Gur, R. E., Shapiro, R. M., Moberg, P. J., et al. (1995). Smaller neuron size in schizophrenia in hippocampal subfields that mediate cortical-hippocampal interactions. *Am. J. Psychiatry* 152, 738–748.

Ashburner, J., and Friston, K. J. (2005). Unified segmentation. *Neuroimage* 26, 839–851. doi:10.1016/j.neuroimage.2005.02.018

Benes, F. M., Sorensen, I., and Bird, E. D. (1991). Reduced neuronal size in posterior hippocampus of schizophrenic patients. *Schizophr. Bull.* 17, 597–608. doi:10.1093/schbul/17.4.597

Bogerts, B., Falkai, P., Haupts, M., Greve, B., Ernst, S., Tapernon-Franz, U., et al. (1990). Post-mortem volume measurements of limbic system and basal ganglia structures in chronic schizophrenics. Initial results from a new brain collection. *Schizophr. Res.* 3, 295–301. doi:10.1016/0920-9964(90)90013-W

Bohbot, V. D., Iaria, G., and Petrides, M. (2004). Hippocampal function and spatial memory: evidence from functional neuroimaging in healthy participants and performance of patients with medial temporal lobe resections. *Neuropsychology* 18, 418–425. doi:10.1037/0894-4105.18.3.418

Bohbot, V. D., Kalina, M., Stepankova, K., Spackova, N., Petrides, M., and Nadel, L. (1998). Spatial memory deficits in patients with lesions to the right hippocampus and to the right parahippocampal cortex. *Neuropsychologia* 36, 1217–1238. doi:10.1016/S0028-3932(97)00161-9

Bohbot, V. D., Lerch, J., Thorndycraft, B., Iaria, G., and Zijdenbos, A. P. (2007). Gray matter differences correlate with spontaneous strategies in a human virtual navigation task. *J. Neurosci.* 27, 10078–10083. doi:10.1523/JNEUROSCI.1763-07.2007

Boyer, P., Phillips, J. L., Rousseau, F. L., and Ilivitsky, S. (2007). Hippocampal abnormalities and memory deficits: new evidence of a strong pathophysiological link in schizophrenia. *Brain Res. Rev.* 54, 92–112. doi:10.1016/j.brainresrev.2006.12.008

Burgess, N., Maguire, E. A., and O'Keefe, J. (2002). The human hippocampus and spatial and episodic memory. *Neuron* 35, 625–641. doi:10.1016/S0896-6273(02)00830-9

Burgess, N., Maguire, E. A., Spiers, H. J., and O'Keefe, J. (2001). A temporoparietal and prefrontal network for retrieving the spatial context of lifelike events. *Neuroimage* 14, 439–453. doi:10.1006/nimg.2001.0806

Clark, D. L., Boutros, N. N., and Mendez, M. F. (2010). *The Brain and Behavior: An Introduction to Behavioral Neuroanatomy.* New York: Cambridge University Press.

Clarke, J. R., Cammarota, M., Gruart, A., Izquierdo, I., and Delgado-García, J. M. (2010). Plastic modifications induced by object recognition memory processing. *Proc. Natl. Acad. Sci. U.S.A.* 107, 2652–2657. doi:10.1073/pnas.0915059107

Eichenbaum, H., Sauvage, M., Fortin, N., Komorowski, R., and Lipton, P. (2012). Towards a functional organization of episodic memory in the medial temporal lobe. *Neurosci. Biobeh. Rev.* 36, 1597–1608. doi:10.1016/j.neubiorev.2011.07.006

Etchamendy, N., and Bohbot, V. D. (2007). Spontaneous navigational strategies and performance in the virtual town. *Hippocampus* 17, 595–599. doi:10.1002/hipo.20303

Gruart, A., Muñoz, M. D., and Delgado-García, J. M. (2006). Involvement of the CA3-CA1 synapse in the acquisition of associative learning in behaving mice. *J. Neurosci.* 26, 1077–1087. doi:10.1523/JNEUROSCI.2834-05.2006

Hamilton, M. (1960). A rating scale for depression. *J. Neurol. Neurosurg. Psychiatry* 23, 56–62. doi:10.1136/jnnp.23.1.56

Hartley, T., Maguire, E. A., Spiers, H. J., and Burgess, N. (2003). The well-worn route and the path less traveled: distinct neural bases of route following and wayfinding in humans. *Neuron* 37, 877–888. doi:10.1016/S0896-6273(03)00095-3

Head, D., and Isom, M. (2010). Age effects on wayfinding and route learning skills. *Behav. Brain Res.* 209, 49–58. doi:10.1016/j.bbr.2010.01.012

Iaria, G., Petrides, M., Dagher, A., Pike, B., and Bohbot, V. D. (2003). Cognitive strategies dependent on the hippocampus and caudate nucleus in human navigation: variability and change with practice. *J. Neurosci.* 23, 5945–5952.

Kay, S. R., Fiszbein, A., and Opler, L. A. (1987). The positive and negative syndrome scale (PANSS) for schizophrenia. *Schizophr. Bull.* 13, 261–276. doi:10.1093/schbul/13.2.261

Konishi, K., and Bohbot, V. D. (2013). Spatial navigational strategies correlate with gray matter in the hippocampus of healthy older adults tested in a virtual maze. *Front. Aging Neurosci.* 5:1. doi:10.3389/fnagi.2013.00001

Kovelman, J. A., and Scheibel, A. B. (1984). A neurohistological correlate of schizophrenia. *Biol. Psychiatry* 19, 1601–1621.

Kumaran, D., and Maguire, E. A. (2005). The human hippocampus: cognitive maps or relational memory? *J. Neurosci.* 25, 7254–7259. doi:10.1523/JNEUROSCI.1103-05.2005

Laroche, S., Davis, S., and Jay, T. M. (2000). Plasticity at hippocampal to prefrontal cortex synapses: dual roles in working memory and consolidation. *Hippocampus* 10, 438–446. doi:10.1002/1098-1063(2000)10:4<438::AID-HIPO10>3.0.CO;2-3

Lauer, M., Beckmann, H., and Senitz, D. (2003). Increased frequency of dentate granule cells with basal dendrites in the hippocampal formation of schizophrenics. *Psychiatry Res.* 122, 89–97. doi:10.1016/S0925-4927(02)00122-1

Ledoux, A.-A., Phillips, J. L., Labelle, A., Smith, A., Bohbot, V. D., and Boyer, P. (2013). Decreased fMRI activity in the hippocampus of patients with schizophrenia compared to healthy control participants, tested on a wayfinding task in a virtual town. *Psychiatry Res. Neuroimaging* 211, 47–56. doi:10.1016/j.pscychresns.2012.10.005

Lerch, J. P., Yiu, A. P., Martinez-Canabal, A., Pekar, T., Bohbot, V. D., Frankland, P. W., et al. (2011). Maze training in mice induces MRI-detectable brain shape changes specific to the type of learning. *Neuroimage* 54, 2086–2095. doi:10.1016/j.neuroimage.2010.09.086

Luts, A., Jonsson, S. A., Guldberg-Kjaer, N., and Brun, A. (1998). Uniform abnormalities in the hippocampus of five chronic schizophrenic men compared with age-matched controls. *Acta Psychiatr. Scand.* 98, 60–64. doi:10.1111/j.1600-0447.1998.tb10043.x

Maguire, E. A., Burgess, N., Donnett, J. G., Frackowiak, R. S., Frith, C. D., and O'Keefe, J. (1998). Knowing where and getting there: a human navigation network. *Science* 280, 921–924. doi:10.1126/science.280.5365.921

Maguire, E. A., and Frith, C. D. (2004). The brain network associated with acquiring semantic knowledge. *Neuroimage* 22, 171–178. doi:10.1016/j.neuroimage.2003.12.036

Maguire, E. A., Gadian, D. G., Johnsrude, I. S., Good, C. D., Ashburner, J., Frackowiak, R. S., et al. (2000). Navigation-related structural change in the hippocampi of taxi drivers. *Proc. Natl. Acad. Sci. U.S.A.* 97, 4398–4403. doi:10.1073/pnas.070039597

Maldjian, J. A., Laurienti, P. J., Kraft, R. A., and Burdette, J. H. (2003). An automated method for neuroanatomic and cytoarchitectonic atlas-based interrogation of fMRI data sets. *Neuroimage* 19, 1233–1239. doi:10.1016/S1053-8119(03)00169-1

Morris, R. G., Garrud, P., Rawlins, J. N., and O'keefe, J. (1982). Place navigation impaired in rats with hippocampal lesions. *Nature* 297, 681–683. doi:10.1038/297681a0

Nelson, M. D., Saykin, A. J., Flashman, L. A., and Riordan, H. J. (1998). Hippocampal volume reduction in schizophrenia as assessed by magnetic resonance imaging: a meta-analytic study. *Arch. Gen. Psychiatry* 55, 433–440. doi:10.1001/archpsyc.55.5.433

O'Keefe, J., and Nadel, L. (1978). *The Hippocampus as a Cognitive Map.* Oxford: Oxford University Press.

Oldfield, R. C. (1971). The assessment and analysis of handedness: the Edinburgh inventory. *Neuropsycologia* 9, 97–113. doi:10.1016/0028-3932(71)90067-4

Packard, M. G., Hirsh, R., and White, N. M. (1989). Differential effects of fornix and caudate nucleus lesions on two radial maze tasks: evidence for multiple memory systems. *J. Neurosci.* 9, 1465–1472.

Pantelis, C., Velakoulis, D., McGorry, P. D., Wood, S. J., Suckling, J., Phillips, L. J., et al. (2003). Neuroanatomical abnormalities before and after onset of psychosis: a cross-sectional and longitudinal MRI comparison. *Lancet* 361, 281–288. doi:10.1016/S0140-6736(03)12323-9

Rosoklija, G., Toomayan, G., Ellis, S. P., Keilp, J., Mann, J. J., Latov, N., et al. (2000). Structural abnormalities of subicular dendrites in subjects with schizophrenia and mood disorders: preliminary findings. *Arch. Gen. Psychiatry* 57, 349–356. doi:10.1001/archpsyc.57.4.349

Saunders, J. B., Aasland, O. G., Babor, T. F., de la Fuente, J. R., and Grant, M. (1993). Development of the alcohol use disorders identification test (AUDIT): WHO collaborative project on early detection of persons with harmful alcohol consumption–II. *Addiction* 88, 791–804. doi:10.1111/j.1360-0443.1993.tb00822.x

Shenton, M. E., Gerig, G., McCarley, R. W., Szekely, G., and Kikinis, R. (2002). Amygdala-hippocampal shape differences in schizophrenia: the application of 3D shape models to volumetric MR data. *Psychiatry Res.* 115, 15–35. doi:10.1016/S0925-4927(02)00025-2

Skinner, H. A. (1982). The drug abuse screening test. *Addict. Behav.* 7, 363–371.

SPM8. (2008). *Statistical Parametric Mapping (Version 2008)* [Computer software]. Wellcome – Department of Imaging Neuroscience, London, UK.

SPSS. (2008). *Statistical Package for the Social Sciences (Version 18)* [Computer software]. SPSS, Inc., Chicago, IL.

Steen, R. G., Hamer, R. M., and Lieberman, J. A. (2007). Measuring brain volume by mr imaging: impact of measurement precision and natural variation on sample size requirements. *Am. J. Neuroradiol.* 28, 1119–1125. doi:10.3174/ajnr.A0537

Thierry, A. M., Gioanni, Y., Degenetais, E., and Glowinski, J. (2000). Hippocampo-prefrontal cortex pathway: anatomical and electrophysiological characteristics. *Hippocampus* 10, 411–419. doi:10.1002/1098-1063(2000)10:4<411::AID-HIPO7>3.0.CO;2-A

Tzourio-Mazoyer, N., Landeau, B., Papathanassiou, D., Crivello, F., Etard, O., Delcroix, N., et al. (2002). Automated anatomical labeling of activations in SPM using a macroscopic anatomical parcellation of the MNI MRI single-subject brain. *Neuroimage* 15, 273–289. doi:10.1006/nimg.2001.0978

Wechsler, D. (1987). *Wechsler Memory Scale – Revised Manual.* San Antonio, TX: Psychological Corporation.

Weinberger, D. R., Berman, K. F., Suddath, R., and Torrey, E. F. (1992). Evidence of dysfunction of a prefrontal-limbic network in schizophrenia: a magnetic resonance imaging and regional cerebral blood flow study of discordant monozygotic twins. *Am. J. Psychiatry* 149, 890–897.

Weiss, A. P., Dewitt, I., Goff, D., Ditman, T., and Heckers, S. (2005). Anterior and posterior hippocampal volumes in schizophrenia. *Schizophr. Res.* 73, 103–112. doi:10.1016/j.schres.2004.05.018

4

Bridging disparate symptoms of schizophrenia: a triple network dysfunction theory

Tereza Nekovarova [1,2]*, Iveta Fajnerova [1,3], Jiri Horacek [3] and Filip Spaniel [3]*

[1] Department of Neurophysiology of Memory, Institute of Physiology, Academy of Sciences of the Czech Republic, Prague, Czech Republic
[2] Ecology and Ethology Research Group, Department of Zoology, Faculty of Science, Charles University in Prague, Prague, Czech Republic
[3] Prague Psychiatric Center, Prague, Czech Republic

Edited by:
Tomiki Sumiyoshi, National Center of Neurology and Psychiatry, Japan

***Correspondence:**
Tereza Nekovarova, Department of Neurophysiology of Memory, Institute of Physiology, Academy of Sciences of the Czech Republic, Vídeňská 1083, Prague 4, 142 00, Czech Republic
e-mail: tnt@biomed.cas.cz; nekovarova.tereza@gmail.com
Filip Spaniel, Prague Psychiatric Center, Ústavní 91, Prague 8, 181 03, Czech Republic
e-mail: filip.spaniel@nudz.cz

Schizophrenia is a complex neuropsychiatric disorder with variable symptomatology, traditionally divided into positive and negative symptoms, and cognitive deficits. However, the etiology of this disorder has yet to be fully understood. Recent findings suggest that alteration of the basic sense of self-awareness may be an essential distortion of schizophrenia spectrum disorders. In addition, extensive research of social and mentalizing abilities has stressed the role of distortion of social skills in schizophrenia. This article aims to propose and support a concept of a triple brain network model of the dysfunctional switching between default mode and central executive network (CEN) related to the aberrant activity of the salience network. This model could represent a unitary mechanism of a wide array of symptom domains present in schizophrenia including the deficit of self (self-awareness and self-representation) and theory of mind (ToM) dysfunctions along with the traditional positive, negative and cognitive domains. We review previous studies which document the dysfunctions of self and ToM in schizophrenia together with neuroimaging data that support the triple brain network model as a common neuronal substrate of this dysfunction.

Keywords: schizophrenia, self, theory of mind, forward model, default mode network, salience network, central executive network

INTRODUCTION: PHENOMENOLOGICAL DOMAINS OF SCHIZOPHRENIA

Schizophrenia is a severe neuropsychiatric disorder with complex manifestations expressed in a wide variety of symptoms traditionally divided into positive and negative symptoms, and cognitive deficits (Crow, 1985; Andreasen, 1999; Sass and Parnas, 2003). Positive symptoms refer to phenomena exceeding normal mental functions, such as conceptual disorganization, abnormal thought contents and hallucinations. Negative symptoms are characterized by a decline in normal functioning, flattened emotions, decrease of social behavior and anhedonia. Cognition is affected in several domains such as attention/vigilance, psychomotor speed, cognitive coordination, visual and verbal learning and memory, working memory, executive functions and social cognition (Green et al., 2004). However, the common etiology of these disparate symptoms remains elusive.

Recent phenomenological research indicates that disturbance of the basic sense of self-awareness (core self) may be a core phenotypic marker of schizophrenia spectrum disorders (Nelson et al., 2013, 2014). Self-awareness is an essential component of more complex self-referential systems (self-representation). The term "self" refers traditionally to the human phenomenon of one's own experience including perceptions, thoughts, and emotions (Vogeley and Fink, 2003). This intrinsic representation (or meta-representation) of mental states as one's own mental states is paralleled by the representation of others, again in terms of cognitive content (perceptions and thoughts) and emotions (Vogeley et al., 2001). These cognitive and emotional representations of others are linked to two domains of social cognition, cognitively targeted "theory of mind" (ToM) and empathy. To capture more clearly the dynamic features of a complex self-concept, a two dimensional model of a human mind's representation could be delineated. The first dimension of this model refers to the self-other distinction, and the second represents the cognitive and emotional distinction (**Figure 1**). In this context, we use the term "cognitive" for all processes related to monitoring the perceptions, thoughts, planning and action performance of ourselves or others. The term "emotional" refers to the monitoring of motivational, positive and negative (aversive) hedonic values automatically assigned to a current situation or mental content. This model groups together four domains (self, ToM, empathy and hedonic evaluation) with one common denominator: meta-representation of the mind (**Figure 1**).

Interestingly, all of these four categories have been identified as dysfunctional in schizophrenia and represent an alternative approach to schizophrenia phenomenology. It is tentative to speculate that a common denominator could be a candidate

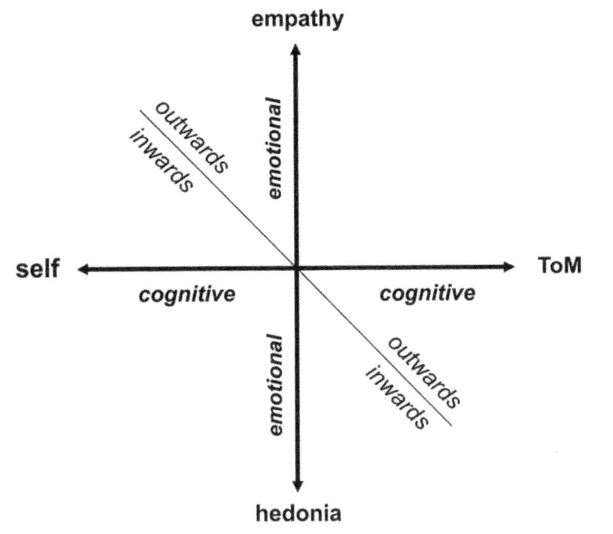

FIGURE 1 | Model of a human mind's representation (inwards/outwards). The horizontal axis refers to "cognitive" dimension, whereas the vertical axis refers to "emotional" dimension with stronger motivational accent. We assume that these two axes can create a mental representation of human mind, that can be focused outwards or inwards, forming four domains: self, ToM, empathy and hedonic evaluation.

for a unified neurobiological mechanism underlying the wide range of schizophrenia symptom manifestations. As we show further in this paper, recent advances in neuroimaging have proven that the array of bizarre perceptual experiences inherent to schizophrenia, i.e., pathological beliefs and cognitive deficits are part of the same core abnormality—prominent disturbance in the orchestration of large-scale brain networks that are conversely related to social cognition and emotional valence evaluation (ToM and empathy) and self-attribution. In order to explain co-occurrence of disparate symptoms of schizophrenia, encompassing broad range phenomenological domains, we have further elaborated the previously postulated theory of the triple network dysfunctional theory (Menon, 2011).

In this article we focus on the disturbance of the cognitive capability to represent ourselves/others as an unifying "super-domain" in schizophrenia (**Figure 1**). The emotional domain will be elaborated in a separate article. However, it is necessary to stress that the disturbances of the poles of the emotional axis belong to emotional flattening, a core negative symptom of schizophrenia differing in an inward (anhedonia) and outward (poor rapport or lack of empathy) perspective of reference.

This article aims to propose and advocate a concept of a common neurobiological substrate for self and ToM and to document its disturbance in schizophrenia. In the first two sections we review previous studies which refer to the dysfunction of self and ToM in schizophrenia together with neuroimaging data elucidating the neuronal substrate of this dysfunction. Secondly, we propose a triple network dysfunction as a candidate mechanism for the deficit of self-awareness, autobiographical self and ToM dysfunctions. Then, from this neurobiological perspective, we provide support for the assumption that the disruption in the orchestration of the triple network may underlie other prominent domains of schizophrenia phenomonology as well.

SELF: SELF-MONITORING AND SELF-DISTURBANCE

In general, self is defined as an essential human phenomenon—an intrinsic meta-representation of bodily and mental states (perceptions, sensations, emotions and thoughts) that are experienced as one's own (Newen and Vogeley, 2003). Literature offers various concepts of self, suggesting a plurality of this phenomenon. Gallagher (2013) proposed a "pattern theory of self", an approach allowing different aspects of self to coexist in parallel, in a "pattern", not exclusively. We use the term "self" as a denomination of the phenomenon itself. It is the most general term, linking and including all other aspects of self.

For the purpose of this article we recognize self-awareness, called "minimal" or "core self" (also called "ipseity" from Latin word ipse for "self" or "itself"), which refers to the fundamental sense of self-presence, to the "center of existence as an independent self-aware being", to the ability to separate oneself from others and to take a first person perspective (Sass and Parnas, 2003; Vogeley and Fink, 2003). Such perception of oneself as an active agent of one's own action is a central part of self-consciousness (David et al., 2008).

In contrast, we use term "autobiographical self" (Damasio, 1999) for a more complex phenomenon, based on autobiographical memory and on anticipation of a future, developing and maturing gradually throughout a lifetime. It also underlies representations of one's own mental states, a process parallel to the representation of the mental states of others (ToM). Newen and Vogeley (2003) propose five different levels of complexity of self-consciousness and emphasize the involvement of the minimal self in each of them. Accordingly, we consider self-awareness (minimal self) to be an intrinsic and essential component (prerequisite) of autobiographical self, allowing the first-person perspective to be taken in the representational processes.

The self-disorder or so-called ipseity-disturbance or ego-disturbance is hypothesized to be a core impairment in schizophrenia (Sass and Parnas, 2003; Sass, 2014). Self-awareness disturbances (passivity phenomena), one of the hallmarks of schizophrenia, are accompanied by a feeling of loss of one's own control and of being controlled by an external agent. This is common in patients suffering from false perception (hallucinations) or from false beliefs (delusions).

Nevertheless, it has been suggested that a deficit in self-monitoring could underlie abnormal perceptions and beliefs behind other positive symptoms in schizophrenia, beyond the scope of Schneider's symptoms (Fletcher and Frith, 2009). Recent evidence at a meta-analytical level has shown that a deficit in self-monitoring is associated with auditory hallucinations *per se* (Waters et al., 2012). Congruently, the impairment in the sense of agency is present in schizophrenia patients even without first-rank symptoms (Franck et al., 2001). Anomalous self-related experiences frequently precede the onset of psychosis by many years (Schultze-Lutter, 2009). In addition, self-monitoring deficit is detectable also in unaffected siblings of patients with schizophrenia (Hommes et al., 2012). Those findings indicate that the deficit in this domain would belong to the endophenotype of schizophrenia.

It has previously been proposed that self-disturbance phenomena—delusions of alien control and thought insertion—can be caused by a distraction of the so called "forward model" (Frith et al., 2000; Frith, 2005; Leube et al., 2008). The forward circuit is a mechanism that allows us to distinguish between our own actions and actions initiated by an external source. The concept has been initially documented in motor-system control, in which two complementary elements were identified. The inverse model ("controller") provides motor commands to perform a sequence of actions determined by an intended goal. The forward model ("predictor") allows us to represent predicted consequences of actions. It creates an "efference copy" processed in parallel with the motor action (Wolpert and Kawato, 1998; Blakemore et al., 2000; Frith et al., 2000; Leube et al., 2008). In healthy subjects, self-monitoring could be based on a comparatory system computing the deviation between the predicted and the perceived consequences of both physical and mental actions. If there is no deviation between predicted and perceived, the action is experienced as self-initiated. Patients with self-awareness-disturbances have problems to correctly comparing predicted and perceived consequences and therefore they misidentify their own acts as external intervention (Leube et al., 2008).

Several brain regions have been assigned a role in this automatic self-referencing mechanism. Functional brain imaging studies confirmed that self-related processing may be specifically mediated by cortical midline structures (CMS) and insula. Several meta-analyses have demonstrated a predominant involvement of the anterior and posterior CMS (anterior and posterior cingulate, precuneus, the hubs of the default mode network (DMN)) in the processing of self-specific stimuli that occur across various functional domains in healthy subjects (Vogeley et al., 2001; Northoff et al., 2006; van der Meer et al., 2010; Qin and Northoff, 2011; Murray et al., 2012).

Although neuroimaging data of self-processing in schizophrenia are sparse, Farrer et al. (2004) demonstrated clear functional differences between schizophrenia patients with positive symptoms and healthy subjects in the action-attribution test. In this task the level of the subject's control of a virtual hand on a computer screen could be modulated by the experimenter. Positron emission tomography showed that the activity of the insular cortex along with right angular gyrus in healthy subjects correlated with the individual's control of a movement of the virtual hand. In contrast, schizophrenia patients did not show such a pattern of activity (Farrer et al., 2004).

In addition to forward system theory, some authors proposed an alternative explanation of the self-disturbance in schizophrenia. Three complementary aspects that manifest differently in the disease have been suggested (Sass and Parnas, 2003; Sass, 2014): (a) "Hyper-reflexivity" relates to an exaggerated form of self-consciousness. The subject can project some aspects of self-awareness onto external objects. (b) "Diminished self-affection" in the sense of a decreased experience of existing as an independent subject of awareness. This could be a source of disruption of the first-person perspective in some cases of schizophrenia disorder. (c) "Disturbed hold of the world" refers to the "disturbance of the spatiotemporal pattern of the world". This disturbance could affect the organization and structure of the field of awareness and a discrepancy between the perceived, remembered and imagined (Sass and Parnas, 2003; Sass, 2014).

Sass and Parnas (2003) assume that the sense of self is a deeply implicit phenomenon of the human mind and that there is no need for a "separate channel of self-monitoring or a second self-directed act of reflection", as was proposed by Frith (1992). Therefore, explicitly focused attention on an implicit experience could paradoxically lead to a sense of "alienation" that is often present in schizophrenia.

THEORY OF MIND

Humans have adopted the strategy to represent, anticipate and think about the mental states of others. This ability, referred to as the ToM or mentalizing, allows us to attribute and model the mental states (perceptions, motivations, knowledge, beliefs, emotions) of others and to predict their behavior. The term "theory of mind" was first introduced by Premack and Woodruff (1978). Initially, this term comprised the representation of the mental states of both ourselves and others. However, there is still an on-going and widespread discussion about the relation between self, a meta-representation of our own mental states (Vogeley et al., 2001), and ToM; and to what extent self is involved in the modeling of the mental states of others and vice versa (Brüne and Brüne-Cohrs, 2006).

Despite the variability in studies of ToM related neuronal activation and its abnormalities in schizophrenia, the most frequently replicated findings of these studies involve regions of the prefrontal area, the temporo-parietal junction and the middle brain structures (for review see Bosia et al., 2012).

In addition, Vogeley et al. (2001) demonstrated that ToM (representation of other's mental states) and SELF (representation of one's own mental states, a process parallel to ToM) capacities rely on both different and common neuronal mechanisms. While the ToM capacity predominantly activates mPFC along with the anterior cingulate cortex (ACC), the SELF capacity particularly activates the precuneus, bilaterally. In addition, an area within the right prefrontal cortex is particularly activated during conditions when an integration of ToM and SELF is demanded. Although ToM and SELF tasks also partly activate different brain regions, common brain areas are involved in both tasks.

It was demonstrated that the CMS including the medial prefrontal cortex (mPFC) and ACC are mainly activated in both processes, i.e., during self-referential processing (evaluation of one's personality traits) as well as during third-person perspective taking or meta-cognitive representations ("thinking about thinking") (Amodio and Frith, 2006; D'Argembeau et al., 2007). Interestingly, the degree to which the rostral part of mPFC was activated while processing others' personality traits correlated with the degree of similarity perceived between one's own and others' characteristics (Benoit et al., 2010). Mars et al. demonstrated in their meta-analysis that the brain regions involved in higher-order social tasks overlapped partly with the DMN, which is connected with self-referential processes.

These findings support the concept that self-referential (self-reflection) processes are employed also while thinking about other persons, where own person is used as a model for the evaluation of others. Mitchell et al. (2005) suggest that self-reflection is used to infer the mental states of others when they are sufficiently similar to one's own. This "social loop" is closed with the second level of self-referencing, when thinking about our reputation, which requires us to produce a representation of attributes that others apply to us (Amodio and Frith, 2006).

Essentially, regardless of the mechanism involved, available evidence suggests the importance of self-awareness processes in the representation of one's own mind (self) as well as in the representation of the minds of others (ToM). This concept parallels the fact that self-awareness, as a main component of self and also self-recognition (Irani et al., 2006), together with ToM are comparably affected in schizophrenia (horizontal axis of **Figure 1**).

ToM abnormalities were monitored in schizophrenia over the last few decades based on the difficulties in evaluating the mental states of others involved in the communication process, observed in some schizophrenia patients. Today, nobody argues the presence of the mentalizing deficit in schizophrenia, which was confirmed using various methodological approaches that can be divided into three categories: (a) verbal paradigms—indirect speech utterances (Corcoran et al., 1995), verbal jokes (Corcoran et al., 1997) and storytelling tasks involving false beliefs or deception (Andreasen et al., 2008); (b) nonverbal paradigms—comics strips or cartoon tasks (Sarfati et al., 1997), Mind in the Eyes test (Irani et al., 2006; Pentaraki et al., 2012) and false-belief picture sequencing task (Langdon and Coltheart, 1999; Brüne, 2003); or (c) combined methods—movies with actors for the assessment of social cognition (Montag et al., 2011), moving shapes paradigm, where the visual observations of actions are described verbally (Koelkebeck et al., 2010; Das et al., 2012; Pedersen et al., 2012) or verbal ToM stories presented simultaneously with cartoons that display the action occurring in the stories (Mazza et al., 2001).

Nevertheless, apparent variability in the applied methods has led to high heterogeneity in the obtained findings, making the investigation of the complex ToM deficit very problematic. The large degree of heterogeneity of ToM findings could be explained by the state variables and task differences, as was shown in a meta-analysis (Bora and Pantelis, 2013). In addition, it was demonstrated that the ToM deficit is not uniform in individual patients and is distributed varyingly among different components of ToM (Bosco et al., 2009). This opens the question of possible associations between the ToM impairment and psychopathology and/or cognitive functioning in schizophrenia. Nevertheless, the persistence of the ToM deficits in remitted patients (even less pronounced than in non-remitted ones) suggests that there are traits related to mentalizing impairments in schizophrenia as well as some potential effects of residual symptoms (Bora and Pantelis, 2013).

Several studies reported symptom specific ToM deficits by dividing the symptomatology into three subgroups according to the triadic domains model of schizophrenia (psychomotor poverty/negative symptoms, disorganization and reality distortion symptoms) (e.g., Mazza et al., 2001). Most studies observed a more prominent ToM deficit in patients with severe negative symptomatology or disorganization of thought and speech (Sarfati et al., 1997; Sarfati and Hardy-Bayle, 1999; Mazza et al., 2001). It was also demonstrated that some reality distortions, especially persecutory delusions, could be related to the ToM deficit (Corcoran et al., 1995; Mazza et al., 2001; Pousa et al., 2008). A current study showed that while negative symptoms are associated with a lack of mentalizing, positive symptoms such as delusions were associated with another type of error, overmentalizing (Montag et al., 2011). Importantly, patients without symptoms present at the time of testing showed normal ToM performance levels (Corcoran et al., 1997).

Interestingly, some studies focusing on schizotypal traits in clinical and non-clinical populations found the ToM deficit in a healthy population with higher schizotypy (Langdon and Coltheart, 1999). In addition, high levels of schizotypal traits (such as social anxiety, constricted affect and no close friends) have been shown to be important for the ToM performance in schizophrenia patients (Irani et al., 2007) which is more prominent than in their first-degree relatives (Irani et al., 2006).

Since mentalizing abilities demand some level of intact cognitive processes, several studies are focused on clarification of the relationship between the ToM deficit and a deficit in cognitive functioning present in schizophrenia. The poor ToM performance was demonstrated to be strongly associated with Intelligence Quotient (IQ) and measured cognitive performance, especially executive abilities (Abdel-Hamid et al., 2009) or working memory load (Brüne, 2003). However, importantly, some studies controlled for cognitive performance and IQ levels showed that the ToM deficit cannot be completely explained by the impairment of cognitive functioning in schizophrenia itself (Brüne, 2003; Bozikas et al., 2011; Montag et al., 2011; Pentaraki et al., 2012). A systematic review of the relationship between ToM and executive functions confirms the idea that the impairments in ToM and executive functions are independent of one another (Pickup, 2008).

TRIPLE NETWORK DYSFUNCTION: A CORE OF SCHIZOPHRENIA?

Over the past few years the focus of neuroimaging research has shifted from the localization of task-related neural activity towards functional connectivity within and between organized cerebral networks. A wealth of data based on temporal coupling of fMRI responses during rest and context/stimulus-dependent activations has identified a triple large-scale brain network model consisting of the default mode network (DMN), salience network (SN) and central executive network (CEN; Menon, 2011; **Figure 2**). It is widely accepted that coordination of these networks plays a key regulatory role in organizing neural responses underlying fundamental brain functions.

The DMN shows decreased activation during cognitive task performance relative to resting-state or internally focused tasks and is implicated in self-referential internal mentation (Andrews-Hanna, 2012). Its subsystems include CMS, i.e., mPFC, posterior cingulate cortex and adjacent ventral precuneus, along with the medial, lateral and inferior parietal cortex and a part of the medial temporal lobe. The second

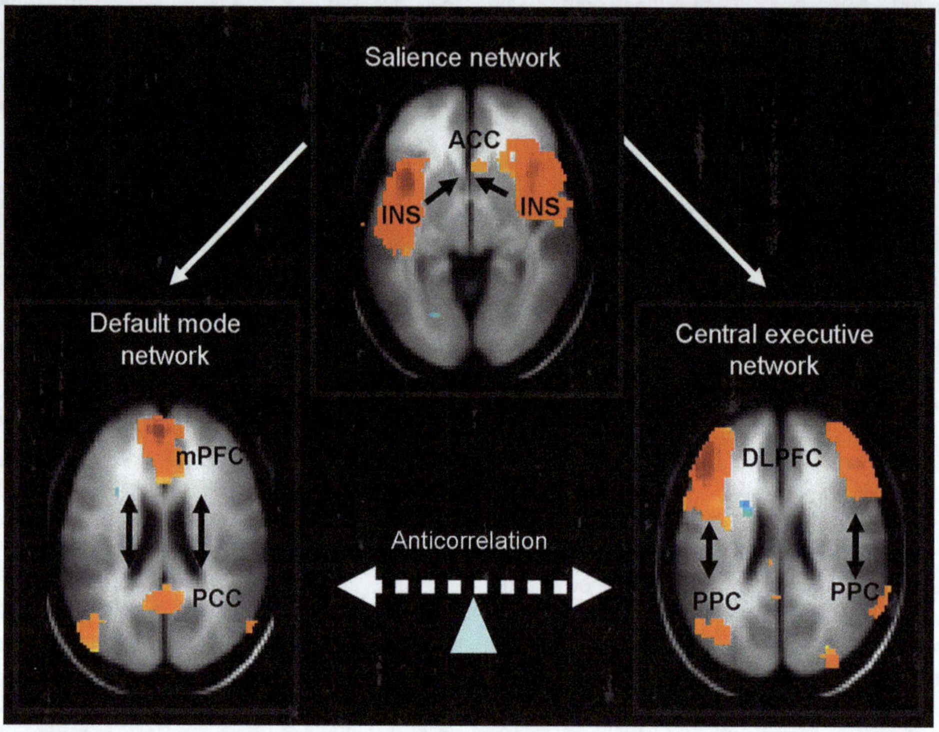

FIGURE 2 | Schematic figure of the triple network model consisting of the default mode network (DMN), salience network (SN) and central executive network (CEN). According to this model, the anterior insula (belonging to the salience network) activates the CEN and deactivates the DMN in response to the salient stimuli. Legend: ACC: anterior cingulated cortex, DPLFC: dorsolateral prefrontal cortex, PPC: posterior parietal cortex, mPFC: medial prefrontal cortex, PPC: posterior cingulate cortex, INS: anterior insula. Adapted from Menon and Uddin (2010); Sridharan et al. (2008), the images of networks derived from our in house resting fMRI sample, *n* = 20.

network—CEN—engaged in externally oriented attention during demanding cognitive tasks, includes primarily the dorsolateral prefrontal cortex (DLPFC), and posterior parietal cortex (PPC; Menon and Uddin, 2010). In general, cognitive states that activate the DMN typically deactivate the CEN and a vice versa. The last large-scale SN, composed of the anterior cingulate and the anterior insula, mediates selection of salient external and interoceptive signals (Sridharan et al., 2008; Menon and Uddin, 2010).

Accumulating evidence from neuroimaging studies in healthy individuals indicates that SN causally influences anticorrelated activation of DMN and CEN. The existing evidence supports a general role for the SN in switching between these two networks upon salient stimuli mediated by midbrain dopaminergic input (Menon and Uddin, 2010). The aberrant orchestration within the triple network model has been suggested as a backbone for some clinical and cognitive features of various psychiatric and neurological disorders (Menon, 2011).

In this section, we examine how large-scale brain networks provide integrative albeit rather mechanistic models of schizophrenia psychopathology, traditionally clustered into positive, negative and cognitive domains. Furthermore, we emphasize a great deal of evidence accumulated over the last decade suggesting that insula/ACC i.e., SN dysfunction is a unified cause of brain-network disturbances observed in schizophrenia. Finally, we propose that deficits in coordination of these neurocognitive networks in schizophrenia may underlie a disruption in self-related functions that causes and also antecedes a disparate assortment of signs and symptoms encompassing such distant phenomena as first rank symptoms and impaired social cognition.

As a starting point, we take into consideration numerous resting-state and stimulus-evoked fMRI measurements in patients with schizophrenia compared to healthy controls that repeatedly showed aberrant functional connectivity within and between DMN, SN and CEN (White et al., 2010; Camchong et al., 2011; Kasparek et al., 2013; Moran et al., 2013; Orliac et al., 2013; Palaniyappan et al., 2013; Guo et al., 2014a; Manoliu et al., 2014).

Those results converge on the conclusion that SN dysfunction may be causative to triple network dysfunction inherent to the illness (Palaniyappan et al., 2012b). Indeed, based on non-psychiatric lesion studies, it was clearly shown that structural SN integrity plays a crucial role in the fine-tuned orchestration of the other two major brain networks (Zhou et al., 2010; Bonnelle et al., 2012). This gains particular importance considering concentration of the most often reproduced structural deviations in schizophrenia in regions of insula and ACC, which represent key hubs of SN. A prominent gray matter reduction within these structures has been consistently and robustly reported in the meta-analyses of morphometric MRI studies (Glahn et al., 2008; Ellison-Wright and Bullmore, 2010; Bora et al., 2011;

Shepherd et al., 2012). ACC and insula gray matter volume reduction precede the occurrence of the first psychotic symptoms and thus represent candidates for trait symptoms of the disease. A transition to psychosis and further chronicity is associated with additional morphological changes in the adjacent regions of the mediofrontal cortex and the temporal lobe. (Chan et al., 2011).

Further, an impaired anti-correlated relationship between task-positive CEN and task-negative DMN due to SN malfunction may be phenotypically expressed as major symptoms of schizophrenia. Firstly, the existing data provide an explanation of a fundamental representation of positive symptoms: auditory verbal hallucinations (AVH). Data obtained from a resting state fMRI in schizophrenia patients suggest aberrant functional connectivity between the DMN and CEN as a denominator of AVH severity (Manoliu et al., 2014). Additionally, one recent fMRI study showed aberrant down-regulation of the DMN during a resting state that was concomitant with spontaneous hallucinations in schizophrenia, whereas overall spatial and temporal instabilities of the DMN correlated with the severity of hallucinatory experience (Jardri et al., 2013). This is of particular importance, since, as noted above, a large number of studies using both resting-state and task-related fMRI studies in healthy human subjects implicate the main hubs of DMN as being key structures for "self" as opposed to "other" discrimination (van der Meer et al., 2010; Qin and Northoff, 2011).

Therefore, keeping in line with this, the phasic hallucinations may emerge from a spontaneous switching off of the dysregulated and unstable DMN, secondary to SN dysfunction (Northoff and Qin, 2011). This may result in a malfunction of this self-attributional tagging system with a consequent misattribution of internal mental states to an external source. Along a somewhat different line, both structural and functional changes within the SN key node, the insular region, correlate with the occurrence of AVH in schizophrenia (Jardri et al., 2011; Palaniyappan et al., 2012a) and positive symptoms in general (Moran et al., 2014).

Correspondingly, a putative consequence of SN dysfunction, i.e., instability of DMN hub, correlates with overall positive symptom severity in schizophrenic patients (Rotarska-Jagiela et al., 2010). Correlation between illness duration, positive and negative symptom severity and an altered DMN cortical midline system has been further confirmed by combined resting-state fMRI and voxel-based morphometry (Guo et al., 2014b).

That is to say that a precise interlink between a triple network dysfunction and occurrence of positive symptoms, namely those beyond boundaries of first-rank symptoms, remains unclear. However, preliminary evidence suggests that the theoretical account presented herein may be complementary with the previously postulated alteration of the dopamine-dependent process of salience attribution in a psychotic state (Howes and Kapur, 2009).

Dopamine-mediated salience dysfunction hypothesis in a psychotic state has been suggested as an underlying cause for highly prevalent non-ego-disorder delusions, such as persecutory delusions and delusions of reference, whereas the theory appears at first sight less applicable to ego-disturbances inherent to first-rank symptoms in schizophrenia. Nevertheless, those disparate delusional phenomena may share the same mechanism. In a fMRI study, heightened self-relevance to ambiguous stimuli in patients with schizophrenia with delusions of reference compared to controls was associated with an increased blood-oxygen-level dependent (BOLD) contrast imaging response in DMN hubs as well as insula (SN) and midbrain dopaminergic regions (Menon et al., 2011). This finding suggests a direct link between dopamine-dependent aberrant salience and recruitment of main DMN cortical midline regions in heightened self-relevance that is thought to underlie delusions of reference. On top of that, the activity in insula and ventral striatum correlated with the strength of this particular type of delusions in patients.

It is tempting to conclude that following a continuum model approach, the same neural dysregulation within large scale brain networks may, on the one hand, underlie the sensation of delusions of reference and, on the other hand, lead—on its extreme end delusional alienation—to mental processes resulting in first rank symptoms of schizophrenia. This assumption is in accordance with the recent shift from a categorical to a dimensional concept of schizophrenia. It is in a general agreement with a factor analysis carried out in a large cohort of psychotic patients (Peralta and Cuesta, 2005). Based on this study, schizophrenia may be viewed as the "end-stage" disease or the extreme pole of the psychotic continuum. This and other evidence underline a dimensional construct of schizophrenia and support the continuum hypothesis of the psychotic illness.

Although the triple network theory provides a conceptual framework for an integrative psychophysiological approach for the study of a wide scope of positive symptoms, in the time being it is unable to provide significant additional explanatory power to the broadest context of schizophrenia-related variables, e.g., formal thought disorder, disorganized or catatonic behavior. On the other hand it is capable of providing a theoretical ground for a cognitive dimension of schizophrenia (Elvevåg and Goldberg, 2000).

It has been suggested that a lack of optimal DMN suppression during cognitive task engagement may be a source of the general cognitive impairment (Anticevic et al., 2012). In previous literature it has been proven that in healthy controls the magnitude of task-induced deactivation within the DMN positively correlates with cognitive performance (McKiernan et al., 2003; Li et al., 2007). In schizophrenia, reduced suppression of the DMN during various cognitive tasks represents a constant finding (Meyer-Lindenberg et al., 2005; Garrity et al., 2007; Harrison et al., 2007; Pomarol-Clotet et al., 2008; Whitfield-Gabrieli et al., 2009; Nygård et al., 2012; Anticevic et al., 2013; Fryer et al., 2013). Therefore, a breakdown in coordinated suppression of DMN activity may impair the overall performance across various cognitive domains in schizophrenia.

In line with the proposed role of SN structures in pathophysiological processes related to cognitive dysfunction in schizophrenia, there is a direct interlink between morphology of insula and inferior frontal gyrus (IFG) and a dysfunctional pattern of CEN activation and DMN deactivation during working memory in patients (Pujol et al., 2013). This is also in accordance with our findings (Horacek et al., 2005) which suggest that the medial forebrain pathways and cingulum bundle underlie the activity of cortical structures required for Stroop test processing.

Thirdly, deficits in social cognition (including ToM abilities) have been well documented in schizophrenia using a wide variety of tasks. Numerous studies suggested that brain areas associated with the DMN, namely mPFC, are involved in this cognitive faculty that includes also ToM (Amodio and Frith, 2006; Schilbach et al., 2006). This has been recently confirmed by an extensive study that compared resting-state networks in healthy participants with brain areas showing consistent co-activation during various task-based neuroimaging experiments archived in the BrainMap database. The DMN was heavily tasked exclusively with ToM and social cognition tasks (Laird et al., 2011). Concurrently, the reverse approach has been applied in additional meta-analyses of fMRI studies using the BrainMap database and likelihood estimations of functional brain activity associated with either rest or social cognition. Again, it has been shown that there is an overlap between the "social brain network" activated during ToM tasks and the DMN, both at the network level and at the level of individual brain regions (Mars et al., 2012).

Further direct evidence of the crucial involvement of DMN in theory of mind comes from a review performing a quantitative meta-analysis of neuroimaging studies of ToM, using the activation-likelihood estimation (ALE) approach (Mars, 2011).

Fourthly, an aberrant synchronization of large-scale networks may underlie even a negative symptom dimension. Both functional connectivity within and between distinct subsystems of the DMN, SN and CEN were calculated and correlated in a resting-state fMRI study. Internal functional connectivity between the SN and CEN correlated with the severity of negative symptoms in patients with schizophrenia (Bosia et al., 2012; Manoliu et al., 2013).

To sum up, meta-analyses targeting consistent activations across studies exploring the neural correlates of self (self-awareness and self-representation) and social cognition, namely ToM revealed shared activations within CMS. This finding parallels the simulation theory of social cognition based on the assumption that the same neural networks support thinking about self and other people.

Additionally, a recent large meta-analysis aimed at the identification of brain regions, which consistently show activations during social cognition, emotional processing and resting state showed a close convergence within CMS as well (Schilbach et al., 2012).

This study provides robust evidence for a shared neural network consisting of mPFC and precuneus that underlies activations during various emotional and social cognition tasks along with deactivations across different types of experimental paradigms. Identification of a common neural denominator of those seemingly disparate faculties brings some support to the above-mentioned two dimensional model of a human mind's representation.

In cognitive terms a commonality may exist between all three types of states, which could be termed "introspective processing". This specific mental faculty may represent a prerequisite for the processing either of one's own or other people's states on both a cognitive and an emotional level.

In schizophrenia, dynamic dysregulation of the CMS, which is considered the strongest part of the DMN, may substantially impair translation of cognitive processes from an internal to an external focus. This might explain schizophrenia symptoms related to defective self-monitoring, such as AVH or other ego-disturbances represented by thought insertion or thought withdrawal.

Nevertheless, an out of control increase in DMN activity or a failure of DMN deactivation may underlie a wide array of other schizophrenia symptoms, including non-ego-disorder positive symptoms, overall cognitive dysfunction and negative symptoms. Taken together, available evidence suggests a testable hypothesis that on the neural level, impaired self-monitoring, social and affective processing in schizophrenia converge and rely upon an aberrant recruitment of large scale brain networks. Principal causes may plausibly include impaired regulating machinery underlying the fine-tuned orchestration of those neural networks.

CONCLUSIONS AND FUTURE DIRECTIONS

This article aims to emphasize the concept of common self and ToM mechanisms and their disturbances as a marker of schizophrenia. We recognize the speculative nature of our hypotheses. Our goal is to provide future directions for neurobiological research in schizophrenia that extend beyond traditionally studied phenomenological dimensions and regional specific functional deviations. We propose an experimental approach addressing behavioral and neuronal features in both self and ToM paradigms in schizophrenia. This perspective provides us a novel direction to study not only brain and behavioral alternations in schizophrenia but also mutual relations between self and theory of mind, e.g., the possible role of the forward system in more complex processes. This approach reflects cumulating evidence of a disordered integration of large-scale brain networks as a critical pathophysiological mechanism underlying heterogeneous symptomatology in schizophrenia.

AUTHOR CONTRIBUTIONS

The main idea behind this work was courtesy of Filip Spaniel. All of the authors contributed to the final version of the paper equally and have approved it.

ACKNOWLEDGMENTS

The study was supported by IGA MZ CR grants No. NT14291, NT13843 and NT13386, GACR grant P303/12/1464, 14-03627S and by CSF Project of excellence in the field of neuroscience (GBP304/12/G069). The institutional support from the Prague Psychiatric Center by MH CZ—DRO (PCP, 00023752) and from the Academy of Sciences of the Czech Republic (RVO: 67985823) covered the salaries and other institutional costs.

REFERENCES

Abdel-Hamid, M., Lehmkamper, C., Sonntag, C., Juckel, G., Daum, I., and Brune, M. (2009). Theory of mind in schizophrenia: the role of clinical symptomatology and neurocognition in understanding other people's thoughts and intentions. *Psychiatry Res.* 165, 19–26. doi: 10.1016/j.psychres.2007.10.021

Amodio, D. M., and Frith, C. D. (2006). Meeting of minds: the medial frontal cortex and social cognition. *Nat. Rev. Neurosci.* 7, 268–277. doi: 10.1038/nrn1884

Andreasen, N. C. (1999). A unitary model of schizophrenia: bleuler's "fragmented phrene" as schizencephaly. *Arch. Gen. Psychiatry* 56, 781–787. doi: 10.1001/archpsyc.56.9.781

Andreasen, N. C., Calarge, C. A., and O'Leary, D. S. (2008). Theory of mind and schizophrenia: a positron emission tomography study of medication-free patients. *Schizophr. Bull.* 34, 708–719. doi: 10.1093/schbul/sbn034

Andrews-Hanna, J. R. (2012). The brain's default network and its adaptive role in internal mentation. *Neuroscientist* 18, 251–270. doi: 10.1177/1073858411403316

Anticevic, A., Cole, M. W., Murray, J. D., Corlett, P. R., Wang, X. J., and Krystal, J. H. (2012). The role of default network deactivation in cognition and disease. *Trends Cogn. Sci.* 16, 584–592. doi: 10.1016/j.tics.2012.10.008

Anticevic, A., Repovs, G., and Barch, D. M. (2013). Working memory encoding and maintenance deficits in schizophrenia: neural evidence for activation and deactivation abnormalities. *Schizophr. Bull.* 39, 168–178. doi: 10.1093/schbul/sbr107

Benoit, R. G., Gilbert, S. J., Volle, E., and Burgess, P. W. (2010). When I think about me and simulate you: medial rostral prefrontal cortex and self-referential processes. *Neuroimage* 50, 1340–1349. doi: 10.1016/j.neuroimage.2009.12.091

Blakemore, S. J., Wolpert, D., and Frith, C. (2000). Why can't you tickle yourself? *Neuroreport* 11, R11–R16. doi: 10.1097/00001756-200008030-00002

Bonnelle, V., Ham, T. E., Leech, R., Kinnunen, K. M., Mehta, M. A., Greenwood, R. J., et al. (2012). Salience network integrity predicts default mode network function after traumatic brain injury. *Proc. Natl. Acad. Sci. U S A* 109, 4690–4695. doi: 10.1073/pnas.1113455109

Bora, E., Fornito, A., Radua, J., Walterfang, M., Seal, M., Wood, S. J., et al. (2011). Neuroanatomical abnormalities in schizophrenia: a multimodal voxelwise meta-analysis and meta-regression analysis. *Schizophr. Res.* 127, 46–57. doi: 10.1016/j.schres.2010.12.020

Bora, E., and Pantelis, C. (2013). Theory of mind impairments in first-episode psychosis, individuals at ultra-high risk for psychosis and in first-degree relatives of schizophrenia: systematic review and meta-analysis. *Schizophr. Res.* 144, 31–36. doi: 10.1016/j.schres.2012.12.013

Bosco, F. M., Colle, L., De, F. S., Bono, A., Ruberti, S., and Tirassa, M. (2009). Th.o.m.a.s.: an exploratory assessment of Theory of Mind in schizophrenic subjects. *Conscious. Cogn.* 18, 306–319. doi: 10.1016/j.concog.2008.06.006

Bosia, M., Riccaboni, R., and Poletti, S. (2012). Neurofunctional correlates of theory of mind deficits in schizophrenia. *Curr. Top. Med. Chem.* 12, 2284–2302. doi: 10.2174/156802661121221002

Bozikas, V. P., Giannakou, M., Kosmidis, M. H., Kargopoulos, P., Kioseoglou, G., Liolios, D., et al. (2011). Insights into theory of mind in schizophrenia: the impact of cognitive impairment. *Schizophr. Res.* 130, 130–136. doi: 10.1016/j.schres.2011.04.025

Brüne, M. (2003). Theory of mind and the role of IQ in chronic disorganized schizophrenia. *Schizophr. Res.* 60, 57–64. doi: 10.1016/s0920-9964(02)00162-7

Brüne, M., and Brüne-Cohrs, U. (2006). Theory of mind—evolution, ontogeny, brain mechanisms and psychopathology. *Neurosci. Biobehav. Rev.* 30, 437–455. doi: 10.1016/j.neubiorev.2005.08.001

Camchong, J., MacDonald, A. W., III, Bell, C., Mueller, B. A., and Lim, K. O. (2011). Altered functional and anatomical connectivity in schizophrenia. *Schizophr. Bull.* 37, 640–650. doi: 10.1093/schbul/sbp131

Chan, R. C., Di, X., McAlonan, G. M., and Gong, Q. Y. (2011). Brain anatomical abnormalities in high-risk individuals, first-episode and chronic schizophrenia: an activation likelihood estimation meta-analysis of illness progression. *Schizophr. Bull.* 37, 177–188. doi: 10.1093/schbul/sbp073

Corcoran, R., Cahill, C., and Frith, C. D. (1997). The appreciation of visual jokes in people with schizophrenia: a study of 'mentalizing' ability. *Schizophr. Res.* 24, 319–327. doi: 10.1016/s0920-9964(96)00117-x

Corcoran, R., Mercer, G., and Frith, C. D. (1995). Schizophrenia, symptomatology and social inference: investigating "theory of mind" in people with schizophrenia. *Schizophr. Res.* 17, 5–13. doi: 10.1016/0920-9964(95)00024-g

Crow, T. J. (1985). The two-syndrome concept: origins and current status. *Schizophr. Bull.* 11, 471–486. doi: 10.1093/schbul/11.3.471

D'Argembeau, A., Ruby, P., Collette, F., Degueldre, C., Balteau, E., Luxen, A., et al. (2007). Distinct regions of the medial prefrontal cortex are associated with self-referential processing and perspective taking. *J. Cogn. Neurosci.* 19, 935–944. doi: 10.1162/jocn.2007.19.6.935

Damasio, A. (1999). *The Feeling of What Happens: Body and Emotion in the Making of Consciousness.* United Kingdom: William Heinemann, 386.

Das, P., Lagopoulos, J., Coulston, C. M., Henderson, A. F., and Malhi, G. S. (2012). Mentalizing impairment in schizophrenia: a functional MRI study. *Schizophr. Res.* 134, 158–164. doi: 10.1016/j.schres.2011.08.019

David, N., Newen, A., and Vogeley, K. (2008). The "sense of agency" and its underlying cognitive and neural mechanisms. *Conscious. Cogn.* 17, 523–534. doi: 10.1016/j.concog.2008.03.004

Ellison-Wright, I., and Bullmore, E. (2010). Anatomy of bipolar disorder and schizophrenia: a meta-analysis. *Schizophr. Res.* 117, 1–12. doi: 10.1016/j.schres.2009.12.022

Elvevåg, B., and Goldberg, T. E. (2000). Cognitive impairment in schizophrenia is the core of the disorder. *Crit. Rev. Neurobiol.* 14, 1–21. doi: 10.1615/critrevneurobiol.v14.i1.10

Farrer, C., Franck, N., Frith, C. D., Decety, J., Georgieff, N., d'Amato, T., et al. (2004). Neural correlates of action attribution in schizophrenia. *Psychiatry Res.* 131, 31–44. doi: 10.1016/j.pscychresns.2004.02.004

Fletcher, P. C., and Frith, C. D. (2009). Perceiving is believing: a Bayesian approach to explaining the positive symptoms of schizophrenia. *Nat. Rev. Neurosci.* 10, 48–58. doi: 10.1038/nrn2536

Franck, N., Farrer, C., Georgieff, N., Marie-Cardine, M., Dalery, J., d'Amato, T., et al. (2001). Defective recognition of one's own actions in patients with schizophrenia. *Am. J. Psychiatry* 158, 454–459. doi: 10.1176/appi.ajp.158.3.454

Frith, C. (2005). The neural basis of hallucinations and delusions. *C. R. Biol.* 328, 169–175. doi: 10.1016/j.crvi.2004.10.012

Frith, C. D. (1992). *The Cognitive Neuropsychology of Schizophrenia.* Hove, UK: Lawrence Erlbaum.

Frith, C. D., Blakemore, S., and Wolpert, D. M. (2000). Explaining the symptoms of schizophrenia: abnormalities in the awareness of action. *Brain Res. Brain Res. Rev.* 31, 357–363. doi: 10.1016/s0165-0173(99)00052-1

Fryer, S. L., Woods, S. W., Kiehl, K. A., Calhoun, V. D., Pearlson, G. D., Roach, B. J., et al. (2013). Deficient Suppression of Default Mode Regions during Working Memory in Individuals with Early Psychosis and at Clinical High-Risk for Psychosis. *Front. Psychiatry* 4:92. doi: 10.3389/fpsyt.2013.00092

Gallagher, S. (2013). A pattern theory of self. *Front. Hum. Neurosci.* 7:443. doi: 10.3389/fnhum.2013.00443

Garrity, A. G., Pearlson, G. D., McKiernan, K., Lloyd, D., Kiehl, K. A., and Calhoun, V. D. (2007). Aberrant "default mode" functional connectivity in schizophrenia. *Am. J. Psychiatry* 164, 450–457. doi: 10.1176/appi.ajp.164.3.450

Glahn, D. C., Laird, A. R., Ellison-Wright, I., Thelen, S. M., Robinson, J. L., Lancaster, J. L., et al. (2008). Meta-analysis of gray matter anomalies in schizophrenia: application of anatomic likelihood estimation and network analysis. *Biol. Psychiatry* 64, 774–781. doi: 10.1016/j.biopsych.2008.03.031

Green, M. F., Nuechterlein, K. H., Gold, J. M., Barch, D. M., Cohen, J., Essock, S., et al. (2004). Approaching a consensus cognitive battery for clinical trials in schizophrenia: the NIMH-MATRICS conference to select cognitive domains and test criteria. *Biol. Psychiatry* 56, 301–307. doi: 10.1016/j.biopsych.2004.06.023

Guo, W., Yao, D., Jiang, J., Su, Q., Zhang, Z., Zhang, J., et al. (2014a). Abnormal default-mode network homogeneity in first-episode, drug-naive schizophrenia at rest. *Prog. Neuropsychopharmacol. Biol. Psychiatry* 49, 16–20. doi: 10.1016/j.pnpbp.2013.10.021

Guo, S., Kendrick, K. M., Yu, R., Wang, H. L., and Feng, J. (2014b). Key functional circuitry altered in schizophrenia involves parietal regions associated with sense of self. *Hum. Brain Mapp.* 35, 123–139. doi: 10.1002/hbm.22162

Harrison, B. J., Yucel, M., Pujol, J., and Pantelis, C. (2007). Task-induced deactivation of midline cortical regions in schizophrenia assessed with fMRI. *Schizophr. Res.* 91, 82–86. doi: 10.1016/j.schres.2006.12.027

Hommes, J., Krabbendam, L., Versmissen, D., Kircher, T., van Os, J., and van, W. R. (2012). Self-monitoring as a familial vulnerability marker for psychosis: an analysis of patients, unaffected siblings and healthy controls. *Psychol. Med.* 42, 235–245. doi: 10.1017/S0033291711001152

Horacek, J., Zavesicka, L., Tintera, J., Dockery, C., Platilova, V., Kopecek, M., et al. (2005). The effect of tryptophan depletion on brain activation measured by functional magnetic resonance imaging during the Stroop test in healthy subjects. *Physiol. Res.* 54, 235–244.

Howes, O. D., and Kapur, S. (2009). The Dopamine Hypothesis of Schizophrenia: version III—the final common pathway. *Schizophr. Bull.* 35, 549–562. doi: 10.1093/schbul/sbp006

Irani, F., Platek, S. M., Bunce, S., Ruocco, A. C., and Chute, D. (2007). Functional near infrared spectroscopy (fNIRS): an emerging neuroimaging technology with important applications for the study of brain disorders. *Clin. Neuropsychol.* 21, 9–37. doi: 10.1080/13854040600910018

Irani, F., Platek, S. M., Panyavin, I. S., Calkins, M. E., Kohler, C., Siegel, S. J., et al. (2006). Self-face recognition and theory of mind in patients with schizophrenia and first-degree relatives. *Schizophr. Res.* 88, 151–160. doi: 10.1016/j.schres.2006.07.016

Jardri, R., Pouchet, A., Pins, D., and Thomas, P. (2011). Cortical activations during auditory verbal hallucinations in schizophrenia: a coordinate-based meta-analysis. *Am. J. Psychiatry* 168, 73–81. doi: 10.1176/appi.ajp.2010.09101522

Jardri, R., Thomas, P., Delmaire, C., Delion, P., and Pins, D. (2013). The neurodynamic organization of modality-dependent hallucinations. *Cereb. Cortex* 23, 1108–1117. doi: 10.1093/cercor/bhs082

Kasparek, T., Prikryl, R., Rehulova, J., Marecek, R., Mikl, M., Prikrylova, H., et al. (2013). Brain functional connectivity of male patients in remission after the first episode of schizophrenia. *Hum. Brain Mapp.* 34, 726–737. doi: 10.1002/hbm.21469

Koelkebeck, K., Pedersen, A., Suslow, T., Kueppers, K. A., Arolt, V., and Ohrmann, P. (2010). Theory of Mind in first-episode schizophrenia patients: correlations with cognition and personality traits. *Schizophr. Res.* 119, 115–123. doi: 10.1016/j.schres.2009.12.015

Laird, A. R., Fox, P. M., Eickhoff, S. B., Turner, J. A., Ray, K. L., McKay, D. R., et al. (2011). Behavioral interpretations of intrinsic connectivity networks. *J. Cogn. Neurosci.* 23, 4022–4037. doi: 10.1162/jocn_a_00077

Langdon, R., and Coltheart, M. (1999). Mentalising, schizotypy and schizophrenia. *Cognition* 71, 43–71. doi: 10.1016/s0010-0277(99)00018-9

Leube, D., Whitney, C., and Kircher, T. (2008). The neural correlates of ego-disturbances (passivity phenomena) and formal thought disorder in schizophrenia. *Eur. Arch. Psychiatry Clin. Neurosci.* 258(Suppl. 5), 22–27. doi: 10.1007/s00406-008-5017-z

Li, C. S., Yan, P., Bergquist, K. L., and Sinha, R. (2007). Greater activation of the "default" brain regions predicts stop signal errors. *Neuroimage* 38, 640–648. doi: 10.1016/j.neuroimage.2007.07.021

Manoliu, A., Riedl, V., Doll, A., Bauml, J. G., Muhlau, M., Schwerthoffer, D., et al. (2013). Insular dysfunction reflects altered between-network connectivity and severity of negative symptoms in schizophrenia during psychotic remission. *Front. Hum. Neurosci.* 7:216. doi: 10.3389/fnhum.2013.00216

Manoliu, A., Riedl, V., Zherdin, A., Muhlau, M., Schwerthoffer, D., Scherr, M., et al. (2014). Aberrant dependence of default mode/central executive network interactions on anterior insular salience network activity in schizophrenia. *Schizophr. Bull.* 40, 428–437. doi: 10.1093/schbul/sbt037

Mars, R. A. (2011). The neural bases of social cognition and story comprehension. *Annu. Rev. Psychol.* 62, 103–134. doi: 10.1146/annurev-psych-120709-145406

Mars, R. B., Neubert, F. X., Noonan, M. P., Sallet, J., Toni, I., and Rushworth, M. F. (2012). On the relationship between the "default mode network" and the "social brain". *Front. Hum. Neurosci.* 6:189. doi: 10.3389/fnhum.2012.00189

Mazza, M., De, R. A., Surian, L., Roncone, R., and Casacchia, M. (2001). Selective impairments of theory of mind in people with schizophrenia. *Schizophr. Res.* 47, 299–308. doi: 10.1016/s0920-9964(00)00157-2

McKiernan, K. A., Kaufman, J. N., Kucera-Thompson, J., and Binder, J. R. (2003). A parametric manipulation of factors affecting task-induced deactivation in functional neuroimaging. *J. Cogn. Neurosci.* 15, 394–408. doi: 10.1162/089892903321593117

Menon, M., Schmitz, T. W., Anderson, A. K., Graff, A., Korostil, M., Mamo, D., et al. (2011). Exploring the neural correlates of delusions of reference. *Biol. Psychiatry* 70, 1127–1233. doi: 10.1016/j.biopsych.2011.05.037

Menon, V. (2011). Large-scale brain networks and psychopathology: a unifying triple network model. *Trends Cogn. Sci.* 15, 483–506. doi: 10.1016/j.tics.2011.08.003

Menon, V., and Uddin, L. Q. (2010). Saliency, switching, attention and control: a network model of insula function. *Brain Struct. Funct.* 214, 655–667. doi: 10.1007/s00429-010-0262-0

Meyer-Lindenberg, A. S., Olsen, R. K., Kohn, P. D., Brown, T., Egan, M. F., Weinberger, D. R., et al. (2005). Regionally specific disturbance of dorsolateral prefrontal-hippocampal functional connectivity in schizophrenia. *Arch. Gen. Psychiatry* 62, 379–386. doi: 10.1001/archpsyc.62.4.379

Mitchell, J. P., Banaji, M. R., and Macrae, C. N. (2005). The link between social cognition and self-referential thought in the medial prefrontal cortex. *J. Cogn. Neurosci.* 17, 1306–1315. doi: 10.1162/0898929055002418

Montag, C., Dziobek, I., Richter, I. S., Neuhaus, K., Lehmann, A., Sylla, R., et al. (2011). Different aspects of theory of mind in paranoid schizophrenia: evidence from a video-based assessment. *Psychiatry Res.* 186, 203–209. doi: 10.1016/j.psychres.2010.09.006

Moran, L. V., Tagamets, M. A., Sampath, H., O'Donnell, A., Stein, E. A., Kochunov, P., et al. (2013). Disruption of anterior insula modulation of large-scale brain networks in schizophrenia. *Biol. Psychiatry* 74, 467–474. doi: 10.1016/j.biopsych.2013.02.029

Moran, M. E., Weisinger, B., Ludovici, K., McAdams, H., Greenstein, D., Gochman, P., et al. (2014). At the boundary of the self: the insular cortex in patients with childhood-onset schizophrenia, their healthy siblings and normal volunteers. *Int. J. Dev. Neurosci.* 32, 58–63. doi: 10.1016/j.ijdevneu.2013.05.010

Murray, R. J., Schaer, M., and Debbane, M. (2012). Degrees of separation: a quantitative neuroimaging meta-analysis investigating self-specificity and shared neural activation between self- and other-reflection. *Neurosci. Biobehav. Rev.* 36, 1043–1059. doi: 10.1016/j.neubiorev.2011.12.013

Nelson, B., Thompson, A., Chanen, A. M., Amminger, G. P., and Yung, A. R. (2013). Is basic self-disturbance in ultra-high risk for psychosis ('prodromal') patients associated with borderline personality pathology? *Early Interv. Psychiatry* 7, 306–310. doi: 10.1111/eip.12011

Nelson, B., Whitford, T. J., Lavoie, S., and Sass, L. A. (2014). What are the neurocognitive correlates of basic self-disturbance in schizophrenia?: integrating phenomenology and neurocognition. Part 1 (Source monitoring deficits). *Schizophr. Res.* 152, 12–19. doi: 10.1016/j.schres.2013.06.022

Newen, A., and Vogeley, K. (2003). Self-representation: searching for a neural signature of self-consciousness. *Conscious. Cogn.* 12, 529–543. doi: 10.1016/s1053-8100(03)00080-1

Northoff, G., and Qin, P. (2011). How can the brain's resting state activity generate hallucinations? A 'resting state hypothesis' of auditory verbal hallucinations. *Schizophr. Res.* 127, 202–214. doi: 10.1016/j.schres.2010.11.009

Northoff, G., Heinzel, A., de, G. M., Bermpohl, F., Dobrowolny, H., and Panksepp, J. (2006). Self-referential processing in our brain–a meta-analysis of imaging studies on the self. *Neuroimage* 31, 440–457. doi: 10.1016/j.neuroimage.2005.12.002

Nygård, M., Eichele, T., Loberg, E. M., Jorgensen, H. A., Johnsen, E., Kroken, R. A., et al. (2012). Patients with schizophrenia fail to up-regulate task-positive and down-regulate task-negative brain networks: an fMRI study using an ICA analysis approach. *Front. Hum. Neurosci.* 6:149. doi: 10.3389/fnhum.2012.00149

Orliac, F., Naveau, M., Joliot, M., Delcroix, N., Razafimandimby, A., Brazo, P., et al. (2013). Links among resting-state default-mode network, salience network and symptomatology in schizophrenia. *Schizophr. Res.* 148, 74–80. doi: 10.1016/j.schres.2013.05.007

Palaniyappan, L., Balain, V., Radua, J., and Liddle, P. F. (2012a). Structural correlates of auditory hallucinations in schizophrenia: a meta-analysis. *Schizophr. Res.* 137, 169–173. doi: 10.1016/j.schres.2012.01.038

Palaniyappan, L., Simmonite, M., White, T. P., Liddle, E. B., and Liddle, P. F. (2013). Neural primacy of the salience processing system in schizophrenia. *Neuron* 79, 814–828. doi: 10.1016/j.neuron.2013.06.027

Palaniyappan, L., White, T. P., and Liddle, P. F. (2012b). The concept of salience network dysfunction in schizophrenia: from neuroimaging observations to therapeutic opportunities. *Curr. Top. Med. Chem.* 12, 2324–2338. doi: 10.2174/1568026611212210005

Pedersen, A., Koelkebeck, K., Brandt, M., Wee, M., Kueppers, K. A., Kugel, H., et al. (2012). Theory of mind in patients with schizophrenia: is mentalizing delayed? *Schizophr. Res.* 137, 224–229. doi: 10.1016/j.schres.2012.02.022

Pentaraki, A. D., Stefanis, N. C., Stahl, D., Theleritis, C., Toulopoulou, T., Roukas, D., et al. (2012). Theory of Mind as a potential trait marker of schizophrenia: a family study. *Cogn. Neuropsychiatry* 17, 64–89. doi: 10.1080/13546805.2011.568289

Peralta, V., and Cuesta, M. J. (2005). The underlying structure of diagnostic systems of schizophrenia: a comprehensive polydiagnostic approach. *Schizophr. Res.* 79, 217–229. doi: 10.1016/j.schres.2005.05.003

Pickup, G. J. (2008). Relationship between Theory of Mind and executive function in schizophrenia: a systematic review. *Psychopathology* 41, 206–213. doi: 10.1159/000125554

Pomarol-Clotet, E., Salvador, R., Sarro, S., Gomar, J., Vila, F., Martinez, A., et al. (2008). Failure to deactivate in the prefrontal cortex in schizophrenia: dysfunction of the default mode network? *Psychol. Med.* 38, 1185–1193. doi: 10.1017/s0033291708003565

Pousa, E., Duno, R., Blas, N. J., Ruiz, A. I., Obiols, J. E., and David, A. S. (2008). Exploratory study of the association between insight and Theory of Mind (ToM) in stable schizophrenia patients. *Cogn. Neuropsychiatry* 13, 210–232. doi: 10.1016/s0920-9964(08)70381-5

Premack, D., and Woodruff, G. (1978). Chimpanzee problem-solving: a test for comprehension. *Science* 202, 532–535. doi: 10.1126/science.705342

Pujol, N., Penades, R., Rametti, G., Catalan, R., Vidal-Pineiro, D., Palacios, E., et al. (2013). Inferior frontal and insular cortical thinning is related to dysfunctional brain activation/deactivation during working memory task in schizophrenic patients. *Psychiatry Res.* 214, 94–101. doi: 10.1016/j.pscychresns.2013.06.008

Qin, P., and Northoff, G. (2011). How is our self related to midline regions and the default-mode network? *Neuroimage* 57, 1221–1233. doi: 10.1016/j.neuroimage.2011.05.028

Rotarska-Jagiela, A., van de Ven, D., Oertel-Knochel, V., Uhlhaas, P. J., Vogeley, K., and Linden, D. E. (2010). Resting-state functional network correlates of psychotic symptoms in schizophrenia. *Schizophr. Res.* 117, 21–30. doi: 10.1016/j.schres.2010.01.001

Sarfati, Y., and Hardy-Bayle, M. C. (1999). How do people with schizophrenia explain the behaviour of others? A study of theory of mind and its relationship to thought and speech disorganization in schizophrenia. *Psychol. Med.* 29, 613–620. doi: 10.1017/s0033291799008326

Sarfati, Y., Hardy-Bayle, M. C., Besche, C., and Widlocher, D. (1997). Attribution of intentions to others in people with schizophrenia: a non-verbal exploration with comic strips. *Schizophr. Res.* 25, 199–209. doi: 10.1016/s0920-9964(97)00025-x

Sass, L. A. (2014). Self-disturbance and schizophrenia: structure, specificity, pathogenesis (Current issues, New directions). *Schizophr. Res.* 152, 5–11. doi: 10.1016/j.schres.2013.05.017

Sass, L. A., and Parnas, J. (2003). Schizophrenia, consciousness and the self. *Schizophr. Bull.* 29, 427–444. doi: 10.1093/oxfordjournals.schbul.a007017

Schilbach, L., Bzdok, D., Timmermans, B., Fox, P. T., Laird, A. R., Vogeley, K., et al. (2012). Introspective minds: using ALE meta-analyses to study commonalities in the neural correlates of emotional processing, social & unconstrained cognition. *PLoS One* 7:e30920. doi: 10.1371/journal.pone.0030920

Schilbach, L., Wohlschlaeger, A. M., Kraemer, N. C., Newen, A., Shah, N. J., Fink, G. R., et al. (2006). Being with virtual others: neural correlates of social interaction. *Neuropsychologia* 44, 718–730. doi: 10.1016/j.neuropsychologia.2005.07.017

Shepherd, A. M., Laurens, K. R., Matheson, S. L., Carr, V. J., and Green, M. J. (2012). Systematic meta-review and quality assessment of the structural brain alterations in schizophrenia. *Neurosci. Biobehav. Rev.* 36, 1342–1356. doi: 10.1016/j.neubiorev.2011.12.015

Sridharan, D., Levitin, D. J., and Menon, V. (2008). A critical role for the right fronto-insular cortex in switching between central-executive and default-mode networks. *Proc. Natl. Acad. Sci. U S A* 105, 12569–12574. doi: 10.1073/pnas.0800005105

van der Meer, L., Costafreda, S., Aleman, A., and David, A. S. (2010). Self-reflection and the brain: a theoretical review and meta-analysis of neuroimaging studies with implications for schizophrenia. *Neurosci. Biobehav. Rev.* 34, 935–946. doi: 10.1016/j.neubiorev.2009.12.004

Vogeley, K., and Fink, G. R. (2003). Neural correlates of the first-person-perspective. *Trends Cogn. Sci.* 7, 38–42. doi: 10.1016/s1364-6613(02)00003-7

Vogeley, K., Bussfeld, P., Newen, A., Herrmann, S., Happe, F., Falkai, P., et al. (2001). Mind reading: neural mechanisms of theory of mind and self-perspective. *Neuroimage* 14, 170–181. doi: 10.1006/nimg.2001.0789

Waters, F., Woodward, T., Allen, P., Aleman, A., and Sommer, I. (2012). Self-recognition deficits in schizophrenia patients with auditory hallucinations: a meta-analysis of the literature. *Schizophr. Bull.* 38, 741–750. doi: 10.1093/schbul/sbQ114

White, T. P., Joseph, V., Francis, S. T., and Liddle, P. F. (2010). Aberrant salience network (bilateral insula and anterior cingulate cortex) connectivity during information processing in schizophrenia. *Schizophr. Res.* 123, 105–115. doi: 10.1016/j.schres.2010.07.020

Whitfield-Gabrieli, S., Thermenos, H. W., Milanovic, S., Tsuang, M. T., Faraone, S. V., McCarley, R. W., et al. (2009). Hyperactivity and hyperconnectivity of the default network in schizophrenia and in first-degree relatives of persons with schizophrenia. *Proc. Natl. Acad. Sci. U S A* 106, 1279–1284. doi: 10.1073/pnas.0900938106

Wolpert, D. M., and Kawato, M. (1998). Multiple paired forward and inverse models for motor control. *Neural Netw.* 11, 1317–1329. doi: 10.1016/s0893-6080(98)00066-5

Zhou, J., Greicius, M. D., Gennatas, E. D., Growdon, M. E., Jang, J. Y., Rabinovici, G. D., et al. (2010). Divergent network connectivity changes in behavioural variant frontotemporal dementia and Alzheimer's disease. *Brain* 133, 1352–1367. doi: 10.1093/brain/awq075

5

Tandospirone, a 5-HT_{1A} partial agonist, ameliorates aberrant lactate production in the prefrontal cortex of rats exposed to blockade of N-methy-D-aspartate receptors; toward the therapeutics of cognitive impairment of schizophrenia

Takashi Uehara[1]*, Tadasu Matsuoka[2] and Tomiki Sumiyoshi[3]

[1] Department of Neuropsychiatry, Kanazawa Medical University, Ucninada-cho, Ishikawa, Japan
[2] Department of Psychiatry, Matsuoka Hospital, Oyabe, Toyama, Japan
[3] Department of Clinical Research Promotion, National Center Hospital, National Center of Neurology and Psychiatry, Tokyo, Japan

Edited by:
Ales Stuchlik, Institute of Physiology Academy of Sciences of the Czech Republic, Czech Republic

****Correspondence:***
Takashi Uehara, Department of Neuropsychiatry, Kanazawa Medical University, 1-1 Daigaku, Uchinada-cho, Ishikawa 920-0293, Japan
e-mail: uehara@kanazawa-med.ac.jp

Rationale: Augmentation therapy with serotonin-1A (5-HT_{1A}) receptor partial agonists has been suggested to improve cognitive impairment in patients with schizophrenia. Decreased activity of prefrontal cortex may provide a basis for cognitive deficits of the disease. Lactate plays a significant role in the supply of energy to the brain, and glutamatergic neurotransmission contributes to lactate production.

Objectives and methods: The purposes of this study were to examine the effect of repeated administration (once a daily for 4 days) of tandospirone (0.05 or 5 mg/kg) on brain energy metabolism, as represented by extracellular lactate concentration (eLAC) in the medial prefrontal cortex (mPFC) of a rat model of schizophrenia.

Results: Four-day treatment with MK-801, an NMDA-R antagonist, prolonged eLAC elevation induced by foot-shock stress (FS). Co-administration with the high-dose tandospirone suppressed prolonged FS-induced eLAC elevation in rats receiving MK-801, whereas tandospirone by itself did not affected eLAC increment.

Conclusions: These results suggest that stimulation of 5-HT_{1A} receptors ameliorates abnormalities of energy metabolism in the mPFC due to blockade of NMDA receptors. These findings provide a possible mechanism, based on brain energy metabolism, by which 5-HT_{1A} agonism improve cognitive impairment of schizophrenia and related disorders.

Keywords: 5-HT_{1A}, cognition, schizophrenia, lactate, microdialysis, glutamate, NMDA receptor, animal model

INTRODUCTION

Disturbances of cognitive function, evaluated by psychological and neurophysiological methods, have been shown to predict social outcome in patients with schizophrenia (Meltzer and McGurk, 1999; McGurk and Meltzer, 2000). There is much attention to the role of psychotropic compounds acting on serotonin (5-HT) receptors in ameliorating cognitive deficits of the disease. Among the 5-HT receptor subtypes, the 5-HT_{1A} receptor is attracting particular interests as a potential target for enhancing cognition (Newman-Tancredi and Albert, 2012; Ohno et al., 2012; Sumiyoshi and Higuchi, 2013; Sumiyoshi et al., 2013). It is reported that adjunctive treatment with selective 5-HT_{1A} receptor (partial) agonists, e.g., tandospirone or buspirone, was associated with improvements in some types of cognitive function in patients with schizophrenia (Sumiyoshi et al., 2001b, 2007; Sumiyoshi and Higuchi, 2013). These observations provide the basis for the ability of 5-HT_{1A} receptor stimulation to enhance cognition, a therapeutic approach that have promoted the development of novel antipsychotic drugs (Sumiyoshi, 2013; Sumiyoshi et al., 2013).

The development of animal models of schizophrenia is important to clarify the pathophysiology of the illness and facilitate the development of novel therapeutics. Non-competitive antagonists at the N-methyl-D-asparate receptor (NMDA-R) have been shown to induce schizophrenia-like symptoms, i.e., positive and negative symptoms, as well as cognitive dysfunction in normal subjects (Jentsch and Roth, 1999). Numerous studies reported that NMDA-R antagonists, such as phencyclidine (PCP), MK-801 and ketamine, produce hyperlocomotion, stereotypy, information processing deficits, impairments of cognitive functions and social interactions, behavioral changes reminiscent of symptoms of schizophrenia (Breese et al., 2002; Moghaddam and Jackson, 2003; Bubenikova-Valesova et al., 2008; Jones et al., 2011).

Four-day treatment with MK-801 changed behaviors and expression of NMDA-Rs in a way that mimicked chronic treatment (Bubenikova-Valesova et al., 2010). Especially, prepulse inhibition (PPI) was impaired, while locomotion was decreased (Bubenikova-Valesova et al., 2010). PPI deficits are one of the most widely used neurophysiological markers of the pathophysiology of schizophrenia, and have been suggested to represent an aspect of cognitive deficits (Geyer, 2006; Singer et al., 2013). Especially, a specific correlative link between working memory and PPI has been reported in rodents (Singer et al., 2013). On the other hand, the mPFC was the target brain region in the current study because our aim was to clarify the mechanisms underlying cognitive enhancement by 5-HT_{1A} receptor stimulation. Functional abnormality of the frontal cortex has been associated with negative symptoms and cognitive deficits (Volk and Lewis, 2002). Specifically, performance on the cognitive tasks governed by the prefrontal cortex (PFC), e.g., working memory and executive function, has been consistently reported in patients with schizophrenia (Tamminga et al., 1992; Volz et al., 1999; Hazlett et al., 2000; Ragland et al., 2007).

Since the proposal of the astrocyte-neuron lactate shuttle (ANLS) hypothesis (Pellerin and Magistretti, 1994), lactate has been found to play a crucial role in energy metabolism in the brain (Tsacopoulos and Magistretti, 1996; Pellerin and Magistretti, 2012). According to this hypothesis, lactate is produced in a neural activity-dependent and glutamate-mediated manner in astrocytes, and is transferred to active neurons (Pellerin et al., 1998, 2007; Pellerin, 2003; Uehara et al., 2008). Moreover, it has been shown that lactate *is* a primary substrate for energy metabolism in the brain of humans (Smith et al., 2003) or rodents (Wyss et al., 2011) under working conditions if both lactate and glucose is sufficiently available, as demonstrated by *in vivo* studies (Wyss et al., 2011).

Whether or not abnormality of lactate metabolism exists in the brain of schizophrenia patients remains to be discussed. A postmortem study reports altered transcription of genes in a large number of metabolic pathways and increased lactate levels in the PFC of patients with schizophrenia (Prabakaran et al., 2004). However, another report argued that these changes are associated with decreased pH, and are possibly related to antipsychotic treatment rather than a primary metabolic abnormality (Halim et al., 2008).

In this study, we investigated the effect of repeated (four consecutive days) administration of MK-801, a non-competitive NMDA-R antagonist, on energy metabolism indicated by extracellular lactate concentration (eLAC) in the medial prefrontal cortex (mPFC) of rats using microdialysis technique. Then, we determined whether co-administration of low and high doses (0.05 or 5 mg/kg) tandospirone affect lactate metabolism in the MK-801 treated animals.

MATERIALS AND METHODS

ANIMALS

Adult male Wistar rats (Japan SLC Inc., Hamamatsu, Japan) weighing 280–300 g (8 weeks postnatal) for microdialysis experiments were housed 4–5 in a standard cage at 24 ± 2°C under a 12-h light (07:00–19:00 h) 12-h dark cycle. The procedures complied with the National Institutes of Health guide for the care and use of Laboratory animals. All experiments were reviewed and approved by the Committee of Animal Research, University of Toyama.

DRUGS

Tandospirone was provided from Dainippon Sumitomo Pharmaceuticals (Tokyo, Japan).

The treatment regimen with MK-801 (dizocilpine, 0.1 mg/kg, Sigma-Aldrich, St. Louis, MO) and/or tandospirone was based on a previous report (Bubenikova-Valesova et al., 2010) with minor modifications. First, to evaluate the effect of 4 days treatment with MK-801 on eLAC in the mPFC, rats received an intraperitoneal (i.p.) injection of MK-801 (0.1 mg/kg) at a volume of 2 ml/kg (MK-801 group, $n = 6$), or the equal volume of saline (saline group, $n = 5$) once daily for 4 days. Second, to access the effect of tandospirone on FS-induced eLAC changes, rats received a subcutaneous (s.c.) injection of tandospirone at 0.05 mg/kg (low-T) or 5.0 mg/kg (high-T) at a volume of 2 ml/kg or the equal volume of saline. This yielded the following 6 groups: saline-saline group ($n = 5$); saline-low-T group ($n = 5$); saline-high-T group ($n = 5$); MK-801-saline group ($n = 5$); MK-801-low-T group (n–5); MK-801-high-T group ($n = 5$). The last injection was administered 10 min before the start of foot-shock (FS) stress (**Figure 1**).

SURGERY

Extracellular lactate concentrations were measured by *in vivo* microdialysis technique with an enzyme reactor/fluorometric detector according to the method previously reported (Uehara et al., 2003, 2005, 2006, 2007a). The animals were anesthetized with pentobarbital sodium (Nembutal, Abbott Laboratories, IL, USA) (40 mg/kg, i.p.), and were mounted on a stereotaxic apparatus. A dialysis probe (molecular weight cutoff 10,000; 200 μm in outer diameter) was implanted into the left mPFC according to the atlas of Paxinos and Watson (1998), and was secured with skull screws and dental acrylate. The exposed tip length of the probe was 1.5 mm. Coordinates were A 3.2 mm, L 0.6 mm, V 5.2 mm from bregma for the mPFC. Following the surgery, the rats were housed in individual cages with free access to food and water.

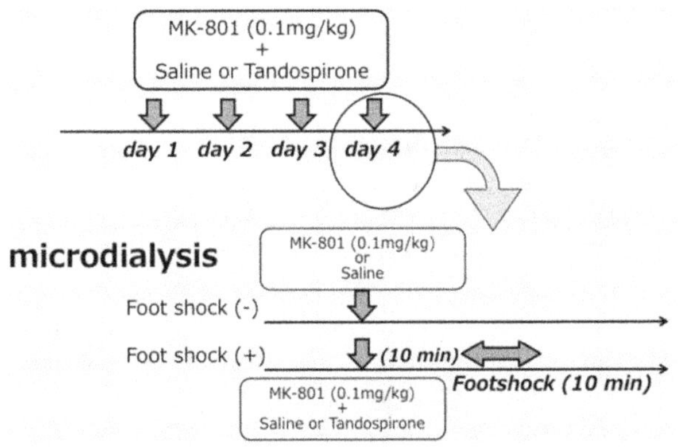

FIGURE 1 | Schematic representation of the experimental protocol for microdialysis experiments. Upper parts in each figure reveals drug treatment for 4 days and lower parts time course in the 4th day (experiment day).

Forty-two to 48 h after surgery, the dialysis experiment was carried out on the freely moving rats. Microdialysis experiments were performed between 08:00 and 16:00. Artificial CSF (consisting of 147 mmol/l NaCl, 3 mmol/l KCl, 1.2 mmol/l $CaCl_2$, 1.2 mmol/l $MgSO_4$, 0.4 mmol/l NaH_2PO_2, pH 7.40) was perfused at a rate of 5.0 μl/min into the dialysis probe. The dialysates were mixed on-line with an enzyme solution containing L-lactate dehydrogenase and NAD^+ in a T-tube. The enzyme solution consisted of 5.0 μg/ml LDH (L-Malate: NAD oxidoreductase, E.C.1.1.1.27; isolated from pig heart, specific activity ca.300 U/mg; Roche Diagnostics GmbH, Mannheim, Germany) and 0.5 mmol/l NAD^+ (Roche Diagnostics GmbH, Mannheim, Germany) in a carbonate buffer (62.5 mmol/l, adjusted to pH 9.4 with NaOH). The solution was pumped using a Model 22 microdialysis pump (Harvard Apparatus, Inc. Massachusetts, USA) at the flow rate of 20 μl/min. The mixture from the T-tube was passed for 20 min reaction before reaching a fluorometer equipped with a 12 μl flow-cell (Shimazu RF-530, Kyoto, Japan). During transport to the fluorometer, lactate was enzymatically oxidized, and the fluorescence of the formed nicotinamid adenosine dinucleotide diphosphate (NADH) was continuously measured with excitation at 340 nm and emission at 450 nm. A standard solution of 100 μmol/l lactate was used for calibration.

FOOT-SHOCK STRESS

Foot-shock (FS) stress was administered using a plastic communication box (CB5, MATYS, Toyama, Japan), according to the method reported previously (Uehara et al., 2012a). The box (L 51 × W 51 × H 40 cm) was equipped with a grid floor composed of stainless steel rods (6-mm in diameter) placed 16 mm apart. The box was subdivided into nine compartments (17 × 17 cm) by transparent plastic walls. In this study, we used 4 compartments areas (34 × 34 cm) for the field of free moving and FS administration. The communication box was connected to a shock-generator (MSG-001, MATYS, Toyama, Japan) and a timer-box (MTB-001, MATYS, Toyama, Japan) to deliver FS as described below. Each FS session consisted of a scramble shock of 0.3 mA for 5 s administered every 30 s for 10 min.

At the end of the experimental sessions, all rats were deeply anesthetized with pentobarbital sodium, and were sacrificed by decapitation. The position of dialysis probes was verified microscopically for all rats.

PRESENTATION OF THE RESULTS AND STATISTICS

Data were analyzed by analysis of variance (ANOVA) using SPSS software (version 19.0 J for Mac; IBM, Tokyo, Japan).

Lactate levels in the dialysates are expressed as μmol/l calculated by a standard solution of 100 μmol/l lactate. The average of the eLAC during the period preceding the last injection (four measurements performed every 5 min) was used as the basal concentrations of lactate. To access the effects of MK-801 and tandospirone on basal lactate levels, two-way ANOVA were carried out with MK-801 treatment (saline, MK-801) as one factor and tandospirone treatment (saline, low-T, high-T) as the second factor. Data from MK-801 administration was analyzed using repeated measure ANOVA. MK-801 treatment (saline, MK-801). Time was treated as repeated measures variable. Data from FS stress procedures were analyzed using two-way repeated measure ANOVA. MK-801 treatment (saline, MK-801) and tandospirone treatment (saline, low-T, high-T) were treated as between-group variable. Time was treated as repeated measures variable. Thereafter, two-way repeated measures ANOVA were performed for each group. Data were analyzed by Kruskal-Wallis test at each time point, and statistical significance was further examined by Mann-Whitney test for multiple comparisons.

To compare the results of with and without FS experiments, we analyzed total increase amount of lactate after last injection in each groups calculated by sum of eLAC data subtractiong the basal concentration of eLAC from eLAC concentration at each time point (from time 0 to time 110). These data were analyzed using one-factor ANOVA (8 groups; saline group without FS, MK-801 group without FS, saline-saline group, saline-low-T group, saline-high-T group, MK-801-saline group, MK-801-low-T group, MK-801-high-T group) followed by *post-hoc* Bonferroni test. A probability (P) of less than 0.05 was considered to be significant.

RESULTS

BASAL LACTATE LEVELS

The basal concentrations of lactate in 8 groups (with or without FS experiments) were shown in **Table 1**. There were no significant interaction [$F_{(2,35)} = 0.48$, $P = 0.62$], main effect of MK-801 treatment [$F_{(1,35)} = 0.48$, $P = 0.49$] and tandospirone treatment [$F_{(2,35)} = 0.19$, $P = 0.83$].

EFFECT OF MK-801 ADMINISTRATION ON eLAC

Repeated measures ANOVA demonstrated that MK-801 treatment increased eLAC in the mPFC [MK-801 x time interaction, $F_{(22,198)} = 5.73$, $P < 0.001$]. MK-801 administration increased eLAC from 35 to 45 min (**Figure 2**).

EFFECT OF MK-801 AND TANDOSPIRONE COMBINATION ON FS-INDUCED eLAC ELEVATION

Two-way ANOVA revealed that both MK-801 treatment x time interaction and tandospirone treatment x time interaction were significant [$F_{(22,528)} = 10.31$, $P < 0.001$; $F_{(44,528)} = 5.65$, $P < 0.001$; respectively]. These results indicated that

Table 1 | The basal concentrations of lactate in dailysates in each grop.

	Foot-shock stress(−)	Foot-shock stress (+)		
		Saline	Tandospirone	
			Low (0.05 mg/kg)	High (5.0 mg/kg)
Saline	50.92 ± 4.99	47.26 ± 4.99	51.46 ± 2.44	50.44 ± 2.63
MK-801	50.47 ± 1.20	47.62 ± 5.12	48.23 ± 2.5	43.96 ± 7.26

The basal concentrations of lactate in daily sates were presented the average of the eLAC during the period preceding the last injection (four measurements performed every 5 min). Values are expressed as mean ± SE, μmol/L.

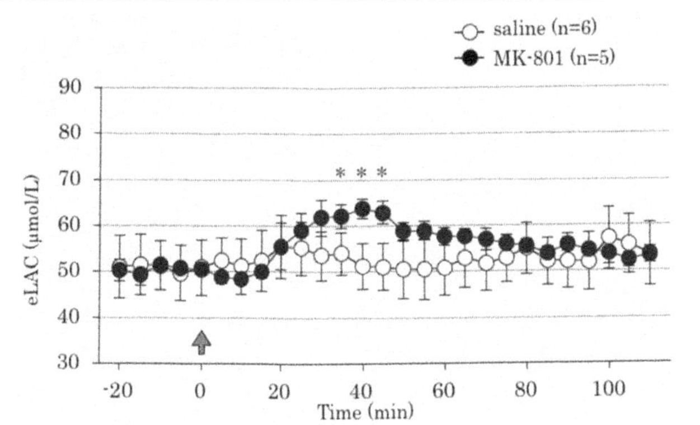

FIGURE 2 | Time course of the effect of 4 days treatment of MK-801 on the extracellular lactate concentrations (eLAC) in the medial prefrontal cortex. Rats were treated with saline (saline group, $n = 6$; open circle) or MK-801 (MK-801 group, $n = 5$; closed circle). Lactate levels in the dialysates are expressed as μmol/l calculated by a standard solution of 100 μmol/l lactate. Data are mean ± s.e.m. The arrow indicates the timing of the last injection. Asterisk showed $p < 0.05$ vs. saline group in each time point.

MK-801 treatment produced prolonged FS-induced eLAC elevation (**Figure 3A**), and that co-administration with tandospirone (5.0 mg/kg) abolished this change (**Figure 3C**) but not tandospirone (0.05 mg/kg) (**Figure 3B**). At each time point data analysis, there were significant eLAC differences between MK-801 and saline group at 70, 75, and 85 min after the last injection in low-dose tandospirone administration group (**Figure 3B**), whereas no significant differences at each time point in saline or high-dose tandospirone administration group (**Figures 3A,C**).

EFFECT OF TANDOSPIRONE ON FS-INDUCED eLAC ELEVATION IN SALINE TREATMENT GROUP

Two-way ANOVA revealed no significant tandospirone treatment x time interaction [$F_{(44,264)} = 1.90$, $P = 0.08$]. This result demonstrated that 4 days treatment with tandospirone did not affected on FS-induced eLAC elevation in the mPFC (**Figures 3A,C**).

TOTAL INCREASE AMOUNT OF LACTATE AFTER LAST INJECTION

One-factor ANOVA demonstrated significant differences among 8 groups [$F_{(7,33)} = 6.01$, $P < 0.001$]. *Post-hoc* Bonferroni test showed significant differences between saline group without FS and MK-801-saline group, saline group without FS and MK-801-low-T group, MK-801 group without FS and MK-801-low-T group, saline-high-T group and MK-801-low-T group (**Figure 4**). These results indicated that repeated MK-801 administration by itself have a temporary effect on eLAC changes in the mPFC.

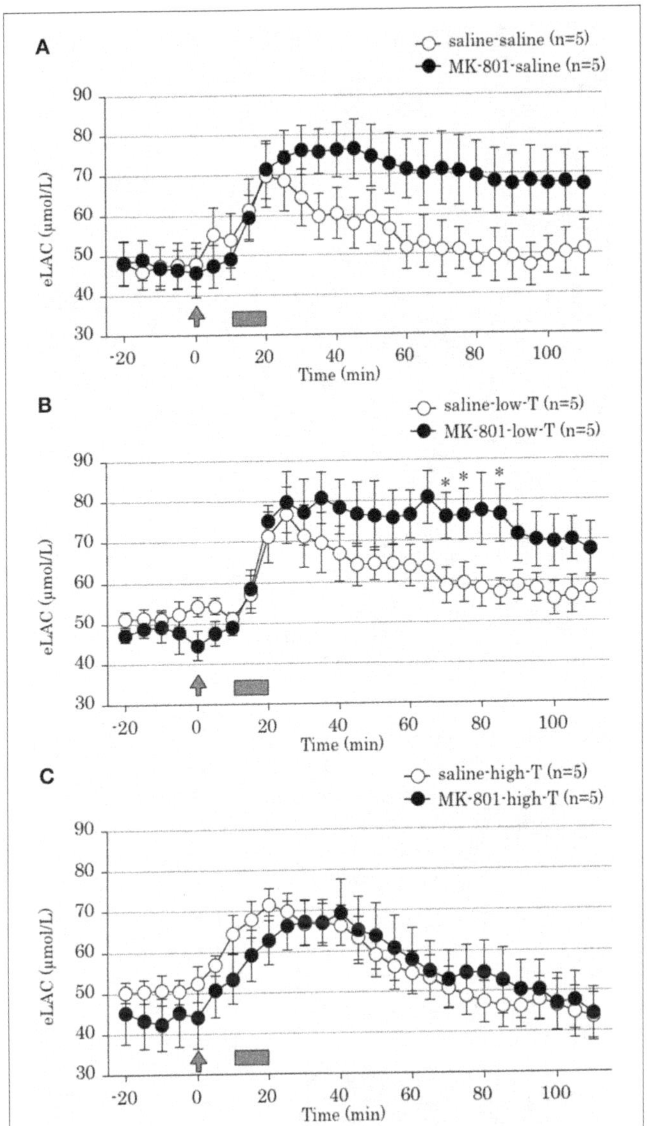

FIGURE 3 | Effect of tandospirone on foot-shock stress-induced increment of the extracellular lactate concentrations (eLAC) in the medial prefrontal cortex in rats treated with (A) saline (saline-saline group, $n = 5$; MK-801-saline group, $n = 5$), (B) tandospirone 0.05 mg/kg (saline-low-T group, $n = 5$; MK-801-low-T group, n-5) and (C) 5.0 mg/kg tandospirone (saline-high-T group, $n = 5$; MK-801-high-T group, $n = 5$). Rats were simultaneously treated with saline (open circle) or MK-801 (closed circle), respectively. Lactate levels in the dialysates are expressed as μmol/l calculated by a standard solution of 100 μmol/l lactate. Data are mean ± s.e.m. The arrow indicates the timing of the last injection. Foot-shock is indicated by solid bars. Asterisk showed $p < 0.05$ vs. saline group in each time point.

DISCUSSION

This study obtained results showing; (1) acute treatment with MK-801 in the 4th day increased eLAC to around 65 μmol/L above the base line level, and 4-day treatment with MK-801 prolonged eLAC elevation induced by FS in the mPFC, whereas its effect was temporary, and (2) co-administration with high-dose tandospirone abolished the effect of MK-801 treatment on prolonged eLAC elevation.

Four-day treatment with MK-801 at the young adult stage resulted in increasing of eLAC after FS (**Figure 3**), while repeated MK-801 treatment by itself may have little effect on total increase amount of lactate (**Figure 4**). This finding is consistent with a postmortem study reporting an increase in lactate levels in the PFC of patients with schizophrenia (Prabakaran et al., 2004). Possible mechanisms include glutamatergic neurotransmissions, because eLAC has been suggested to be linked to them (Uehara

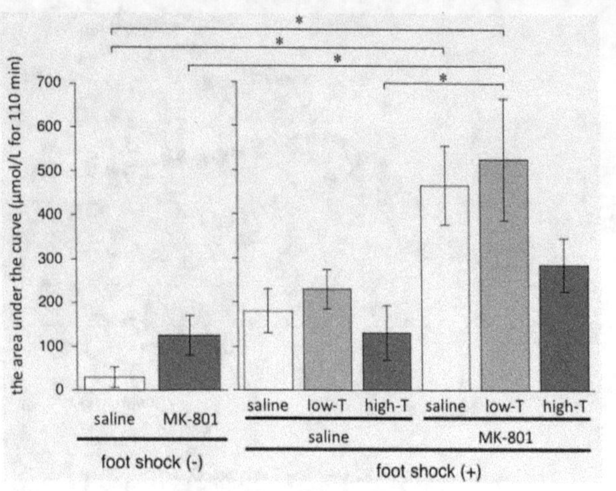

FIGURE 4 | Total increase of lactate after injection (from time 0 to time 110 min) calculated by sum of (each eLAC concentration—basal concentration of eLAC). Basal concentration of eLAC is the average of eLAC during the period preceding the last injection (four measurements performed every 5 min). Asterisk showed $p < 0.05$ between groups.

et al., 2008). Thus, glutamate taken up into astrocytes through glutamate transporters (GLT) after synaptic release stimulates glycolysis and lactate production in astrocytes. In this process, glutamate uptake into astrocytes and the resulting increase in intracellular Na^+ have been identified as a key signal coupling excitatory neural activity to increased glucose utilization (Magistretti et al., 1999; Chatton et al., 2000). Moreover, glutamate stimulates aerobic glycolysis in astrocytes (Pellerin and Magistretti, 1994). This metabolic action of glutamate is mediated by glutamate transporters, and involves the activity of Na^+/K^+ ATPase in astrocytes (Pellerin and Magistretti, 1997). In fact, local perfusion of the glutamate reuptake inhibitor dihydrokainate (DHK) has been reported to attenuated FS-induced increment eLAC in the mPFC (Uehara et al., 2007b). On the other hand, activation of NMDA-Rs increases eLAC in the mPFC of rodents (Kuhr and Korf, 1988; Schasfoort et al., 1988). These authors reported that infusion of NMDA (10 mM) or kainic acid (0.5 mM) for 1 min resulted in an transient increase in extracellular lactate concentrations, which lasted several minutes longer than the drug administration period. Furthermore, MK-801, as well as other NMDA-R antagonists, may produce disinhibition of glutamate and γ-aminobutyric acid (GABA) or other inhibitory inputs to the glutamate-containing neurons, thereby enhancing the firing rate of these glutamatergic neurons. Such disinhibition may occur locally at the PFC and/or at regions with ascending glutamatergic projections to the PFC (Moghaddam et al., 1997). These findings suggest that systemic MK-801 administration increases glutamate levels in the synaptic cleft, and prolong eLAC elevation in the mPFC.

We previously reported that the long-term effect of transient MK-801 treatment in neonatal periods on lactate metabolism in the mPFC of young adult rats (Uehara et al., 2012a). According to the study, transient MK-801 treatment in neonatal stage suppressed FS stress-induced eLAC elevation in the mPFC without changes in the basal levels. Moreover, Neonatal NMDA-R blockade-induced attenuation of lactate response was ameliorated by 5-HT_{1A} receptor stimulations for 14 days in young adult stage. These findings were completely *opposite* effect to young adult rats treated repeatedly with MK-801 in this study. It is possible that the opposite effect on eLAC reactions to FS was based on the timing of MK-801 administration. Administration of NMDA-R antagonists in the late fetal or early postnatal periods enhances neuronal apoptosis (Ikonomidou et al., 1999; Beninger et al., 2002; Harris et al., 2003). PCP administration in the neonatal stage has been shown to induce apoptotic changes, gliosis (Wang et al., 2001, 2003) and to reduce spine density (Nakatani-Pawlak et al., 2009) in the frontal cortex. These findings suggest that neonatal blockade of NMDA-R produced morphological changes and then reduction of the production source and/or dysfunction of the astrocyte-neuron lactate shuttle system. Furthermore, neonatal blockade of the NMDA-R led to up-regulation of the NR1 receptor subunit in the frontal cortex (Wang et al., 1999, 2001; Du Bois and Huang, 2007). We reported neonatal MK-801 administration reduced the number of parvalbumin-positive GABA interneurons in the mPFC (Uehara et al., 2012b,c). Based on these findings, it is possible that neonatal MK-801 treatment decreased glutamate release in the mPFC, leading to the reduction of eLAC. On the other hand, low doses of MK-801 (<3 mg/kg) induced transient vacuolization in cortical layers III and IV of adult rodents, which was maximal 12 h after the drug and then gradually disappeared during the next 12–18 h (Olney et al., 1989). Therefore, it is assumed that the dose of MK-801 (0.1 mg/kg) in this study may have produced little morphological changes.

Co-administration of tandospirone, a 5-HT_{1A} receptor partial agonist, attenuated prolonged eLAC elevation in the mPFC induced by MK-801 (**Figure 3C**). Acute treatment with tandospirone has been shown to attenuate the eLAC elevation by FS (Uehara et al., 2006). 5-HT_{1A} agonists have been shown to inhibit potassium-evoked glutamate release *in vitro* (Mauler et al., 2001) while MK-801 increases glutamate in the mPFC *in vivo* (Lopez-Gil et al., 2009). 5-HT_{1A} receptors are also involved in the modulation of excitatory glutamatergic neurotransmission, since their activation reduces NMDA-mediated currents in PFC neurons (Zhong et al., 2008). Moreover, 5-HT_{1A} agonists block the MK-801-induced increase in 5-HT concentrations in the mPFC (Lopez-Gil et al., 2009). Therefore, it is possible that tandospirone shortens the period of eLAC elevation through inhibition of glutamate release and serotonergic transmissions.

Unexpectedly, 4-day treatment with tandospirone (5.0 mg/kg/day, i.p.) did not suppress FS-induced eLAC elevation in the mPFC of saline-treated rats, in contrast to our previous observation with tandospirone at 2.0 mg/kg (Uehara et al., 2006). Moreover, the drug at 0.1, 1.0, or 5.0 mg/kg attenuated FS-induced eLAC increment (Uehara et al., 2012a), although last injection was 24 h before eLAC measurement.

Chronic administration of 5-HT_{1A} agonists has been shown to desensitize 5-HT_{1A} auto receptors in the raphe nucleus, but not frontal cortex (Sim-Selley et al., 2000; Hensler et al., 2003). After sustained treatment with these agents, 5-HT neurons in the raphe nucleus gradually recover their baseline firing rates and become normalized in 14 days (Blier and De Montigny, 1987;

Godbout et al., 1991; Blier and Ward, 2003). Treatment with tandospirone for 2 days (10 mg/kg/day, s.c.), markedly reduces the firing activity of 5-HT neurons of the dorsal raphe, followed by partial recovery after 7 days and complete recovery after 14 days of tandospirone administration (Godbout et al., 1991). Therefore, 4-day treatment with tandospirone may decrease 5-HT release into the synaptic cleft in the mPFC. On the other hand, postsynaptic 5-HT_{1A} receptor stimulation inhibits NMDA antagonist-induced glutamate release in the mPFC (Calcagno et al., 2006) and potassium-evoked lactate release *in vitro* (Mauler et al., 2001). Taken together, the discrepant results in our reports, above, may be explained by the balance between autoreceptor desensitization in the raphe nucleus and intensity of stimulation of post-synaptic receptors in the mPFC.

In summary, stimulation of 5-HT_{1A} receptors normalized changes of lactate metabolism in the mPFC of rats exposed to repeated NMDA-R injections. Our findings provide a possible mechanism underlying the clinical observations that tandospirone improves cognitive deficits in patients with schizophrenia (Sumiyoshi et al., 2000, 2001a,b). Importantly, lactate metabolism may provide a novel probe for the development of therapeutics for cognitive impairment of schizophrenia (Uehara and Sumiyoshi, 2013).

AUTHOR CONTRIBUTIONS

Takashi Uehara and Tomiki Sumiyoshi designed the study and wrote the protocol. Takashi Uehara and Tomiki Sumiyoshi oversaw data collection. Takashi Uehara and Tadasu Matsuoka made animal models. Takashi Uehara undertook analysis of microdialysis data. Tomiki Sumiyoshi provided consultation regarding all aspects of the study. Takashi Uehara wrote the first draft of the manuscript. All authors contributed to and have approved the final manuscript.

ACKNOWLEDGMENTS

This study was funded by Takeda Science Foundation, Excellent Young Researchers Overseas Visit Program, and grant from Smoking Research Foundation to Takashi Uehara, as well as Japan Society for the Promotion of Science (No. 26461761), Health and Labour Sciences Research Grants for Comprehensive Research on Disability, Health, and Welfare (H24-Seishin-Ippan-002 and H26-Seishin-Ippan-011), and SENSHIN Medical Research Foundation to Tomiki Sumiyoshi. The authors thank Drs. Masayoshi Kurachi and Koichi Kurata for fruitful discussions. Dedicated support by Ms. Hiroko Itoh is greatly appreciated.

REFERENCES

Beninger, R. J., Jhamandas, A., Aujla, H., Xue, L., Dagnone, R. V., Boegman, R. J., et al. (2002). Neonatal exposure to the glutamate receptor antagonist MK-801: effects on locomotor activity and pre-pulse inhibition before and after sexual maturity in rats. *Neurotox. Res.* 4, 477–488. doi: 10.1080/10298420290031414

Blier, P., and De Montigny, C. (1987). Modification of 5-HT neuron properties by sustained administration of the 5-HT1A agonist gepirone: electrophysiological studies in the rat brain. *Synapse* 1, 470–480. doi: 10.1002/syn.890010511

Blier, P., and Ward, N. M. (2003). Is there a role for 5-HT1A agonists in the treatment of depression? *Biol. Psychiatry* 53, 193–203. doi: 10.1016/S0006-3223(02)01643-8

Breese, G. R., Knapp, D. J., and Moy, S. S. (2002). Integrative role for serotonergic and glutamatergic receptor mechanisms in the action of NMDA antagonists: potential relationships to antipsychotic drug actions on NMDA antagonist responsiveness. *Neurosci. Biobehav. Rev.* 26, 441–455. doi: 10.1016/S0149-7634(02)00011-8

Bubenikova-Valesova, V., Horacek, J., Vrajova, M., and Hoschl, C. (2008). Models of schizophrenia in humans and animals based on inhibition of NMDA receptors. *Neurosci. Biobehav. Rev.* 32, 1014–1023. doi: 10.1016/j.neubiorev.2008.03.012

Bubenikova-Valesova, V., Svoboda, J., Horacek, J., and Sumiyoshi, T. (2010). Effect of tandospirone, a serotonin-1A receptor partial agonist, on information processing and locomotion in dizocilpine-treated rats. *Psychopharmacology (Berl).* 212, 267–276. doi: 10.1007/s00213-010-1951-3

Calcagno, E., Carli, M., and Invernizzi, R. W. (2006). The 5-HT(1A) receptor agonist 8-OH-DPAT prevents prefrontocortical glutamate and serotonin release in response to blockade of cortical NMDA receptors. *J. Neurochem.* 96, 853–860. doi: 10.1111/j.1471-4159.2005.03600.x

Chatton, J. Y., Marquet, P., and Magistretti, P. J. (2000). A quantitative analysis of L-glutamate-regulated Na+ dynamics in mouse cortical astrocytes: implications for cellular bioenergetics. *Eur. J. Neurosci.* 12, 3843–3853. doi: 10.1046/j.1460-9568.2000.00269.x

Du Bois, T. M., and Huang, X. F. (2007). Early brain development disruption from NMDA receptor hypofunction: relevance to schizophrenia. *Brain Res. Rev.* 53, 260–270. doi: 10.1016/j.brainresrev.2006.09.001

Geyer, M. A. (2006). Are cross-species measures of sensorimotor gating useful for the discovery of procognitive cotreatments for schizophrenia? *Dialogues Clin. Neurosci.* 8, 9–16.

Godbout, R., Chaput, Y., Blier, P., and De Montigny, C. (1991). Tandospirone and its metabolite, 1-(2-pyrimidinyl)-piperazine–I. Effects of acute and long-term administration of tandospirone on serotonin neurotransmission. *Neuropharmacology* 30, 679–690. doi: 10.1016/0028-3908(91)90175-B

Halim, N. D., Lipska, B. K., Hyde, T. M., Deep-Soboslay, A., Saylor, E. M., Herman, M. M., et al. (2008). Increased lactate levels and reduced pH in postmortem brains of schizophrenics: medication confounds. *J. Neurosci. Methods* 169, 208–213. doi: 10.1016/j.jneumeth.2007.11.017

Harris, L. W., Sharp, T., Gartlon, J., Jones, D. N., and Harrison, P. J. (2003). Long-term behavioural, molecular and morphological effects of neonatal NMDA receptor antagonism. *Eur. J. Neurosci.* 18, 1706–1710. doi: 10.1046/j.1460-9568.2003.02902.x

Hazlett, E. A., Buchsbaum, M. S., Jeu, L. A., Nenadic, I., Fleischman, M. B., Shihabuddin, L., et al. (2000). Hypofrontality in unmedicated schizophrenia patients studied with PET during performance of a serial verbal learning task. *Schizophr. Res.* 43, 33–46. doi: 10.1016/S0920-9964(99)00178-4

Hensler, J. G., Ladenheim, E. E., and Lyons, W. E. (2003). Ethanol consumption and serotonin-1A (5-HT1A) receptor function in heterozygous BDNF (+/−) mice. *J. Neurochem.* 85, 1139–1147. doi: 10.1046/j.1471-4159.2003.01748.x

Ikonomidou, C., Bosch, F., Miksa, M., Bittigau, P., Vockler, J., Dikranian, K., et al. (1999). Blockade of NMDA receptors and apoptotic neurodegeneration in the developing brain. *Science* 283, 70–74. doi: 10.1126/science.283.5398.70

Jentsch, J. D., and Roth, R. H. (1999). The neuropsychopharmacology of phencyclidine: from NMDA receptor hypofunction to the dopamine hypothesis of schizophrenia. *Neuropsychopharmacology* 20, 201–225. doi: 10.1016/S0893-133X(98)00060-8

Jones, C. A., Watson, D. J., and Fone, K. C. (2011). Animal models of schizophrenia. *Br. J. Pharmacol.* 164, 1162–1194. doi: 10.1111/j.1476-5381.2011.01386.x

Kuhr, W. G., and Korf, J. (1988). N-methyl-D-aspartate receptor involvement in lactate production following ischemia or convulsion in rats. *Eur. J. Pharmacol.* 155, 145–149. doi: 10.1016/0014-2999(88)90412-8

Lopez-Gil, X., Artigas, F., and Adell, A. (2009). Role of different monoamine receptors controlling MK-801-induced release of serotonin and glutamate in the medial prefrontal cortex: relevance for antipsychotic action. *Int. J. Neuropsychopharmacol.* 12, 487–499. doi: 10.1017/S1461145708009267

Magistretti, P. J., Pellerin, L., Rothman, D. L., and Shulman, R. G. (1999). Energy on demand. *Science* 283, 496–497. doi: 10.1126/science.283.5401.496

Mauler, F., Fahrig, T., Horvath, E., and Jork, R. (2001). Inhibition of evoked glutamate release by the neuroprotective 5-HT(1A) receptor agonist BAY x 3702 *in vitro* and *in vivo*. *Brain Res.* 888, 150–157. doi: 10.1016/S0006-8993(00)03074-2

McGurk, S. R., and Meltzer, H. Y. (2000). The role of cognition in vocational functioning in schizophrenia. *Schizophr. Res.* 45, 175–184. doi: 10.1016/S0920-9964(99)00198-X

Meltzer, H. Y., and McGurk, S. R. (1999). The effects of clozapine, risperidone, and olanzapine on cognitive function in schizophrenia. *Schizophr. Bull.* 25, 233–255. doi: 10.1093/oxfordjournals.schbul.a033376

Moghaddam, B., Adams, B., Verma, A., and Daly, D. (1997). Activation of glutamatergic neurotransmission by ketamine: a novel step in the pathway from NMDA receptor blockade to dopaminergic and cognitive disruptions associated with the prefrontal cortex. *J. Neurosci.* 17, 2921–2927.

Moghaddam, B., and Jackson, M. E. (2003). Glutamatergic animal models of schizophrenia. *Ann. N.Y. Acad. Sci.* 1003, 131–137. doi: 10.1196/annals.1300.065

Nakatani-Pawlak, A., Yamaguchi, K., Tatsumi, Y., Mizoguchi, H., and Yoneda, Y. (2009). Neonatal phencyclidine treatment in mice induces behavioral, histological and neurochemical abnormalities in adulthood. *Biol. Pharm. Bull.* 32, 1576–1583. doi: 10.1248/bpb.32.1576

Newman-Tancredi, A., and Albert, P. R. (2012). "Gene polymorphism at serotonin 5-HT1A receptors: moving towards personalized medicine for psychosis and mood deficits?," in *Schizophrenia Research: Recent Advances,* ed T. Sumiyoshi (New York, NY: Nova Science Publisher), 337–358.

Ohno, Y., Tatara, A., Shimizu, S., and Sasa, M. (2012). "Management of cognitive impairments in schizophrenia: the therapeutic role of 5-HT receptors," in *Schizophrenia Research: Recent Advances,* ed. T. Sumiyoshi (New York, NY: Nova Science Publishers), 321–335.

Olney, J. W., Labruyere, J., and Price, M. T. (1989). Pathological changes induced in cerebrocortical neurons by phencyclidine and related drugs. *Science* 244, 1360–1362. doi: 10.1126/science.2660263

Paxinos, G., and Watson, C. (1998). *The Rat Brain in Stereotaxic Coordinates.* Sydney: Academic Press.

Pellerin, L. (2003). Lactate as a pivotal element in neuron-glia metabolic cooperation. *Neurochem. Int.* 43, 331–338. doi: 10.1016/S0197-0186(03)00020-2

Pellerin, L., Bouzier-Sore, A. K., Aubert, A., Serres, S., Merle, M., Costalat, R., et al. (2007). Activity-dependent regulation of energy metabolism by astrocytes: an update. *Glia* 55, 1251–1262. doi: 10.1002/glia.20528

Pellerin, L., and Magistretti, P. J. (1994). Glutamate uptake into astrocytes stimulates aerobic glycolysis: a mechanism coupling neuronal activity to glucose utilization. *Proc. Natl. Acad. Sci. U.S.A.* 91, 10625–10629. doi: 10.1073/pnas.91.22.10625

Pellerin, L., and Magistretti, P. J. (1997). Glutamate uptake stimulates Na+,K+−ATPase activity in astrocytes via activation of a distinct subunit highly sensitive to ouabain. *J. Neurochem.* 69, 2132–2137. doi: 10.1046/j.1471-4159.1997.69052132.x

Pellerin, L., and Magistretti, P. J. (2012). Sweet sixteen for ANLS. *J. Cereb. Blood Flow Metab.* 32, 1152–1166. doi: 10.1038/jcbfm.2011.149

Pellerin, L., Pellegri, G., Bittar, P. G., Charnay, Y., Bouras, C., Martin, J. L., et al. (1998). Evidence supporting the existence of an activity-dependent astrocyte-neuron lactate shuttle. *Dev. Neurosci.* 20, 291–299. doi: 10.1159/000017324

Prabakaran, S., Swatton, J. E., Ryan, M. M., Huffaker, S. J., Huang, J. T., Griffin, J. L., et al. (2004). Mitochondrial dysfunction in schizophrenia: evidence for compromised brain metabolism and oxidative stress. *Mol. Psychiatry* 9, 684–697, 643. doi: 10.1038/sj.mp.4001532

Ragland, J. D., Yoon, J., Minzenberg, M. J., and Carter, C. S. (2007). Neuroimaging of cognitive disability in schizophrenia: search for a pathophysiological mechanism. *Int. Rev. Psychiatry* 19, 417–427. doi: 10.1080/09540260701486365

Schasfoort, E. M., De Bruin, L. A., and Korf, J. (1988). Mild stress stimulates rat hippocampal glucose utilization transiently via NMDA receptors, as assessed by lactography. *Brain Res.* 475, 58–63. doi: 10.1016/0006-8993(88)90198-9

Sim-Selley, L. J., Vogt, L. J., Xiao, R., Childers, S. R., and Selley, D. E. (2000). Region-specific changes in 5-HT(1A) receptor-activated G-proteins in rat brain following chronic buspirone. *Eur. J. Pharmacol.* 389, 147–153. doi: 10.1016/S0014-2999(99)00875-4

Singer, P., Hauser, J., Llano Lopez, L., Peleg-Raibstein, D., Feldon, J., Gargiulo, P. A., et al. (2013). Prepulse inhibition predicts working memory performance whilst startle habituation predicts spatial reference memory retention in C57BL/6 mice. *Behav. Brain Res.* 242, 166–177. doi: 10.1016/j.bbr.2012.12.011

Smith, D., Pernet, A., Hallett, W. A., Bingham, E., Marsden, P. K., and Amiel, S. A. (2003). Lactate: a preferred fuel for human brain metabolism *in vivo*. *J. Cereb. Blood Flow Metab.* 23, 658–664. doi: 10.1097/01.WCB.0000063991.19746.11

Sumiyoshi, T. (2013). Antipsychotic treatments: focus on lurasidone. *Front. Pharmacol.* 4:102. doi: 10.3389/fphar.2013.00102

Sumiyoshi, T., and Higuchi, Y. (2013). Facilitative effect of serotonin(1A) receptor agonists on cognition in patients with schizophrenia. *Curr. Med. Chem.* 20, 357–362. doi: 10.2174/0929867311320030006

Sumiyoshi, T., Higuchi, Y., and Uehara, T. (2013). Neural basis for the ability of atypical antipsychotic drugs to improve cognition in schizophrenia. *Front. Behav. Neurosci.* 7:140. doi: 10.3389/fnbeh.2013.00140

Sumiyoshi, T., Matsui, M., Nohara, S., Yamashita, I., Kurachi, M., Sumiyoshi, C., et al. (2001a). Enhancement of cognitive performance in schizophrenia by addition of tandospirone to neuroleptic treatment. *Am. J. Psychiatry* 158, 1722–1725. doi: 10.1176/appi.ajp.158.10.1722

Sumiyoshi, T., Matsui, M., Yamashita, I., Nohara, S., Kurachi, M., Uehara, T., et al. (2001b). The effect of tandospirone, a serotonin(1A) agonist, on memory function in schizophrenia. *Biol. Psychiatry* 49, 861–868. doi: 10.1016/S0006-3223(00)01025-8

Sumiyoshi, T., Matsui, M., Yamashita, I., Nohara, S., Uehara, T., Kurachi, M., et al. (2000). Effect of adjunctive treatment with serotonin-1A agonist tandospirone on memory functions in schizophrenia. *J. Clin. Psychopharmacol.* 20, 386–388. doi: 10.1097/00004714-200006000-00019

Sumiyoshi, T., Park, S., Jayathilake, K., Roy, A., Ertugrul, A., and Meltzer, H. Y. (2007). Effect of buspirone, a serotonin1A partial agonist, on cognitive function in schizophrenia: a randomized, double-blind, placebo-controlled study. *Schizophr. Res.* 95, 158–168. doi: 10.1016/j.schres.2007.06.008

Tamminga, C. A., Thaker, G. K., Buchanan, R., Kirkpatrick, B., Alphs, L. D., Chase, T. N., et al. (1992). Limbic system abnormalities identified in schizophrenia using positron emission tomography with fluorodeoxyglucose and neocortical alterations with deficit syndrome. *Arch. Gen. Psychiatry* 49, 522–530. doi: 10.1001/archpsyc.1992.01820070016003

Tsacopoulos, M., and Magistretti, P. J. (1996). Metabolic coupling between glia and neurons. *J. Neurosci.* 16, 877–885.

Uehara, T., Itoh, H., Matsuoka, T., Rujescu, D., Genius, J., Seo, T., et al. (2012a). Effect of transient blockade of N-methyl-D-aspartate receptors at neonatal stage on stress-induced lactate metabolism in the medial prefrontal cortex of adult rats: role of 5-HT1A receptor agonism. *Synapse* 66, 408–417. doi: 10.1002/syn.21529

Uehara, T., Kurata, K., Sumiyoshi, T., and Kurachi, M. (2003). Immobilization stress-induced increment of lactate metabolism in the basolateral amygdaloid nucleus is attenuated by diazepam in the rat. *Eur. J. Pharmacol.* 459, 211–215. doi: 10.1016/S0014-2999(02)02871-6

Uehara, T., and Sumiyoshi, T. (2013). "Lactate metabolism as a new target for the therapeutics of schizophrenia," in *Frontiers in Clinical Drug Research-CNS and Neurological Disorders,* ed A. U. Rahman (Sharjah: Bentham Science Publishers), 135–148.

Uehara, T., Sumiyoshi, T., Hattori, H., Itoh, H., Matsuoka, T., Iwakami, N., et al. (2012b). T-817MA, a novel neurotrophic agent, ameliorates loss of GABAergic parvalbumin-positive neurons and sensorimotor gating deficits in rats transiently exposed to MK-801 in the neonatal period. *J. Psychiatr. Res.* 46, 622–629. doi: 10.1016/j.jpsychires.2012.01.022

Uehara, T., Sumiyoshi, T., Itoh, H., and Kurachi, M. (2007a). Dopamine D1 and D2 receptors regulate extracellular lactate and glucose concentrations in the nucleus accumbens. *Brain Res.* 1133, 193–199. doi: 10.1016/j.brainres.2006.11.040

Uehara, T., Sumiyoshi, T., Itoh, H., and Kurachi, M. (2007b). Role of glutamate transporter in the modulation of stress-induced lactate metabolism in the rat brain. *Psychopharmacology (Berl).* 195, 297–302. doi: 10.1007/s00213-007-0881-1

Uehara, T., Sumiyoshi, T., Itoh, H., and Kurata, K. (2008). Lactate production and neurotransmitters; evidence from microdialysis studies. *Pharmacol. Biochem. Behav.* 90, 273–281. doi: 10.1016/j.pbb.2008.04.001

Uehara, T., Sumiyoshi, T., Matsuoka, T., Itoh, H., and Kurachi, M. (2006). Role of 5-HT(1A) receptors in the modulation of stress-induced lactate metabolism in the medial prefrontal cortex and basolateral amygdala. *Psychopharmacology (Berl).* 186, 218–225. doi: 10.1007/s00213-006-0370-y

Uehara, T., Sumiyoshi, T., Matsuoka, T., Tanaka, K., Tsunoda, M., Itoh, H., et al. (2005). Enhancement of lactate metabolism in the basolateral amygdala by physical and psychological stress: role of benzodiazepine receptors. *Brain Res.* 1065, 86–91. doi: 10.1016/j.brainres.2005.10.035

Uehara, T., Sumiyoshi, T., Seo, T., Matsuoka, T., Itoh, H., and Kurachi, M. (2012c). T-817MA, but not haloperidol and risperidone, restores parvalbumin-positive gamma -aminobutyric acid neurons in the prefrontal cortex and hippocampus of rats transiently exposed to MK-801 at the neonatal period. *ISRN Psychiatry* 2012:947149. doi: 10.5402/2012/947149

Volk, D. W., and Lewis, D. A. (2002). Impaired prefrontal inhibition in schizophrenia: relevance for cognitive dysfunction. *Physiol. Behav.* 77, 501–505. doi: 10.1016/S0031-9384(02)00936-8

Volz, H., Gaser, C., Hager, F., Rzanny, R., Ponisch, J., Mentzel, H., et al. (1999). Decreased frontal activation in schizophrenics during stimulation with the continuous performance test–a functional magnetic resonance imaging study. *Eur. Psychiatry* 14, 17–24. doi: 10.1016/S0924-9338(99)80711-1

Wang, C., McInnis, J., Ross-Sanchez, M., Shinnick-Gallagher, P., Wiley, J. L., and Johnson, K. M. (2001). Long-term behavioral and neurodegenerative effects of perinatal phencyclidine administration: implications for schizophrenia. *Neuroscience* 107, 535–550. doi: 10.1016/S0306-4522(01)00384-0

Wang, C., McInnis, J., West, J. B., Bao, J., Anastasio, N., Guidry, J. A., et al. (2003). Blockade of phencyclidine-induced cortical apoptosis and deficits in prepulse inhibition by M40403, a superoxide dismutase mimetic. *J. Pharmacol. Exp. Ther.* 304, 266–271. doi: 10.1124/jpet.102.041798

Wang, C., Showalter, V. M., Hillman, G. R., and Johnson, K. M. (1999). Chronic phencyclidine increases NMDA receptor NR1 subunit mRNA in rat forebrain. *J. Neurosci. Res.* 55, 762–769. doi: 10.1002/(SICI)1097-4547(19990315)55:6<762::AID-JNR10>3.0.CO;2-E

Wyss, M. T., Jolivet, R., Buck, A., Magistretti, P. J., and Weber, B. (2011). *In vivo* evidence for lactate as a neuronal energy source. *J. Neurosci.* 31, 7477–7485. doi: 10.1523/JNEUROSCI.0415-11.2011

Zhong, P., Yuen, E. Y., and Yan, Z. (2008). Modulation of neuronal excitability by serotonin-NMDA interactions in prefrontal cortex. *Mol. Cell. Neurosci.* 38, 290–299. doi: 10.1016/j.mcn.2008.03.003

6

Mismatch negativity and P3a/reorienting complex in subjects with schizophrenia or at-risk mental state

Yuko Higuchi[1], Tomonori Seo[1], Tomohiro Miyanishi[1], Yasuhiro Kawasaki[2], Michio Suzuki[1] and Tomiki Sumiyoshi[3]*

[1] Department of Neuropsychiatry, University of Toyama Graduate School of Medicine and Pharmaceutical Science, Toyama, Japan
[2] Department of Neuropsychiatry, Kanazawa Medical University, Ishikawa, Japan
[3] Department of Clinical Research Promotion, National Center Hospital, National Center of Neurology and Psychiatry, Tokyo, Japan

Edited by:
Ales Stuchlik, Academy of Sciences of the Czech Republic, Czech Republic

***Correspondence:**
Tomiki Sumiyoshi, Department of Clinical Research Promotion, National Center of Neurology and Psychiatry, 4-1-1 Ogawahigashi, Kodaira, Tokyo 187-8551, Japan
e-mail: sumiyot@ncnp.go.jp

Introduction: We measured duration mismatch negativity (dMMN), P3a, and reorienting negativity (RON) in subjects with at-risk mental state (ARMS), patients with first-episode or chronic schizophrenia, and healthy volunteers. The main interest was to determine if these event-related potentials provide a biomarker associated with progression to overt schizophrenia in ARMS subjects.

Methods: Nineteen ARMS subjects meeting the criteria of the Comprehensive Assessment of ARMS, 38 patients with schizophrenia (19 first-episode and 19 chronic), and 19 healthy controls participated in the study. dMMN, P3a, and RON were measured with an auditory odd-ball paradigm at baseline.

Results: During the follow-up period (2.2 years), 4 out of the 19 ARMS subjects transitioned to schizophrenia (Converters) while 15 did not (non-Converters). dMMN amplitudes of Converters were significantly smaller than those of non-Converters at frontal and central electrodes before onset of illness. dMMN amplitudes of non-Converters did not differ from those of healthy controls, while Converters showed significantly smaller dMMN amplitudes compared to control subjects. RON amplitudes were also reduced at frontal and central electrodes in subjects with schizophrenia, but not ARMS. Converter subjects tended to show smaller RON amplitudes compared to non-Converters.

Conclusions: Our data confirm that diminished dMMN amplitudes provide a biomarker, which is present before and after the development of psychosis. In this respect, RON amplitudes may also be useful, as suggested for the first time based on longitudinal observations.

Keywords: mismatch negativity, reorienting negativity, event-related potentials, prodromal, schizophrenia

INTRODUCTION

Schizophrenia is a disorder characterized by positive symptoms (hallucination, delusion, thought disturbance, etc.), negative symptoms (blunted affect, lack of volition, social withdrawal, etc.), and a range of disturbances of cognitive functions (Heinrichs and Zakzanis, 1998; Sumiyoshi et al., 2003; Harvey et al., 2004). In particular, cognitive impairment of schizophrenia is considered to largely determine the outcome of patients, including quality of life and social function (Green, 1996).

Prolonged duration of untreated psychosis (DUP) has been associated with poor long-term outcome, including work function, communication skills, and longer hospitalization (Loebel et al., 1992; Edwards et al., 1999; Malla et al., 2004; Melle et al., 2008; Yamazawa et al., 2008; Chang et al., 2011; Galderisi et al., 2012). On the other hand, shorter DUP has been related with a greater response to antipsychotic drugs in terms of symptoms and quality of life (Perkins et al., 2005). For these reasons, early detection, intervention, and treatment of schizophrenia are needed. In this context, it was reasonable that recent efforts have been directed to subjects with "at-risk mental state (ARMS)" or "ultra-high-risk patients" (McGorry et al., 2009).

The criteria for ARMS require that a young person aged between 14 and 30 years being referred for mental health difficulties met criteria for one or more of the following groups: (i) attenuated psychotic symptoms group (APS): have experienced sub-threshold, attenuated positive psychotic symptoms during the past year; (ii) brief limited intermittent psychotic symptoms group (BLIPS): have experienced episodes of frank psychotic symptoms that have not lasted longer than a week and have spontaneously abated; or (iii) trait and state risk factor group: have a first-degree relative with a psychotic disorder or the identified client has a schizotypal personality disorder, and they have experienced a significant decrease in functioning during the previous year (Yung et al., 1996; Broome et al., 2005).

To promote early diagnosis, objective markers, particularly those based on brain morphology, neurophysiology, and neuropsychology, have been reported to provide useful information (Nakamura et al., 2004; Kawasaki et al., 2007b; Higuchi et al., 2008, 2013b; Takahashi et al., 2011; Takayanagi et al., 2011; Lin et al., 2012). Accordingly, event-related potentials (ERPs) have been suggested to provide a biomarker for cognitive impairment of schizophrenia.

P300 (P3a and P3b) and mismatch negativity (MMN) have been widely used for this purpose. Specifically, patients with schizophrenia have been reported to show smaller P300 amplitudes compared with normal control subjects (Roth et al., 1980; Kawasaki et al., 1997; Bruder et al., 1998). Also, P300 amplitudes have been shown to be reduced in subjects with ARMS (Ozgurdal et al., 2008). On the other hand, P300 is affected by various factors, including medication (Umbricht et al., 1998; Higuchi et al., 2008, 2013a; Sumiyoshi et al., 2009), suggesting the utility as a state marker of psychotic disorders.

Mismatch negativity is another component of ERPs generated in response to occasional variations (e.g., duration, frequency, intensity) of acoustic stimuli, which occurs about 100–200 ms after the onset of deviant stimulation, with peak amplitudes at fronto-central leads (Naatanen et al., 2007, 2012). MMN amplitudes have been suggested to reflect pre-attentive cognitive operations, and decreased in patients with schizophrenia, as indicated by a recent meta-analysis reporting a large effect size (Umbricht and Krljes, 2005). Unlike the case with P300, MMN amplitudes are generally not affected by psychotropic drugs, for example, benzodiazepines (Kasai et al., 2002) and dopamine antagonists (Leung et al., 2007). For these reasons, MMN is considered to provide a trait marker for schizophrenia.

Duration mismatch negativity (dMMN) amplitudes have been shown to be reduced already in the prodromal stage of the illness (Bodatsch et al., 2011; Jahshan et al., 2012; Shaikh et al., 2012; Higuchi et al., 2013b). Furthermore, smaller dMMN amplitudes have been reported in subjects with ARMS who later converted to overt psychosis, compared to those who did not (Shaikh et al., 2012; Higuchi et al., 2013b). Thus, reduced dMMN amplitudes are regarded to predict conversion to schizophrenia in at-risk subjects (Sumiyoshi et al., 2013).

P3a is a positive waveform that appears following MMN, i.e., between 250 and 300 ms after the presentation of stimuli. Its amplitudes are largest at fronto-central electrodes. The P3a component is assumed to reflect a pre-attentive index of deviance detection, and represent the involuntary capture of attention (Friedman et al., 2001).

A negative activity reflecting attentional "re"-orienting follows P3a. This component is referred to as reorienting negativity (RON) (Schroger and Wolff, 1998), which peaks at latencies between 400 and 600 ms, and is centered on fronto-central electrodes (Schroger and Wolff, 1998; Otten et al., 2000; Schroger et al., 2000). The MMN/P3a/RON complex has been shown to provide a neurophysiological index of the cascade of three main processes involved in involuntary attention controls (i.e., automatic change detection, orienting of attention, and reorienting of attention), following deviant stimuli (Berti et al., 2004; Horvath et al., 2008).

Investigations into this series of ERP components should provide further insights into cognitive disturbances in schizophrenia spectrum disorders, which have not been satisfactorily addressed. Specifically, there is little information about the RON in schizophrenia spectrum disorders. Jahshan et al. (2012) measured the amplitudes of MMN, P3a, and RON complex, and found reductions of these parameters in schizophrenia patients. Also, amplitudes of MMN and P3a, but not RON were diminished in individuals at-risk for psychosis. In spite of the above cross-sectional study, further work is needed to test the utility of the ERP complex for predicting progression to schizophrenia in vulnerable individuals.

In this study, we measured dMMN, P3a, and RON amplitudes in subjects with ARMS, first-episode schizophrenia (FES), or chronic phase of the illness. These data were compared with those of normal control subjects. We also attempted to determine if these ERP parameters would predict later progression to schizophrenia in ARMS subjects by means of longitudinal observations. Specifically, preliminary data are provided on the evaluation of RON in relation to transition to overt schizophrenia in vulnerable subjects.

MATERIALS AND METHODS

PARTICIPANTS

Diagnosis was made based on the Structured Clinical Interview for DSM-IV (SCID) for schizophrenia and the Comprehensive Assessment of At-Risk Mental State (CAARMS) for ARMS (Yung et al., 2005), by experienced psychiatrists. Most of these subjects were referred from Psychiatric Health and Welfare Center of Toyama (PHWCT), as previously described (Higuchi et al., 2013b). Nineteen ARMS subjects followed at the University of Toyama Hospital participated in this study [male/female = 9/10; mean (SD) age = 19.4 (3.6) years]. Thirty-eight schizophrenia patients also participated in this study. Patients with duration of illness <2 years were defined as FES [$n = 19$; male/female = 9/10; mean (SD) age = 22.8 (5.2) years], while those with duration of illness 2 years or longer were defined as chronic schizophrenia (CS) [$n = 19$; male/female = 9/10; mean (SD) age = 22.9 (3.6) years] (Higuchi et al., 2013b). The patients who allocated "first episode" are defined "single psychotic episode" and "duration of illness is <2 years." CS patients are defined "duration of illness is more than 2 years." Even if patients experienced only one psychotic episode, they allocated to CS group. We recruited normal control subjects from the community by advertisements. They are healthy volunteers [$n = 19$; male/female = 9/10; mean (SD) age = 19.4 (2.5) years] without any personal history of psychiatric illnesses, including schizophrenia or other psychotic disorders. All participants were right-handed. A psychiatric and treatment history was obtained from the subjects, families, and medical records. Subjects with a current history of substance abuse or dependence, seizure, or head injury were excluded from the study. Eligible patients had a complete physical examination and standard laboratory testing was normal. As clinical assessments, the Scale for the Assessment of Positive Symptoms (SAPS) and the Scale for the Assessment of Negative Symptoms (SANS) (Andreasen, 1990) were administered by an experienced psychiatrist. Demographic data at baseline evaluation are shown in **Table 1A**.

At-risk mental state subjects were followed-up at the hospital. Four out of the 19 ARMS subjects transitioned to schizophrenia during the observation period. When DSM-IV criteria were met, e.g., auditory hallucinations persisted or any delusion (for example, disturbance of the self) clearly observed, the subject was regarded to have converted to schizophrenia (Converters; Conv). Subjects who did not develop psychosis were defined as non-converters (Non-C). The average observation period for Non-C subjects was 2.2 ± 1.5 years.

Table 1 | (A) Demographic and clinical data; (B) ERP data.

(A)	Healthy controls ($n=19$)	ARMS ($n=19$)	First-episode schizophrenia ($n=19$)	Chronic schizophrenia ($n=19$)	Group comparison	
Male/female	9/10	9/10	9/10	9/10	n.s.	
Age (years)	19.4 (2.5)	19.4 (3.6)	22.8 (5.2)	22.9 (3.6)	$F(3,74)=4.94$, $p=0.004$	
Age of onset (years)	–	–	22.2 (5.2)	17.9 (3.9)	$p=0.007$	
Duration of illness (years)	–	–	0.7 (0.6)	5.0 (2.3)	–	
Drug dose[a]	–	0.1 (0.4)	1.7 (2.0)	3.7 (4.2)	$F(2,56)=8.54$, $p=0.001$	
SAPS	–	17.3 (7.4)	27.0 (16.9)	19.2 (18.0)	$F(2,56)=2.29$, $p=0.11$	
SANS	–	60.8 (24.3)	60.6 (27.2)	53.3 (22.9)	$F(2,56)=0.52$, $p=0.59$	
(B)	**Healthy controls ($n=19$)**	**ARMS ($n=19$)**	**First-episode schizophrenia ($n=19$)**	**Chronic schizophrenia ($n=19$)**	**Analyze of variance (df=3,75), group effect**	
					F	***p***
dMMN amplitude (μV)						
F3	−6.9 (1.7)	−6.2 (2.0)	−5.0 (1.8)	−4.6 (1.0)	7.505	<0.001**
F4	−7.5 (1.4)	−6.5 (2.2)	−5.2 (2.1)	−4.6 (2.0)	7.767	<0.001**
Fz	−7.4 (1.4)	−6.5 (2.0)	−5.4 (1.9)	−4.8 (1.5)	8.322	<0.001**
Cz	−6.0 (1.4)	−5.6 (2.1)	−4.8 (1.9)	−3.7 (0.9)	6.831	<0.001**
Pz	−4.2 (1.4)	−4.5 (4.0)	−3.3 (1.4)	−2.2 (0.9)	6.240	0.001**
dMMN latency (ms)						
F3	167.3 (15.1)	172.1 (17.5)	173.0 (23.0)	177.8 (30.7)	0.702	0.55
F4	169.1 (15.4)	175.8 (18.3)	172.5 (19.7)	176.6 (24.0)	0.404	0.75
Fz	172.2 (15.6)	177.3 (12.6)	173.0 (19.1)	176.8 (25.6)	0.364	0.77
Cz	168.4 (14.8)	182.3 (18.7)	174.6 (16.7)	177.6 (26.2)	1.675	0.18
Pz	173.0 (15.8)	188.6 (24.4)	178.3 (17.4)	174.8 (30.7)	1.753	0.16
P3a amplitude (μV)						
F3	1.6 (1.8)	1.1 (1.4)	1.3 (2.2)	1.5 (1.3)	0.277	0.84
F4	1.4 (2.3)	1.2 (1.8)	1.6 (2.1)	1.4 (1.4)	0.110	0.95
Fz	2.0 (2.3)	1.7 (1.5)	1.7 (2.2)	1.7 (1.1)	0.179	0.91
Cz	2.4 (2.4)	2.1 (1.6)	2.5 (2.1)	2.1 (1.4)	0.209	0.89
Pz	2.0 (2.2)	1.8 (1.4)	2.3 (1.8)	1.8 (1.3)	0.408	0.74
P3a latency (ms)						
F3	255.6 (23.5)	265.2 (25.0)	264.2 (28.3)	262.8 (23.0)	0.395	0.75
F4	256.9 (20.2)	269.7 (28.0)	262.9 (31.1)	255.2 (30.8)	0.755	0.52
Fz	254.6 (21.5)	268.7 (28.8)	261.8 (30.9)	262.3 (22.3)	0.314	0.81
Cz	255.1 (21.7)	266.0 (25.9)	254.8 (28.7)	262.2 (22.9)	0.509	0.67
Pz	255.7 (19.8)	272.2 (27.2)	254.7 (27.6)	261.4 (19.7)	0.359	0.78
RON amplitude (μV)						
F3	−4.4 (1.7)	−4.1 (1.7)	−3.5 (1.3)	−3.3 (1.3)	2.320	0.08
F4	−5.2 (1.8)	−4.2 (1.5)	−3.6 (1.7)	−3.4 (1.6)	4.191	0.009**
Fz	−5.1 (1.6)	−4.2 (1.8)	−3.9 (1.4)	−3.4 (1.7)	3.143	0.03*
Cz	−4.3 (1.9)	−3.8 (2.1)	−3.6 (1.6)	−3.2 (1.6)	1.143	0.33
Pz	−3.1 (1.8)	−2.7 (1.7)	−2.5 (1.5)	−2.6 (1.6)	0.391	0.76
RON latency (ms)						
F3	396.3 (51.8)	380.7 (49.4)	395.0 (42.7)	389.0 (52.6)	0.395	0.75
F4	392.7 (53.9)	404.0 (54.1)	409.1 (53.1)	385.4 (53.8)	0.755	0.52
Fz	396.2 (50.2)	397.2 (46.8)	409.3 (40.9)	397.7 (53.3)	0.314	0.81
Cz	401.2 (39.0)	398.3 (44.4)	412.5 (40.9)	397.0 (47.4)	0.509	0.67
Pz	409.5 (48.2)	401.7 (45.7)	411.7 (40.7)	397.4 (58.2)	0.359	0.78

Values represent mean (SD).

[a] *Risperidone equivalent (mg/day), ARMS, at-risk mental state; SAPS, Scale for the Assessment of Positive Symptoms; SANS, Scale for the Assessment of Negative Symptoms.*

Values represent mean (SD). ARMS, at-risk mental state.

$^{*}p < 0.05$, $^{**}p < 0.01$.

ELECTROENCEPHALOGRAM RECORDING

Electroencephalograms (EEGs) were recorded based on the previous report from our laboratory (Sumiyoshi et al., 2006, 2009; Kawasaki et al., 2007a; Higuchi et al., 2008, 2010, 2013a,b; Itoh et al., 2011).

A 32-channel DC-amplifier (EEG-2100 version 2.22J, Nihon Kohden Corp., Tokyo, Japan) was used. Recordings were performed using an electro cap (Electrocap Inc., Eaton, OH) in a sound-attenuated room. Data were collected with a sampling rate of 500 Hz. EEG data were collected from 29 scalp electrodes (Fp1, Fp2, F3, F4, F7, F8, FC3, FC4, C3, C4, T3, T4, CP3, CP4, TP7, TP8, P3, P4, T5, T6, O1, O2, FPz, Fz, FCz, Cz, CPz, Pz, and Oz according to the extended International 10–20 system). All electrodes were referred to the average amplitude of the ear electrodes (bandwidth = 0.53–120 Hz, 60 Hz notch filter). Electrode impedance was <5 kΩ.

Measurements of dMMN/P3a/RON complex were based on our previous report (Higuchi et al., 2010). One-thousand auditory stimuli were delivered binaurally through headphones with interstimulus intervals 500 ms. Standard/target tones of 50/100 ms duration were randomly presented with the presentation probability of 0.9/0.1. All tones were 60 dB, 1000 Hz, and with a rise–fall time of 10 ms. The subjects were requested to watch silent animation movie (Tom and Jerry) and pay attention to the monitor and ignore the tones.

Averaging of ERP waves and related procedures were performed using Vital Tracer and EPLYZER II software (Kissei Comtec, Co. Ltd., Nagano, Japan). Epochs were 600 ms, including a 100 ms prestimulus baseline. Eye movement artifacts (blinks and eye movements) were manually rejected. MMN waveforms were obtained by subtract standard waveforms from target ones. MMN, P3a, and RON peaks were identified within the 150–250 ms (minus peak), 200–350 ms (plus peak), and 250–500 ms (minus peak) search windows, respectively.

STATISTICAL METHODS

Statistical analyses were performed using the Statistical Package for Social Sciences (SPSS) version 20 (SPSS Japan Inc., Tokyo, Japan). We performed comparison of age between four groups (HC, ARMS, FES, and CS) by one-way analysis of variance. Onset age and duration of illness of two schizophrenia groups (first-episode and chronic) were compared by independent t-test. Drug dose, SAPS, and SANS score among three groups (ARMS, FES, and CS) were analyzed by one-way ANOVA.

Event-related potential amplitudes and latencies were measured and analyzed at five electrodes; three from frontal lobe (F3, F4, and Fz), and two from midline (Cz and Pz). They are typical electrodes that commonly used on ERP studies. MMN amplitudes are generally largest at frontal electrodes, so we choose three electrodes from frontal lobe. Moreover, grand average waveforms (**Figures 1** and **3**) and scatterplots (**Figures 2** and **4**) were drawn and analyzed by Fz lead as a representative of electrodes because amplitudes ERPs of Fz were largest. Laterality of ERPs was analyzed by F3/F4 comparison as we performed in previous report (Higuchi et al., 2008), but there were no difference in this study (data not shown).

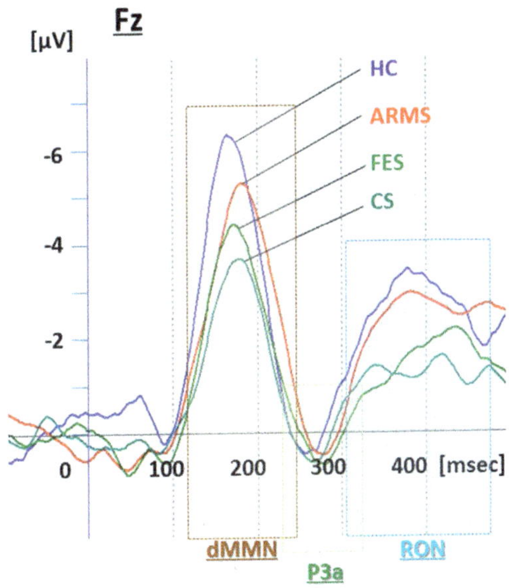

FIGURE 1 | Duration mismatch negativity (dMMN), P3a, and reorienting negativity (RON) complex waveforms at Fz for all subjects. Waveforms are presented for healthy controls (HC, blue line), at-risk mental state (ARMS, red line), first-episode schizophrenia (FES, light green line), and chronic schizophrenia (CS, dark green line).

Two-way ANOVA was conducted on amplitudes and latencies of dMMN, P3a, and RON, with "Stage" (HC, ARMS, FES, and CS) and "Lead" (F3, F4, Fz, Cz, and Pz) as fixed factors. Main effects (of Stage and Lead) were described on **Table 1B** (significant differences were seen in all leads of dMMN amplitude and F4/Fz of RON amplitude). The Stage-by-Lead interactions on amplitudes (dMMN, $F = 1.172$, $p = 0.30$; P3a, $F = 0.511$, $p = 0.90$; RON, $F = 1.024$, $p = 0.42$) and latencies (dMMN, $F = 1.254$, $p = 0.246$; P3a, $F = 1.475$, $p = 0.13$; RON, $F = 0.516$, $p = 0.904$) were not significant.

Gender difference between Conv and Non-C were analyzed by Chi-square test. Other factors (age, drug dose, SAPS, SANS, ERP amplitude, and latency) of them were calculated by independent t-test. All analyses of variance were corrected by Bonferroni correction.

Correlations of symptoms and ERP amplitudes were performed by Pearson product–moment correlation coefficient. SAPS scores (hallucinations, delusions, bizarre behavior, and positive formal thought disorder) and SANS scores (affective flattening/blunting, alogia, avolition-apathy, anhedonia-asociality, and attention) were used.

Raters were not informed of subjects' profiles and diagnosis.

RESULTS

SUBJECTS' PROFILE

Demographic and clinical data of participants are shown in **Tables 1A** and **2**. There was significant group difference in age [$F(3,74) = 4.94, p = 0.004$, ANOVA], and Conv subjects were older than Non-C in age ($p = 0.009$, t-test). Male/female ratio did not differ between of Conv. and Non-C groups [$\chi^2 = 2.47$, $p = 0.3$, Chi-square test].

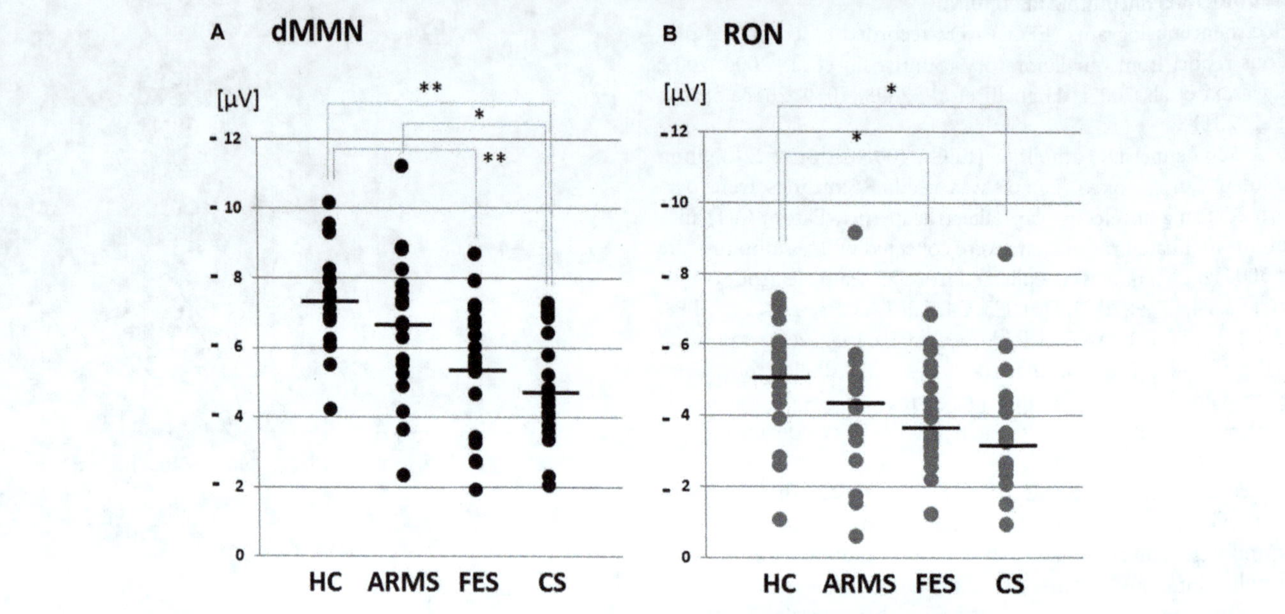

FIGURE 2 | Distribution of amplitudes of duration mismatch negativity [dMMN; (A)] and reorienting negativity [RON; (B)] at Fz for all subjects. Data are presented for healthy controls (HC), ARMS, first-episode schizophrenia (FES), and chronic schizophrenia (CS). *$p < 0.05$, **$p < 0.01$.

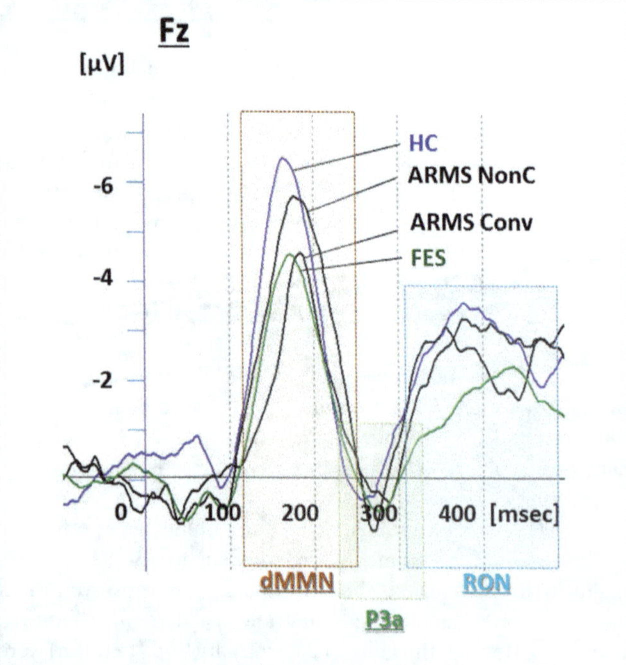

FIGURE 3 | Duration mismatch negativity (dMMN), P3a, and reorienting negativity (RON) complex waveforms at the Fz lead. Waveforms are presented for healthy controls (blue line), ARMS Converters (Conv), and non-Converter (Non-C) (black lines), and FES (green line).

Sixteen out of 19 ARMS subjects were not taking any medication, while three were prescribed a small dose of risperidone (1.5 mg/day), aripiprazole (3 mg/day), and sulpiride (150 mg/day), respectively, for acute psychosis episodes (sometimes with strong agitation), based on the criteria of International Early Psychosis Association Writing Group (2005). MMN recordings for these subjects were conducted immediately after medications were started (9, 15, and 27 days). Two out of the three subjects subsequently developed schizophrenia. Thirteen out of 19 FES patients and 15 out of 19 CS patients were taking antipsychotic medications. There were no significant differences among ARMS, FES, and CS groups in SAPS [$F(2,56) = 2.29$, $p = 0.11$, ANOVA] and SANS [$F(2,56) = 0.52$, $p = 0.59$, ANOVA] scores. Conv and Non-C groups did not differ in the SAPS and SANS scores at baseline ($p = 0.08$, 0.24, respectively, t-test).

COMPARISONS OF ERP BETWEEN HEALTHY CONTROLS VS. ARMS VS. SCHIZOPHRENIA

Grand average ERP waveforms in the Fz lead following deviant stimulation are shown in **Figure 1**. Scatterplots of dMMN and RON amplitudes at Fz lead are shown in **Figures 2A,B**, respectively. P3a did not show any statistical differences so we skipped making scatterplot of P3a. ARMS subjects showed relatively smaller dMMN amplitudes at Fz ($-6.5 \pm 2.0\,\mu V$) compared to those of healthy control subjects ($-7.4 \pm 1.4\,\mu V$), which was not statistically significant ($p = 0.13$, t-test). On the other hand, FES group showed significantly smaller dMMN amplitudes at Fz ($-5.4 \pm 1.9\,\mu V$) compared to healthy control ($p = 0.001$, t-test). Patients with CS showed greater amplitude reductions at Fz ($-4.8 \pm 1.5\,\mu V$) compared to healthy controls ($p = 0.000004$, t-test).

At-risk mental state subjects showed relatively smaller RON amplitudes at Fz ($-4.2 \pm 1.8\,\mu V$) than healthy controls ($-5.1 \pm 1.6\,\mu V$), which was not significant ($p = 0.15$, t-test). On the other hand, FES group showed significantly smaller RON amplitudes at Fz ($-3.9 \pm 1.4\,\mu V$, $p = 0.02$). Patients with CS also elicited significantly smaller RON amplitudes at Fz ($-3.4 \pm 1.7\,\mu V$) compared to healthy controls ($p = 0.005$, t-test).

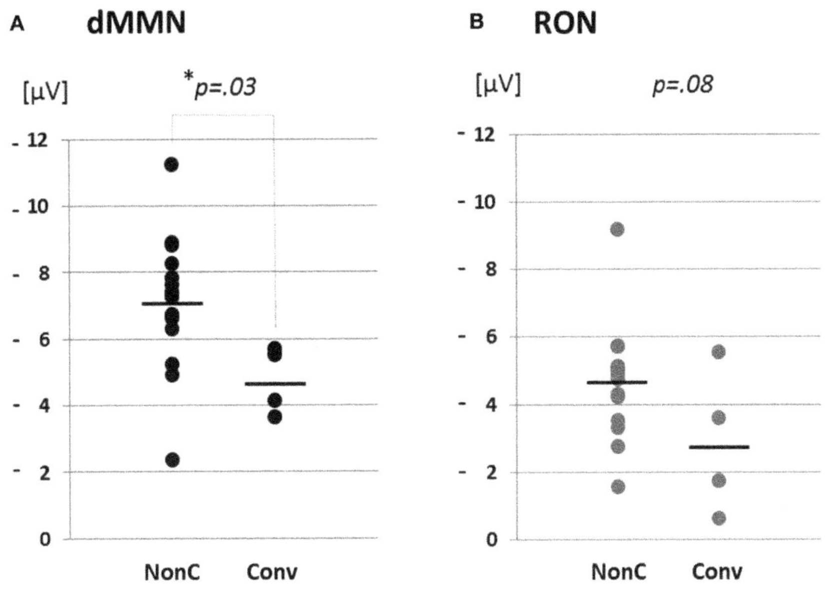

FIGURE 4 | Distribution of amplitudes of duration mismatch negativity [dMMN; (A)] and reorienting negativity [RON, (B)] at Fz for ARMS. Data are presented Converters (Conv) and Non-Converter (Non-C). *$p < 0.05$.

Latencies of dMMN, P3a, and RON at any electrodes did not differ among the four groups (see **Table 1B**).

COMPARISONS BETWEEN CONVERTERS VS. NON-CONVERTERS

Grand average ERP waveforms are shown in **Figure 3**. Scatterplots of dMMN and RON amplitudes at Fz lead are shown in **Figures 4A,B**, respectively. P3a did not show any statistical differences so we skipped making scatterplot of P3a. Waveforms of Conv group were similar to those of FES patients. By contrast, waveforms of Non-C subjects resembled to those of healthy controls. Conv subjects showed significantly smaller dMMN amplitudes at Fz and Cz electrodes compared with Non-C subjects ($p = 0.03$, 0.05 by t-test, respectively, **Table 2**). On the other hand, amplitudes of Non-C did not differ from those of HC ($p = 0.51$ at Fz, t-test, data not shown) and there was no significant difference in dMMN amplitudes between Conv and FES subjects ($p = 0.44$ at Fz, t-test, data not shown). In other electrode of Non-C vs. HC and Conv vs. FES comparisons, differences were smaller and did not reach significance.

Conv subjects tended to show smaller RON amplitudes compared to those of Non-C subjects at Fz and F4 electrodes ($p = 0.08$, $p = 0.08$ by t-test, respectively, **Table 2**). Also, HC group showed relatively larger RON amplitudes at Fz lead compared to Conv subjects, which did not reach significant level ($p = 0.08$, t-test, data not shown). No significant differences were found at any electrode between FES vs Non-C groups (data not shown).

Latencies of dMMN, P3a, and RON at any electrodes did not differ between Conv and Non-C groups (see **Table 2**).

RELATIONSHIP BETWEEN SYMPTOMS AND ERPs

We evaluated the correlations between dMMN, P3a, and RON amplitudes and symptoms (SAPS and SANS) in patients (schizophrenia and ARMS, $n = 57$).

Data are shown in **Table 3**. There were significant correlation between attention disorder score (SANS) and dMMN amplitude at Fz and F3 lead ($r = 0.317$; $p = 0.025$, $r = 0.290$, $p = 0.041$, respectively, by Pearson's correlation). Moreover, there were significant correlation between positive formal thought disorder score (SAPS) and RON amplitude at Fz and F3 lead ($r = 0.280$; $p = 0.049$, $r = 0.346$, $p = 0.014$, respectively, by Pearson's correlation). Thus, reduction of ERPs was correlated with severity of some symptoms.

DISCUSSION

Duration mismatch negativity amplitudes at frontal and central leads were reduced in ARMS subjects who later converted to overt schizophrenia in comparison with non-converters and normal subjects, consistent with previous reports (Bodatsch et al., 2011; Shaikh et al., 2012; Higuchi et al., 2013b). Specifically, the current data from gender matched subjects across groups (**Table 1**) confirmed previous observations in patients with variable demographic backgrounds (Bodatsch et al., 2011; Shaikh et al., 2012; Higuchi et al., 2013b). Importantly, this study is the first to suggest that RON provides a marker for the progression to overt schizophrenia in subjects with ARMS, based on longitudinal observations.

Three out of 4 Conv, 7 out of 15 Non-C, 7 out of 19 FES, 5 out of 19 CS, and 9 out of 19 HC subjects overlapped with subjects in our previous report (Higuchi et al., 2013b). We selected subjects for the current study, according to the following considerations; (1) ARMS subjects with a longer followed-up period, (2) gender-match between HC and schizophrenia patients, (3) younger HC and schizophrenia patients than those used in the previous study. The current one used a longer observation period, and was gender-matched across groups with less variation in age. According to a previous report (Yung et al., 2003), 10–40% of ARMS subjects

Table 2 | Comparison between converters and non-converters of ARMS subjects.

	ARMS ($n = 19$)		Group comparison (p)
	Non-C ($n = 15$)	Conv ($n = 4$)	
Male/female	7/8	3/1	$\chi 2 = 2.47$, $p = 0.3$
Age (years)	18.3 (2.2)	23.4 (4.9)	0.009
Drug dose[a]	0.1 (0.2)	0.4 (0.6)	0.12
SAPS	15.3 (7.0)	22.7 (5.8)	0.08
SANS	56.9 (26.3)	73.7 (9.6)	0.24
dMMN amplitude (μV)			
F3	−6.5 (2.1)	−4.9 (0.6)	0.16
F4	−7.0 (2.2)	−4.6 (0.9)	0.06
Fz	−7.0 (2.0)	−4.7 (1.0)	0.03*
Cz	−6.1 (2.1)	−3.7 (0.6)	0.05*
Pz	−3.8 (2.1)	−3.0 (0.4)	0.48
dMMN latency (ms)			
F3	169.3 (18.5)	182.5 (8.2)	0.19
F4	174.2 (20.1)	182.0 (8.1)	0.47
Fz	176.2 (13.6)	181.5 (8.2)	0.47
Cz	180.2 (19.7)	190.0 (13.3)	0.37
Pz	186.8 (25.2)	195.5 (23.2)	0.54
P3a amplitude (μV)			
F3	1.0 (1.4)	1.5 (1.1)	0.60
F4	1.2 (2.0)	1.2 (1.1)	0.96
Fz	1.6 (1.5)	2.0 (1.2)	0.67
Cz	1.9 (1.6)	2.6 (1.4)	0.47
Pz	2.0 (1.4)	0.7 (0.8)	0.10
P3a latency (ms)			
F3	264.7 (27.9)	267.0 (27.9)	0.88
F4	270.1 (31.3)	268.0 (31.3)	0.90
Fz	269.1 (32.3)	267.5 (32.3)	0.93
Cz	264.8 (28.8)	270.5 (28.8)	0.71
Pz	268.4 (29.0)	286.5 (29.0)	0.26
RON amplitude (μV)			
F3	−4.3 (1.7)	−3.1 (1.2)	0.20
F4	−4.5 (1.4)	−3.1 (1.0)	0.08
Fz	−4.6 (1.6)	−2.8 (2.1)	0.08
Cz	−4.2 (2.1)	−2.5 (1.6)	0.16
Pz	−2.7 (1.8)	−2.7 (1.1)	0.97
RON latency (ms)			
F3	388.0 (51.3)	353.5 (33.4)	0.22
F4	403.6 (51.4)	405.5 (72.0)	0.95
Fz	391.3 (44.8)	419.5 (53.8)	0.29
Cz	399.3 (48.6)	394.5 (28.4)	0.85
Pz	401.8 (51.3)	401.2 (33.4)	0.98

Values represent mean (SD).

[a] *Risperidone equivalent (mg/day).*

ARMS, at-risk mental state; Non-C., ARMS non-Converters; Conv., ARMS Converters; SAPS, Scale for the Assessment of Positive Symptoms; SANS, Scale for the Assessment of Negative Symptoms.

$*p < 0.05$.

later developed schizophrenia, consistent with our observations that 21.0% progressed to the illness.

ARMS subjects as a whole have been reported to demonstrate reduced dMMN amplitudes, but with a lesser degree compared to patients with overt schizophrenia (Bodatsch et al., 2011; Atkinson et al., 2012; Jahshan et al., 2012), consistent with the present results (**Figure 1**). On the other hand, the current data may be partly different from our previous observations indicating the lack of difference in dMMN amplitudes between ARMS subjects as whole and healthy controls (Higuchi et al., 2013b). One of the reasons for this discrepancy may include the difference in age and gender ratio. In fact, as previous reports indicate ERPs amplitudes gradually decrease by age, and male subjects show relatively smaller amplitudes than female because of the difference in skull thickness (Ikezawa et al., 2008; Matsubayashi et al., 2008; Naatanen et al., 2012). Another confounding factor may include the observation periods for follow-up. While our previous report (Higuchi et al., 2013b) employed a relatively short period (mean ± SD = 1.6 ± 0.8 years for non-converters), the present study used a longer period (2.2 ± 1.5 years), similar to those in the literature.

Compared to Non-C, Conv subjects elicited significantly smaller dMMN amplitudes at F4 and Fz leads (**Table 2**). These observations suggest the ability of dMMN amplitudes to differentiate between high-risk individuals who later progress to schizophrenia and those who do not, as has been suggested (Higuchi et al., 2013b; Sumiyoshi et al., 2013).

Little information has been available about the feature of RON in schizophrenia. In this study, RON amplitudes of ARMS subjects as a whole were not different from those of HC subjects, while FES and CS group showed significantly smaller RON amplitudes at Fz and F4 leads compared to the HC group. This finding is consistent with observations by Jahshan et al. (2012). As the results of the current study suggest that RON amplitudes may decrease according to progression of clinical stages of schizophrenia (**Table 1B**; **Figure 1**), they may provide an intermediate phenotype of the illness.

Importantly, RON amplitudes of Conv subjects tended to be smaller than those of Non-C at the Fz and F4 leads (**Figure 4**). The failure to reach statistical significance may be due to the fact that RON waveforms are not stable and smaller compared to dMMN waveforms. Future investigations with a larger number of subjects would be desirable to determine if the combined measurement of RON and dMMN would further facilitate early detection of schizophrenia.

P3a amplitudes were barely detectable in this study (**Figures 1** and **3**). These amplitudes have been reported to be decreased in schizophrenia and ARMS (Friedman et al., 2001; Jahshan et al., 2012; Mondragon-Maya et al., 2013; Nagai et al., 2013). Variations of P3a amplitudes may be large, due, probably, to the difference in measurement.

Limitations of this study include the small sample number, especially in ARMS ($n = 19$) and Conv subjects ($n = 4$). According to the power analysis, at least 26 patients are needed to obtain adequate effect size (i.e., 0.6). Investigations with a larger number of patients will make the data more satisfactory. Second, significant age difference was seen in the ARMS vs. HC and FES

Table 3 | ERP amplitudes and symptoms.

	SAPS							
	Hallucinations		**Delusions**		**Bizarre behavior**		**Positive formal thought disorder**	
	r	*p*	*r*	*p*	*r*	*p*	*r*	*p*
dMMN amplitude (μV)								
F3	0.039	0.786	0.011	0.938	−0.122	0.398	0.086	0.552
F4	0.071	0.625	0.066	0.648	−0.131	0.365	0.076	0.599
Fz	0.021	0.884	−0.016	0.910	−0.199	0.166	0.090	0.536
Cz	−0.021	0.888	−0.036	0.805	−0.108	0.457	0.056	0.697
Pz	−0.163	0.258	−0.178	0.216	−0.225	0.117	−0.069	0.636
P3a amplitude (μV)								
F3	−0.148	0.305	−0.188	0.192	−0.188	0.191	−0.036	0.802
F4	−0.075	0.605	−0.190	0.187	−0.256	0.073	0.029	0.842
Fz	−0.191	0.185	−0.181	0.209	−0.233	0.104	−0.008	0.956
Cz	−0.149	0.302	−0.056	0.701	−0.213	0.138	0.020	0.891
Pz	0.022	0.879	0.046	0.753	−0.023	0.874	−0.117	0.417
RON amplitude (μV)								
F3	0.014	0.926	−0.131	0.363	0.067	0.646	0.280	**0.049***
F4	0.087	0.549	−0.092	0.523	−0.158	0.274	0.244	0.087
Fz	−0.024	0.869	−0.109	0.450	−0.265	0.063	0.346	**0.014***
Cz	−0.033	0.818	−0.214	0.136	−0.081	0.578	0.151	0.295
Pz	0.002	0.990	−0.257	0.071	−0.025	0.861	0.022	0.881

	SANS									
	Affective flattening		**Alogia**		**Avolition-apathy**		**Anhedonia-asociality**		**Attention**	
	r	*p*	*r*	*p*	*r*	*p*	*r*	*p*	*r*	*p*
dMMN amplitude (μV)										
F3	0.109	0.452	0.149	0.301	0.096	0.509	−0.102	0.483	0.317	**0.025***
F4	0.142	0.325	0.122	0.399	0.016	0.910	−0.066	0.650	0.260	0.068
Fz	0.115	0.427	0.165	0.254	−0.014	0.923	−0.081	0.576	0.290	**0.041***
Cz	0.060	0.680	0.147	0.307	0.117	0.420	0.050	0.730	0.262	0.066
Pz	−0.041	0.778	0.066	0.650	0.122	0.400	−0.063	0.666	−0.007	0.963
P3a amplitude (μV)										
F3	−0.029	0.843	−0.034	0.815	0.037	0.796	−0.037	0.796	0.130	0.368
F4	0.021	0.883	0.021	0.885	0.003	0.984	−0.102	0.480	0.148	0.306
Fz	−0.043	0.767	0.032	0.823	−0.032	0.827	−0.090	0.533	0.101	0.487
Cz	−0.066	0.649	−0.029	0.843	0.012	0.934	−0.010	0.943	0.112	0.441
Pz	0.063	0.662	−0.027	0.852	0.108	0.454	−0.046	0.753	0.032	0.827
RON amplitude (μV)										
F3	−0.112	0.438	−0.111	0.441	−0.054	0.712	−0.215	0.134	−0.055	0.704
F4	0.022	0.882	0.039	0.788	−0.089	0.539	−0.103	0.475	−0.050	0.730
Fz	−0.046	0.752	−0.017	0.905	−0.104	0.474	−0.073	0.617	−0.025	0.861
Cz	0.128	0.375	0.210	0.143	−0.040	0.781	0.002	0.988	−0.108	0.455
Pz	0.014	0.922	0.095	0.513	−0.123	0.393	−0.117	0.419	−0.242	0.090

SAPS, Scale for the Assessment of Positive Symptoms; SANS, Scale for the Assessment of Negative Symptoms.

$^*p < 0.05$, *r* = *Pearson product–moment correlation coefficient.*

vs. CS comparisons. Since part of ARMS subjects is regarded as prodromal state of schizophrenia, it is natural that they are mostly younger than schizophrenia patients. Therefore, adjustment of age between FES/CS and ARMS subjects may increase the number of certain type of schizophrenia, e.g., hebephrenic type. Due to an effort to make the FES/CS groups more homogeneous, patients of these groups became somewhat older than the ARMS group. Application of ANCOVA to 19 members may provide over-adjustment. Although MMN amplitudes are reduced gradually by age, the decline is not substantial ($-0.056\,\mu$V/year in schizophrenia and $-0.079\,\mu$V/year in healthy control) (Kiang et al., 2009). ARMS/HC subjects are about 2.5 years younger than FES/CS (**Table 1**). According to this formula, about 0.2 μV amplitude reduction may occur between these two. Differences in our data presented (at Fz lead) were 1.1 μV or greater (ARMS vs. FES groups.), which was sufficiently large. Third, some ARMS subjects and most schizophrenia patients were taking antipsychotic drugs, which may be another limitation of the current study. Fourth, in this study, we measured ERPs at baseline, and did not perform follow-up measurements. Therefore, little information is available about longitudinal data of ERPs parameters.

In conclusions, diminished amplitudes in dMMN/RON may provide a biomarker that is present before and after the development of psychosis. Our results should be interpreted with caution before applying to the at-risk population, especially to avoid over-diagnosis. Ideally, the combination with other cognitive modalities, e.g., neuropsychological tests (Higuchi et al., 2013b), brain morphology, and biochemical markers, would enhance the sensitivity and specificity for early diagnosis. These efforts are expected to help improve functional outcome in subjects with schizophrenia and vulnerable individuals as well.

ACKNOWLEDGMENTS

This study was funded by grants-in-aid for Scientific Research from Japan Society for the Promotion of Science (No. 26461761), Health and Labour Sciences Research Grants for Comprehensive Research on Disability, Health, and Welfare (H23-Seishin-Ippan-002; H24-Seishin-Ippan-002), and SENSHIN Medical Research Foundation.

REFERENCES

Andreasen, N. C. (1990). Methods for assessing positive and negative symptoms. *Mod. Probl. Pharmacopsychiatry* 24, 73–88.

Atkinson, R. J., Michie, P. T., and Schall, U. (2012). Duration mismatch negativity and P3a in first-episode psychosis and individuals at ultra-high risk of psychosis. *Biol. Psychiatry* 71, 98–104. doi:10.1016/j.biopsych.2011.08.023

Berti, S., Roeber, U., and Schroger, E. (2004). Bottom-up influences on working memory: behavioral and electrophysiological distraction varies with distractor strength. *Exp. Psychol.* 51, 249–257. doi:10.1027/1618-3169.51.4.249

Bodatsch, M., Ruhrmann, S., Wagner, M., Muller, R., Schultze-Lutter, F., Frommann, I., et al. (2011). Prediction of psychosis by mismatch negativity. *Biol. Psychiatry* 69, 959–966. doi:10.1016/j.biopsych.2010.09.057

Broome, M. R., Woolley, J. B., Johns, L. C., Valmaggia, L. R., Tabraham, P., Gafoor, R., et al. (2005). Outreach and support in south London (OASIS): implementation of a clinical service for prodromal psychosis and the at risk mental state. *Eur. Psychiatry* 20, 372–378. doi:10.1016/j.eurpsy.2005.03.001

Bruder, G. E., Tenke, C. E., Towey, J. P., Leite, P., Fong, R., Stewart, J. E., et al. (1998). Brain ERPs of depressed patients to complex tones in an oddball task: relation of reduced P3 asymmetry to physical anhedonia. *Psychophysiology* 35, 54–63. doi:10.1111/1469-8986.3510054

Chang, W. C., Hui, C. L., Tang, J. Y., Wong, G. H., Lam, M. M., Chan, S. K., et al. (2011). Persistent negative symptoms in first-episode schizophrenia: a prospective three-year follow-up study. *Schizophr. Res.* 133, 22–28. doi:10.1016/j.schres.2011.09.006

Edwards, J., McGorry, P. D., Waddell, F. M., and Harrigan, S. M. (1999). Enduring negative symptoms in first-episode psychosis: comparison of six methods using follow-up data. *Schizophr. Res.* 40, 147–158. doi:10.1016/S0920-9964(99)00043-2

Friedman, D., Cycowicz, Y. M., and Gaeta, H. (2001). The novelty P3: an event-related brain potential (ERP) sign of the brain's evaluation of novelty. *Neurosci. Biobehav. Rev.* 25, 355–373. doi:10.1016/S0149-7634(01)00019-7

Galderisi, S., Mucci, A., Bitter, I., Libiger, J., Bucci, P., Wolfgang Fleischhacker, W., et al. (2012). Persistent negative symptoms in first episode patients with schizophrenia: results from the European First Episode Schizophrenia Trial. *Eur. Neuropsychopharmacol.* 23, 196–204. doi:10.1016/j.euroneuro.2012.04.019

Green, M. F. (1996). What are the functional consequences of neurocognitive deficits in schizophrenia? *Am. J. Psychiatry* 153, 321–330.

Harvey, P. D., Green, M. F., Keefe, R. S., and Velligan, D. I. (2004). Cognitive functioning in schizophrenia: a consensus statement on its role in the definition and evaluation of effective treatments for the illness. *J. Clin. Psychiatry* 65, 361–372. doi:10.4088/JCP.v65n0312

Heinrichs, R. W., and Zakzanis, K. K. (1998). Neurocognitive deficit in schizophrenia: a quantitative review of the evidence. *Neuropsychology* 12, 426–445. doi:10.1037/0894-4105.12.3.426

Higuchi, Y., Sumiyoshi, T., Ito, T., and Suzuki, M. (2013a). Perospirone normalized P300 and cognitive function in a case of early psychosis. *J. Clin. Psychopharmacol.* 33, 263–266. doi:10.1097/JCP.0b013e318287c527

Higuchi, Y., Sumiyoshi, T., Seo, T., Miyanishi, T., Kawasaki, Y., and Suzuki, M. (2013b). Mismatch negativity and cognitive performance for the prediction of psychosis in subjects with at-risk mental state. *PLoS ONE* 8:e54080. doi:10.1371/journal.pone.0054080

Higuchi, Y., Sumiyoshi, T., Kawasaki, Y., Ito, T., Seo, T., and Suzuki, M. (2010). Effect of tandospirone on mismatch negativity and cognitive performance in schizophrenia: a case report. *J. Clin. Psychopharmacol.* 30, 732–734. doi:10.1097/JCP.0b013e3181faa57d

Higuchi, Y., Sumiyoshi, T., Kawasaki, Y., Matsui, M., Arai, H., and Kurachi, M. (2008). Electrophysiological basis for the ability of olanzapine to improve verbal memory and functional outcome in patients with schizophrenia: a LORETA analysis of P300. *Schizophr. Res.* 101, 320–330. doi:10.1016/j.schres.2008.01.020

Horvath, J., Winkler, I., and Bendixen, A. (2008). Do N1/MMN, P3a, and RON form a strongly coupled chain reflecting the three stages of auditory distraction? *Biol. Psychol.* 79, 139–147. doi:10.1016/j.biopsycho.2008.04.001

Ikezawa, S., Nakagome, K., Mimura, M., Shinoda, J., Itoh, K., Homma, I., et al. (2008). Gender differences in lateralization of mismatch negativity in dichotic listening tasks. *Int. J. Psychophysiol.* 68, 41–50. doi:10.1016/j.ijpsycho.2008.01.006

International Early Psychosis Association Writing Group. (2005). International clinical practice guidelines for early psychosis. *Br. J. Psychiatry Suppl.* 48, s120–s124. doi:10.1192/bjp.187.48.s120

Itoh, T., Sumiyoshi, T., Higuchi, Y., Suzuki, M., and Kawasaki, Y. (2011). LORETA analysis of three-dimensional distribution of delta band activity in schizophrenia: relation to negative symptoms. *Neurosci. Res.* 70, 442–448. doi:10.1016/j.neures.2011.05.003

Jahshan, C., Cadenhead, K. S., Rissling, A. J., Kirihara, K., Braff, D. L., and Light, G. A. (2012). Automatic sensory information processing abnormalities across the illness course of schizophrenia. *Psychol. Med.* 42, 85–97. doi:10.1017/S0033291711001061

Kasai, K., Yamada, H., Kamio, S., Nakagome, K., Iwanami, A., Fukuda, M., et al. (2002). Do high or low doses of anxiolytics and hypnotics affect mismatch negativity in schizophrenic subjects? An EEG and MEG study. *Clin. Neurophysiol.* 113, 141–150. doi:10.1016/S1388-2457(01)00710-6

Kawasaki, Y., Maeda, Y., Higashima, M., Nagasawa, T., Koshino, Y., Suzuki, M., et al. (1997). Reduced auditory P300 amplitude, medial temporal volume reduction and psychopathology in schizophrenia. *Schizophr. Res.* 26, 107–115. doi:10.1016/S0920-9964(97)00055-8

Kawasaki, Y., Sumiyoshi, T., Higuchi, Y., Ito, T., Takeuchi, M., and Kurachi, M. (2007a). Voxel-based analysis of P300 electrophysiological topography associated with positive and negative symptoms of schizophrenia. *Schizophr. Res.* 94, 164–171. doi:10.1016/j.schres.2007.04.015

Kawasaki, Y., Suzuki, M., Kherif, F., Takahashi, T., Zhou, S. Y., Nakamura, K., et al. (2007b). Multivariate voxel-based morphometry successfully differentiates schizophrenia patients from healthy controls. *Neuroimage* 34, 235–242. doi:10.1016/j.neuroimage.2006.08.018

Kiang, M., Braff, D. L., Sprock, J., and Light, G. A. (2009). The relationship between preattentive sensory processing deficits and age in schizophrenia patients. *Clin. Neurophysiol.* 120, 1949–1957. doi:10.1016/j.clinph.2009.08.019

Leung, S., Croft, R. J., Baldeweg, T., and Nathan, P. J. (2007). Acute dopamine D(1) and D(2) receptor stimulation does not modulate mismatch negativity (MMN) in healthy human subjects. *Psychopharmacology (Berl.)* 194, 443–451. doi:10.1007/s00213-007-0865-1

Lin, Y. T., Liu, C. M., Chiu, M. J., Liu, C. C., Chien, Y. L., Hwang, T. J., et al. (2012). Differentiation of schizophrenia patients from healthy subjects by mismatch negativity and neuropsychological tests. *PLoS ONE* 7:e34454. doi:10.1371/journal.pone.0034454

Loebel, A. D., Lieberman, J. A., Alvir, J. M., Mayerhoff, D. I., Geisler, S. H., and Szymanski, S. R. (1992). Duration of psychosis and outcome in first-episode schizophrenia. *Am. J. Psychiatry* 149, 1183–1188.

Malla, A. K., Norman, R. M., Takhar, J., Manchanda, R., Townsend, L., Scholten, D., et al. (2004). Can patients at risk for persistent negative symptoms be identified during their first episode of psychosis? *J. Nerv. Ment. Dis.* 192, 455–463. doi:10.1097/01.nmd.0000131804.34977.c1

Matsubayashi, J., Kawakubo, Y., Suga, M., Takei, Y., Kumano, S., Fukuda, M., et al. (2008). The influence of gender and personality traits on individual difference in auditory mismatch: a magnetoencephalographic (MMNm) study. *Brain Res.* 1236, 159–165. doi:10.1016/j.brainres.2008.07.120

McGorry, P. D., Nelson, B., Amminger, G. P., Bechdolf, A., Francey, S. M., Berger, G., et al. (2009). Intervention in individuals at ultra-high risk for psychosis: a review and future directions. *J. Clin. Psychiatry* 70, 1206–1212. doi:10.4088/JCP.08r04472

Melle, I., Larsen, T. K., Haahr, U., Friis, S., Johannesen, J. O., Opjordsmoen, S., et al. (2008). Prevention of negative symptom psychopathologies in first-episode schizophrenia: two-year effects of reducing the duration of untreated psychosis. *Arch. Gen. Psychiatry* 65, 634–640. doi:10.1001/archpsyc.65.6.634

Mondragon-Maya, A., Solis-Vivanco, R., Leon-Ortiz, P., Rodriguez-Agudelo, Y., Yanez-Tellez, G., Bernal-Hernandez, J., et al. (2013). Reduced P3a amplitudes in antipsychotic naive first-episode psychosis patients and individuals at clinical high-risk for psychosis. *J. Psychiatr. Res.* 47, 755–761. doi:10.1016/j.jpsychires.2012.12.017

Naatanen, R., Kujala, T., Escera, C., Baldeweg, T., Kreegipuu, K., Carlson, S., et al. (2012). The mismatch negativity (MMN) – a unique window to disturbed central auditory processing in ageing and different clinical conditions. *Clin. Neurophysiol.* 123, 424–458. doi:10.1016/j.clinph.2011.09.020

Naatanen, R., Paavilainen, P., Rinne, T., and Alho, K. (2007). The mismatch negativity (MMN) in basic research of central auditory processing: a review. *Clin. Neurophysiol.* 118, 2544–2590. doi:10.1016/j.clinph.2007.04.026

Nagai, T., Tada, M., Kirihara, K., Yahata, N., Hashimoto, R., Araki, T., et al. (2013). Auditory mismatch negativity and P3a in response to duration and frequency changes in the early stages of psychosis. *Schizophr. Res.* 150, 547–554. doi:10.1016/j.schres.2013.08.005

Nakamura, K., Kawasaki, Y., Suzuki, M., Hagino, H., Kurokawa, K., Takahashi, T., et al. (2004). Multiple structural brain measures obtained by three-dimensional magnetic resonance imaging to distinguish between schizophrenia patients and normal subjects. *Schizophr. Bull.* 30, 393–404. doi:10.1093/oxfordjournals.schbul.a007087

Otten, L. J., Alain, C., and Picton, T. W. (2000). Effects of visual attentional load on auditory processing. *Neuroreport* 11, 875–880. doi:10.1097/00001756-200003200-00043

Ozgurdal, S., Gudlowski, Y., Witthaus, H., Kawohl, W., Uhl, I., Hauser, M., et al. (2008). Reduction of auditory event-related P300 amplitude in subjects with at-risk mental state for schizophrenia. *Schizophr. Res.* 105, 272–278. doi:10.1016/j.schres.2008.05.017

Perkins, D. O., Gu, H., Boteva, K., and Lieberman, J. A. (2005). Relationship between duration of untreated psychosis and outcome in first-episode schizophrenia: a critical review and meta-analysis. *Am. J. Psychiatry* 162, 1785–1804. doi:10.1176/appi.ajp.162.10.1785

Roth, W. T., Pfefferbaum, A., Horvath, T. B., Berger, P. A., and Kopell, B. S. (1980). P3 reduction in auditory evoked potentials of schizophrenics. *Electroencephalogr. Clin. Neurophysiol.* 49, 497–505. doi:10.1016/0013-4694(80)90392-2

Schroger, E., Giard, M. H., and Wolff, C. (2000). Auditory distraction: event-related potential and behavioral indices. *Clin. Neurophysiol.* 111, 1450–1460. doi:10.1016/S1388-2457(00)00337-0

Schroger, E., and Wolff, C. (1998). Attentional orienting and reorienting is indicated by human event-related brain potentials. *Neuroreport* 9, 3355–3358. doi:10.1097/00001756-199810260-00003

Shaikh, M., Valmaggia, L., Broome, M. R., Dutt, A., Lappin, J., Day, F., et al. (2012). Reduced mismatch negativity predates the onset of psychosis. *Schizophr. Res.* 134, 42–48. doi:10.1016/j.schres.2011.09.022

Sumiyoshi, T., Higuchi, Y., Itoh, T., Matsui, M., Arai, H., Suzuki, M., et al. (2009). Effect of perospirone on P300 electrophysiological activity and social cognition in schizophrenia: a three-dimensional analysis with sloreta. *Psychiatry Res.* 172, 180–183. doi:10.1016/j.pscychresns.2008.07.005

Sumiyoshi, T., Higuchi, Y., Kawasaki, Y., Matsui, M., Kato, K., Yuuki, H., et al. (2006). Electrical brain activity and response to olanzapine in schizophrenia: a study with LORETA images of P300. *Prog. Neuropsychopharmacol. Biol. Psychiatry* 30, 1299–1303. doi:10.1016/j.pnpbp.2006.04.028

Sumiyoshi, T., Jayathilake, K., and Meltzer, H. Y. (2003). The effect of melperone, an atypical antipsychotic drug, on cognitive function in schizophrenia. *Schizophr. Res.* 59, 7–16. doi:10.1016/S0920-9964(01)00329-2

Sumiyoshi, T., Miyanishi, T., Seo, T., and Higuchi, Y. (2013). Electrophysiological and neuropsychological predictors of conversion to schizophrenia in at-risk subjects. *Front. Behav. Neurosci.* 7:148. doi:10.3389/fnbeh.2013.00148

Takahashi, T., Zhou, S. Y., Nakamura, K., Tanino, R., Furuichi, A., Kido, M., et al. (2011). A follow-up MRI study of the fusiform gyrus and middle and inferior temporal gyri in schizophrenia spectrum. *Prog. Neuropsychopharmacol. Biol. Psychiatry* 35, 1957–1964. doi:10.1016/j.pnpbp.2011.07.009

Takayanagi, Y., Takahashi, T., Orikabe, L., Mozue, Y., Kawasaki, Y., Nakamura, K., et al. (2011). Classification of first-episode schizophrenia patients and healthy subjects by automated MRI measures of regional brain volume and cortical thickness. *PLoS ONE* 6:e21047. doi:10.1371/journal.pone.0021047

Umbricht, D., Javitt, D., Novak, G., Bates, J., Pollack, S., Lieberman, J., et al. (1998). Effects of clozapine on auditory event-related potentials in schizophrenia. *Biol. Psychiatry* 44, 716–725. doi:10.1016/S0006-3223(97)00524-6

Umbricht, D., and Krljes, S. (2005). Mismatch negativity in schizophrenia: a meta-analysis. *Schizophr. Res.* 76, 1–23. doi:10.1016/j.schres.2004.12.002

Yamazawa, R., Nemoto, T., Kobayashi, H., Chino, B., Kashima, H., and Mizuno, M. (2008). Association between duration of untreated psychosis, premorbid functioning, and cognitive performance and the outcome of first-episode schizophrenia in Japanese patients: prospective study. *Aust. N. Z. J. Psychiatry* 42, 159–165. doi:10.1080/00048670701787537

Yung, A. R., McGorry, P. D., McFarlane, C. A., Jackson, H. J., Patton, G. C., and Rakkar, A. (1996). Monitoring and care of young people at incipient risk of psychosis. *Schizophr. Bull.* 22, 283–303. doi:10.1093/schbul/22.2.353

Yung, A. R., Phillips, L. J., Yuen, H. P., Francey, S. M., McFarlane, C. A., Hallgren, M., et al. (2003). Psychosis prediction: 12-month follow up of a high-risk (prodromal) group. *Schizophr. Res.* 60, 21–32. doi:10.1016/S0920-9964(03)80061-0

Yung, A. R., Yuen, H. P., McGorry, P. D., Phillips, L. J., Kelly, D., Dell'Olio, M., et al. (2005). Mapping the onset of psychosis: the comprehensive assessment of at-risk mental states. *Aust. N. Z. J. Psychiatry* 39, 964–971. doi:10.1080/j.1440-1614.2005.01714.x

7

Distinct phenotypes of new transmembrane-domain neuregulin 1 mutant mice and the rescue effects of valproate on the observed schizophrenia-related cognitive deficits

Ju-Chun Pei[1], Chih-Min Liu[2] and Wen-Sung Lai[1,3,4]*

[1] Laboratory of Integrated Neuroscience and Ethology, Department of Psychology, National Taiwan University, Taipei, Taiwan
[2] Department of Psychiatry, National Taiwan University Hospital, Taipei, Taiwan
[3] Graduate Institute of Brain and Mind Sciences, National Taiwan University, Taipei, Taiwan
[4] Neurobiology and Cognitive Science Center, National Taiwan University, Taipei, Taiwan

Edited by:
Ales Stuchlik, Institute of Physiology Academy of Sciences of the Czech Republic, Czech Republic

****Correspondence:***
Wen-Sung Lai, Department of Psychology, National Taiwan University, 1 Roosevelt Road, Sec. 4, Taipei 10617, Taiwan
e-mail: wslai@ntu.edu.tw

Accumulating evidence suggests that neuregulin 1 (NRG1) might be involved in the neurodevelopment, neural plasticity, GABAergic neurotransmission, and pathogenesis of schizophrenia. NRG1 is abundantly expressed in the hippocampus, and emerging studies have begun to reveal the link between NRG1 signaling and cognitive deficits in schizophrenic patients. Because the transmembrane domain of NRG1 is vital for both forward and reverse signaling cascades, new Nrg1-deficient mice that carry a truncation of the transmembrane domain of the Nrg1 gene were characterized and used in this study to test a NRG1 loss-of-function hypothesis for schizophrenia. Both male and female Nrg1 heterozygous mutant mice and their wild-type littermates were used in a series of 4 experiments to characterize the impact of Nrg1 on behavioral phenotypes and to determine the importance of Nrg1 in the regulation of hippocampal neuromorphology and local GABAergic interneurons. First, a comprehensive battery of behavioral tasks indicated that male Nrg1-deficient mice exhibited significant impairments in cognitive functions. Second, pharmacological challenges were conducted and revealed that Nrg1 haploinsufficiency altered GABAergic activity in males. Third, although no genotype-specific neuromorphological alterations were found in the hippocampal CA1 pyramidal neurons, significant reductions in the hippocampal expressions of GAD67 and parvalbumin were revealed in the Nrg1-deficient males. Fourth, chronic treatment with valproate rescued the observed behavioral deficits and hippocampal GAD67 reduction in Nrg1-deficient males. Collectively, these results indicate the potential therapeutic effect of valproate and the importance of Nrg1 in the regulation of cognitive functions and hippocampal GABAergic interneurons, especially in males.

Keywords: schizophrenia, transmembrane-domain Nrg1 mutant mice, cognitive function, hippocampus, GABAergic interneuron, valproate

INTRODUCTION

Schizophrenia is a costly and devastating mental disorder that afflicts ~1% of the worldwide population (Insel, 2010). It appears to be a multifactorial disorder with a strong genetic predisposition. Accumulating evidence from human genetic studies suggests that multiple susceptibility genes or loci, including *Neuregulin 1* (*NRG1*) (Schwab and Wildenauer, 2009), might contribute to the pathogenesis of schizophrenia. The association between *NRG1* and schizophrenia was initially revealed in a study of families in Iceland (Stefansson et al., 2002), and the association has been further confirmed in other ethnic groups (Walker et al., 2010). Reduced levels of the expression of NRG1 have also been reported in schizophrenic post-mortem tissues (Bertram et al., 2007; Nicodemus et al., 2009; Parlapani et al., 2010), which indicates that alterations in *NRG1* might contribute to the pathophysiology of schizophrenia.

NRG1, a trophic factor, belongs to the neuregulin family of growth factors, whose effects are mediated via four neuregulin genes (*NRG1-4*) that bind to the ErbB (epidermal growth factor-like receptor) family of tyrosine kinase transmembrane receptors (ErbB1-4) (Harrison and Weinberger, 2005; O'Tuathaigh et al., 2006). As a consequence of multiple promoters and rich alternative splicing, more than 30 different NRG1 isoforms produced from a single *NRG1* gene have been identified to date, and these isoforms have been classified into at least 7 different isoform types (Falls, 2003; Steinthorsdottir et al., 2004; Walss-Bass et al., 2006; Mei and Xiong, 2008). Pro-Neuregulin 1, which contains a transmembrane domain (i.e., the TMc domain, a critical motif for forward and reverse signaling cascades) that forms membrane-anchored precursors, undergoes proteolytic cleavage leading to mature NRG1. NRG1, as a ligand and a receptor for ErbB3 and ErbB4, initiates forward or reverse signaling pathways that have numerous neurotrophic roles (Liu et al., 1998a,b; Bao et al., 2003; Falls, 2003), and NRG1 is abundant in many brain regions, especially in the hippocampus (Law et al., 2004). Numerous roles for NRG1 in CNS development and function have been identified, including synapse formation, neuronal migration, axon guidance, axon myelination, synaptic plasticity, and the regulation of neurotransmitter expression (Harrison and Law, 2006; Mei and Xiong, 2008; Iwakura and Nawa, 2013). The abundant expressions of NRG1 and ErbB and the interactions of these molecules with GABAergic (Yau et al., 2003; Vullhorst et al., 2009; Neddens and Buonanno, 2010), glutamatergic (Hahn et al., 2006; Li et al., 2007), and dopaminergic neurons (Abe et al., 2009; Kato et al., 2011) imply that these molecules have critical roles in the regulation of synaptic plasticity at excitatory and inhibitory synapses that might be involved in the pathogenesis of the cognitive deficits in schizophrenia. Indeed, a novel missense mutation (Val to Leu) in the TMc domain of *NRG1* was reported to be associated with schizophrenia (Walss-Bass et al., 2006), suggesting a potential causal mutations within this gene.

Evidence revealing the link between *Nrg1/ErbB4* and cognitive deficits in patients with schizophrenia has begun to accumulate (Hall et al., 2006; Krug et al., 2010). A number of *Nrg1*-related mutant mice have been generated to further elucidate the role of *Nrg1* in the pathogenesis of schizophrenia-related behavioral and cognitive deficits (O'Tuathaigh et al., 2007; Chen et al., 2008; Ehrlichman et al., 2009; Duffy et al., 2010; Wen et al., 2010; Shamir et al., 2012). For example, Nrg1 heterozygous knockout mice with TMc-domain truncation of exon 11 were first reported in 2002 (Stefansson et al., 2002) and this original TMc-*Nrg1*$^{+/-}$ mutant strain has been reported to exhibit behavioral deficits in locomotor activity, explorative behavior, and anxiety-like behaviors (O'Tuathaigh et al., 2006; Boucher et al., 2007). Age-dependent alterations in locomotor activity and exploratory behavior have also been reported in these original TMc-*Nrg1*$^{+/-}$ mutant mice (Karl et al., 2007). Alterations in social and cognitive function have also been reported in these TMc-*Nrg1*$^{+/-}$ mutant mice, such as increased aggression, increased social recognition, decreased prepulse inhibition, and impaired contextual fear conditioning (Stefansson et al., 2002; O'Tuathaigh et al., 2007; Chesworth et al., 2012; Desbonnet et al., 2012). Furthermore, the involvement of *Nrg1* in the modulation of cognitive functions has been further bolstered by *in vitro* electrophysiological studies in the hippocampus of EGF-like domain *Nrg1*$^{+/-}$ mice (Bjarnadottir et al., 2007). A recent study also indicated that ErbB4-null parvalbumin interneuron-restricted mutant mice and EGF-like domain *Nrg1*$^{+/-}$ mice exhibit increased hippocampal LTP (Shamir et al., 2012). These studies suggest the importance of *Nrg1* in the regulation of basic behavioral functions and hippocampal electrophysiology, which might account for the alterations of cognitive functions in these mice. Although some interesting findings were reported, these previous behavioral phenotyping results appear to be somewhat inconsistent across these *Nrg1*-related mutant mice or even across variants of some lines of *Nrg1* mutant mice from one study to another. It is also difficult to make direct comparisons between different lines of mutant mice because different gene targeting strategies were used in different studies and because the expression levels of Nrg1 protein in these haploinsufficient mice are not available due to the lack of antibodies that are capable of recognizing the different isoforms. Besides, in the past decade, most of Nrg1-related mouse studies were conducted in male mice and only a few studies used either female mice or both male and female mice. Interestingly, sex-specific effects were reported. For example, using both male and female TMc-*Nrg1*$^{+/-}$ mutant mice, it was previously found that only male mutant mice had impaired performance in Barnes maze (O'Tuathaigh et al., 2007) and only female mutant mice had reduced grooming behavior (O'Tuathaigh et al., 2006). It is of interest to further compare sex-specific effect on different behavioral tasks in Nrg1-related mutant mice.

To further characterize the effects of *Nrg1* haploinsufficiency and to validate the impact of the complete truncation of the *Nrg1* TMc-domain on cognitive functioning and its behavioral consequences in both males and females, a novel line of TMc-domain *Nrg1*$^{+/-}$ mutant mice with a truncation from exon 9 was obtained and used in this study. A set of four experiments was designed. Because sex (or sex hormones) might have differential effects on NRG/ErbB via glial-neuronal signaling in schizophrenic patients (Lacroix-Fralish et al., 2006; Wong and Weickert, 2009) and because sex-specific effects of Nrg1 on behavioral phenotypes have not been well characterized in mice, both male and female mice were used in Experiments 1–3. In Experiment 1, a comprehensive battery of cognitive-related tasks (Experiment 1A) and basic behavioral tasks (Experiment 1B) was applied to evaluate the behavioral phenotype of the novel TMc-*Nrg1*$^{+/-}$ mutant mice. Experiments 2 and 3 were conducted to facilitate the interpretation of the behavioral deficits observed in Experiment 1. Accordingly, in Experiment 2, MK-801 (an NMDA receptor antagonist), methamphetamine (a potent psychostimulant that increases the amount of extracellular dopamine), and pentylenetetrazol (PTZ, a $GABA_A$ receptor antagonist) were used to induce behavioral alterations and to reveal which neurotransmitters were more vulnerable in these novel TMc-*Nrg1*$^{+/-}$ mutant mice. Neuromorphological and neurochemical alterations in the hippocampi of these mutant mice were further examined in Experiments 3A and 3B, respectively. Based on the findings from the first 3 experiments, an effective and useful procedure of valproate (a *GABA* transaminase inhibitor) treatment (Guidotti et al., 2009) was used to evaluate whether rescue of the observed cognitive deficits in these novel TMc-*Nrg1*$^{+/-}$ mice was possible.

MATERIALS AND METHODS

ANIMALS

All *neuregulin 1* heterozygous mutant mice (*Nrg1*$^{+/-}$) and wild-type (WT) littermate mice used in this study were generated from *Nrg1*$^{+/-}$ breeding pairs with C57BL/6J genetic backgrounds ($n > 10$). Only *Nrg1*$^{+/-}$ mice were used because *Nrg1* homozygous embryos die due to cardiac defects around E10.5–E11.5 (Gassmann et al., 1995; Meyer and Birchmeier, 1995; Kramer et al., 1996). *Nrg1*$^{+/-}$ mice were healthy, and basic physical examination revealed no observable physical damage. Mice were weaned at 4 weeks and separated by sex. Littermates of the same sex were caged separately and maintained in groups of 3–5 mice per cage. For behavioral testing, each mouse was housed individually 1 week before behavioral testing. All mice were housed, with food and water provided *ad libitum*, in individually ventilated polysulfone cages (Alternative design Inc., U.S.A.) within the animal rooms of the Psychology Department of National Taiwan University. All animals used in this study were adult mice (at least 2 months of age). They were handled and weighed daily for at least 1 week prior to each experiment. All behavioral and pharmacological experiments were conducted in the dark phase. Minimal numbers of mice were used to meet the 3R reduction principle of animal use. All animal procedures were performed according to protocols approved by the Animal Care and Use Committee of National Taiwan University. Adequate measures were taken to minimize potential pain and discomfort that the mice used in this study may have experienced.

OBTAINMENT AND VALIDATION OF THE NOVEL TMc-*Nrg1*$^{+/-}$ MICE

Given the fact that the TMc domain of NRG1 is a critical motif for NRG1 forward and reverse signaling cascades and that reduced levels of the expression of NRG1 have been reported in some schizophrenic post-mortem tissues, the validation of this novel TMc-*Nrg1* mutant mouse strain is important and this mouse strain is beneficial to study the effect of TMc domain of *Nrg1* in the pathogenesis of schizophrenia-related symptoms. In complementary to other Nrg1-related mouse strains, this novel strain of mice is also helpful to elucidate the functional consequences of TMc domain ablation and the impact of *Nrg1* TMc-domain complete truncation on behavioral functions. The novel TMc-*Nrg1* mutant mice were originally generated by Lexicon Genetics (NIH-0932, LEXKO-1007) using pKOS-53 with LacZ/Neo cassettes. Using homologous recombination, exon 9 of *Nrg1,* where it was translated into the TMc domain, were targeted and truncated by the LacZ/Neo cassettes. Further information about this mouse has been described previously (http://www.informatics.jax.org/external/ko/lexicon/4608.html). A schematic diagram of the targeting strategy is depicted in **Figure 1A**. The entire sequence encoding the TMc is encoded by a single exon so that the truncated exon can be referred as the TMc exon. Likely due to differences in exon annotations, the targeted TMc exon was previously referred to as exon 11 in the original TMc-*Nrg1* mutant strain (Stefansson et al., 2002) and it was referred to as exon 9 in our novel TMc-*Nrg1* mutant strain here. The expected sizes of the PCR products for the novel TMc-Nrg1 mice are indicated in **Figure 1A** as well. Genomic DNA isolated from the tails of the mice of the indicated genotypes was submitted to PCR, and WT and recombinant alleles were distinguished with agarose gel electrophoresis (**Figure 1B**). The following primers were used to confirm the genotypes of the mice: 0932-8, 5′-GTCATGAAG CATGCCAGCTG-3′; 0932-10, 5′-GTATTACTCAGTCGGGAAC-3′; and Neo3a, 5′-GCAGCGCATCGCCTTCTATC-3′ (**Figure 1**). The TMc domain of *Nrg1* was truncated by the target vector, which resulted in the lack of a C-terminal on Nrg1 and a resistance to proteolytic release. The deletion included the sequence VLTITGICIALLVVGIMCVVAY, which has been described previously as the TMc domain of *Nrg1* (Walss-Bass et al., 2006). The truncated region starts with a hydrophilic part and the majority in this region appears to be hydrophobic (average hydrophobicity = 1.233; >1 means this region is hydrophobic) based on analyses with SOSUI (i.e., a classification and secondary structure prediction system for membrane proteins) (Hirokawa et al., 1998). The result of hydrophobicity analysis predicts that this region is in the very 5′ region of the TMc-domain of Nrg1 and it is translated as a hydrophobic protein structure because most of the amino acids in the TMc-domain are hydrophobic. The expression of Nrg1 protein in the cerebral cortex of the novel TMc-*Nrg1*$^{+/-}$mutant mice was further validated using Western blot with a *Nrg1* C-terminal antibody (Neuregulin-1α/β1/2, 1:500, sc348, Santa Cruz Biotechnology). As indicated in **Figure 1C**, compared to WT littermate controls, a significant (~37%) reduction of Nrg1 protein (~51 kDa) was found in the brains of the novel TMc-*Nrg1*$^{+/-}$ mice [WT: 1 ± 0.013; *Nrg1*$^{+/-}$: 0.628 ± 0.110; $t_{(4)} = 3.373$; $p = 0.027$].

EXPERIMENT 1: EXAMINATION OF THE COGNITIVE AND BASIC BEHAVIORAL FUNCTIONING OF THE NOVEL TMc-*Nrg1*$^{+/-}$ MUTANT MICE

Two cohorts of male and female adult TMc-*Nrg1*$^{+/-}$ mice and their WT littermates were used in this experiment. Two series of experiments were conducted to examine the effects of Nrg1 haploinsufficiency on the cognitive functions (Experiment 1A) and the basic behaviors (Experiment 1B) in these mice. Cognitive function-related behavioral tasks used in this experiment included the object recognition task, contextual and cued fear conditioning, the Morris water maze task, prepulse inhibition, and social preference and recognition task. The object recognition task, contextual fear conditioning, Morris water maze, and social recognition task are considered to be related to hippocampus-dependent function. Cued fear conditioning is considered to rely heavily upon the amygdala. Prepulse inhibition was performed to measure sensorimotor gating function in these mice. Basic behaviors (Experiment 1B) were evaluated with a battery of behavioral tasks that consisted of an open-field locomotor assay, a hole board task, an elevated plus maze task, a sucrose preference task, and a hot plate task. Because it has been reported that some basic behaviors might be age-dependent in the original TMc-*Nrg1* mutant mice (Karl et al., 2007), both novel TMc-*Nrg1*$^{+/-}$ and WT mice were tested twice at ages close to 2 and 6 months for basic behavioral phenotyping and clarification of age-dependent effects. Two cohorts of mice were used. The first cohort of mice ($n = 12$ each) was sequentially tested with the novel object recognition task on post-natal days 63–65 (PND 63–65), with the fear conditioning task on PND 66–70 and with the Morris water maze on PND 90–110. The other cohort of mice (male = 12; female = 10) was tested with the open field task on PND 63 and PND 189, with the hole board task on PND 65 and PND 191, the elevated plus maze task on PND 67 and PND 193, the social preference and recognition task on PND 71, the sucrose preference task on PND 72–75 and PND 199–202, and the prepulse inhibition task on PND 78. The details of the behavioral tasks are briefly described in the Supplementary Materials. These behavioral tasks have been evaluated with varying degrees of test validities for assessing schizophrenia-relevant behavioral deficits in mice (Brooks and Dunnett, 2009; Lai et al., 2014).

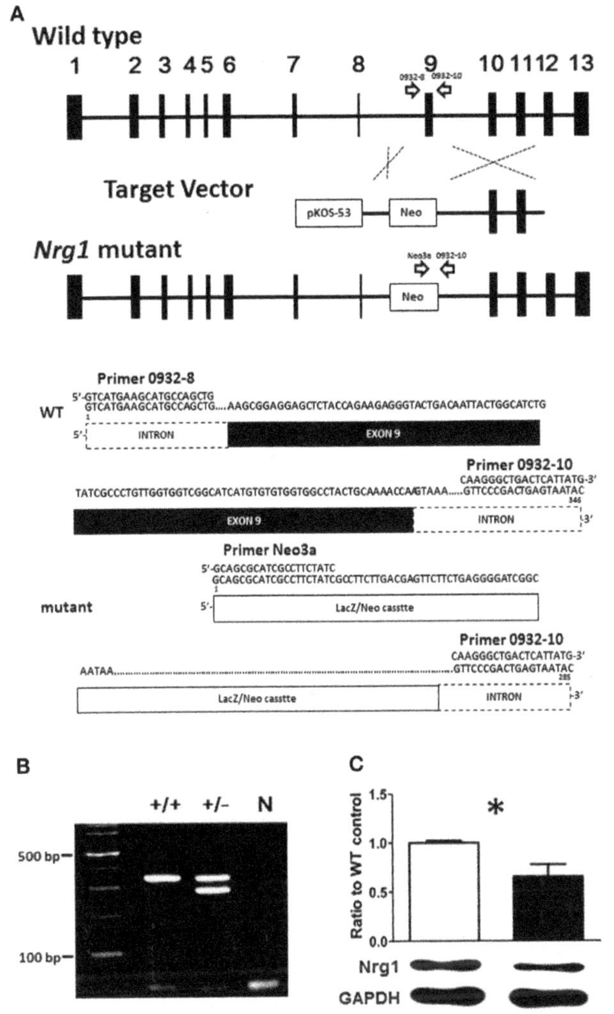

FIGURE 1 | (A) Schematic diagram of the targeting strategy for the novel TMc-*Nrg1*$^{+/-}$ mutant mice. Upper panel, wild type (WT) *Nrg1* locus including 13 exons, shown as black boxes. The target vector, pKOS-53 with a LacZ/Neo cassette, was targeted to exon 9 of *Nrg1* by homologous recombination. Lower panel, primer 0932-8, primer 0932-10, and primer Neo3a were used to distinguish WT alleles (346 bps) from mutant alleles (258 bps). **(B)** Mouse-tail DNA was submitted to PCR analysis. N: negative control. **(C)** The expression level of Nrg1 proteins in the brain of both WT and *Nrg1*$^{+/-}$ mice. *$P < 0.05$ between two genotypes.

EXPERIMENT 2: EVALUATION OF DRUG-INDUCED BEHAVIORAL ALTERATIONS IN THE NOVEL TMc-*Nrg1*$^{+/-}$ MICE

Based on three major neurotransmitter-based hypotheses of schizophrenia (i.e., the dopamine, glutamate, and GABA hypotheses), three related drugs were selected to investigate which neurotransmitter system was most vulnerable to the alterations of behavioral performance observed in our TMc-*Nrg1*$^{+/-}$ mutant mice. Three cohorts of male and female TMc-*Nrg1*$^{+/-}$ and WT adult (2 months of age; $n = 12$ each) mice were used in this experiment. Mice from Experiments 2A–C received an acute administration of MK-801 (an NMDA receptor antagonist, 0.25 mg/kg, i.p.), methamphetamine (a potent psychostimulant, 2 mg/kg, i.p.), or pentylenetetrazol (PTZ, a $GABA_A$ receptor antagonist, 60 mg/kg, s.c.). The volume of administration was 5 ml/kg and the vehicle used in this study was saline (0.9%). The subsequent behaviors of these mice in a polyvinylchloride chamber (48 × 24 × 25 cm) were recorded using an EthoVision video tracking system or ETHOM software (Shih and Mok, 2000). On the day of the measurements, the total distances traveled (cm) by both the male and female mice in the first cohort were recorded in the chamber for 60 min after the administration of saline (0.9%, 5 ml/kg) as a baseline. Then, locomotor activity was recorded for two 60-min periods after the injection of MK-801. For the second cohort of male and female mice, total distances traveled (cm) were also recorded for a 60-min baseline period following the administration of saline and for two 60-min periods following methamphetamine injection. The doses of MK-801 and methamphetamine were chosen to avoid stereotypic behaviors in the open field as described previously (Wu et al., 2005; Van Den Buuse et al., 2009; Chen et al., 2012, 2014). The third cohort of male and female mice received an injection of PTZ to induce a seizure response, and their behaviors were videotaped and recorded in the chamber for 1 h. The dose of PTZ was chosen based on previous dose studies of C57BL/6 mice (Itoh and Watanabe, 2009). The severities of the seizure responses were scored blindly using the following previously described scale: 0, no response; 1, hypoactivity; 2, partial clonus; 3, generalized clonus; and 4, tonic-clonic (maximal) seizure (Ferraro et al., 1999, 2010).

EXPERIMENT 3: EXAMINATION OF THE NEUROMORPHOLOGICAL AND NEUROCHEMICAL ALTERATIONS IN THE HIPPOCAMPI OF THE NOVEL TMc-*Nrg1*$^{+/-}$ MICE

Based on the behavioral deficits observed in Experiment 1A, Experiment 3 concentrated on examination of the neuromorphological alterations of the hippocampi of mutant and WT mice. Based on the findings regarding the drug-induced behavioral alterations of the TMc-*Nrg1*$^{+/-}$ mutant mice in Experiment 2C, we further examined the expression of GABAergic markers in the hippocampi of these mutant mice. Both male and female TMc-*Nrg1*$^{+/-}$ and WT adult (2–4 months of age) mice were used in this experiment. Neuromorphological analyses were first conducted to evaluate whether the haploinsufficieny of Nrg1 resulted in neuromorphological alterations of the pyramidal neurons of the CA1 region of the hippocampus (Experiment 3A). Hippocampal samples from both mutant and WT mice were harvested after behavioral testing to examine protein expression using Western blot (Experiment 3B).

Experiment 3A—neuromorphological analysis of hippocampal CA1 pyramidal neurons

As a follow up to the observations of hippocampal-dependent impairments in the novel TMc-*Nrg1*$^{+/-}$ mutant mice, hippocampi were examined for any neuromorphological alterations in the mutant mice that could partially account for the behavioral deficits. Because pyramidal neurons of the CA1 region of the hippocampus are critical for the afferent and efferent connections of the hippocampus, the C57BL6-*Tg* (GFPm) driven by the Thy1 promoter specific transgenic mouse line was selected and used for analyses of the neuromorphologies of GFP (green fluorescent protein)-labeled CA1 pyramidal neurons of the hippocampus (Feng et al., 2000). The expression patterns of GFP-labeled pyramidal neurons in Thy1-C57BL6-*Tg*(GFPm) transgenic mouse line was reported previously (Feng et al., 2000) and this mouse line has been successfully used to analyze neuromorphological alterations of pyramidal neurons in mutant mice (Lai et al., 2006; Chen and Lai, 2011). Based on the hippocampus-dependent behavioral deficits observed in the novel TMc-$Nrg1^{+/-}$mutant mice, additional male and female subjects generated from our TMc-$Nrg1^{+/-}$ breeding pairs with C57BL6-*Tg* (GFPm) backgrounds were used in this experiment. Adult mice were anesthetized and transcardially perfused with PBS followed by 4% paraformaldehyde in PBS. Fixed brains were sectioned coronally using a vibratome. A series of 150-μm coronal sections were collected and mounted on slides for scanning. Confocal microscopy stack images of GFP-labeled neurons were obtained at intervals of 0.4 μm using 20×, 40×-oil, and 63×-oil objectives from a Leica TCS SP5 confocal microsystem (Leica, Taipei, Taiwan). The Neurolucida software (MicroBrightField Incorporated, Williston, VT, USA) was used to trace and reconstruct the neurons in 3 dimensions. GFP labeling was nearly exclusively restricted to the cell bodies and dendritic trees of CA1 pyramidal neurons of both mutant mice and their littermate controls. Using Neurolucida software, morphometric analyses of the GFP-labeled pyramidal neurons (between Bregma −1.46 and −2.80 mm) of the TMc-$Nrg1^{+/-}$ mice and WT littermate controls were performed (total $n \geqq 4$ each group) to reveal the neuromorphological differences between genotypes. The following 14 morphological variables were chosen based on previous studies (Lai et al., 2006; Chen and Lai, 2011): (1) soma size (cell soma sizes were obtained by outlining cell somas and automatically calculating the pixel areas in μm^2); (2) the distance to apical bifurcation (base of the apical tuft) measured from the cell body to the major branch point of the apical dendrite; (3) the number of branches on the apical branches; (4) the number of apical tips; (5) the total length of the apical tuft, which was taken as the sum of the lengths of the apical stem and the branches that formed the tuft; (6) the apical dendritic field area (ADFA), which measures the area of the dendritic field of a neuron and is calculated as the area enclosed by a polygon that joins the most distal points of the dendritic processes (convex area); (7) the branch angles of the primary apical dendrites (from the distal end of apical bifurcation); (8) the number of primary basal dendrites (not including apical dendrites and axons); (9) the total length of the primary basal dendrites; (10) the number of branches from the basal branches; (11) the number of basal tips; (12) the total length of the basal dendrites; (13) the basal dendritic field area (BDFA), which measures the area of the dendritic field of a neuron and is calculated as the area enclosed by a polygon that joins the most distal points of the dendritic processes (convex area); and (14) Sholl analysis of basal dendritic complexity.

Experiment 3B—examination of the expression of GABAergic markers in the hippocampi of the novel TMc-$Nrg1^{+/-}$ mice

After finishing behavioral testing for cognitive functions in Experiment 1A, some mice from Experiment 1A were randomly selected and used to examine the expression of hippocampal GABAergic markers in this experiment. Hippocampi from both WT and TMc-$Nrg1^{+/-}$ male ($n = 7$ each) and female ($n = 6$ each) adult mice (3–4 months of age) were quickly dissected, frozen in liquid nitrogen, and stored at −80°C. Tissue samples were homogenized in lysis buffer containing 25 mM Tris (pH 8.0), 125 mM NaCl, Protease Inhibitor Cocktail tablets (Roche, Taipei, Taiwan) and Phosphatase Inhibitor Cocktail 1 (P2850, Sigma-Aldrich, St. Louis, MO, USA) and then centrifuged at 12,500 rpm (14324 g) at 4°C for 15 min. The supernatant was then collected. The protein concentrations of the supernatants were measured with the Bradford protein assay (Bio-Rad Laboratories, Tokyo, Japan) and spectrometry at 620 nm. The same amount of protein was separated by 4–10% sodium dodecyl sulfate/polyacrylamide gel electrophoresis (SDS/PAGE) and transferred onto a nitrocellulose membrane (Millipore, Billerica, MA, USA). Ponceau S staining of the membrane was used to ensure successful transfer. Subsequently, the membranes were washed in Tris-buffered saline containing 0.1% Tween-20 (TBST) and blocked in 5% (w/v) skim milk for 1 h at 25°C. The membrane was then incubated in a 5% (w/v) skim milk solution with the appropriate primary antibody overnight at 4°C. The blots were probed with the following antibodies: GAD67 (1:5000, MAB5406, Millipore), calretinin (1:2000, AB5054, Millipore), parvalbumin (1:2000, P3088, Sigma-Aldrich), and GAPDH (1:5000, #2118, Cell Signaling Technology, Inc., Danvers, MA, USA). Immune complexes were visualized using the appropriate peroxidase-conjugated secondary antibodies (Cell Signaling Technology). Bound antibody was detected using an enhanced chemiluminescence (ECL) kit (Millipore), and densitometric analysis was performed using Image J (a Java-based image processing program developed at the National Institutes of Health).

EXPERIMENT 4: EVALUATION OF THE EFFECT OF VALPROATE ON THE RESCUE OF COGNITIVE DEFICITS IN THE NOVEL TMc-$Nrg1^{+/-}$ MALE MICE

Valproate, a *GABAergic* anti-epileptic drug and a potential pharmacoepigenetic agent, has been reported to facilitate GABAergic-promoter demethylation, to inhibit histone deacetylase via chromatin remodeling, and to enhance the expression of GABA-related genes (Guidotti et al., 2009, 2011). To evaluate rescue of the observed behavioral deficits that resulted from GABAergic alternation in young adult (3–4 months of age) TMc-$Nrg1^{+/-}$ male mice, valproate (VPA, 1.5 mmol/kg, s.c.) or vehicle (0.9% saline, 10 ml/kg) was injected into male TMc-$Nrg1^{+/-}$and WT mice twice daily for 17 days (WT/saline: $n = 6$; WT/VPA: $n = 7$; $Nrg1^{+/-}$/saline: $n = 8$; $Nrg1^{+/-}$/VPA: $n = 8$). Based on the findings from Experiment 1A, two behavioral tasks were selected to evaluate the drug's efficacy in rescuing hippocampal function in the mutant mice. The object recognition task was conducted on day 16. Fear conditioning training was conducted on day 16, and contextual/cued tests of fear conditioning were conducted on day 17. Prior to behavioral testing, each subject was left untreated for at least 12 h to exclude any acute effects of daily valproate injection. The behavioral procedures were nearly identical to those described for Experiment 1A, with the exception that the cued fear conditioning tests were conducted 1 h, rather than 1 day, after contextual fear conditioning to reduce the number of testing days. One day after last behavioral testing (on day 18), whole hippocampi from these mice were dissected and processed for Western blotting using GAD67 antibody as described previously in Experiment 3B.

STATISTICAL ANALYSIS

All data are presented as the mean ± standard error of the mean (SEM). Statistical analyses were performed using SPSS 13.0 (SPSS Inc., Chicago, IL, USA), and the data were analyzed with One- or Two-Way ANOVAs or two-sample Student's *t*-tests, where appropriate. *Post-hoc* analyses were performed using Fisher's LSD tests when the *F*-values revealed significant differences. A priori *t*-tests (with Bonferroni adjustments when needed) were conducted to compare genotype-dependent differences and to examine specific hypotheses. *P* values of < 0.05 were considered statistically significant.

RESULTS

EXPERIMENT 1: THE NOVEL TMc-*Nrg1*$^{+/-}$ MICE HAVE NORMAL BASIC BEHAVIORAL FUNCTIONING AND IMPAIRMENTS IN HIPPOCAMPAL-DEPENDENT COGNITIVE FUNCTIONS

Experiment 1A—examination of cognitive-related function

A total of five behavioral tasks were conducted in this experiment. In the object recognition task, a Two-Way ANOVA revealed a significant interaction of genotype and sex [$F_{(1,\ 29)} = 7.222$, $p = 0.012$] on the time spent investigating a novel object. As depicted in **Figures 2A,B**, further statistical analyses reveal a significant simple main effect of genotype for the males ($p = 0.011$) but not the females ($p = 0.309$). Because we intended to examine the sex-specific effects of Nrgl in mice and also because we found a sex difference, the following data analyses were carried out independently for each sex. During fear conditioning, the freezing responses of male TMc-*Nrg1*$^{+/-}$ mice in both contextual [$t_{(22)} = -2.622$, $p = 0.016$; **Figure 2C**] and cued [$t_{(22)} = -2.487$, $p = 0.021$; **Figure 2E**] fear conditioning were significantly reduced compared to WT controls. In contrast, no significant differences due to genotype were found for the female mice (both $p > 0.05$; **Figures 2D,F**). In the Morris water maze, no significant differences due to genotype were found for either the male or female mice during the learning phase (both $p > 0.05$) or the probe phase (both $p > 0.05$), as depicted in **Figures 2G,H.** Regarding sensorimotor gating functions, no genotype-dependent differences were present in either the males ($p > 0.05$; **Figure 2I**) or the females ($p > 0.05$; **Figure 2J**). No genotype-dependent differences were found in their startle response and startle habituation as well. In the social preference and social recognition tasks, no significant genotype-dependent differences were found in either the males ($p > 0.05$; **Figure 2K**) or the females ($p > 0.05$; **Figure 2L**).

Experiment 1B—basic behavioral phenotyping

The basic functioning of the novel TMc-*Nrg1*$^{+/-}$ mice was further examined using a battery of behavioral tasks. As illustrated in **Table 1**, relative to the WT mice, both 2-month-old male and female TMc-*Nrg1*$^{+/-}$ mice displayed normal behavioral profiles across a series of basic behavioral tasks that included the open field, hole board, elevated plus maze, 2% sucrose preference, and hot plate tasks (all *ps* > 0.05). Because age-dependent effects have been previously reported for some *Nrg1* mutant mice, these mice were examined again with the same battery of behavioral tasks at 6 months of age. Again, no genotype-dependent differences were found in either the males or females (**Table 1**).

EXPERIMENT 2: EVALUATION OF DRUG-INDUCED BEHAVIORAL ALTERATIONS IN THE NOVEL TMc-*Nrg1*$^{+/-}$ MICE

Three cohorts of male and female TMc-*Nrg1*$^{+/-}$ and WT adult mice were used to evaluate MK-801-, methamphetamine-, and PTZ-induced behavioral alterations in Experiments 2A–C, respectively. In Experiment 2A, a significant MK-801 treatment effect was found in both males [$F_{(2,\ 44)} = 15.505$, $p < 0.001$] and females [$F_{(2,\ 44)} = 5.188$, $p = 0.009$]. But no significant genotype-dependent differences were found in either the 60-min baseline activity or MK-801-induced hyperlocomotion in either the male (**Figure 3A**) or female mice (**Figure 3B**). Similarly, in Experiment 2B, a significant methamphetamine treatment effect was found in both males [$F_{(2,\ 44)} = 59.680$, $p < 0.001$] and females [$F_{(2,\ 44)} = 126.353$, $p < 0.001$]. But no significant genotype-dependent differences were found in either the 60-min baseline activity or methamphetamine-induced hyperlocomotion in either the male (**Figure 3C**) or female mice (**Figure 3D**). In contrast to the results of Experiments 2A and 2B, the severities of PTZ-induced seizures were significantly greater in male TMc-*Nrg1*$^{+/-}$ mice [$t_{(22)} = -2.288$, $p = 0.032$; **Figure 3E**] but not in female TMc-*Nrg1*$^{+/-}$ mutant mice compared their respective WT controls. This genotype-dependent deficit of the males is further illustrated in **Figure 3F**, which shows the distributions of PTZ-induced seizure scores (**Figure 3F**).

EXPERIMENT 3: EXAMINATION OF NEUROMORPHOLOGICAL AND NEUROCHEMICAL ALTERATIONS IN THE HIPPOCAMPI OF THE NOVEL TMc-*Nrg1*$^{+/-}$ MICE

Experiment 3A—neuromorphological analysis

Based on the cognitive deficits observed in Experiment 1A, the neuronal architectures of the GFP-labeled CA1 pyramidal neurons in the hippocampus were examined. The neuromorphological results are summarized in **Table 2.** Neither the male nor the female mice exhibited any significant genotype-dependent differences in GFP-labeled pyramidal neurons in the CA1 region of hippocampus in any of the morphological variables that we examined.

Experiment 3B—examination of the expression of GABAergic markers in the hippocampus

The protein expression levels of GAD67, parvalbumin (PV), and calretinin were examined in the hippocampi of both male and female mice. Representative images of protein expressions are shown in **Figures 4A,B.** Compared to WT controls, a significant reduction of GAD67 expression was found in our TMc-*Nrg1*$^{+/-}$males [$t_{(12)} = 2.245$, $p = 0.044$; **Figure 4C**] but not in females (**Figure 4D**). Regarding calretinin, no genotype-dependent differences were found in either males or females (**Figures 4E,F**). Regarding parvalbumin, TMc-*Nrg1*$^{+/-}$ males displayed a significant reduction of parvalbumin expression [$t_{(10)} = 2.253$, $p = 0.048$; **Figure 4G**] compared to WT controls,

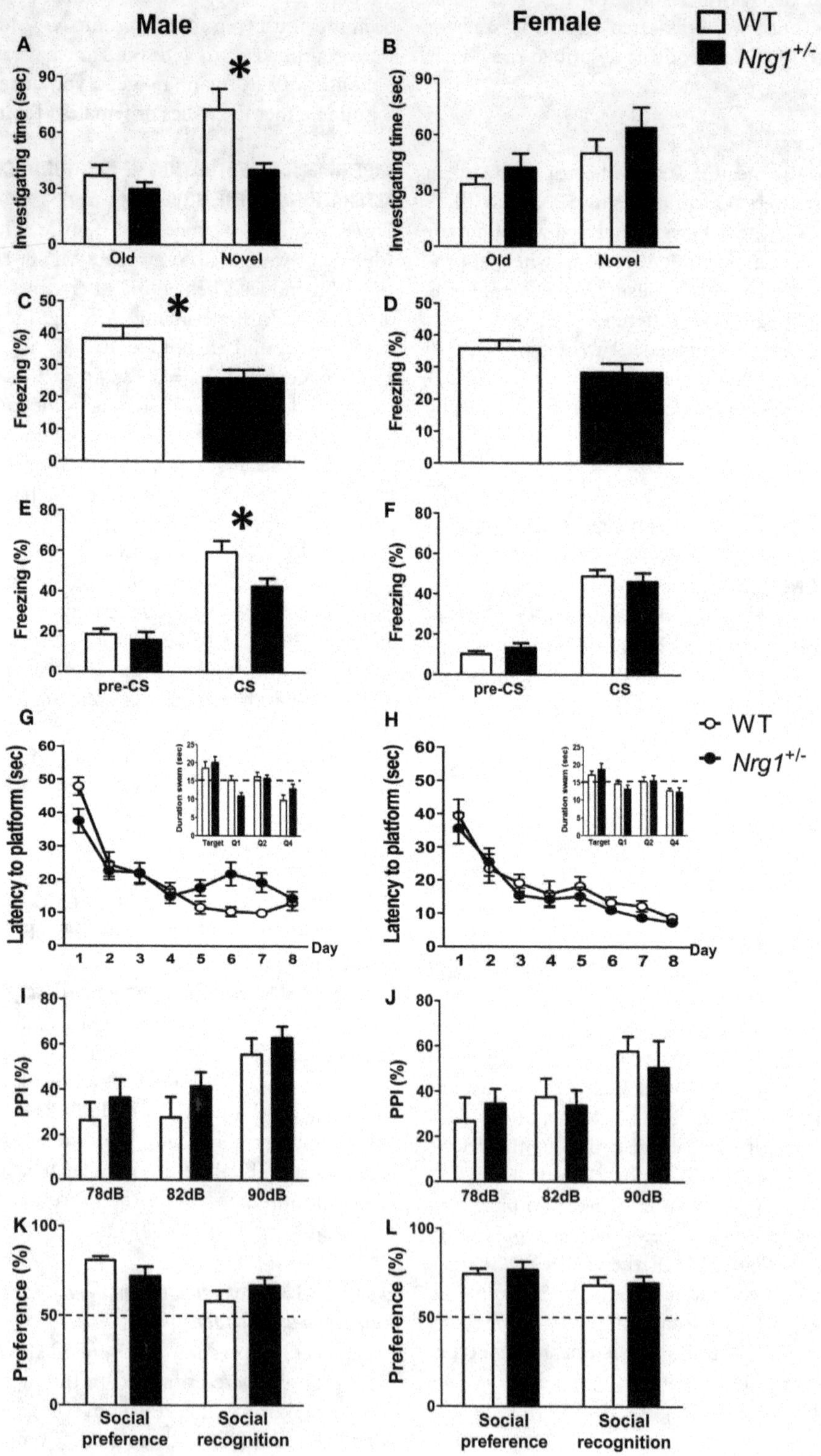

FIGURE 2 | The cognitive functions (mean + s.e.m.) of both male and female TMc-*Nrg1*$^{+/-}$ mutant mice (black bars) and their wild-type littermate controls (WT, white bars) were evaluated in the Experiment 1 of this study. (A,B) In the object recognition task, a reduction in investigation time (s) of the novel object was observed in male, but not female, TMc-*Nrg1*$^{+/-}$ mice. **(C,D)** In the contextual fear conditioning task, a reduction in freezing time percentage was observed in male, but not female, TMc-*Nrg1*$^{+/-}$ mice. **(E,F)** In the cued fear conditioning task, a reduction in freezing time percentage (%) was found in male, but not female, TMc-*Nrg1*$^{+/-}$ mice. In contrast, no significant genotype-dependent differences were found in the Morris water maze, prepulse inhibition task, or the social task in either males **(G,I,K)** or females **(H,J,L)**, respectively. Dash lines indicate chance level. $*P < 0.05$ between two genotypes.

Table 1 | A summary of the basic behavioral phenotyping and statistical analyses (mean ± s.e.m) in the novel TMc-*Nrg1*$^{+/-}$ (*Nrg1*$^{+/-}$) mutant mice and their wild-type (WT) littermates.

Behavioral task	2-month-old				6-month-old			
	Male		Female		Male		Female	
	WT	*Nrg1*$^{+/-}$	WT	*Nrg1*$^{+/-}$	WT	*Nrg1*$^{+/-}$	WT	*Nrg1*$^{+/-}$
Open field	PND 63		PND 63		PND 189		PND 189	
Aversive ratio (central zone/total duration)	0.10 ± 0.12	0.27 ± 0.08	0.11 ± 0.01	0.18 ± 0.08	0.15 ± 0.02	0.21 ± 0.06	0.13 ± 0.01	0.23 ± 0.07
Travel distance (cm)	19350.85 ± 759.67	20391.52 ± 1107.93	17909.69 ± 1688.31	19105.10 ± 1904.06	21729.07 ± 1115.63	22962.49 ± 1272.84	19410.62 ± 1368.97	22920.24 ± 1834.40
Travel distance habituation								
First 10-min (cm)	4774.00 ± 268.28	4931.53 ± 226.45	4470.28 ± 390.28	4844.71 ± 390.78	4560.65 ± 250.31	4915.65 ± 254.11	4261.78 ± 311.75	5216.76 ± 419.29
Second 10-min (cm)	3509.14 ± 219.53	3786.85 ± 283.86	3104.64 ± 374.80	3071.39 ± 440.58	3617.72 ± 251.13	4073.96 ± 191.76	3158.06 ± 267.98	3853.18 ± 335.61
Third 10-min (cm)	3344.77 ± 243.33	3263.94 ± 358.69	2732.59 ± 307.71	2905.19 ± 432.88	3679.20 ± 178.48	3679.68 ± 255.05	3239.92 ± 260.67	3596.45 ± 290.17
Fourth 10-min (cm)	2847.36 ± 159.58	2939.80 ± 197.43	2636.30 ± 272.01	3549.86 ± 547.15	3508.67 ± 253.71	3549.91 ± 254.77	3039.12 ± 257.56	3680.28 ± 290.03
Fifth 10-min (cm)	2564.62 ± 186.07	2946.20 ± 237.96	2671.88 ± 286.70	2419.68 ± 299.39	3417.01 ± 176.23	3408.28 ± 293.49	2905.29 ± 244.49	3376.65 ± 326.67
Sixth 10-min (cm)	2310.97 ± 147.14	2523.20 ± 170.86	2294.01 ± 361.53	2314.27 ± 414.70	2945.82 ± 181.92	3335.02 ± 233.27	2806.45 ± 260.11	3196.92 ± 314.25
Hole board	PND 65		PND 65		PND 191		PND 191	
Number of head dipping (#)	201.67 ± 25.95	189.17 ± 35.00	233.80 ± 52.52	238.90 ± 38.37	124.33 ± 20.19	140.67 ± 21.37	153.40 ± 18.11	180.40 ± 18.01
Travel distance (cm)	6508.39 ± 289.29	6866.35 ± 243.81	6343.31 ± 353.52	7127.08 ± 337.22	6457.39 ± 239.37	6487.12 ± 364.16	6090.96 ± 236.28	7112.74 ± 318.51
Head dipping habituation								
First 5-min (#)	40.75 ± 5.09	36.50 ± 5.58	51.80 ± 10.50	51.50 ± 6.37	21.75 ± 3.29	28.58 ± 4.78	30.20 ± 4.44	42.00 ± 5.63
Second 5-min (#)	39.67 ± 5.38	36.25 ± 6.42	44.90 ± 10.39	48.30 ± 8.27	24.17 ± 4.92	27.92 ± 5.76	30.60 ± 3.79	32.30 ± 4.48
Third 5-min (#)	36.08 ± 5.75	30.00 ± 5.85	37.90 ± 8.48	40.80 ± 6.68	20.42 ± 3.43	22.00 ± 3.05	24.70 ± 3.93	30.10 ± 3.39
Fourth 5-min (#)	30.75 ± 4.76	31.83 ± 7.01	38.80 ± 13.00	37.60 ± 8.48	19.67 ± 5.67	22.00 ± 3.06	24.30 ± 4.73	26.00 ± 3.35
Fifth 5-min (#)	29.00 ± 4.78	28.17 ± 6.30	32.70 ± 7.69	32.80 ± 7.39	20.58 ± 3.74	23.00 ± 4.69	24.10 ± 4.96	26.90 ± 4.25
Sixth 5-min (#)	25.42 ± 4.18	26.42 ± 5.70	27.70 ± 5.01	27.90 ± 4.54	17.75 ± 3.14	17.17 ± 3.73	19.50 ± 3.62	23.10 ± 2.77
Travel distance habituation								
First 5-min (cm)	1269.49 ± 40.78	1357.08 ± 65.25	1289.60 ± 69.55	1392.35 ± 61.02	1330.91 ± 55.53	1328.89 ± 88.20	1282.37 ± 33.57	1381.22 ± 83.26
Second 5-min (cm)	1132.73 ± 44.03	1215.48 ± 62.73	1130.86 ± 68.89	1246.50 ± 49.04	1119.68 ± 43.96	1108.36 ± 81.33	1061.13 ± 37.29	1184.67 ± 55.76
Third 5-min (cm)	1070.93 ± 40.15	1097.51 ± 44.89	1055.56 ± 64.15	1178.20 ± 59.55	1044.60 ± 44.07	1082.08 ± 59.39	943.84 ± 52.58	1184.59 ± 73.09
Fourth 5-min (cm)	1093.80 ± 52.36	1116.40 ± 41.85	977.99 ± 61.45	1115.24 ± 82.81	1045.09 ± 57.52	1030.64 ± 66.32	996.34 ± 42.75	1174.38 ± 63.02
Fifth 5-min (cm)	995.75 ± 68.49	1075.98 ± 39.52	998.38 ± 66.39	1163.19 ± 103.82	985.70 ± 35.07	963.88 ± 45.66	920.71 ± 45.97	1065.95 ± 76.68
Sixth 5-min (cm)	945.69 ± 75.63	1003.89 ± 43.86	890.92 ± 90.25	1031.60 ± 61.97	931.41 ± 57.90	973.27 ± 75.32	886.57 ± 69.46	1121.93 ± 62.33
Elevated plus maze	PND 67		PND 67		PND 193		PND 193	
Aversive ratio (open arm/total duration)	0.20 ± 0.03	0.29 ± 0.05	0.23 ± 0.04	0.29 ± 0.03	0.18 ± 0.06	0.21 ± 0.05	0.17 ± 0.03	0.25 ± 0.05
Number of head dipping (#)	11.92 ± 2.05	15.83 ± 1.99	15.40 ± 2.54	15.80 ± 1.45	10.17 ± 2.50	9.58 ± 1.91	10.20 ± 1.30	12.10 ± 2.16
Number of rearing (#)	10.42 ± 1.10	13.42 ± 2.05	13.00 ± 2.16	12.10 ± 1.91	11.58 ± 1.76	14.00 ± 1.86	15.10 ± 2.05	13.90 ± 2.34

(Continued)

Table 1 | Continued

Behavioral task	2-month-old				6-month-old			
	Male		Female		Male		Female	
	WT	$Nrg1^{+/-}$	WT	$Nrg1^{+/-}$	WT	$Nrg1^{+/-}$	WT	$Nrg1^{+/-}$
Sucrose preference	PND 72–75		PND 72–75		PND 199–202		PND 199–202	
2% sucrose preference (%)	78.78 ± 2.10	80.32 ± 1.80	82.21 ± 1.74	81.59 ± 2.14	81.07 ± 1.94	80.35 ± 3.56	83.96 ± 3.28	78.03 ± 3.31
2% sucrose preference habituation								
Day 1 sucrose preference (%)	75.68 ± 2.19	81.66 ± 1.97	81.12 ± 1.97	76.87 ± 5.58	81.98 ± 2.23	74.41 ± 5.85	78.49 ± 5.65	71.36 ± 8.27
Day 2 sucrose preference (%)	77.42 ± 4.95	82.54 ± 1.24	80.60 ± 4.72	83.77 ± 2.10	80.40 ± 3.71	79.43 ± 5.77	83.95 ± 7.26	78.94 ± 4.65
Day 3 sucrose preference (%)	83.25 ± 1.27	76.77 ± 5.77	84.83 ± 3.02	84.14 ± 1.41	80.84 ± 4.54	87.20 ± 2.35	87.73 ± 2.12	83.81 ± 3.59

A series of four basic behavioral tests (left column, from top to bottom), including the open-field task, the hole board task, the elevated plus maze, and the sucrose preference task, were conducted repeatedly at ages close to 2 and 6 months in these mice. There were no significant differences between genotypes in either sex at any age. PND, post-natal day.

whereas the females did not exhibit this reduction (**Figure 4H**). The sex-specific reductions of hippocampal GAD67 and parvalbumin expression found in the TMc-*Nrg1*$^{+/-}$ males of this experiment might be responsible for the observed cognitive deficits of these mice.

EXPERIMENT 4: EVALUATION OF THE EFFECT OF VALPROATE ON THE RESCUE OF COGNITIVE DEFICITS IN THE NOVEL TMc-*Nrg1*$^{+/-}$ MALE MICE

Based on the findings of Experiments 1A, 2, and 3B, chronic administration of valproate was used to evaluate the effects of valproate on the rescue of the cognitive deficits that were observed in the male TMc-*Nrg1*$^{+/-}$ mice. As reported in Experiment 1A, significant genotype-dependent reductions in behavioral performance on the object recognition task [$t_{(12)} = 2.351$, $p = 0.037$; **Figure 5A**], the contextual fear conditioning task [$t_{(12)} = 2.556$, $p = 0.025$; **Figure 5B**], and the cued fear conditioning task [$t_{(12)} = 2.469$, $p = 0.029$; **Figure 5C**] were found in the male TMc-*Nrg1*$^{+/-}$mice that received chronic saline injections. In contrast, after chronic injections of valproate, male TMc-*Nrg1*$^{+/-}$mice did not display any significant deficits in these tasks compared to WT control males (all $p > 0.05$; **Figures 5A–C**). For the expression of GAD67 in the hippocampus, a significant genotype-dependent reduction (~26%) of GAD67 was found in mice that received chronic saline treatment [$t_{(10)} = 2.651$; $p = 0.024$; **Figure 5D**]. In contrast, no significant reduction was found in the TMc-*Nrg1*$^{+/-}$ male mice that received chronic valproate injections compared to their WT controls.

DISCUSSION

The use of genetically modified mice that carry a truncated TMc domain-*Nrg1* gene as an experimental tool offers an alternative model with which to mimic a NRG1 deficiency in some schizophrenic patients and to test a NRG1 loss-of-function hypothesis for schizophrenia. In complementary to the original TMc-Nrg1 mutant strain and other mutant strains, the impact of TMc exon ablation can be studied in both sexes using this novel TMc-*Nrg1*$^{+/-}$ mouse strain and its functional consequences can be compared with findings in other Nrg1-related mouse strains. A significant reduction of Nrg1 proteins was also confirmed in the brain of this novel mutant strain. This novel TMc-*Nrg1*$^{+/-}$ mouse strain provides a feasible model for the characterization of the roles of the TMc domain of *Nrg1* in basic behaviors and cognitive functions. In Experiment 1, we found that both male and female TMc-*Nrg1*$^{+/-}$ mice displayed normal profiles of basic behaviors but were impaired in cognition-related functions. In Experiment 2, we found that, compared to WT controls, the injection of PTZ induced significant behavioral alterations in male (but not female) TMc-*Nrg1*$^{+/-}$mice, whereas the other two drugs we tested had no effect. In Experiment 3, neuromorphological analyses failed to reveal any *Nrg1* genotype-dependent effects on the neuronal architecture of the GFP-labeled CA1 pyramidal neurons in the hippocampi of either male or female mice. However, reductions of GAD67 and parvalbumin expression were found in the hippocampi of male TMc-*Nrg1*$^{+/-}$ mice, and females did not exhibit these reductions. In Experiment 4, the chronic administration of valproate successfully rescued the observed cognitive

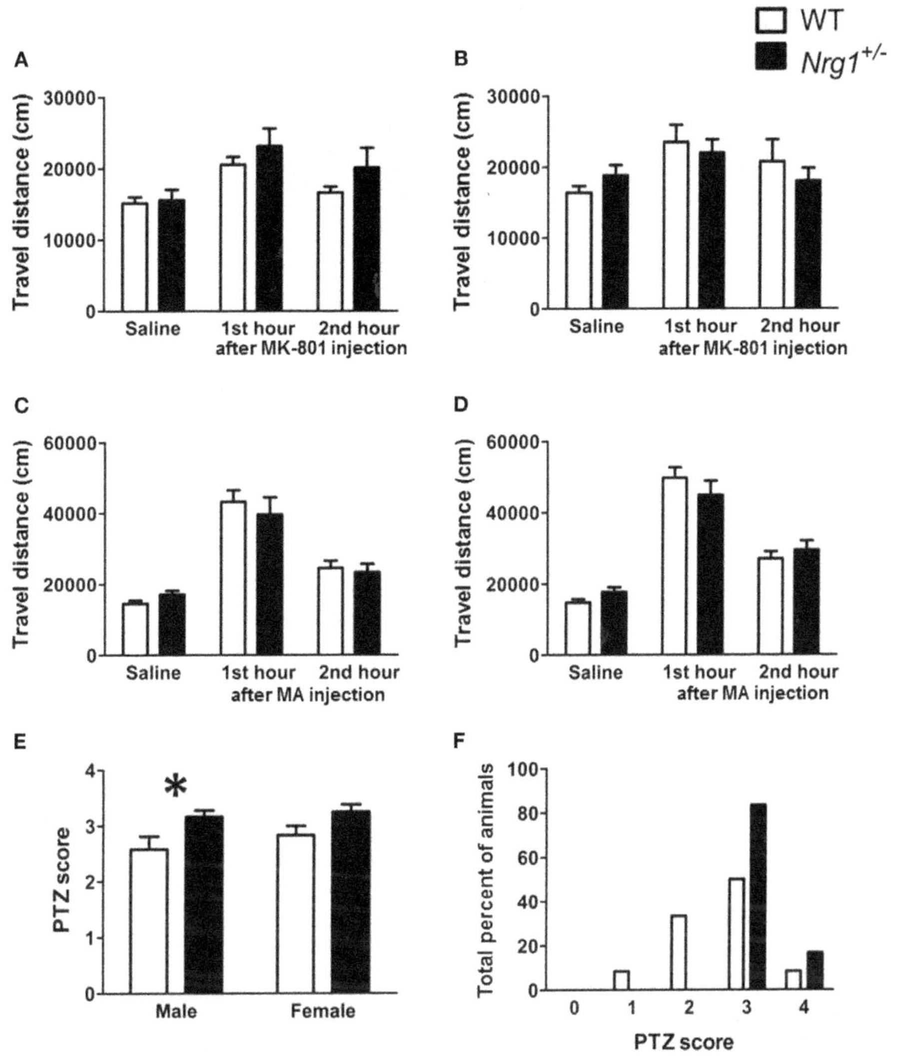

FIGURE 3 | Drug-induced behavioral alterations (mean + s.e.m.) in the novel TMc-*Nrg1*$^{+/-}$ mice (black bars) and their wild-type controls (WT, white bars) (n = 12 each group) of this study. (A,B) Total travel distances for the two groups of male and female mice during the 1-h saline baseline and the 1st and 2nd 1-h periods after the injection of MK-801 (0.25 mg/kg, i.p.). **(C,D)** Total travel distances (mean + s.e.m.) for the two groups of male and female mice during the 1-h saline baseline and during the 1st and 2nd 1-h periods after the injection of methamphetamine (MA, 2 mg/kg i.p.). **(E)** PTZ (60 mg/kg, s.c.)-induced seizure severity scores [from 0 (no response) to 4 (maximal seizure)] for both male and female mice. **(F)** Distributions of PTZ-induced seizure severity scores for male mice (%). $^*P < 0.05$ between two genotypes.

deficits of male TMc-*Nrg1*$^{+/-}$ mice and hippocampal GAD67 expression.

To the best of our knowledge, this study is the first to characterize behavioral phenotypes of this novel TMc-*Nrg1*$^{+/-}$ mutant strain. We also illustrated and verified that the truncated region had a hydrophobic protein structure that was located in the TMc of Nrg1. In complementary to those existing Nrg1-related mutant mouse strains, this novel mouse strain used in this study can be referred as a novel TMc-Nrg1 mutant strain. Our behavioral phenotyping data indicated that the truncation of the TMc domain in our TMc-Nrg1 mutant mice affected some cognitive functions but apparently did not have any effect on basic behaviors. The basic behavioral data reported in the present study, along with data regarding the basic behavioral phenotypes that have been reported for different lines of *Nrg1*-related mutant mice, are summarized in **Table 3**. There are several inconsistencies in this dataset; for example, PPI deficits have been observed in studies of type III Nrg1 mutant mice (Chen et al., 2008), *ErbB4* mutant mice (Shamir et al., 2012), ErbB2/4 mutant mice (Barros et al., 2009), and NRG1-overexpressing transgenic mice (Deakin et al., 2009; Kato et al., 2010), and in some (but not all) studies of the original TMc-*Nrg1* mutant mice (Stefansson et al., 2002; Desbonnet et al., 2012). These original TMc-*Nrg1*$^{+/-}$ mutant mice have been widely used in recent years. It is of great interest to compare the behavioral phenotypes of these original TMc-Nrg1 mutant mice with those of our novel TMc-*Nrg1* mutant mice. As indicated in **Table 3**, the behavioral phenotypes of the original TMc-*Nrg1*$^{+/-}$ mutant mice seem to vary somewhat across studies. Generally,

Table 2 | Neuromorphological analyses (mean ± s.e.m.) of GFP-labeled pyramidal neurons in the hippocampi of male and female TMc-*Nrg1*$^{+/-}$ (*Nrg1*$^{+/-}$) mice and their wild-type (WT) littermate controls.

		Male		Female	
		WT	***Nrg1***$^{+/-}$	**WT**	***Nrg1***$^{+/-}$
Soma size (μm^2)		92.090 ± 4.974	86.850 ± 5.725	86.270 ± 4.278	80.190 ± 6.040
Distance to apical bifurcation (μm)		241.100 ± 55.430	265.200 ± 66.730	257.100 ± 57.750	249.200 ± 65.130
Number of branches of apical branches		19.000 ± 2.781	18.170 ± 1.249	19.880 ± 2.356	19.500 ± 1.268
Number of apical tips		20.000 ± 2.781	18.830 ± 1.138	20.630 ± 2.412	20.380 ± 1.322
Total length of the apical tuft (μm)		3009.000 ± 397.700	2621.000 ± 465.900	2973.000 ± 370.100	2593.000 ± 348.000
Apical dendritic field area (ADFA) (× 1000 μm^2)		11.100 ± 1.644	9.512 ± 2.588	10.850 ± 1.493	9.532 ± 1.980
Branch angle of primary apical dendrites (°)		49.270 ± 4.899	68.800 ± 13.010	69.650 ± 11.360	48.420 ± 7.560
Number of primary basal dendrites		3.444 ± 0.242	3.900 ± 0.315	3.286 ± 0.360	3.400 ± 0.221
The total length of primary basal dendrites (μm)		79.310 ± 16.820	87.610 ± 13.460	95.000 ± 30.090	69.120 ± 13.810
Number of branches of basal branches		20.110 ± 1.989	19.400 ± 0.957	22.430 ± 1.757	21.900 ± 1.980
Number of basal tips		22.780 ± 1.722	23.000 ± 1.000	25.000 ± 1.464	24.900 ± 1.894
The total length of basal dendrites (μm)		3301.000 ± 293.600	3001.000 ± 294.600	3590.000 ± 317.500	3179.000 ± 429.300
Basal dendritic field area (BDFA) (× 1000 μm^2)		10.230 ± 1.309	8.047 ± 1.077	10.690 ± 1.284	10.720 ± 1.893
Sholl analysis of basal dendritic complexity					
Distance to soma (μm)	10	0.444 ± 0.342	1.900 ± 0.795	0.429 ± 0.578	1.300 ± 0.297
	20	4.222 ± 0.946	4.800 ± 0.712	3.571 ± 0.563	4.500 ± 0.429
	30	5.333 ± 1.108	7.100 ± 1.016	5.429 ± 0.674	7.100 ± 0.841
	40	7.333 ± 1.308	9.900 ± 1.394	10.140 ± 0.702	9.600 ± 0.829
	50	10.110 ± 0.955	12.400 ± 1.376	12.290 ± 0.605	11.900 ± 0.680
	60	12.000 ± 1.065	13.200 ± 1.083	13.570 ± 0.359	13.200 ± 0.841
	70	13.110 ± 0.872	14.500 ± 0.860	15.860 ± 0.716	14.300 ± 0.857
	80	14.110 ± 1.138	15.800 ± 0.554	17.000 ± 1.024	14.600 ± 0.951
	90	15.000 ± 1.065	16.400 ± 0.806	16.570 ± 1.016	15.100 ± 0.896
	100	14.780 ± 1.265	15.800 ± 0.827	16.570 ± 1.083	15.200 ± 1.088
	>100	9.127 ± 0.632	8.756 ± 0.725	9.108 ± 1.076	8.335 ± 0.509

this line of mutant mice has been reported to exhibit behavioral deficits in some behavioral tasks, such as the PPI, social recognition, and open field tasks (Stefansson et al., 2002; O'Tuathaigh et al., 2006, 2007; Boucher et al., 2007; Karl et al., 2007; Van Den Buuse et al., 2009; Chesworth et al., 2012; Desbonnet et al., 2012). However, our novel TMc-*Nrg1*$^{+/-}$ mutant mice did not exhibit any significant impairment in these behavioral tasks. We also found no age-dependent effects in our novel TMc-Nrg1 mutant mice after examination at 2 and 6 months of age; this result is similar to reports that the age of onset is not associated with the NRG1 genotype in patients with schizophrenia (Kampman et al., 2004; Voineskos et al., 2009). In contrast, Karl et al. reported that the original TMc-*Nrg1*$^{+/-}$ mutant mice do not display age-dependent hyperlocomotion until the age of 4.5 months (Karl et al., 2007), but these mice have been found to exhibit hyperlocomotion at 3 month of age in other studies (Van Den Buuse et al., 2009). Different targeting strategies were used to generate our new TMc-*Nrg1* mutant mice and the original TMc-*Nrg1* mutant mice. But as we described previously, it is possible that both TMc-*Nrg1* mutant mouse strains are targeting the same TMc exon due to differences in exon annotation. To further verify this possibility, we conducted a nucleotide BLAST search using our primer set and the forward primer sequence reported previously (Liu et al., 1998a; Lai et al., 2010). Based on the location of the forward primer and the size of PCR product, we found that the forward primer used for the original TMc-Nrg1 mutant mice located ~951 bps upstream of the forward primer used for our new TMc-Nrg1 mutant mice, suggesting both TMc-*Nrg1* mutant mouse strains are targeting the same exon. However, it should be noted that different targeting strategies can result in different biological functions. As far as we can tell from previous literatures (Liu et al., 1998a; Lai et al., 2010), the original TMc-*Nrg1* mutant strain was designed to generate most soluble forms of Nrg1 by replacing the TMc exon with a mini-exon that introduces stop codons right upstream of the TMc. In contrast, our new TMc-*Nrg1* mutant mice have no such added stop codons and are more likely to result in complete functional knockout of all Nrg1 isoforms except for those that naturally terminate before the TMc (such as SMDF). In addition to biological difference, above-mentioned discrepancy could be due to different experimental designs, different experimental procedures (Van Den Buuse et al., 2009; Karl et al., 2011), age differences, or genetic background differences. As indicated in **Table 3**, differences in gene targeting strategy and the truncation of different domains or exon location in *Nrg1* gene appear to have differential effects on behavioral performance.

A sex-specific effect of Nrg1 on cognitive function was found in Experiment 1 of this study. Our male TMc-*Nrg1*$^{+/-}$ mutant mice exhibited behavioral deficits in the novel object recognition task, contextual fear conditioning task, and cued fear

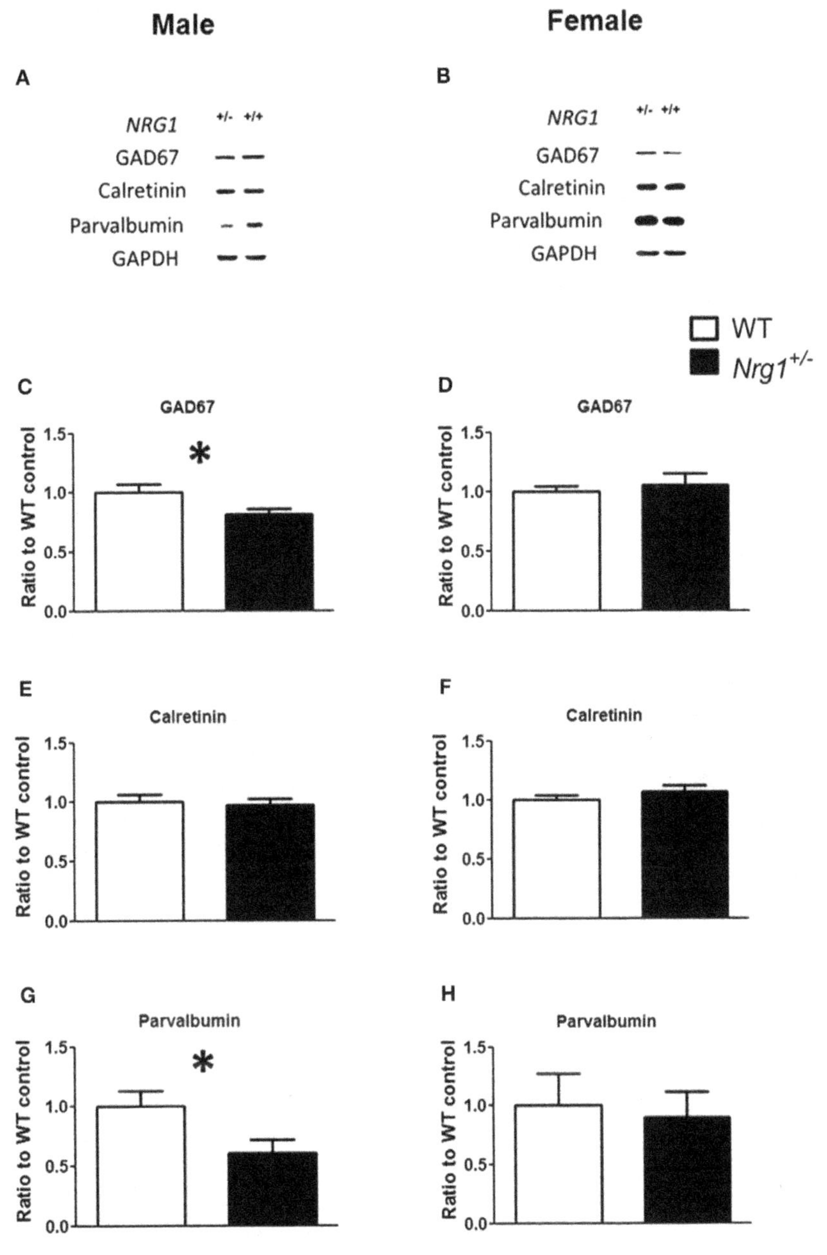

FIGURE 4 | The neurochemical analysis of the expression of GABAergic markers in the hippocampi of the novel TMc-*Nrg1*$^{+/-}$mutant mice (black bars) and their wild-type controls (WT, white bars) determined by Western blot. (A,B) Representative Western blots of hippocampal tissue (30 μg/lane) with GAD67 (67 kDa), calretinin (29 kDa), parvalbumin (12 kDa), and GAPDH (37 kDa) from males and females. **(C–H)** Quantification of the data revealed reductions in GAD67 and parvalbumin expression levels in the hippocampi of male **(C,E,G)**, but not female **(D,F,H)**, TMc-*Nrg1*$^{+/-}$mice. Data are presented as the mean + s.e.m. *$P < 0.05$ between two genotypes.

conditioning task, whereas females did not display these impairments. As indicated in **Table 3**, many *Nrg1*-related studies have only been conducted on male mice. Interestingly, either haploinsufficiency of Nrgl or overexpression of Nrgl (Deakin et al., 2009, 2012; Kato et al., 2010) in mice can result in some types of cognitive deficits, which implies a possible U-shaped relationship between Nrgl expression and cognitive function, which has been reported for the *COMT* gene (Honea et al., 2009). Few studies have examined female mice, and these studies have reported that the original TMc-*Nrg1*$^{+/-}$ mutant female mice exhibit hyperlocomotion, altered social recognition, and impaired contextual and cued fear conditioning (O'Tuathaigh et al., 2006, 2007; Chesworth et al., 2012). In contrast, both male and female TMc-*Nrg1*$^{+/-}$ mutants and their WT littermates were examined in this study. The basic and cognitive functions of our novel TMc-*Nrg1*$^{+/-}$ mutant female mice seemed to be largely unaffected when compared to their female WT controls. The sex-specific alterations of cognitive function observed in our

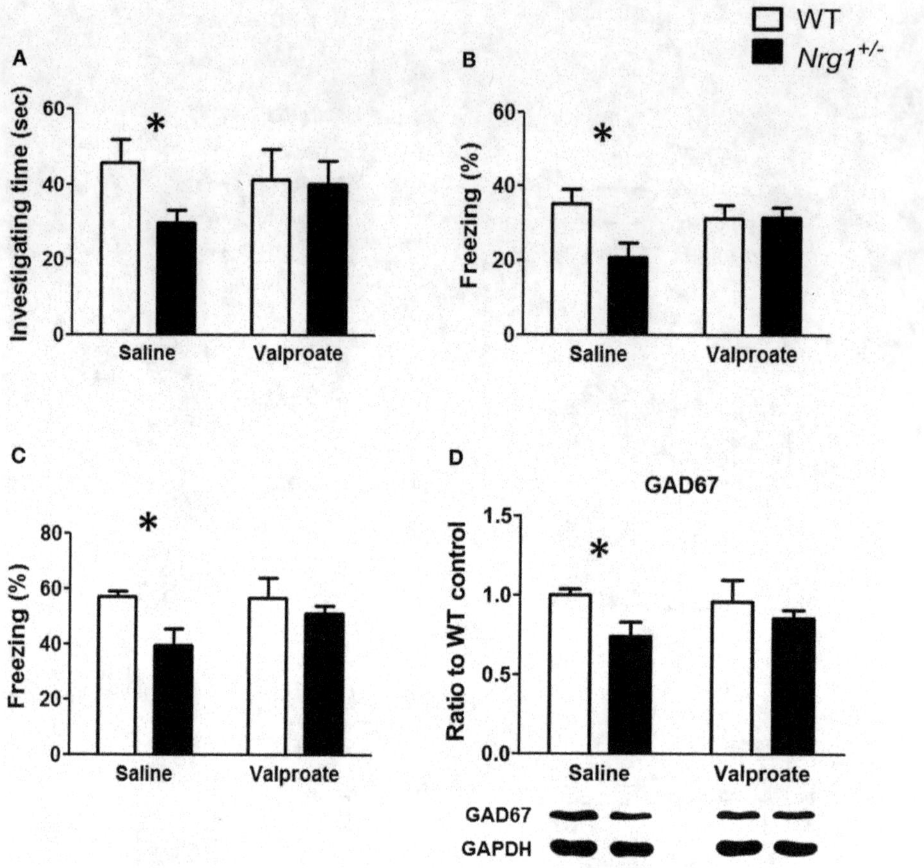

FIGURE 5 | The effect of chronic valproate treatment on the rescue of cognitive deficits in male wild-type (WT, white bars) and TMc-*Nrg1*$^{+/-}$ mutant (black bars) mice. Three cognitive tasks, including **(A)** an object recognition task, **(B)** a contextual fear conditioning task, and **(C)** a cued fear conditioning task, were conducted. Either valproate (1.5 mmol/kg, s.c.) or 0.9% saline was injected twice a day for 17 days. The object recognition task was conducted on day 16,and the contextual/cued tests of fear conditioning were performed on day 17. **(D)** The expression of GAD67 in the hippocampus of both WT and TMc-*Nrg1*$^{+/-}$ mice after chronic injections of either saline or valproate. Data are presented as the mean + s.e.m. $*P < 0.05$ between two genotypes.

male TMc-*Nrg1*$^{+/-}$mutant mice are somewhat consistent with the gender-specific differences in patients with schizophrenia (Kulkarni et al., 2012). This finding also suggests a potential interaction between NRG1/ErbB signaling and sex hormones (e.g., estrogen) in the regulation of schizophrenia-related cognitive deficits; a similar interaction has been described in human studies (Wong and Weickert, 2009; Agim et al., 2013). Examination of the protective effects of estrogen (i.e., the estrogen protection hypothesis of schizophrenia) in our TMc-*Nrg1* mutant mice is warranted.

In Experiment 2, based upon major neurotransmitter-based hypothesis of schizophrenia, 3 related drugs were chosen to evaluate drug-induced behavioral alterations in our novel TMc-*Nrg1*$^{+/-}$mutant mice. Our behavioral data revealed a sex-specific effect of PTZ (but not MK-801 or methamphetamine) on PTZ-induced responses in male TMc-*Nrg1*$^{+/-}$mutant mice. It has been reported that Nrg1 interacts with NMDA receptors through Fyn kinase and Pyk2 (proline-rich tyrosine kinase 2) and that attenuated Nrg1 signaling affects the phosphorylation of NR2B receptors in *Nrg1*$^{+/-}$mutant mice with either TMc-domain truncation or EGF-like domain truncation (Bjarnadottir et al., 2007). Moreover, subchronic injections of MK-801 (0.2 mg/kg, s.c.) disrupt sociability and social novelty preference in the original TMc-*Nrg1*$^{+/-}$mutant mice (O'Tuathaigh et al., 2010). However, compared with WT controls, different doses of MK-801 (0.01, 0.05, 0.25 mg/kg, i.p.) did not affect MK-801-induced hyperlocomotion in the original TMc-*Nrg1*$^{+/-}$ mutant mice (Van Den Buuse et al., 2009), which is consistent with our current findings in the new TMc-*Nrg1*$^{+/-}$mutant mice. Additionally, no significant differences were found in [^{3}H]MK-801 and [^{3}H]kainate binding levels with Nrg1 status in the brains of the original TMc-*Nrg1*$^{+/-}$ mutant mice using *in situ* radioligand binding (Dean et al., 2008). Glutamate and GABA concentrations in the brains of these original TMc-*Nrg1*$^{+/-}$ mutant mice also did not differ from those of WT mice (O'Tuathaigh et al., 2010). In contrast, alteration of GABAergic neurons is considered as one of the most reliable abnormalities found in post-mortem analyses of the schizophrenic brain (Lewis et al., 2005). Accumulating evidence emerging from human genetic studies suggests the involvement of GABA-A receptor subunit genes in schizophrenia (Lewis et al., 2003) and the genetic link between GAD67 and early-onset schizophrenia (Addington et al., 2005). Dysfunction of cerebral

Table 3 | Summary of the behavioral phenotypes and comparison of the different lines of *Nrg1*-related mutant mice.

Genetic mouse model for	Behavioral phenotype						
	Learning and memory	Sensorimotor gating and information processing	Social	Motor function and locomotor activity	Explorative behavior	Anxiety-like behavior	Hedonia
TM domain (exon 9, the novel TMc-Nrg1 mutant mice) Background: C57BL/6	Object recognition ♂↓ Contextual FC ♂↓ Cued FC ♂↓ WMW =	PPI =	Preference = Recognition =	OF = HB =	HB = EPM =	EPM =	Sucrose =
TM domain (exon 11, the original TMc-Nrg1 mutant mice) Background: C57BL/6	Object recognition ↓ Contextual FC ↓ Passive avoidance = (Duffy et al., 2010) ♀(Chesworth et al., 2012) Cued FC = (Duffy et al., 2010) Cued FC ↓ ♀(Chesworth et al., 2012) Radial arm maze = (Duffy et al., 2010) Y-maze = ♂♀(O'Tuathaigh et al., 2007) (Duffy et al., 2010) ♀(Desbonnet et al., 2012) Barnes maze ↓ ♂(O'Tuathaigh et al., 2007) Cheeseboard = ♀ (Chesworth et al., 2012)	PPI = (Boucher et al., 2007) (Van Den Buuse et al., 2009) PPI ↓ (Stefansson et al., 2002) (Desbonnet et al., 2012) Startle = (Boucher et al., 2007) Startle ↓ (Desbonnet et al., 2012)	Preference = Recognition ↓ (O'Tuathaigh et al., 2007) (Desbonnet et al., 2012) Interaction = (Boucher et al., 2007) (Desbonnet et al., 2012) Aggression ↑ ♂♀(O'Tuathaigh et al., 2007) (O'Tuathaigh et al., 2008) Aggression = Agonistic behavior ↑ (Desbonnet et al., 2012) Agonistic behavior = (Boucher et al., 2007) (O'Tuathaigh et al., 2008)	OF ↑ (Stefansson et al., 2002) ♂♀(O'Tuathaigh et al., 2006) (Boucher et al., 2007) PND 138 (Karl et al., 2007) 15-week-old ♀(Chesworth et al., 2012) 3-month-old (Van Den Buuse et al., 2009) OF = PND 91 (Karl et al., 2007) 7–8-month-old (Van Den Buuse et al., 2009)	Explorative behavior ↑ ♀ (O'Tuathaigh et al., 2006) HB ↑ LD ↑ (vertical activity) (Boucher et al., 2007) (Karl et al., 2007) LD = (Karl et al., 2007)	OF = (Boucher et al., 2007) OF ↓ (PND138; 60) (Karl et al., 2007) (Desbonnet et al., 2012) EPM ↓ LD ↑ (Boucher et al., 2007) EPM = LD = (Karl et al., 2007) (O'Tuathaigh et al., 2008)	Sucrose = (Desbonnet et al., 2012)

(Continued)

Table 3 | Continued

Genetic mouse model for	Behavioral phenotype						
	Learning and memory	**Sensorimotor gating and information processing**	**Social**	**Motor function and locomotor activity**	**Explorative behavior**	**Anxiety-like behavior**	**Hedonia**
EGF-like Domain (exon 6) Background: C57BL/6 (Duffy et al., 2008)	Contextual FC ↓ Object recognition = (Ehrlichman et al., 2009)	PPI = (Duffy et al., 2008) (Ehrlichman et al., 2009)	Recognition ↓ (Ehrlichman et al., 2009)	OF ↑ LD ↑ Marble burying = (Duffy et al., 2008)	HB = (Duffy et al., 2008)	OF ↓ EPM = LD = (Duffy et al., 2008)	
C57BL/6 × 129/SVEV (Ehrlichman et al., 2009)	Cross maze = (Duffy et al., 2008)	MMN ↓ P20 = P40 = (Ehrlichman et al., 2009)		OF= (Ehrlichman et al., 2009) Bar test = Rotard rod = (Michailov et al., 2004)			
Ig-like domain (exon 3) Background: C57BL/6	T maze = Latent inhibition ↓ (Rimer et al., 2005)			Running wheel = (Rimer et al., 2005)			
Type III Background: C57BL/6	DNMS ↓ (Chen et al., 2008)	PPI ↓ (Chen et al., 2008)		OF = (Chen et al., 2008)			
ErbB4$^{+/-}$ Background: C57BL/6		PPI = (Stefansson et al., 2002)		OF ↑ (Stefansson et al., 2002)			
CNS-specific ErbB4 KO Background: C57BL/6	MWM ♂↓ (Golub et al., 2004)			OF ↓ delayed motor development (Golub et al., 2004)			
Heart-rescued ErbB4 KO Background: C57BL/6	Cued FC ↓ Contextual FC ↓ (Shamir et al., 2012)	PPI ↓ (Shamir et al., 2012)		OF ↓ (Shamir et al., 2012)		EPM ↓ (Shamir et al., 2012)	
PV-Cre; ErbB4 Background: C57BL/6 × 129/SVEV	Cued FC = Contextual FC = (Shamir et al., 2012) Radial arm maze ↓ (Wen et al., 2010)	PPI ↓ (Shamir et al., 2012)		OF ↑ (Shamir et al., 2012)		EPM = (Shamir et al., 2012)	

(Continued)

Table 3 | Continued

Genetic mouse model for	Behavioral phenotype						
	Learning and memory	Sensorimotor gating and information processing	Social	Motor function and locomotor activity	Explorative behavior	Anxiety-like behavior	Hedonia
CNS-specific ErbB2/4 KO Background: FVB		PPI ↓ (Barros et al., 2009)	Aggressive ↑ (Barros et al., 2009)			OF ↓ (Barros et al., 2009)	
Transgenic NRG1 Background: not described	Contextual FC ↓ Cued FC = (Kato et al., 2010)	PPI ↓ (Kato et al., 2010)	Interaction ↑ Aggression ↑ (Kato et al., 2010)	OF ↑ (Kato et al., 2010)			
Transgenic Type I Background: C57BL/6	Y-maze = (11 month) DNMS = (3 month) DNMS ↓ (10 month) (Deakin et al., 2012)	%PPI ↓ ASR ↑ (Deakin et al., 2012)		OF = (5, 7.5, 10 month) OF ↑ (12.5 month) (Deakin et al., 2012) Rotard rod = (Michailov et al., 2004) Rotard rod ↓ Nesting ↓ Burrowing ↓ (Deakin et al., 2009)			

A comparison of the behavioral phenotypes of different mutants (left column, from top to bottom), including the novel TMc- Nrg1$^{+/-}$ mutant mice, the original TMc-Nrg1$^{+/-}$ mutant mice, Nrg1 heterozygous knockout mice with an EFG-like domain truncation of exon 6, Nrg1 heterozygous knockout mice with an Ig-like domain truncation (type I and II) of exon 3, Type III (CRD-domain) Nrg1 mutant mice, ErbB4 mutant mice, CNS-specific ErbB4 knock-out mice, ErbB4 knock-out mice that were rescued from embryonic lethality by reexpression of ErbB4 in the heart, parvalbumin-positive-specific ErbB4 knock-out mice, CNS-specific ErbB2/4 knock-out mice, Nrg1 overexpression transgenic mice, and type I Nrg1 overexpression transgenic mice. All studies summarized in this table were conducted in only male Nrg1-related mice except one study used only female mice and two studies used both male and female mice. Among these 3 studies, ♂ indicates that only male (but not female) mutants showed behavioral deficits, and ♀ indicates that only female (but not male) mutants showed behavioral impairments. Behavioral phenotypes are divided based on tasks (top row, from left to right) into categories that include learning and memory, sensorimotor gating, information processing, social function, motor function and locomotor activity, explorative behavior, anxiety-like behavior, and hedonia. NORT, novel object recognition task; FC, fear conditioning task; MWM, Morris water maze; DNMS, delay non-match to sample tasks; PPI, prepulse inhibition; ASR, auditory brain response; startle, startle response; MMN, mismatch negativity; P20, P20 event-related potential (ERP); P40, P40 ERP; OF, open field task; LD, light-dark chamber task; HB, hole broad task; EPM, elevated plus maze task; sucrose, sucrose preference task; ↑, increased in mutant mice compared to wild type littermates; ↓, decreased in mutant mice compared to wild type littermates; =, no difference between mutant mice and wild type littermates.

cortex (especially PFC) and hippocampus in schizophrenia is also thought to include alteration in GABAergic, inhibitory neurotransmission (Guidotti et al., 2005; Lewis et al., 2005). Although PTZ is usually considered as a convulsant drug and has less face validity to schizophrenia compared to MK-801 and methamphetamine, the well-established PTZ-induced responses appear to be a useful index for evaluating the vulnerability of GABAergic system in mutant mice with reasonable construct validity and predictive validity. Our data suggest that the GABA transmission of our male TMc-*Nrg1*$^{+/-}$ mutant mice was affected to a greater extent than glutamatergic and dopaminergic transmission. The truncation of different loci of Nrg1 might have differential effects compared to other Nrg1-related mutant mice.

Furthermore, because both Nrg1 and ErbB4 are highly abundant in the hippocampus (Corfas et al., 1995; Law et al., 2004; Vullhorst et al., 2009) and also because some hippocampus-dependent cognitive deficits were observed in Experiment 1, we examined GFP-labeled CA1 pyramidal neurons to elucidate any neuromorphological alterations of excitatory neurons in the hippocampus. This study might be the first to analyze morphometric alterations of CA1 pyramidal neurons in TMc-related *Nrg1*$^{+/-}$ mutant mice. However, no significant genotype-dependent neuromorphological alterations were found in either the males or females in any of the morphological variables we examined, suggesting that the neuromorphology and function of these hippocampal excitatory units may be intact in our TMc-*Nrg1*$^{+/-}$mutant mice. Our current results suggest that the GABAergic system is affected to a greater extent than either the glutamatergic or dopaminergic systems in the brains of our mutant mice, especially the males. It has been proposed that NRG1 has both forward and reverse functions in ErbB/NRG1 signaling. The forward signaling via ErbBs promotes the formation of the excitatory and inhibitory synapses of interneurons. The reverse signaling is ErbBs-independent; Nrg1 is cleaved by gamma-secretase to release the intracellular domain (NRG1-ICD), which is important for the development of cortical pyramidal neurons (Chen et al., 2008, 2010; Fazzari et al., 2010; Pedrique and Fazzari, 2010). Although more work needs to be performed to elucidate the role of NRG1-ICD in the hippocampus, our current data suggest that the deficiency of TMc domain might have a minor impact on reverse signaling that alters the neuromorphology of CA1 pyramidal neurons, whereas this haploinsufficiency might have a major impact on the development and neuroplasticity of interneuron that is mediated through forward signaling; these suppositions are also supported by the PTZ-induced behavioral alterations we observed in our TMc-*Nrg1*$^{+/-}$ mutant mice.

Additionally, further evidence arose from Experiment 3B, in which we found sex-specific reductions on GAD67 and parvalbumin expression in the hippocampi of our TMc-*Nrg1*$^{+/-}$ mutant mice. Indeed, it has been reported that Nrg1 and ErbB4 signaling controls the development of inhibitory circuitries in the mammalian cerebral cortex through GABAergic interneurons (Barros et al., 2009; Vullhorst et al., 2009; Pedrique and Fazzari, 2010; Wen et al., 2010; Cahill et al., 2012) and that Nrg1 treatment has a synaptogenic effect, which is possibly mediated by the stabilization of PSD-95 on GABAergic interneurons, but not glutamatergic neurons (Ting et al., 2011). A genetic association between ErbB4 and human cortical GABA levels has also been reported (Marenco et al., 2011). Besides, exogenous NRG1 down-regulated the expression of $GABA_A$ receptors in hippocampal CA1 pyramidal neurons (Okada and Corfas, 2004). Our findings from Experiment 3B are concordant with these findings and indicate the importance of Nrg1 in the regulation of GAD67 and parvalbumin expression in the hippocampus. Thus, haploinsufficiency of Nrg1 resulted in reductions in hippocampal GAD67 and parvalbumin expression, which may have caused alterations in the inhibitory interneuron networks by desynchronizing gamma oscillations [as has been proposed previously (Gonzalez-Burgos and Lewis, 2008; Del Pino et al., 2013)] and caused the cognitive impairments we observed in male Nrg1 mutant mice. This mechanism may contribute to the pathogenesis of some cognitive deficits in some patients with schizophrenia and *Nrg1* alterations.

The effect of valproate on the rescue of the cognitive deficits observed in our male TMc-*Nrg1* mutant mice should be of great interest to researchers. Valproate is a pharmacoepigenomic agent that has epigenetic effects on the modification of GABAergic interneurons (Csoka and Szyf, 2009). Valproate has been reported to ameliorate cognitive impairments in adult mice via demethylation of GABAergic-promotors (Tremolizzo et al., 2002, 2005; Matrisciano et al., 2013), inhibition of histone deacetylases (Phiel et al., 2001), and enhancement of central GABAergic tone that is mediated through an inhibition of GABA-transaminase (Johannessen, 2000). The reciprocal interaction between defects of NRG1 and hypermethylation of GABAergic promotors remains unclear. Our findings indicate that deficiencies of Nrg1 resulted in reductions of hippocampal GAD67 and parvalbumin expression, which might affect hippocampus-related cognitive functions. Interestingly, protracted treatment with valproate ameliorated observed cognitive deficits and the reduction of hippocampal GAD67 expression in our male TMc-*Nrg1* mutant mice. It has also been reported that protracted valproate treatment increased GAD67 mRNA expression in the brain, which likely facilitated GABAergic neurotransmission (Loscher, 1999; Tremolizzo et al., 2002, 2005). Notably, in terms of the pharmacokinetics of valproate, the dose we used has been shown to be comparable to the effective concentrations (0.15–0.30 mmol/kg) of valproate that are administered to psychiatric patients (Tremolizzo et al., 2005). Accordingly, the observed cognitive deficits that resulted from the haploinsufficiency of Nrg1 and the reduction of GABAergic transmission in our male TMc-*Nrg1* mutant mice were likely to be ameliorated by the upregulation of the GABAergic system due to chronic valproate injections. It is of interest to confirm hippocampal GAD67 and parvalbumin expressions in a new batch of valproate-treated Nrg1 mutant mice that did not receive any behavioral testing and further examine its epigenetic effect. Although the underlying mechanisms require further investigation, our data suggest that valproate has great potential for improving cognitive deficits in patients with schizophrenia, especially males with NRG1 haploinsufficiency. Further studies are greatly needed.

ACKNOWLEDGMENTS

This research was supported by grant numbers 102-2420-H-002-008-MY2 and 102-2628-H-002-003-MY3 to Wen-Sung Lai from the Ministry of Science and Technology in Taiwan, grant numbers 101-042 and 102-053 from National Taiwan University Hospital, and grant support from the Drunken Moon Lake Integrated Scientific Research Platform and Aim for Top University Project at National Taiwan University. We thank Dr. Hai-Gwo Hwu, Dr. Keng-Chen Liang, and Dr. Chih-Cheng Chen for their generous help and support. We also thank all members at the Laboratory of Integrated Neuroscience and Ethology (LINE) in the Department of Psychology, National Taiwan University for their assistance and contributions.

REFERENCES

Abe, Y., Namba, H., Zheng, Y., and Nawa, H. (2009). *In situ* hybridization reveals developmental regulation of ErbB1-4 mRNA expression in mouse midbrain: implication of ErbB receptors for dopaminergic neurons. *Neuroscience* 161, 95–110. doi: 10.1016/j.neuroscience.2009.03.022

Addington, A. M., Gornick, M., Duckworth, J., Sporn, A., Gogtay, N., Bobb, A., et al. (2005). GAD1 (2q31.1), which encodes glutamic acid decarboxylase (GAD67), is associated with childhood-onset schizophrenia and cortical gray matter volume loss. *Mol. Psychiatry* 10, 581–588. doi: 10.1038/sj.mp.4001599

Agim, Z. S., Esendal, M., Briollais, L., Uyan, O., Meschian, M., Martinez, L. A., et al. (2013). Discovery, validation and characterization of Erbb4 and Nrg1 haplotypes using data from three genome-wide association studies of schizophrenia. *PLoS ONE* 8:e53042. doi: 10.1371/journal.pone.0053042

Bao, J., Wolpowitz, D., Role, L. W., and Talmage, D. A. (2003). Back signaling by the Nrg-1 intracellular domain. *J. Cell Biol.* 161, 1133–1141. doi: 10.1083/jcb.200212085

Barros, C. S., Calabrese, B., Chamero, P., Roberts, A. J., Korzus, E., Lloyd, K., et al. (2009). Impaired maturation of dendritic spines without disorganization of cortical cell layers in mice lacking NRG1/ErbB signaling in the central nervous system. *Proc. Natl. Acad. Sci. U.S.A.* 106, 4507–4512. doi: 10.1073/pnas.0900355106

Bertram, I., Bernstein, H. G., Lendeckel, U., Bukowska, A., Dobrowolny, H., Keilhoff, G., et al. (2007). Immunohistochemical evidence for impaired neuregulin-1 signaling in the prefrontal cortex in schizophrenia and in unipolar depression. *Ann. N.Y. Acad. Sci.* 1096, 147–156. doi: 10.1196/annals.1397.080

Bjarnadottir, M., Misner, D. L., Haverfield-Gross, S., Bruun, S., Helgason, V. G., Stefansson, H., et al. (2007). Neuregulin1 (NRG1) signaling through Fyn modulates NMDA receptor phosphorylation: differential synaptic function in NRG1$^{+/-}$ knock-outs compared with wild-type mice. *J. Neurosci.* 27, 4519–4529. doi: 10.1523/JNEUROSCI.4314-06.2007

Boucher, A. A., Arnold, J. C., Duffy, L., Schofield, P. R., Micheau, J., and Karl, T. (2007). Heterozygous neuregulin 1 mice are more sensitive to the behavioural effects of Delta9-tetrahydrocannabinol. *Psychopharmacology (Berl.)* 192, 325–336. doi: 10.1007/s00213-007-0721-3

Brooks, S. P., and Dunnett, S. B. (2009). Tests to assess motor phenotype in mice: a user's guide. *Nat. Rev. Neurosci.* 10, 519–529. doi:10.1038/nrn2652

Cahill, M. E., Jones, K. A., Rafalovich, I., Xie, Z., Barros, C. S., Muller, U., et al. (2012). Control of interneuron dendritic growth through NRG1/erbB4-mediated kalirin-7 disinhibition. *Mol. Psychiatry* 17, 99–107. doi: 10.1038/mp.2011.35

Chen, Y., Hancock, M. L., Role, L. W., and Talmage, D. A. (2010). Intramembranous valine linked to schizophrenia is required for neuregulin 1 regulation of the morphological development of cortical neurons. *J. Neurosci.* 30, 9199–9208. doi: 10.1523/JNEUROSCI.0605-10.2010

Chen, Y. C., Chen, Y. W., Hsu, Y. F., Chang, W. T., Hsiao, C. K., Min, M. Y., et al. (2012). Akt1 deficiency modulates reward learning and reward prediction error in mice. *Genes Brain Behav.* 11, 157–169. doi: 10.1111/j.1601-183X.2011.00759.x

Chen, Y. J., Johnson, M. A., Lieberman, M. D., Goodchild, R. E., Schobel, S., Lewandowski, N., et al. (2008). Type III neuregulin-1 is required for normal sensorimotor gating, memory-related behaviors, and corticostriatal circuit components. *J. Neurosci.* 28, 6872–6883. doi: 10.1523/JNEUROSCI.1815-08.2008

Chen, Y. W., Kao, H. Y., Min, M. Y., and Lai, W. S. (2014). A sex- and region-specific role of Akt1 in the modulation of methamphetamine-induced hyperlocomotion and striatal neuronal activity: implications in schizophrenia and methamphetamine-induced psychosis. *Schizophr. Bull.* 40, 388–398. doi: 10.1093/schbul/sbt031

Chen, Y. W., and Lai, W. S. (2011). Behavioral phenotyping of v-akt murine thymoma viral oncogene homolog 1-deficient mice reveals a sex-specific prepulse inhibition deficit in females that can be partially alleviated by glycogen synthase kinase-3 inhibitors but not by antipsychotics. *Neuroscience* 174, 178–189. doi: 10.1016/j.neuroscience.2010.09.056

Chesworth, R., Downey, L., Logge, W., Killcross, S., and Karl, T. (2012). Cognition in female transmembrane domain neuregulin 1 mutant mice. *Behav. Brain Res.* 226, 218–223. doi: 10.1016/j.bbr.2011.09.019

Corfas, G., Rosen, K. M., Aratake, H., Krauss, R., and Fischbach, G. D. (1995). Differential expression of ARIA isoforms in the rat brain. *Neuron* 14, 103–115. doi: 10.1016/0896-6273(95)90244-9

Csoka, A. B., and Szyf, M. (2009). Epigenetic side-effects of common pharmaceuticals: a potential new field in medicine and pharmacology. *Med. Hypotheses* 73, 770–780. doi: 10.1016/j.mehy.2008.10.039

Deakin, I. H., Law, A. J., Oliver, P. L., Schwab, M. H., Nave, K. A., Harrison, P. J., et al. (2009). Behavioural characterization of neuregulin 1 type I overexpressing transgenic mice. *Neuroreport* 20, 1523–1528. doi: 10.1097/WNR.0b013e328330f6e7

Deakin, I. H., Nissen, W., Law, A. J., Lane, T., Kanso, R., Schwab, M. H., et al. (2012). Transgenic overexpression of the type I isoform of neuregulin 1 affects working memory and hippocampal oscillations but not long-term potentiation. *Cereb. Cortex* 22, 1520–1529. doi: 10.1093/cercor/bhr223

Dean, B., Karl, T., Pavey, G., Boer, S., Duffy, L., and Scarr, E. (2008). Increased levels of serotonin 2A receptors and serotonin transporter in the CNS of neuregulin 1 hypomorphic/mutant mice. *Schizophr. Res.* 99, 341–349. doi: 10.1016/j.schres.2007.10.013

Del Pino, I., Garcia-Frigola, C., Dehorter, N., Brotons-Mas, J. R., Alvarez-Salvado, E., Martinez De Lagran, M., et al. (2013). Erbb4 deletion from fast-spiking interneurons causes schizophrenia-like phenotypes. *Neuron* 79, 1152–1168. doi: 10.1016/j.neuron.2013.07.010

Desbonnet, L., O'Tuathaigh, C., Clarke, G., O'Leary, C., Petit, E., Clarke, N., et al. (2012). Phenotypic effects of repeated psychosocial stress during adolescence in mice mutant for the schizophrenia risk gene neuregulin-1: a putative model of gene x environment interaction. *Brain Behav. Immun.* 26, 660–671. doi: 10.1016/j.bbi.2012.02.010

Duffy, L., Cappas, E., Lai, D., Boucher, A. A., and Karl, T. (2010). Cognition in transmembrane domain neuregulin 1 mutant mice. *Neuroscience* 170, 800–807. doi: 10.1016/j.neuroscience.2010.07.042

Duffy, L., Cappas, E., Scimone, A., Schofield, P. R., and Karl, T. (2008). Behavioral profile of a heterozygous mutant mouse model for EGF-like domain neuregulin 1. *Behav. Neurosci.* 122, 748–759. doi: 10.1037/0735-7044.122.4.748

Ehrlichman, R. S., Luminais, S. N., White, S. L., Rudnick, N. D., Ma, N., Dow, H. C., et al. (2009). Neuregulin 1 transgenic mice display reduced mismatch negativity, contextual fear conditioning and social interactions. *Brain Res.* 1294, 116–127. doi: 10.1016/j.brainres.2009.07.065

Falls, D. L. (2003). Neuregulins: functions, forms, and signaling strategies. *Exp. Cell Res.* 284, 14–30. doi: 10.1016/S0014-4827(02)00102-7

Fazzari, P., Paternain, A. V., Valiente, M., Pla, R., Lujan, R., Lloyd, K., et al. (2010). Control of cortical GABA circuitry development by Nrg1 and ErbB4 signalling. *Nature* 464, 1376–1380. doi: 10.1038/nature08928

Feng, G., Mellor, R. H., Bernstein, M., Keller-Peck, C., Nguyen, Q. T., Wallace, M., et al. (2000). Imaging neuronal subsets in transgenic mice expressing multiple spectral variants of GFP. *Neuron* 28, 41–51. doi: 10.1016/S0896-6273(00)00084-2

Ferraro, T. N., Golden, G. T., Smith, G. G., St. Jean, P., Schork, N. J., Mulholland, N., et al. (1999). Mapping loci for pentylenetetrazol-induced seizure susceptibility in mice. *J. Neurosci.* 19, 6733–6739.

Ferraro, T. N., Smith, G. G., Schwebel, C. L., Doyle, G. A., Ruiz, S. E., Oleynick, J. U., et al. (2010). Confirmation of multiple seizure susceptibility QTLs on chromosome 15 in C57BL/6J and DBA/2J inbred mice. *Physiol. Genomics* 42A, 1–7. doi: 10.1152/physiolgenomics.00096.2010

Gassmann, M., Casagranda, F., Orioli, D., Simon, H., Lai, C., Klein, R., et al. (1995). Aberrant neural and cardiac development in mice lacking the ErbB4 neuregulin receptor. *Nature* 378, 390–394. doi: 10.1038/378390a0

Golub, M. S., Germann, S. L., and Lloyd, K. C. (2004). Behavioral characteristics of a nervous system-specific erbB4 knock-out mouse. *Behav. Brain Res.* 153, 159–170. doi: 10.1016/j.bbr.2003.11.010

Gonzalez-Burgos, G., and Lewis, D. A. (2008). GABA neurons and the mechanisms of network oscillations: implications for understanding cortical dysfunction in schizophrenia. *Schizophr. Bull.* 34, 944–961. doi: 10.1093/schbul/sbn070

Guidotti, A., Auta, J., Chen, Y., Davis, J. M., Dong, E., Gavin, D. P., et al. (2011). Epigenetic GABAergic targets in schizophrenia and bipolar disorder. *Neuropharmacology* 60, 1007–1016. doi: 10.1016/j.neuropharm.2010.10.021

Guidotti, A., Auta, J., Davis, J. M., Dong, E., Grayson, D. R., Veldic, M., et al. (2005). GABAergic dysfunction in schizophrenia: new treatment strategies on the horizon. *Psychopharmacology (Berl.)* 180, 191–205. doi: 10.1007/s00213-005-2212-8

Guidotti, A., Dong, E., Kundakovic, M., Satta, R., Grayson, D. R., and Costa, E. (2009). Characterization of the action of antipsychotic subtypes on valproate-induced chromatin remodeling. *Trends Pharmacol. Sci.* 30, 55–60. doi: 10.1016/j.tips.2008.10.010

Hahn, C. G., Wang, H. Y., Cho, D. S., Talbot, K., Gur, R. E., Berrettini, W. H., et al. (2006). Altered neuregulin 1-erbB4 signaling contributes to NMDA receptor hypofunction in schizophrenia. *Nat. Med.* 12, 824–828. doi: 10.1038/nm1418

Hall, J., Whalley, H. C., Job, D. E., Baig, B. J., McIntosh, A. M., Evans, K. L., et al. (2006). A neuregulin 1 variant associated with abnormal cortical function and psychotic symptoms. *Nat. Neurosci.* 9, 1477–1478. doi: 10.1038/nn1795

Harrison, P. J., and Law, A. J. (2006). Neuregulin 1 and schizophrenia: genetics, gene expression, and neurobiology. *Biol. Psychiatry* 60, 132–140. doi: 10.1016/j.biopsych.2005.11.002

Harrison, P. J., and Weinberger, D. R. (2005). Schizophrenia genes, gene expression, and neuropathology: on the matter of their convergence. *Mol. Psychiatry* 10, 40–68; image 45. doi: 10.1038/sj.mp.4001558

Hirokawa, T., Boon-Chieng, S., and Mitaku, S. (1998). SOSUI: classification and secondary structure prediction system for membrane proteins. *Bioinformatics* 14, 378–379. doi: 10.1093/bioinformatics/14.4.378

Honea, R., Verchinski, B. A., Pezawas, L., Kolachana, B. S., Callicott, J. H., Mattay, V. S., et al. (2009). Impact of interacting functional variants in COMT on regional gray matter volume in human brain. *Neuroimage* 45, 44–51. doi: 10.1016/j.neuroimage.2008.10.064

Insel, T. R. (2010). Rethinking schizophrenia. *Nature* 468, 187–193. doi: 10.1038/nature09552

Itoh, K., and Watanabe, M. (2009). Paradoxical facilitation of pentylenetetrazole-induced convulsion susceptibility in mice lacking neuronal nitric oxide synthase. *Neuroscience* 159, 735–743. doi: 10.1016/j.neuroscience.2008.12.040

Iwakura, Y., and Nawa, H. (2013). ErbB1-4-dependent EGF/neuregulin signals and their cross talk in the central nervous system: pathological implications in schizophrenia and Parkinson's disease. *Front. Cell. Neurosci.* 7:4. doi: 10.3389/fncel.2013.00004

Johannessen, C. U. (2000). Mechanisms of action of valproate: a commentatory. *Neurochem. Int.* 37, 103–110. doi: 10.1016/S0197-0186(00)00013-9

Kampman, O., Anttila, S., Illi, A., Saarela, M., Rontu, R., Mattila, K. M., et al. (2004). Neuregulin genotype and medication response in Finnish patients with schizophrenia. *Neuroreport* 15, 2517–2520. doi: 10.1097/00001756-200411150-00017

Karl, T., Burne, T. H., Van Den Buuse, M., and Chesworth, R. (2011). Do transmembrane domain neuregulin 1 mutant mice exhibit a reliable sensorimotor gating deficit? *Behav. Brain Res.* 223, 336–341. doi: 10.1016/j.bbr.2011.04.051

Karl, T., Duffy, L., Scimone, A., Harvey, R. P., and Schofield, P. R. (2007). Altered motor activity, exploration and anxiety in heterozygous neuregulin 1 mutant mice: implications for understanding schizophrenia. *Genes Brain Behav.* 6, 677–687. doi: 10.1111/j.1601-183X.2006.00298.x

Kato, T., Abe, Y., Sotoyama, H., Kakita, A., Kominami, R., Hirokawa, S., et al. (2011). Transient exposure of neonatal mice to neuregulin-1 results in hyperdopaminergic states in adulthood: implication in neurodevelopmental hypothesis for schizophrenia. *Mol. Psychiatry* 16, 307–320. doi: 10.1038/mp.2010.10

Kato, T., Kasai, A., Mizuno, M., Fengyi, L., Shintani, N., Maeda, S., et al. (2010). Phenotypic characterization of transgenic mice overexpressing neuregulin-1. *PLoS ONE* 5:e14185. doi: 10.1371/journal.pone.0014185

Kramer, R., Bucay, N., Kane, D. J., Martin, L. E., Tarpley, J. E., and Theill, L. E. (1996). Neuregulins with an Ig-like domain are essential for mouse myocardial and neuronal development. *Proc. Natl. Acad. Sci. U.S.A.* 93, 4833–4838. doi: 10.1073/pnas.93.10.4833

Krug, A., Markov, V., Krach, S., Jansen, A., Zerres, K., Eggermann, T., et al. (2010). The effect of Neuregulin 1 on neural correlates of episodic memory encoding and retrieval. *Neuroimage* 53, 985–991. doi: 10.1016/j.neuroimage.2009.12.062

Kulkarni, J., Hayes, E., and Gavrilidis, E. (2012). Hormones and schizophrenia. *Curr. Opin. Psychiatry* 25, 89–95. doi: 10.1097/YCO.0b013e328350360e

Lacroix-Fralish, M. L., Tawfik, V. L., Nutile-McMenemy, N., Harris, B. T., and Deleo, J. A. (2006). Differential regulation of neuregulin 1 expression by progesterone in astrocytes and neurons. *Neuron Glia Biol.* 2, 227–234. doi: 10.1017/S1740925X07000385

Lai, D., Liu, X. F., Forrai, A., Wolstein, O., Michalicek, J., Ahmed, I., et al. (2010). Neuregulin 1 sustains the gene regulatory network in both trabecular and nontrabecular myocardium. *Circ. Res.* 107, 715–U774. doi: 10.1161/Circresaha.110.218693

Lai, W. S., Chang, C. Y., Wong, W. R., Pei, J. C., Chen, Y. S., and Hung, W. L. (2014). Assessing schizophrenia-relevant cognitive and social deficits in mice: a selection of mouse behavioral tasks and potential therapeutic compounds. *Curr. Pharm. Des.* doi: 10.2174/13816128196661401101 22750. [Epub ahead of print].

Lai, W. S., Xu, B., Westphal, K. G., Paterlini, M., Olivier, B., Pavlidis, P., et al. (2006). Akt1 deficiency affects neuronal morphology and predisposes to abnormalities in prefrontal cortex functioning. *Proc. Natl. Acad. Sci. U.S.A.* 103, 16906–16911. doi: 10.1073/pnas.0604994103

Law, A. J., Shannon Weickert, C., Hyde, T. M., Kleinman, J. E., and Harrison, P. J. (2004). Neuregulin-1 (NRG-1) mRNA and protein in the adult human brain. *Neuroscience* 127, 125–136. doi: 10.1016/j.neuroscience.2004.04.026

Lewis, C. M., Levinson, D. F., Wise, L. H., Delisi, L. E., Straub, R. E., Hovatta, I., et al. (2003). Genome scan meta-analysis of schizophrenia and bipolar disorder, part II: schizophrenia. *Am. J. Hum. Genet.* 73, 34–48. doi: 10.1086/376549

Lewis, D. A., Hashimoto, T., and Volk, D. W. (2005). Cortical inhibitory neurons and schizophrenia. *Nat. Rev. Neurosci.* 6, 312–324. doi: 10.1038/nrn1648

Li, B., Woo, R. S., Mei, L., and Malinow, R. (2007). The neuregulin-1 receptor erbB4 controls glutamatergic synapse maturation and plasticity. *Neuron* 54, 583–597. doi: 10.1016/j.neuron.2007.03.028

Liu, X., Hwang, H., Cao, L., Buckland, M., Cunningham, A., Chen, J., et al. (1998a). Domain-specific gene disruption reveals critical regulation of neuregulin signaling by its cytoplasmic tail. *Proc. Natl. Acad. Sci. U.S.A.* 95, 13024–13029. doi: 10.1073/pnas.95.22.13024

Liu, X., Hwang, H., Cao, L., Wen, D., Liu, N., Graham, R. M., et al. (1998b). Release of the neuregulin functional polypeptide requires its cytoplasmic tail. *J. Biol. Chem.* 273, 34335–34340. doi: 10.1074/jbc.273.51.34335

Loscher, W. (1999). Valproate: a reappraisal of its pharmacodynamic properties and mechanisms of action. *Prog. Neurobiol.* 58, 31–59. doi: 10.1016/S0301-0082(98)00075-6

Marenco, S., Geramita, M., Van Der Veen, J. W., Barnett, A. S., Kolachana, B., Shen, J., et al. (2011). Genetic association of ErbB4 and human cortical GABA levels *in vivo*. *J. Neurosci.* 31, 11628–11632. doi: 10.1523/JNEUROSCI.1529-11.2011

Matrisciano, F., Tueting, P., Dalal, I., Kadriu, B., Grayson, D. R., Davis, J. M., et al. (2013). Epigenetic modifications of GABAergic interneurons are associated with the schizophrenia-like phenotype induced by prenatal stress in mice. *Neuropharmacology* 68, 184–194. doi: 10.1016/j.neuropharm.2012.04.013

Mei, L., and Xiong, W. C. (2008). Neuregulin 1 in neural development, synaptic plasticity and schizophrenia. *Nat. Rev. Neurosci.* 9, 437–452. doi: 10.1038/nrn2392

Meyer, D., and Birchmeier, C. (1995). Multiple essential functions of neuregulin in development. *Nature* 378, 386–390. doi: 10.1038/378386a0

Michailov, G. V., Sereda, M. W., Brinkmann, B. G., Fischer, T. M., Haug, B., Birchmeier, C., et al. (2004). Axonal neuregulin-1 regulates myelin sheath thickness. *Science* 304, 700–703. doi: 10.1126/science.1095862

Neddens, J., and Buonanno, A. (2010). Selective populations of hippocampal interneurons express ErbB4 and their number and distribution is altered in ErbB4 knockout mice. *Hippocampus* 20, 724–744. doi: 10.1002/hipo.20675

Nicodemus, K. K., Law, A. J., Luna, A., Vakkalanka, R., Straub, R. E., Kleinman, J. E., et al. (2009). A 5′ promoter region SNP in NRG1 is associated with schizophrenia risk and type III isoform expression. *Mol. Psychiatry* 14, 741–743. doi: 10.1038/mp.2008.150

Okada, M., and Corfas, G. (2004). Neuregulin1 downregulates postsynaptic GABAA receptors at the hippocampal inhibitory synapse. *Hippocampus* 14, 337–344. doi: 10.1002/hipo.10185

O'Tuathaigh, C. M., Babovic, D., O'Sullivan, G. J., Clifford, J. J., Tighe, O., Croke, D. T., et al. (2007). Phenotypic characterization of spatial cognition and social behavior in mice with "knockout" of the schizophrenia risk gene neuregulin 1. *Neuroscience* 147, 18–27. doi: 10.1016/j.neuroscience.2007.03.051

O'Tuathaigh, C. M., Harte, M., O'Leary, C., O'Sullivan, G. J., Blau, C., Lai, D., et al. (2010). Schizophrenia-related endophenotypes in heterozygous neuregulin-1 "knockout" mice. *Eur. J. Neurosci.* 31, 349–358. doi: 10.1111/j.1460-9568.2009.07069.x

O'Tuathaigh, C. M., O'Connor, A. M., O'Sullivan, G. J., Lai, D., Harvey, R., Croke, D. T., et al. (2008). Disruption to social dyadic interactions but not emotional/anxiety-related behaviour in mice with heterozygous "knockout" of the schizophrenia risk gene neuregulin-1. *Prog. Neuropsychopharmacol. Biol. Psychiatry* 32, 462–466. doi: 10.1016/j.pnpbp.2007.09.018

O'Tuathaigh, C. M., O'Sullivan, G. J., Kinsella, A., Harvey, R. P., Tighe, O., Croke, D. T., et al. (2006). Sexually dimorphic changes in the exploratory and habituation profiles of heterozygous neuregulin-1 knockout mice. *Neuroreport* 17, 79–83. doi: 10.1097/01.wnr.0000192738.31029.0a

Parlapani, E., Schmitt, A., Wirths, O., Bauer, M., Sommer, C., Rueb, U., et al. (2010). Gene expression of neuregulin-1 isoforms in different brain regions of elderly schizophrenia patients. *World J. Biol. Psychiatry* 11, 243–250. doi: 10.3109/15622970802022376

Pedrique, S. P., and Fazzari, P. (2010). Nrg1 reverse signaling in cortical pyramidal neurons. *J. Neurosci.* 30, 15005–15006. doi: 10.1523/JNEUROSCI.4669-10.2010

Phiel, C. J., Zhang, F., Huang, E. Y., Guenther, M. G., Lazar, M. A., and Klein, P. S. (2001). Histone deacetylase is a direct target of valproic acid, a potent anticonvulsant, mood stabilizer, and teratogen. *J. Biol. Chem.* 276, 36734–36741. doi: 10.1074/jbc.M101287200

Rimer, M., Barrett, D. W., Maldonado, M. A., Vock, V. M., and Gonzalez-Lima, F. (2005). Neuregulin-1 immunoglobulin-like domain mutant mice: clozapine sensitivity and impaired latent inhibition. *Neuroreport* 16, 271–275. doi: 10.1097/00001756-200502280-00014

Schwab, S. G., and Wildenauer, D. B. (2009). Update on key previously proposed candidate genes for schizophrenia. *Curr. Opin. Psychiatry* 22, 147–153. doi: 10.1097/YCO.0b013e328325a598

Shamir, A., Kwon, O. B., Karavanova, I., Vullhorst, D., Leiva-Salcedo, E., Janssen, M. J., et al. (2012). The importance of the NRG-1/ErbB4 pathway for synaptic plasticity and behaviors associated with psychiatric disorders. *J. Neurosci.* 32, 2988–2997. doi: 10.1523/JNEUROSCI.1899-11.2012

Shih, H. T., and Mok, H. K. (2000). ETHOM: event-recording computer software for the study of animal behavior. *Acta Zool. Taiwan.* 11, 47–61.

Stefansson, H., Sigurdsson, E., Steinthorsdottir, V., Bjornsdottir, S., Sigmundsson, T., Ghosh, S., et al. (2002). Neuregulin 1 and susceptibility to schizophrenia. *Am. J. Hum. Genet.* 71, 877–892. doi: 10.1086/342734

Ting, A. K., Chen, Y., Wen, L., Yin, D. M., Shen, C., Tao, Y., et al. (2011). Neuregulin 1 promotes excitatory synapse development and function in GABAergic interneurons. *J. Neurosci.* 31, 15–25. doi: 10.1523/jneurosci.2538-10.2011

Tremolizzo, L., Carboni, G., Ruzicka, W. B., Mitchell, C. P., Sugaya, I., Tueting, P., et al. (2002). An epigenetic mouse model for molecular and behavioral neuropathologies related to schizophrenia vulnerability. *Proc. Natl. Acad. Sci. U.S.A.* 99, 17095–17100. doi: 10.1073/pnas.262658999

Tremolizzo, L., Doueiri, M. S., Dong, E., Grayson, D. R., Davis, J., Pinna, G., et al. (2005). Valproate corrects the schizophrenia-like epigenetic behavioral modifications induced by methionine in mice. *Biol. Psychiatry* 57, 500–509. doi: 10.1016/j.biopsych.2004.11.046

Van Den Buuse, M., Wischhof, L., Lee, R. X., Martin, S., and Karl, T. (2009). Neuregulin 1 hypomorphic mutant mice: enhanced baseline locomotor activity but normal psychotropic drug-induced hyperlocomotion and prepulse inhibition regulation. *Int. J. Neuropsychopharmacol.* 12, 1383–1393. doi: 10.1017/S1461145709000388

Voineskos, D., De Luca, V., Macgregor, S., Likhodi, O., Miller, L., Voineskos, A. N., et al. (2009). Neuregulin 1 and age of onset in the major psychoses. *J. Neural Transm.* 116, 479–486. doi: 10.1007/s00702-008-0182-9

Vullhorst, D., Neddens, J., Karavanova, I., Tricoire, L., Petralia, R. S., McBain, C. J., et al. (2009). Selective expression of ErbB4 in interneurons, but not pyramidal cells, of the rodent hippocampus. *J. Neurosci.* 29, 12255–12264. doi: 10.1523/JNEUROSCI.2454-09.2009

Walker, R. M., Christoforou, A., Thomson, P. A., McGhee, K. A., Maclean, A., Muhleisen, T. W., et al. (2010). Association analysis of Neuregulin 1 candidate regions in schizophrenia and bipolar disorder. *Neurosci. Lett.* 478, 9–13. doi: 10.1016/j.neulet.2010.04.056

Walss-Bass, C., Liu, W., Lew, D. F., Villegas, R., Montero, P., Dassori, A., et al. (2006). A novel missense mutation in the transmembrane domain of neuregulin 1 is associated with schizophrenia. *Biol. Psychiatry* 60, 548–553. doi: 10.1016/j.biopsych.2006.03.017

Wen, L., Lu, Y. S., Zhu, X. H., Li, X. M., Woo, R. S., Chen, Y. J., et al. (2010). Neuregulin 1 regulates pyramidal neuron activity via ErbB4 in parvalbumin-positive interneurons. *Proc. Natl. Acad. Sci. U.S.A.* 107, 1211–1216. doi: 10.1073/pnas.0910302107

Wong, J., and Weickert, C. S. (2009). Transcriptional interaction of an estrogen receptor splice variant and ErbB4 suggests convergence in gene susceptibility pathways in schizophrenia. *J. Biol. Chem.* 284, 18824–18832. doi: 10.1074/jbc.M109.013243

Wu, J., Zou, H., Strong, J. A., Yu, J., Zhou, X., Xie, Q., et al. (2005). Bimodal effects of MK-801 on locomotion and stereotypy in C57BL/6 mice. *Psychopharmacology* 177, 256–263. doi: 10.1007/s00213-004-1944-1

Yau, H. J., Wang, H. F., Lai, C., and Liu, F. C. (2003). Neural development of the neuregulin receptor ErbB4 in the cerebral cortex and the hippocampus: preferential expression by interneurons tangentially migrating from the ganglionic eminences. *Cereb. Cortex* 13, 252–264. doi: 10.1093/cercor/13.3.252

8

The effect of psilocin on memory acquisition, retrieval, and consolidation in the rat

Lukas Rambousek[1]*, Tomas Palenicek[2], Karel Vales[1] and Ales Stuchlik[1]*

[1] *Institute of Physiology, Academy of Sciences of the Czech Republic, Prague, Czech Republic*
[2] *Prague Psychiatric Center, Prague, Czech Republic*

Edited by:
Tomiki Sumiyoshi, National Center of Neurology and Psychiatry, Japan

***Correspondence:**
Lukas Rambousek and Ales Stuchlik, Department of Neurophysiology of Memory, Institute of Physiology, Academy of Sciences of the Czech Republic, Videnska 1083, Prague 4 142 20, Czech Republic
e-mail: rambousek@biomed.cas.cz; stuchlik@biomed.cas.cz

The involvement of the serotonin system in the pathophysiology of schizophrenia has been elucidated by experiments with hallucinogens. Application of a hallucinogen to humans leads to changes in perception, cognition, emotions, and induction of psychotic-like symptoms that resemble symptoms of schizophrenia. In rodent studies, their acute administration affects sensorimotor gating, locomotor activity, social behavior, and cognition including working memory, the phenotypes are considered as an animal model of schizophrenia. The complexity and singularity of human cognition raises questions about the validity of animal models utilizing agonists of 5-HT_{2A} receptors. The present study thus investigated the effect of psilocin on memory acquisition, reinforced retrieval, and memory consolidation in rats. Psilocin is a main metabolite of psilocybin acting as an agonist at 5-HT_{2A} receptors with a contribution of 5-HT_{2C} and 5-HT_{1A} receptors. First, we tested the effect of psilocin on the acquisition of a Carousel maze, a spatial task requiring navigation using distal cues, attention, and cognitive coordination. Psilocin significantly impaired the acquisition of the Carousel maze at both doses (1 and 4 mg/kg). The higher dose of psilocin blocked the learning processes even in an additional session when the rats received only saline. Next, we examined the effect of psilocin on reinforced retrieval and consolidation in the Morris water maze (MWM). The dose of 4 mg/kg disrupted reinforced retrieval in the MWM. However, the application of a lower dose was without any significant effect. Finally, neither the low nor high dose of psilocin injected post-training caused a deficit in memory consolidation in the MWM. Taken together, the psilocin dose dependently impaired the acquisition of the Carousel maze and reinforced retrieval in MWM; however, it had no effect on memory consolidation.

Keywords: psilocin, spatial memory, Carousel maze, Morris water maze, allocentric navigation, hallucinogenic alkaloids, learning, memory

INTRODUCTION

Psilocybin (*O*-phosphoryl-4-hydroxy-*N,N*-dimethyltryptamine) and its active metabolite psilocin (4-hydroxy-*N,N*-dimethyltrypt amine) are the main psychoactive indolealkylamines contained in hallucinogenic mushrooms (Hasler et al., 1997; Passie et al., 2002; Tyls et al., 2013). They act as agonists at serotonin receptors, mainly 5-$HT_{2A/C}$ and 5-HT_{1A} subtypes (for a review, see Tyls et al., 2013). Recently, affinities to other than serotonergic receptors have also been reported (e.g., D1 and D3 receptors); however, their role in the neurobiology of psilocin's and psilocybin's action is disputable (Ray, 2010). Nevertheless, most of the evidence agrees that hallucinogenic effects are mediated mainly via agonism at postsynaptic 5-HT_{2A} receptors with a contribution of 5-HT_{2C} and 5-HT_{1A} receptors (Nichols, 2004). A secondary role of the activated limbic dopaminergic system also seems to be responsible for some of its effects (Vollenweider et al., 1999).

The acute effects of psilocybin in humans are characterized by changes in perception, cognition, emotions, and induction of psychotic-like symptoms that resemble early stages of schizophrenia (Vollenweider et al., 1998). Psilocybin also attenuates neurocognitive parameters in humans (e.g., disrupted sustained attention and altered visual information processing) and disrupts sensorimotor processing (Tyls et al., 2013), effects that are also typically disrupted in psychotic patients (Park and Holzman, 1992; Vollenweider et al., 1997, 1998; Geyer, 1998). Due to this phenomenological resemblance of acute intoxication with psychosis and its long history of safe clinical use (including psychiatric treatment) it is, nowadays, the most frequently used serotonergic model of psychosis in humans (Tyls et al., 2013). Furthermore, the therapeutic potential of psilocin/psilocybin has been recently investigated in several psychiatric disorders such as obsessive–compulsive disorder, anxiety, and addiction (Moreno et al., 2006; Grob et al., 2011; Bogenschutz and Pommy, 2012; Stebelska, 2013; dos Santos, 2014). Despite the evidence of how psilocybin changes cognitive performance in humans, little is known about its effects on cognition in animals.

To further investigate the effect of psilocin on cognition in animals we decided to test spatial memory using two spatial paradigms: the Morris water maze (MWM) and the Carousel maze.

Spatial navigation as a behavioral manifestation of knowledge of the environment (i.e., cognitive map; Tolman, 1948) is considered as a useful and experimentally well-accessible animal analogy of declarative memory (O'Keefe and Nadel, 1978; Eichenbaum, 2001; Morris, 2013). Testing of spatial navigation requires sensitive spatial paradigms, such as the MWM (Morris, 1981; Morris et al., 1982; Stuchlik et al., 2007). This test can be used in many configurations, allowing testing of reference and working memory acquisition, consolidation, and retrieval. The water maze typically requires so-called allocentric spatial memory, i.e., guidance of navigation by spatial relationships of the distal visual cues located in the experimental room. Another powerful and relatively novel spatial paradigm is active place avoidance in a Carousel maze, previously also referred to as active allothetic place avoidance (AAPA) (Cimadevilla et al., 2000, 2001; Stuchlik et al., 2004; Wesierska et al., 2005). In this test, animals walking on a slowly rotating arena are required to avoid a sector located in a stable position of the room. It was demonstrated that rats avoiding places remember the arena- and room-based frames of reference (Fenton et al., 1998), which are continuously dissociated by the rotation of the arena. In its active place avoidance version, animals must, besides allocentric mapping, segregate spatial information into coherent representations of the room and arena frames and to select the room frame as the only one relevant for navigation. This ability was shown to strictly require hippocampus and termed cognitive coordination (Wesierska et al., 2005). Importantly, this task was demonstrated to require the presence of visual extra-arena information in the room frame (Fajnerova et al., 2014) as well as vestibular inertial stimulation caused by continuous arena rotation, which likely enhances the attention of the rats to distal visual cues (Blahna et al., 2011).

The aim of the present study is to test the hypothesis that psilocin attenuates acquisition of the Carousel maze (demanding mainly cognitive coordination) and reinforced retrieval and memory consolidation in the MWM (demanding allocentric memory). The effect of psilocin on the locomotor activity was assessed in the Carousel maze in order to dissociate effects upon cognition and/or motor and motivational functions.

MATERIALS AND METHODS

ANIMALS

All experimental procedures complied with the Animal Protection Code of the Czech Republic, the appropriate directive of the European Union (2010/63/EC) and NIH guidelines. Male adult Wistar rats (12–14 weeks, weighing 250–350 g) were obtained from the Institute's accredited breeding colony. Animals were housed in pairs in 30 cm × 30 cm × 40 cm transparent plastic cages in a laboratory air-conditioned animal facility with a constant temperature (21°C) and 12:12 light/dark cycle with lights on at 7:00. Water and food were available *ad libitum* throughout the experiments. In all experiments, eight animals were used per group. Seventy-two animals were used in total.

DRUGS

Psilocin 1 and 4 mg/kg (synthesized at Pharmaceutical Faculty of Charles University in Prague, the structure was confirmed by mass spectroscopy and nuclear magnetic resonance techniques) was dissolved in saline (0.9% NaCl) acidified with 10 μl of glacial acetic acid. All injections were administered subcutaneously (s.c.) at a volume of 2 ml/kg. Fresh solutions were prepared every day, stored at 4°C and were protected from light.

EXPERIMENTAL APPARATUSES AND BEHAVIORAL PROCEDURES

Carousel maze

The Carousel maze apparatus was described in detail in our previous study (Stuchlik et al., 2007, 2013). Briefly, it consisted of a smooth metallic circular arena (82 cm in diameter), enclosed with a 30-cm high transparent Plexiglas wall and elevated 1 m above the floor of a 4 m × 5 m room. The room contained an abundance of extra-maze landmarks. The rats were initially placed in the arena rotating at 1 rpm in a place directly opposite to the shock sector. Animals had to avoid a directly imperceptible 60° sector, defined in the North of the four arbitrary cardinal compass directions. The sector was identifiable solely by its relationships to distal room cues. A latex harness was attached between the shoulders of the rats, which carried an infrared light-emitting diode (LED). A computer-based tracking system (iTrack; Biosignal Group, USA) was located in an adjacent room. The tracking system recorded the rat's position every 40 ms. Position time series were stored for off-line analyses (Track Analysis; Biosignal Group, USA). Whenever the rat entered the to-be-avoided sector for more than 0.5 s, the tracking system delivered a shock and counted an entrance. If the rat did not leave the sector, additional shocks were given every 1.4 s, but no more entrances were counted until the rat left the sector for more than 0.5 s. Mild shocks (50 Hz, 0.5 s, 0.4–0.7 mA) were administered from a computer-driven shock generator through the implanted low-impedance hypodermic needle implanted on the rats' backs and through the contact between the rats' keratinized paws and the grounded arena floor. Since the voltage drop is highest at the contact between rats' paws and the floor, the rats "feel" the shock most likely in their feet. We avoided using a grid because in the Carousel maze it is necessary to allow accumulation of scent marks on the floor in order to generate a conflict between the arena and the room frames. The exact shock current, ranging between 0.4 and 0.7 mA, was adjusted for each rat to elicit a rapid escape response but not freezing. Rats were trained 4 days, 30 min after psilocin injection in four acquisition sessions of Carousel maze. On the fifth day, animals were tested without the presence of the drug (after-session). While the first four sessions evaluate the learning capacity, the last session would correspond to the short-term memory. The sector position was kept constant on the North compass direction throughout the training. The interval between sessions was 24 h. Eight animals were used in each group (24 rats in total).

Morris water maze

The MWM consisted of a blue-painted metallic circular tank (180 cm in diameter, 50 cm high) filled with water (20°C, 40 cm deep). A small, transparent Plexiglas escape platform (10 cm in diameter) was placed in the center of an arbitrarily defined Northeast (NE) quadrant of the pool and submerged 1.5 cm below the water surface. Rats were released facing the wall from the four cardinal compass directions (N, W, S, and E) in a quasi-random order. A trial stopped when the rat found the escape platform and climbed upon it. If the rat failed to find the escape platform in

60 s, the trial was stopped (recording latency of 60 s), and the rat was gently guided to the platform by the experimenter. The escape latency was recorded by the experimenter using a stopwatch. The rat was allowed to stay on the platform for 10 s and then it was placed to a waiting cage. One daily session consisted of eight swims (trials).

In the reinforced retrieval experiment four acquisition sessions (each consisting of eight swims) were conducted without the drug. On Day 5, psilocin was applied s.c. (1 or 4 mg/kg) 30 min prior to testing and the rats were released again for eight swims under the influence of the drug with the platform present in the same location of the pool (reinforced retrieval). Reinforced retrieval (actually re-acquisition) was chosen over a classical probe trial to also investigate re-acquisition under the drug. Five days later, drug-free animals underwent another re-acquisition with the platform present. Eight animals were used in each group (24 rats in total).

The experiment dedicated to testing the effect of psilocin on memory consolidation consisted of an initial 16 trials in the first session (Day 1) followed by psilocin injection immediately after the last swim at doses of 1 or 4 mg/kg, s.c. On the subsequent day (Day 2), the animals were released again for eight trials (swims) without any injections and the platform was again present in the same position (NE). Eight animals were used in each group (24 rats in total).

DATA ANALYSIS AND STATISTICS

The total distance traveled in a session (measured in the arena frame) reflected active locomotor activity without the contribution of the passive arena rotation. The distance was measured by the off-line tracking system by summing linear distances of points recorded each 1 s (the sampling frequency was 40 Hz). This sampling eliminated non-locomotor movements of the rat such as shivering. The number of entrances into the to-be-avoided sector (number of errors) measured the efficiency of avoidance in the Carousel maze. Another measure of the spatial performance within the session was the maximum time between the two entrances in a session (maximum time avoided). Results were analyzed using a two-way ANOVA (Groups × Sessions) with repeated measures on sessions, and Tukey's HSD test was used when appropriate. Significance was accepted at $P < 0.05$.

In the MWM, we recorded the latency to find the platform as a measure of spatial memory (Morris, 1981; Stuchlik et al., 2007) and analyzed it with a two-way ANOVA (Groups × Sessions) with repeated measures on sessions. Tukey's HSD test was used as *post hoc* when appropriate. We were not able to track the trajectories of the animals in this MWM experiment (however, locomotion was assessed in the Carousel maze; see the previous paragraph).

RESULTS

EFFECT OF PSILOCIN ON THE ACQUISITION OF THE CAROUSEL MAZE

The animals did not exhibit any signs of stress or excessive discomfort during or after the drug injections. All data are summarized in **Figure 1**. First, we analyzed the locomotor activity, which was different between 1 mg/kg of psilocin, 4 mg/kg of psilocin, and the control group. A two-way ANOVA with repeated measures on sessions revealed a significant main effect of group [$F(2, 22) = 8.51$; $P < 0.001$] and sessions [$F(4, 88) = 44.4$; $P < 0.0001$] and interaction between the two factors [$F(8, 88) = 3.47$; $P < 0.001$]. The locomotor activity of the control group increased during the first three sessions and then stabilized to a constant level. There was no significant difference between the control group and the group treated with 1 mg/kg of psilocin ($P > 0.05$) during all five sessions. The group treated with 4 mg/kg of psilocin significantly differed from the control group only during the first three sessions ($P < 0.05$). These results show that

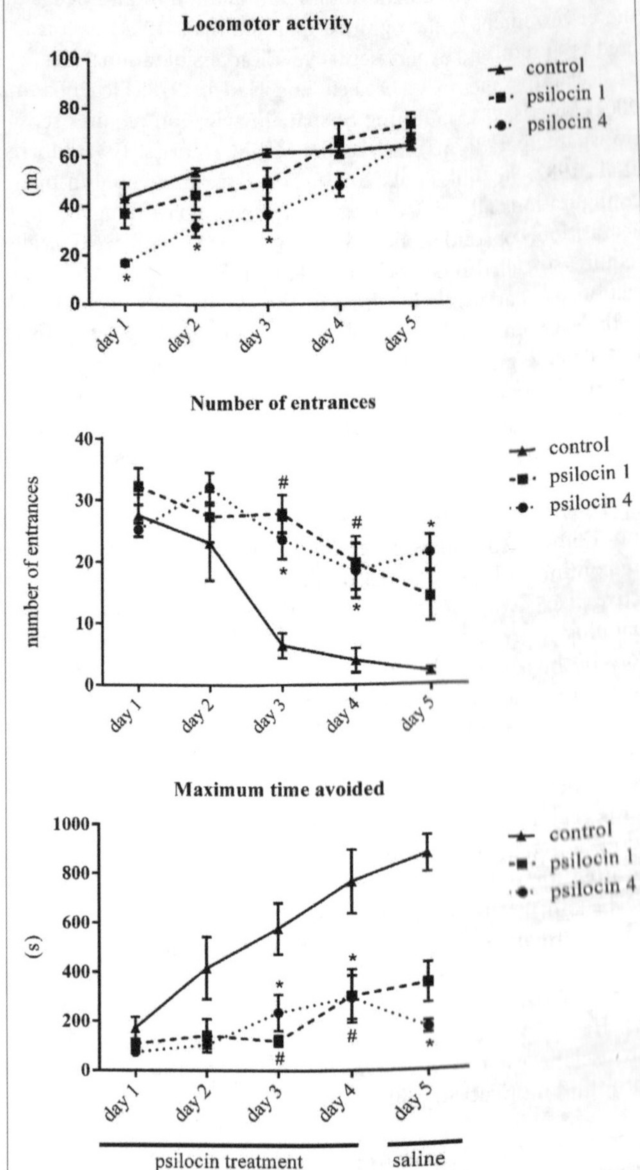

FIGURE 1 | The effect of psilocin on locomotor activity, number of entrances, and maximum time avoided in the Carousel maze. Psilocin impaired spatial memory acquisition (higher number of entrances) at both doses. #$P < 0.05$, psilocin 1 group (1 mg/kg, s.c.) compared to the control group on the same day. *$P < 0.05$, psilocin 4 group (4 mg/kg, s.c.) compared to the control group on the same day.

a dose of 4 mg/kg of psilocin induced a decrease in locomotor activity but the locomotion of this group still increased with the training. This increasing trend persisted even in session 5 (the day without the application of psilocin), the locomotor activity was significantly higher in session 5 than in session 4 ($P < 0.01$). These results show that the dose of 4 mg/kg of psilocin impaired locomotor activity in the Carousel maze, whilst the dose of 1 mg/kg did not affect it.

The analysis of the number of entrances into the shock sector revealed differences between the studied groups. The two-way ANOVA showed a significant main effect of groups [$F(2, 20) = 6.86$; $P < 0.01$] and a main effect of sessions [$F(4, 80) = 20.64$; $P < 0.0001$]. There was also an effect of the interaction between these two factors [$F(8, 80) = 3.95$; $P < 0.001$]. A *post hoc* analysis of the factor of sessions showed that in the control group performance was better in sessions 3–5 compared to the first session ($P < 0.05$). The group treated with the low dose of psilocin (1 mg/kg) showed significant impairment in solving the Carousel maze task in sessions 3 and 4. The group treated with the higher dose of psilocin 4 mg/kg showed significant impairment in solving the Carousel maze in sessions 3 through 5. The higher dose of psilocin 4 mg/kg blocked the learning processes even in session 5 when the rats received saline instead of psilocin, although state-dependent learning might explain the impairment on the last day of training.

The maximum time avoided is generally strongly inversely correlated with the number of errors. Accordingly, analysis of this parameter also revealed differences between the studied groups. The two-way ANOVA showed a significant main effect of groups [$F(2, 20) = 15.7$; $P < 0.0001$] and a main effect of sessions [$F(4, 80) = 12.5$; $P < 0.0001$]. There was also an effect of the interaction between these two factors [$F(8, 80) = 3.38$; $P < 0.01$]. A *post hoc* comparison between the groups revealed that the control group exhibited a higher maximum time avoided in session 4 than the two groups treated with psilocin (1 and 4 mg/kg). There were no significant differences between the group treated with psilocin 1 and 4 mg/kg.

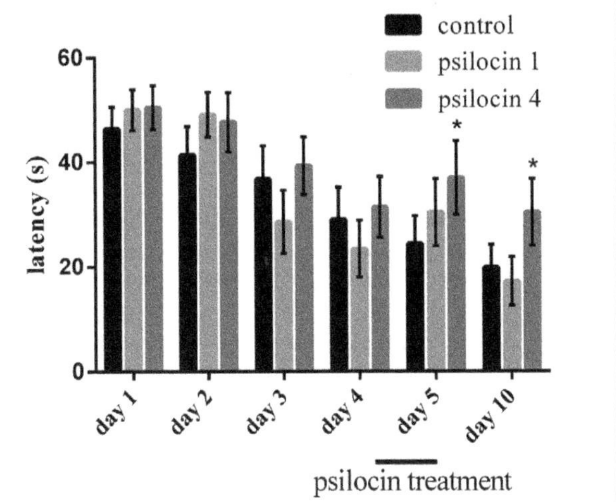

FIGURE 2 | Psilocin treatment (4 mg/kg) disrupted memory retrieval in the MWM after 4 days of pre-training and also impaired memory retrieval 5 days later (Day 10) without the presence of the drug.
$*P < 0.05$, compared to the control group on the same day.

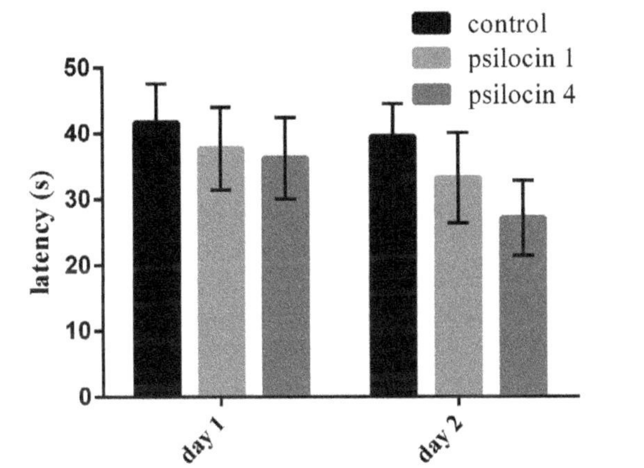

FIGURE 3 | Psilocin injected after training on Day 1 had no effect on memory consolidation at both doses (1 or 4 mg/kg) in the MWM.

EFFECT OF PSILOCIN ON MEMORY RETRIEVAL IN THE MWM

We analyzed the behavioral parameter related to performance in the MWM, escape latency (**Figure 2**). Animals from all groups were pre-trained in the reference memory version of the MWM for 4 days without drug injections; the performance was similar across all of the groups [no significant effect between groups on Day 1–4 $F(2, 20) = 2.1$; $P = 0.14$]. There was a significant effect of days on all measures [$F(2, 20) = 7.77$; $P < 0.0031$]. On Day 5, memory retrieval was tested under the influence of psilocin (1 or 4 mg/kg, s.c). There was significant effect of days and sessions [$F(2, 20) = 4.88$; $P < 0.01$; $F(7, 140) = 4.7$; $P < 0.0001$]. *Post hoc* tests indicated that the retrieval was impaired in the group treated with a 4-mg/kg dose ($P < 0.01$). We found an effect of groups and sessions [$F(2, 20) = 5.91$; $P < 0.01$; $F(7, 140) = 6.46$; $P < 0.0001$] 5 days after the psilocin treatment. A control retrieval experiment was pursued without injections; surprisingly, the group with the previously administered high dose of psilocin was impaired again ($P < 0.01$).

EFFECT OF PSILOCIN ON MEMORY CONSOLIDATION IN THE MWM

The animals were trained for 16 trials without drug injection on the first day (Day 1); subsequently, psilocin was injected (1 or 4 mg/kg) to investigate its effect of memory consolidation. On the next (Day 2), the animals were re-tested in the MWM with the same platform position. Psilocin did not affect the consolidation in the MWM. We found no effect of groups and sessions [$F(2, 42) = 1.110$; $P = 0.3390$; $F(1, 42) = 1.163$; $P = 0.2870$]. **Figure 3** shows slightly better cognitive performance than on Day 1, but no significant between-group differences.

DISCUSSION

Our findings indicate that psilocin affects learning and memory acquisition necessary for spatial navigation and that it also has a disruptive effect on memory retrieval in MWM. Previous reports on the effects of psilocin/psilocybin on cognition in animals are very sparse, use different paradigms and did not bring uniform results, which make them difficult to compare. One study in rats reported impaired acquisition of a conditioned avoidance response (Sugrue, 1969) while another one in mice did not find any effect on the acquisition of an escape avoidance conditioning task (Collins et al., 1966). However, both studies were conducted with very high doses of psilocin/psilocybin. Furthermore, opposing effects of low psilocin doses on memory consolidation were found in two different mice strains when psilocin was injected immediately after each training session in a light–dark discrimination task (Castellano, 1978). On the other hand, most of the studies with other hallucinogens congruently found a disruption of cognitive performance. Similar findings to ours were shown for 2,5-dimethoxy-4-iodoamphetamine (DOI) in a special water maze, where this compound worsened the performance during acute intoxication as well as when subsequently tested without the influence of the drug (Kant et al., 1998). Early studies with LSD and mescaline congruently found disruption of spatial navigation, exploration, and discrimination within different frameworks in T-maze/Y-maze (Castellano, 1971; Davies and Redfern, 1973; Molinengo et al., 1986; Koupilova et al., 1989, 1999). LSD and other hallucinogens also induced errors in swimming through an underwater maze and increased starting latency of swimming through the maze (Uyeno, 1969, 1986). Recently, the use of a translational touch-screen based approach also showed alterations in visuo-spatial learning after acute LSD treatment in rats (Talpos et al., 2014). Finally, chronic mescaline treatment completely blocked the ability to switch between learned trials during operant conditioning (food reinforcement) (Fundaro et al., 1986).

There are two main aspects that have a crucial role in psilocin induced changes. Firstly, psilocybin, like other hallucinogens, had an inhibitory effect on locomotor and exploratory activity with the higher dose used (Collins et al., 1966; Halberstadt et al., 2011; Palenicek et al., 2012, 2013). However, we believe that the main effect of locomotor inhibition can be excluded, since the lower psilocin dose in the Carousel maze did not significantly differ from the controls during any of the sessions even though it induced the deficit in this task. Furthermore, the higher dose during session 4, when the animals showed peak performance, did not induce any significant locomotor inhibition. The psilocin-treated animals also showed a trend toward an increase in their locomotion within every session similarly to the control group, suggesting either developing tolerance to the drug or task sensitization. On the other hand, such an increase might also be attributable to the gradual acquisition of an avoidance strategy, which requires a highly coordinated spatiotemporal locomotion pattern in order to avoid a sector.

Secondly, since active avoidance in the Carousel maze as well as the MWM are spatial tasks requiring extra-maze cue orientation for successful acquisition, altered spatiotemporal perception (hallucinatory effects) can definitely contribute/underlie these changes. Unlike human studies on psilocybin (for a review, see Tyls et al., 2013); unfortunately, we are unable to directly confirm hallucinatory effects in rats in our setting. However, previous studies in rodents found an attenuation of time perception after hallucinogens (Hanks and González-Maeso, 2013) and studies in primates also support hallucinogenic effects in these species (Uyeno, 1969; Fantegrossi et al., 2004). Therefore, we might expect temporal and visual perceptual alterations to be present also in our setting. Indeed, it is well known that psilocin induces attention distraction (Hasler et al., 2004; Carter et al., 2005), which can also underlie the learning deficits. Interestingly, learning in the Carousal maze was also disrupted in the after-session, with no exposition to psilocin, indicating that psilocin blocked the learning process until the last session. Also, the higher dose of psilocin disrupted memory retrieval in the MWM, an effect that persisted for another 5 days. In other words, the rats that received psilocin during the retrieval trial did not improve their performance during this task, contrary to the control group, suggesting that not only retrieval but also re-acquisition was corrupted. This supports the idea that psilocin also had amnestic effects.

It is well known from the literature that psilocin effects are mainly mediated through 5-$HT_{2A/C}$ and 5-HT_{1A} receptors (Tyls et al., 2013). These receptors are widely distributed in the neocortex, basal ganglia, limbic system, and hippocampus and in the case of 5-HT_{1A} also in rapheal nuclei (Barnes and Sharp, 1999). All of these areas are known to be involved in cognitive processes and memory. It is well known that 5-$HT_{2A/C}$ receptors in particular are rapidly downregulated/desensitized after stimulation (Roth et al., 1990, 1995, 1998). This can explain the loss of the locomotor inhibitory effect observed in the Carousel maze. Since systemic administration of 5-HT_{2A} receptor antagonists induces cognitive deficit in rats (Ma and Yu, 1993; Fedotova and Ordyan, 2010) the down-regulation/desensitization of 5-$HT_{2A/C}$ receptors after repeated administration of psilocin might also yield some of the effects observed in our setting. It is of interest that stimulation of 5-HT_{1A} and 5-HT_{1B} receptors is also known to impair acquisition of spatial memory tasks (Buhot et al., 1995; Herremans et al., 1995; Koenig et al., 2008). Nevertheless, further experiments are needed to explain the receptor mechanisms underlying these changes.

In conclusion, our study demonstrated that 5-$HT_{2A/C}$ and 5-HT_{1A} agonist psilocin impaired spatial learning in the Carousel maze and it also had an amnestic effect in the MWM. On the other hand, it had no effect on memory consolidation.

ACKNOWLEDGMENTS

This study was supported by the projects IGA MHCR NT/13897, MICR VG20122015080, VG20122015075, MH CZ – DRO (PCP, 00023752), PRVOUK P34, NIMH-CZ 1.05/2.1.00/03.0078 and the European Regional Development Fund. Scientists from the Institute of Physiology Academy of Sciences were supported by GACR grants 14-03627S, 14-20613S, and GACR P304-12-G069. We also declare support of IGA MZ CR NT13386. We thank Craig Hampson B.Sc. (Hons) for his helpful comments and language correction.

REFERENCES

Barnes, N. M., and Sharp, T. (1999). Review of central 5-HT receptors and their function. *Neuropharmacology* 28, 1083–1152. doi:10.1016/S0028-3908(99)00010-6

Blahna, K., Svoboda, J., Telensky, P., and Klement, D. (2011). Inertial stimuli generated by arena rotation are important for acquisition of the active place avoidance task. *Behav. Brain Res.* 216, 207–213. doi:10.1016/j.bbr.2010.07.038

Bogenschutz, M. P., and Pommy, J. M. (2012). Therapeutic mechanisms of classic hallucinogens in the treatment of addictions: from indirect evidence to testable hypotheses. *Drug Test. Anal.* 4, 543–555. doi:10.1002/dta.1376

Buhot, M. C., Patra, S. K., and Naïli, S. (1995). Spatial memory deficits following stimulation of hippocampal 5-HT1B receptors in the rat. *Eur. J. Pharmacol.* 285, 221–228. doi:10.1016/0014-2999(95)00407-C

Carter, O. L., Pettigrew, J. D., Hasler, F., Wallis, G. M., Liu, G. B., Hell, D., et al. (2005). Modulating the rate and rhythmicity of perceptual rivalry alternations with the mixed 5-HT2A and 5-HT1A agonist psilocybin. *Neuropsychopharmacology* 30, 1154–1162. doi:10.1038/sj.npp.1300621

Castellano, C. (1971). Lysergic acid diethylamide, amphetamine and chlorpromazine on water maze discrimination in mice. *Psychopharmacologia* 19, 16–25. doi:10.1007/BF00403698

Castellano, C. (1978). Effects of mescaline and psilocin on acquisition, consolidation, and performance of light-dark discrimination in two inbred strains of mice. *Psychopharmacology (Berl.)* 59, 129–137. doi:10.1007/BF00427746

Cimadevilla, J. M., Fenton, A. A., and Bures, J. (2001). New spatial cognition tests for mice: passive place avoidance on stable and active place avoidance on rotating arenas. *Brain Res. Bull.* 54, 559–563. doi:10.1016/S0361-9230(01)00448-8

Cimadevilla, J. M., Kaminsky, Y., Fenton, A., and Bures, J. (2000). Passive and active place avoidance as a tool of spatial memory research in rats. *J. Neurosci. Methods* 102, 155–164. doi:10.1016/S0165-0270(00)00288-0

Collins, R. L., Ordy, J. M., and Samorajski, T. (1966). Psilocin: effects on behaviour and brain serotonin in mice. *Nature* 209, 785–787. doi:10.1038/209785a0

Davies, J. A., and Redfern, P. H. (1973). The effects of hallucinogenic drugs on maze exploration in the rat over a 24 hour period. *Br. J. Pharmacol.* 49, 121–127. doi:10.1111/j.1476-5381.1973.tb08274.x

dos Santos, R. G. (2014). Potential therapeutic effects of psilocybin/psilocin are minimized while possible adverse reactions are overrated. *Ther. Drug Monit.* 36, 131–132. doi:10.1097/FTD.0000000000000028

Eichenbaum, H. (2001). The hippocampus and declarative memory: cognitive mechanisms and neural codes. *Behav. Brain Res.* 127, 199–207. doi:10.1016/S0166-4328(01)00365-5

Fajnerova, I., Kenney, J., Lobellova, V., Okrouhlicova, S., Stuchlik, A., Klement, D. (2014). Can rats solve the active place avoidance task without the room-bound cues? *Behav. Brain Res.* 267, 126–132. doi:10.1016/j.bbr.2014.03.028

Fantegrossi, W. E., Woods, J. H., and Winger, G. (2004). Transient reinforcing effects of phenylisopropylamine and indolealkylamine hallucinogens in rhesus monkeys. *Behav. Pharmacol.* 15, 149–157. doi:10.1097/00008877-200403000-00007

Fedotova, Y. O., and Ordyan, N. E. (2010). Blockade of 5-HT2A/2C-type receptors impairs learning in female rats in the course of estrous cycle. *Bull. Exp. Biol. Med.* 150, 6–8. doi:10.1007/s10517-010-1053-6

Fenton, A. A., Wesierska, M., Kaminsky, Y., and Bures, J. (1998). Both here and there: simultaneous expression of autonomous spatial memories in rats. *Proc. Natl. Acad. Sci. U.S.A.* 1998, 11493–11498. doi:10.1073/pnas.95.19.11493

Fundaro, A., Molinengo, L., Cassone, M. C., and Orsetti, M. (1986). Action of a chronic administration of mescaline in dynamic behavioural situations. *Prog. Neuropsychopharmacol. Biol. Psychiatry* 10, 41–48. doi:10.1016/0278-5846(86)90042-4

Geyer, M. A. (1998). Behavioral studies of hallucinogenic drugs in animals: implications for schizophrenia research. *Pharmacopsychiatry* 2, 73–79. doi:10.1055/s-2007-979350

Grob, C. S., Danforth, A. L., Chopra, G. S., Hagerty, M., McKay, C. R., Halberstadt, A. L., et al. (2011). Pilot study of psilocybin treatment for anxiety in patients with advanced-stage cancer. *Arch. Gen. Psychiatry* 68, 71–78. doi:10.1001/archgenpsychiatry.2010.116

Halberstadt, A. L., Koedood, L., Powell, S. B., and Geyer, M. A. (2011). Differential contributions of serotonin receptors to the behavioral effects of indoleamine hallucinogens in mice. *J. Psychopharmacol.* 25, 1548–1561. doi:10.1177/0269881110388326

Hanks, J. B., and González-Maeso, J. (2013). Animal models of serotonergic psychedelics. *ACS Chem. Neurosci.* 4, 33–42. doi:10.1021/cn300138m

Hasler, F., Bourquin, D., Brenneisen, R., Bär, T., and Vollenweider, F. X. (1997). Determination of psilocin and 4-hydroxyindole-3-acetic acid in plasma by HPLC-ECD and pharmacokinetic profiles of oral and intravenous psilocybin in man. *Pharm. Acta Helv.* 72, 175–184. doi:10.1016/S0031-6865(97)00014-9

Hasler, F., Grimberg, U., Benz, M. A., Huber, T., and Vollenweider, F. X. (2004). Acute psychological and physiological effects of psilocybin in healthy humans: a double-blind, placebo-controlled dose-effect study. *Psychopharmacology (Berl.)* 172, 145–156. doi:10.1007/s00213-003-1640-6

Herremans, A. H., Hijzen, T. H., Olivier, B., and Slangen, J. L. (1995). Serotonergic drug effects on a delayed conditional discrimination task in the rat; involvement of the 5-HT1A receptor in working memory. *J. Psychopharmacol.* 9, 242–250. doi:10.1177/026988119500900307

Kant, G. J., Wylie, R. M., Chu, K., and Ghosh, S. (1998). Effects of the serotonin agonists 8-OH-DPAT, buspirone, and DOI on water maze performance. *Pharmacol. Biochem. Behav.* 59, 729–735. doi:10.1016/S0091-3057(97)00553-4

Koenig, J., Cosquer, B., and Cassel, J. C. (2008). Activation of septal 5-HT1A receptors alters spatial memory encoding, interferes with consolidation, but does not affect retrieval in rats subjected to a water-maze task. *Hippocampus* 18, 99–118. doi:10.1002/hipo.20368

Koupilova, M., Herink, J., and Hrdina, V. (1989). The effect of local mescaline application on learning and memory in rats. *Physiol. Bohemoslov.* 38, 497–502.

Koupilova, M., Herink, J., and Krs, O. (1999). Influencing of spatial memory in rats by DSP-4 and mescaline. *Acta Med. (Hradec Kralove)* 42, 69–72.

Ma, T. C., and Yu, Q. H. (1993). Effect of 20 (S)-ginsenoside-Rg2 and cyproheptadine on two-way active avoidance learning and memory in rats. *Arzneimittelforschung* 43, 1049–1052.

Molinengo, L., Cassone, M. C., Baroli, A., and Orsetti, M. (1986). Mescaline action on "memory decay" and "problem solving" behavior in the rat. *Prog. Neuropsychopharmacol. Biol. Psychiatry* 10, 709–715. doi:10.1016/0278-5846(86)90055-2

Moreno, F. A., Wiegand, C. B., Taitano, E. K., and Delgado, P. L. (2006). Safety, tolerability, and efficacy of psilocybin in 9 patients with obsessive-compulsive disorder. *J. Clin. Psychiatry* 67, 1735–1740. doi:10.4088/JCP.v67n1110

Morris, R. G. M. (1981). Spatial localization does not require the presence of local cues. *Learn. Motiv.* 12, 239–261. doi:10.1016/0023-9690(81)90020-5

Morris, R. G. M., Garrud, P., Rawlings, J., and O'Keefe, J. (1982). Place navigation impaired in rats with hippocampal lesions. *Nature* 297, 681–683. doi:10.1038/297681a0

Morris, R. (2013). "Neurobiology of learning and memory" in *Neuroscience in the 21st Century*, ed. D. W. Pfaff (New York: Springer), 2173–2211. doi:10.1007/978-1-4614-1997-6

Nichols, D. E. (2004). Hallucinogens. *Pharmacol. Ther.* 101, 131–181. doi:10.1016/j.pharmthera.2003.11.002

O'Keefe, J., and Nadel, L. (1978). *The Hippocampus as a Cognitive Map.* New York: Oxford University Press.

Palenicek, T., Fujakova, M., Brunovsky, M., Horacek, J., Gorman, I., Balikova, M., et al. (2013). Behavioral, neurochemical and pharmaco-EEG profiles of the psychedelic drug 4-bromo-2,5-dimethoxyphenethylamine (2C-B) in rats. *Psychopharmacology (Berl.)* 225, 75–93. doi:10.1007/s00213-012-2797-7

Palenicek, T., Hlinak, Z., Bubenikova-Valesova, V., Novak, T., and Horacek, J. (2012). Sex differences in the effects of N,N-diethyllysergamide (LSD) on behavioural activity and prepulse inhibition. *Prog. Neuropsychopharmacol. Biol. Psychiatry* 34, 588–596. doi:10.1016/j.pnpbp.2010.02.008

Park, S., and Holzman, P. S. (1992). Schizophrenics show spatial working memory deficits. *Arch. Gen. Psychiatry* 49, 975–982. doi:10.1001/archpsyc.1992.01820120063009

Passie, T., Seifert, J., Schneider, U., and Emrich, H. M. (2002). The pharmacology of psilocybin. *Addict. Biol.* 7, 357–364. doi:10.1080/1355621021000005937

Ray, T. S. (2010). Psychedelics and the human receptorome. *PLoS ONE* 5:e9019. doi:10.1371/journal.pone.0009019

Roth, B. L., Berry, S. A., Kroeze, W. K., Willins, D. L., and Kristiansen, K. (1998). Serotonin 5-HT2A receptors: molecular biology and mechanisms of regulation. *Crit. Rev. Neurobiol.* 12, 319–338. doi:10.1615/CritRevNeurobiol.v12.i4.30

Roth, B. L., Hamblin, M., and Ciaranello, R. D. (1990). Regulation of 5-HT2 and 5-HT1C serotonin receptor levels. Methodology and mechanisms. *Neuropsychopharmacology* 3, 427–433.

Roth, B. L., Palvimaki, E. P., Berry, S., Khan, N., Sachs, N., Uluer, A., et al. (1995). 5-Hydroxytryptamine2A (5-HT2A) receptor desensitization can occur without down-regulation. *J. Pharmacol. Exp. Ther.* 275, 1638–1646.

Stebelska, K. (2013). Fungal hallucinogens psilocin, ibotenic acid, and muscimol: analytical methods and biologic activities. *Ther. Drug Monit.* 35, 420–442. doi:10.1097/FTD.0b013e31828741a5

Stuchlik, A., Petrasek, T., Prokopova, I., Holubova, K., Hatalova, H., Vales, K., et al. (2013). Place avoidance tasks as tools in the behavioral neuroscience of learning and memory. *Physiol. Res.* 1, 1–19.

Stuchlik, A., Rehakova, L., Telensky, P., and Vales, K. (2007). Morris water maze learning in Long-Evans rats is differentially affected by blockade of D1-like and

D2-like dopamine receptors. *Neurosci. Lett.* 422, 169–174. doi:10.1016/j.neulet.2007.06.012

Stuchlik, A., Rezacova, L., Vales, K., Bubenikova, V., and Kubik, S. (2004). Application of a novel active allothetic place avoidance task (AAPA) in testing a pharmacological model of psychosis in rats: comparison with the Morris water maze. *Neurosci. Lett.* 366, 162–166. doi:10.1016/j.neulet.2004.05.037

Sugrue, M. F. (1969). A study of the role of noradrenaline in behavioral changes produced in the rat by psychotomimetic drugs. *Br. J. Pharmacol.* 35, 243–252. doi:10.1111/j.1476-5381.1969.tb07983.x

Talpos, J. C., Aerts, N., Fellini, L., and Steckler, T. (2014). A touch-screen based paired-associates learning (PAL) task for the rat may provide a translatable pharmacological model of human cognitive impairment. *Pharmacol. Biochem. Behav.* 122C, 97–106. doi:10.1016/j.pbb.2014.03.014

Tolman, E. C. (1948). Cognitive maps in rats and men. *Psychol. Rev.* 55, 189–208. doi:10.1037/h0061626

Tyls, F., Palenicek, T., and Horacek, J. (2013). Psilocybin – summary of knowledge and new perspectives. *Eur. Neuropsychopharmacol.* 24, 342–356. doi:10.1016/j.euroneuro.2013.12.006

Uyeno, E. T. (1969). Alteration of a learned response of the squirrel monkey by hallucinogens. *Int. J. Neuropharmacol.* 8, 245–253. doi:10.1016/0028-3908(69)90045-8

Uyeno, E. T. (1986). Hallucinogenic compounds and swimming response. *J. Pharmacol. Exp. Ther.* 159, 216–221.

Vollenweider, F. X., Leenders, K. L., Scharfetter, C., Maguire, P., Stadelmann, O., and Angst, J. (1997). Positron emission tomography and fluorodeoxyglucose studies of metabolic hyperfrontality and psychopathology in the psilocybin model of psychosis. *Neuropsychopharmacology* 16, 357–372. doi:10.1016/S0893-133X(96)00246-1

Vollenweider, F. X., Vollenweider-Scherpenhuyzen, M. F., Bäbler, A., Vogel, H., and Hell, D. (1998). Psilocybin induces schizophrenia-like psychosis in humans via a serotonin-2 agonist action. *Neuroreport* 9, 3897–3902. doi:10.1097/00001756-199812010-00024

Vollenweider, F. X., Vontobel, P., Hell, D., and Leenders, K. L. (1999). 5-HT modulation of dopamine release in basal ganglia in psilocybin-induced psychosis in man – a PET study with [11C]raclopride. *Neuropsychopharmacology* 20, 424–433. doi:10.1016/S0893-133X(98)00108-0

Wesierska, M., Dockery, C., and Fenton, A. A. (2005). Beyond memory, navigation, and inhibition: behavioral evidence for hippocampus-dependent cognitive coordination in the rat. *J. Neurosci.* 25, 2413–2419. doi:10.1523/JNEUROSCI.3962-04.2005

9

MK-801 impairs cognitive coordination on a rotating arena (Carousel) and contextual specificity of hippocampal immediate-early gene expression in a rat model of psychosis

Štěpán Kubík *, Helena Buchtová, Karel Valeš and Aleš Stuchlík

Neurophysiology of Memory, Institute of Physiology, Academy of Sciences of the Czech Republic, Prague, Czech Republic

Edited by:
Tomiki Sumiyoshi, National Center of Neurology and Psychiatry, Japan

****Correspondence:***
Štěpán Kubík, Neurophysiology of Memory, Institute of Physiology, Academy of Sciences of the Czech Republic, Videnska 1083, CZ-14220 Prague 4, Czech Republic
e-mail: kubik@biomed.cas.cz

Flexible behavior in dynamic, real-world environments requires more than static spatial learning and memory. Discordant and unstable cues must be organized in coherent subsets to give rise to meaningful spatial representations. We model this form of cognitive coordination on a rotating arena – Carousel where arena- and room-bound spatial cues are dissociated. Hippocampal neuronal ensemble activity can repeatedly switch between multiple representations of such an environment. Injection of tetrodotoxin into one hippocampus prevents cognitive coordination during avoidance of a stationary room-defined place on the Carousel and increases coactivity of previously unrelated neurons in the uninjected hippocampus. Place avoidance on the Carousel is impaired after systemic administration of non-competitive NMDAr blockers (MK-801) used to model schizophrenia in animals and people. We tested if this effect is due to cognitive disorganization or other effect of NMDAr antagonism such as hyperlocomotion, spatial memory impairment, or general learning deficit. We also examined if the same dose of MK-801 alters patterns of immediate-early gene (IEG) expression in the hippocampus. IEG expression is triggered in neuronal nuclei in a context-specific manner after behavioral exploration and it is used to map activity in neuronal populations. IEG expression is critical for maintenance of synaptic plasticity and memory consolidation. We show that the same dose of MK-801 that impairs spatial coordination of rats on the Carousel also eliminates contextual specificity of IEG expression in hippocampal CA1 ensembles. This effect is due to increased similarity between ensembles activated in different environments, consistent with the idea that it is caused by increased coactivity between neurons, which did not previously fire together. Our data support the proposition of the Hypersynchrony theory that cognitive disorganization in psychosis is due to increased coactivity between unrelated neurons.

Keywords: hippocampus, arc, homer 1a, place avoidance, rotating arena, carousel, cognitive coordination, schizophrenia

INTRODUCTION

Dynamic environments in the real world often involve multiple reference frames without stable mutual relationships. Drivers need to keep control of their cars and attend to the road at the same time. Similarly, animals need to keep track of their positions within a group of conspecifics as well as within ambient environment. Elements of experience must be segregated into coherent, meaningful representations to support context-relevant behavioral responses (**Figures 1A,C**). Impairment of this cognitive coordination could be responsible for cognitive disorganization in psychosis including inappropriate associations, deficits in contextual binding, and impaired discrimination between relevant and irrelevant information (Ellenbroek and Cools, 1990; Silverstein et al., 2000; Phillips and Silverstein, 2003; Uhlhaas et al., 2004; Hemsley, 2005). Spatial, contextual, and episodic-like memory critically depends on the hippocampus (Moscovitch et al., 2006) and hippocampal pathology (Harrison, 2004; Tamminga et al., 2012; Ledoux et al., 2013) and episodic memory deficits are common in schizophrenia (Weiss et al., 2003; Barch, 2005; Boyer et al., 2007; Ranganath et al., 2008). However, most laboratory tests of hippocampal function occur in static environments or involve only one-off changes or between-session alternations.

During place avoidance (PA) on a continuously rotating circular arena (Carousel), rats have to avoid a place hidden in either

---

Abbreviations: Arc/Arg 3.1, activity-regulated cytoskeleton-associated protein/RNA; CC, caged controls; D, total distance actively traveled during the session; DAPI, 4′,6-diamidino-2-phenylindole; DG, dentate gyrus; E, the number of entrances; ED, the number of entrances per unit distance; FAB, fragment antigen-binding; FISH, fluorescence *in situ* hybridization; GABA, gamma-aminobutyric acid; HRP, horseradish peroxidase; IEG, immediate-early gene; MaxT, maximum avoidance time (duration); NMDA(r), *N*-methyl D-aspartate (receptor); OCT, optimal cutting temperature freezing medium; PA, place avoidance; PV, parvalbumin; pTime, shock zone occupancy; TSA, tyramide signal amplification; TTX, tetrodotoxin; UTR, untranslated region.

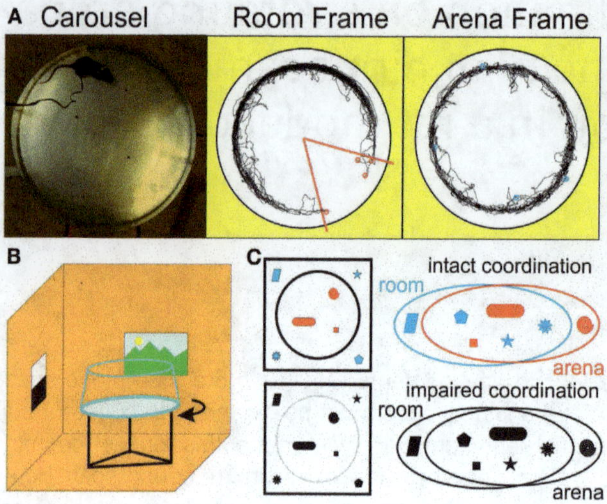

FIGURE 1 | Dissociated reference frames on the Carousel. (A) A photograph of the Carousel arena (left) and example trajectories in the stationary Room frame (middle), where the shock zone (red) is defined and in the rotating Arena frame (right) during a room-defined place avoidance session. Red and blue circles mark locations where shocks were administered in the Room and Arena frames, respectively. **(B)** Schematics of the rotating arena in a stationary room. Continuous rotation of the arena dissociates spatial reference frames of the stationary room and the rotating arena **(C)** Illustration of the cognitive coordination function in a color model, where cue color facilitates discrimination between two sets of cues. When color is lost, discrimination becomes more difficult. The two cue sets are still clearly delineated from the top view (left), but the distinction is much less clear from the perspective of the animal, let alone a multi-modal spatial representation system in the hippocampus (right).

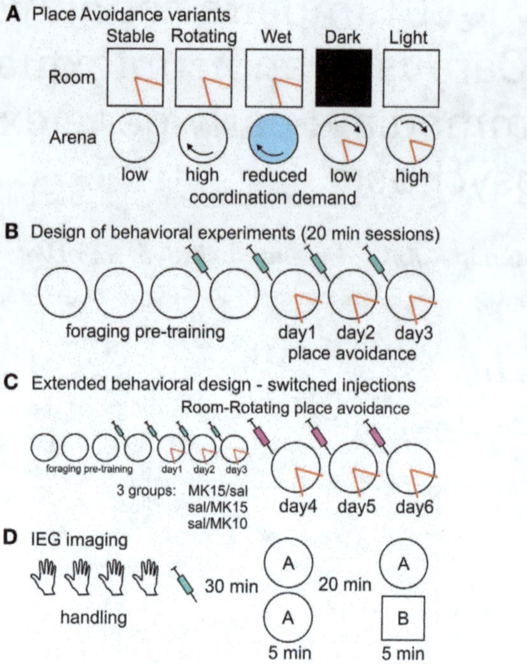

FIGURE 2 | Experimental design (A). A schematic of five versions of the place avoidance task. All spatial cues are relevant and the demand for cognitive coordination is low during room-defined avoidance on the Stable arena when the arena rotation is off. In contrast, the room and arena cues are dissociated on the Rotating arena resulting in a high coordination demand. Cues on the arena surface are hidden by shallow water, but the arena-bound idiothetic cues can still interfere with the avoidance, and the demand for coordination is reduced on the Wet arena. The cognitive coordination demand during arena-based avoidance is low when irrelevant room cues are hidden by Darkness and high when they are available in Light. The shock zone (red) is defined in one reference frame **(B)**. Design of the place avoidance experiments. The rats were pre-trained to forage on the arena prior to the place avoidance training. Saline or MK-801 was administered 30 min before the session starting from the last day of foraging **(C)**. Extended place avoidance training design. After 3 days of Room-Rotating training, injections were switched so that rats initially trained with MK-801 (0.15 mg/kg) received saline (MK15/sal) and rats initially trained with saline received MK-801 at 0.15 mg/kg (sal/MK15) or 0.10 mg/kg (sal/MK10). The extended training continued for 3 days. **(D)**. Design of the IEG imaging experiment. Rats received four handling sessions (5 min), an injection of saline or MK-801, and two exploration sessions in environment **(A)** or in environments **(A,B)**.

the stationary room or the rotating arena frame (**Figures 1A,B**; Cimadevilla et al., 2001). They have to selectively attend to cues from the relevant frame and ignore the others to avoid the shock effectively. Inactivation of one hippocampus by tetrodotoxin (TTX) increased coactivity of previously uncorrelated CA1 neurons in the uninjected hippocampus (Olypher et al., 2006) and impaired cognitive coordination on the Carousel (Wesierska et al., 2005). PA on the Carousel is also impaired after systemic administration of dizocilpine (MK-801; Stuchlík et al., 2004; Stuchlík and Valeš, 2005; Valeš et al., 2006; Bubeníková-Valešová et al., 2008b). Non-competitive NMDA receptor antagonists such as MK-801 are used to model schizophrenia in animals (Deutsch et al., 2002; Powel and Geyer, 2007; Bubeníková-Valešová et al., 2008a; Adell et al., 2012), because they elicit psychosis in people (Newcomer and Krystal, 2001). We tested if the PA deficit on the Carousel is due to MK-801-induced cognitive disorganization or another effect of NMDAr antagonism such as hyperlocomotion (Martin et al., 1997) or spatial navigation and memory deficits (Stuchlík et al., 2004; van der Staay et al., 2011). We compared the effect of MK-801 on PA in five versions of the task, which differed in the amount of misleading information from the irrelevant spatial frame left to interfere with the PA (**Figure 2A**).

Behavioral activity triggers immediate-early gene (IEGs) expression in hippocampal and cortical neurons (Kubik et al., 2007, 2012). Precise temporal regulation of transcription and intracellular distribution of RNA for IEG *Arc/Arg3.1* (Link et al., 1995; Lyford et al., 1995) has been used to map activity history of hippocampal pyramidal neurons during two distinct behavioral epochs (Guzowski et al., 1999). Intranuclear foci expression of *Arc* marked neurons activated immediately before the sacrifice, whereas cytoplasmic signal marked neurons activated ~25 min earlier. Although the IEGs *Arc* and *Homer1a* are co-expressed in the same neurons, the signal from riboprobes targeting the 3′ UTR of the long (~40 kb) primary transcript of *Homer 1a* only appears in the nuclei ~25 min after the induction and can be used to replace the diffuse cytoplasmic *Arc* signal (Vazdarjanova et al., 2002).

Proportions of hippocampal neurons expressing *Arc* or *Homer 1a* after exploration of an environment (Guzowski et al., 1999;

Vazdarjanova and Guzowski, 2004) are similar to proportions of neurons displaying place cell activity in an environment (Lee et al., 2004; Leutgeb et al., 2004). Both IEG expression and place cell activity occur in an environment-specific manner suggesting that IEG expression is triggered in place cells displaying firing fields during behavioral exploration. The Hypersynchrony theory posits that increased coactivity selectively between previously non-coactive neurons disrupts cognitive coordination and causes cognitive disorganization in psychosis (Fenton, 2009). Neurons active in the same environment are more likely to be coactive than neurons active in different environments. Ensembles of hippocampal neurons expressing *Arc* and *Homer 1a* are more similar after repeated exploration of the same environment than after exploration of different environments (Guzowski et al., 1999; Vazdarjanova and Guzowski, 2004). We tested if MK-801 increases similarity between hippocampal ensembles expressing the IEGs in different environments more than between ensembles activated in the same environment.

MATERIALS AND METHODS

SUBJECTS

One hundred and fifty-one young adult (~3 month old) male Long–Evans rats from the Institute of Physiology breeding colony were used in the study. They were housed in pairs in transparent Plexiglas cages and maintained at a 12/12 h light/dark cycle with lights on at 7:00 and water available *ad libitum*. The rats were acclimatized to the laboratory vivarium for 10 days, handled, and habituated to the experimental apparatus prior to the PA training. This design was adopted to reduce learning-related stress later during training. After the conclusion of behavioral procedures, rats were killed by an overdose of Thiopental. Rats used in the IEG imaging experiment ($n = 42$) were housed individually in opaque cages to avoid high IEG expression background resulting from social interactions. The animals were handled for 4 days, but not habituated to the environment prior to behavioral sessions used to trigger IEG expression (see below). All behavioral testing was conducted during the light phase of the day. All animal treatment complied with the Czech Animal Protection Act, EU directive 2010/63/EC, and NIH guidelines.

DRUG TREATMENT

MK-801 [dizocilpine (+)-5-methyl-10,11-dihydro-5*H*-dibenzo cycloheptene-5,10-imine maleate; Sigma] was diluted in sterile physiological saline at a *low* (0.10 mg/kg) or *high* (0.15 mg/kg) dose. Beginning with the last foraging session, rats received daily injections of either MK-801 or saline solution (1 ml/kg, i.p.) 30 min before behavioral testing (**Figures 2B,C**). The first injection allowed rats to habituate to the injection procedure and to the MK-801-induced state before the onset of the PA training. Rats in the IEG imaging experiment received a single injection 30 min prior to the catFISH test sessions (**Figure 2D**).

CAROUSEL

The apparatus was a smooth metallic elevated circular arena (82 cm diameter) equipped with a 5 cm high lip on the perimeter, a detachable transparent plexiglass wall, and a motor, which rotated the arena (1 rpm; **Figure 1B**). The wall consisted of four parts connected by small bolts arranged in four vertical strips and prevented the rats from accidentally or deliberately falling off the arena. This symmetrical design was chosen because it provided less spatial information than asymmetrical single joint strip. The wall was always in the same position relative to the arena surface and as such provided arena-based visual information. The rats wore a harness carrying infrared (IR) LEDs and an alligator clip for shock delivery. A tracking system (iTrack, Biosignal Group, Inc., New York, USA) recorded the rat's position via an overhead IR camera, delivered shocks to reinforce the PA behavior, and stored the data for off-line analysis. The harness was attached to a cable carrying power for the LEDs and the shock current. AC shock current (50 Hz, 0.5 s, 0.5–0.7 mA) was delivered from a constant-current source via the alligator clip connected to a subcutaneously implanted electrode between the rat's shoulders. It was made by piercing the rat's skin by a sterile hypodermic needle and twisting the sharp end to prevent slipping out. This design was adopted to facilitate perception of the shock at the high-impedance (~100 kΩ) contact between the rats body and the grounded arena floor rather than at the low-impedance (~100 Ω) implanted electrode. A second IR LED was fixed to the arena perimeter and used by the tracking system to compute a virtual "arena frame" view of the rotating arena (**Figure 1A**). Indirect light was provided by a 40 W light bulb during all behavioral sessions.

PLACE AVOIDANCE

After food-restriction to 90% of their pre-restriction weight, rats were trained in four foraging sessions with no shocks and subsequently given three PA training sessions on seven consecutive days (**Figure 2B**). Some rats received extended PA training on three more days (**Figure 2C**). Each session lasted 20 min. Cereal cocoa puffs (Nesquik; Nestlé) were dispersed from an overhead feeder to ensure sufficient exploration throughout the experiment and prevent passivity. Importantly, the cocoa puffs remained floating and did not dissolve (Kubik and Fenton, 2005) when the arena was covered with shallow water in one of the experiments (see below). The rats were weighed and their weights recorded daily to maintain constant motivation. During the PA training, a computer-based tracking system (Tracker, Biosignal Group, USA) administered a mild 500 ms shock and counted an entrance whenever the rat entered a 60° shock zone for at least 500 ms. Additional shocks were delivered every 1500 ms until the rat left the shock zone. Additional entrances were counted if the rat left the area for at least 1500 ms. To adjust for variability in shock sensitivity, shock intensity was set individually for each rat to the lowest value sufficient to elicit an escape response, but not freezing. This adjustment was performed on the arena during initial PA training. This design was adopted to enhance comparability between different versions of the PA task by stimulating exploration and discouraging passivity.

EXPERIMENTAL DESIGN

One hundred and nine rats were trained in five different variants of the PA task (**Figure 2A**). Two doses (0.10 and 0.15 mg/kg) of MK-801 were used in the first two experiments. Thirty-one rats (16 saline, 8 low, and 7 high dose of MK-801) were trained to avoid a place defined in the stationary room on a stable (Room-Stable) and 29 rats (15 saline, 7 low, and 7 high dose of MK-801) on a rotating (Room-Rotating) dry arena. The low dose showed no effect on the rotating arena and therefore only the high dose was used in the following experiments. Sixteen rats (eight saline and eight high MK-801) were tested on the rotating arena covered with shallow water (<1 cm; Room-Wet). Twenty-eight rats were trained to avoid a place defined on the rotating arena either in darkness (Arena-Dark; 12 rats; 6 saline and 6 high MK-801) or in the light (Arena-Light; 16 rats; 8 saline and 8 high MK-801). Conditions during foraging pre-training always matched those during avoidance training except that no shocks were delivered. In the Room-Rotating version, the same PA training was *Extended* for three more days (**Figure 2C**), but the injections were switched so that rats initially trained with MK-801 (0.15 mg/kg) received saline (MK15/sal, $n = 7$) and rats trained with saline received either 0.15 mg/kg (sal/MK15, $n = 7$) or 0.10 mg/kg MK-801 (sal/MK10, $n = 7$). Rats in the sal/MK10 group showed asymptotic performance from PA day 3 with no MK-801-induced impairment on day 4 and they were used as controls in this experiment. One of the rats did not complete the extended training and was not included in the analysis.

BEHAVIORAL DATA ANALYSIS

Stored data files were analyzed by Track Analysis (Biosignal Group, Inc.). Data from the 3 days of PA training are reported (**Figure 2B**). The total number of Entrances (E) into the shock zone, the Maximum Avoidance Time (MaxT), and the proportion of Time spent in the shock zone (pTime) per session were used to evaluate the avoidance. The total Distance (D) traveled during a session measured the overall locomotion. To assess the effect of increased locomotion on the avoidance, the number of Entrances per unit Distance was calculated (ED). In experiments on the rotating arena, we obtained a measure of purely active locomotion (without the arena rotation) in a virtual "arena view" calculated by the tracking system using the reference IR LED fixed to the arena. A two-way ANOVA with repeated measures on sessions was used to compare the effect of MK-801 to vehicle controls over multiple days of training in each condition and to examine the effect of arena rotation on control performance. Newman–Keuls *post hoc* tests were used where appropriate. Paired t-tests were used to assess the effect of injection switch within-subject. No specific corrections for multiple comparisons were performed in this study. These corrections involve a trade-off between Type I and II errors and usually require the comparisons to be independent. Bonferroni correction would accept significance at $\alpha = 0.0167$, the less conservative Šidák correction at $\alpha = 0.0170$. Majority of tests reported here are not affected by these adjustments because they yielded much lower p. In notable exceptions (see Discussion and MK-801 Impaired Segregation of Discordant Spatial Information), a Tukey HSD test was used as a weak control for Type I error connected with repeated measures. Given that the repeated measures were not independent, we report uncorrected ANOVA statistics and actual values for all $p > 0.01$ to provide maximum relevant information. Five rats were excluded from the analysis. One rat did not receive the shock properly due to a damaged cable, and four rats (each from a different group) were excluded based on Dixon's Q-test for outliers ($Q = $ gap/range) at 99% confidence (Rorabacher, 1991; Christian, 2003).

IMMEDIATE-EARLY GENE IMAGING

Thirty rats received two 6 min exploration sessions in either the same environment A/A or in two different environments A/B separated by 20 min (**Figure 2D**). Environment A was the Carousel arena described above equipped with three identical objects (dark plastic cylinders 8 cm high 2 cm diameter) whereas environment B was a white square open field of equivalent size (72 cm) with three wooden blocks 3 cm × 6 cm × 6 cm located in a different room. Twelve (four per each treatment) more rats served as caged controls (CC). The rats were injected with saline or MK-801 (0.10 and 0.15 mg/kg) 30 min before the exploration sessions. Immediately after the second session, the rats were deeply anesthetized with isoflurane and decapitated. Their brains were quickly removed, flash-frozen in a dry ice-cooled isopentane bath and stored in a −80°C freezer for later analysis. Four millimeter segments containing the dorsal hippocampus from left hemispheres were arranged in blocks maximizing the number of within-block, between-group comparisons and embedded in optimal cutting temperature medium (OCT; Sakura). The blocks were sectioned at 20 μm in a cryostat (Leica CM 1850, Germany), mounted on gelatine-coated superfrost slides (Fisher), and processed for fluorescence *in situ* hybridization as previously described (Vazdarjanova and Guzowski, 2004; Kubik et al., 2012). Briefly, fluorescein-labeled antisense riboprobes for *Homer 1a* 3′UTR and digoxigenin-labeled *Arc* antisense riboprobes were hybridized overnight in a single hybridization step and then sequentially detected with anti-fluorescein-HRP (Jackson labs) and anti-digoxigenin-HRP FAB fragments (Roche). *Homer 1a* probes were visualized with a tyramide-fluorescein signal amplification system (TSA-Fluorescein) and *Arc* probes with TSA-Cy3 (Perkin-Elmer). Slides were incubated with a nuclear counterstain (DAPI, Invitrogen), coverslipped with antifade media (Vectashield, Vector labs), and sealed with nail polish.

IMAGE DATA ACQUISITION AND ANALYSIS

Confocal stacks from CA1 were acquired on an inverted Leica SP5 laser scanning microscope with apochromatic objectives HCX PL APO 20× (n.a. 0.7) imm corr Lbd. BL and HCX PL APO 10× (n.a. 0.40) CS. The blue signal (DAPI) was imaged using 405 nm excitation and a 415–490 bandpass, the green signal (TSA-Fluorescein) with 488 nm excitation and a 510–550 bandpass, and the orange/red signal (TSA-Cy3) with 561 nm excitation and a 610–680 bandpass. The laser power, gain, and offset were always set for the whole slide. The settings were optimized to obtain bright intranuclear foci of ongoing IEG transcription. Six to eight CA1 images with an average of 570 ± 13 cells were analyzed from each animal. The image data were analyzed by a technician blind to the identity of the samples using a custom macro for ImageJ as described before (Kubik et al., 2012). The proportions of *Homer 1a*+ and *Arc*+ neurons were used to map neuronal ensembles active during the first and second test session, respectively. The similarity of these activated ensembles was evaluated using similarity scores = diff(E1E2)/least epoch − p(E1E2), where E1 and E2 are proportions of *Homer 1a*+ and *Arc*+ neurons, respectively, p(E1E2) is a random overlap = E1*E2, least epoch is the smaller one of E1 and E2, and diff(E1E2) is the difference between the observed proportion of double-labeled neurons (*Arc*&*Homer*

1a)+ and the random overlap (pE1E2) between the two ensembles. A three-way ANOVA with repeated measures on the test sessions (*Arc*+ and *Homer 1a*+), and main factors of treatment (saline, 0.10 and 0.15 mg/kg MK-801), and behavior (A/A, A/B, CC) was used to evaluate the effect of MK-801 on IEG expression as such and specifically after behavioral exploration. A two-way factorial ANOVA on treatment (saline, 0.10 and 0.15 mg/kg MK-801), and behavior (A/A, A/B) as independent variables was used to evaluate the effect of MK-801 on ensemble similarity scores in CA1. Newman–Keuls *post hoc* tests were used when appropriate.

RESULTS

We first compared the effects of two doses of MK-801 (0.10 and 0.15 mg/kg) on PA on a stable (low coordination demand) or a rotating arena (high coordination demand).

ROOM-STABLE: MK-801 (0.15 MG/KG) SPARED PLACE AVOIDANCE IN CONGRUENT SPATIAL FRAMES ON A STABLE ARENA

Place avoidance on a stable arena was spared when the room and arena frames were not dissociated, all cues could be used to support the avoidance, no misleading information was present, and the coordination demand was low (**Figure 3A**). No significant main effect of MK-801 treatment was found on any of the parameters on the stationary arena, but significant interactions on E ($F_{4,56} = 4.64$, $p < 0.005$), ED ($F_{4,56} = 5.10$, $p < 0.005$), and D ($F_{4,56} = 7.23$, $p < 10^{-4}$) pointed to a transient impairment on day 1 after the low (E: $p = 0.025$; ED: $p = 0.023$) and high dose of MK-801 (E: $p = 0.017$). Highly significant effects of days (E: $F_{2,56} = 49.4$, $p < 10^{-6}$; MaxT: $F_{2,56} = 6.26$, $p < 0.005$; pTime: $F_{2,56} = 47.1$, $p < 10^{-6}$; ED: $F_{2,56} = 52.\ 6$, $p < 10^{-6}$) showed robust learning in all rats during training. However, the learning

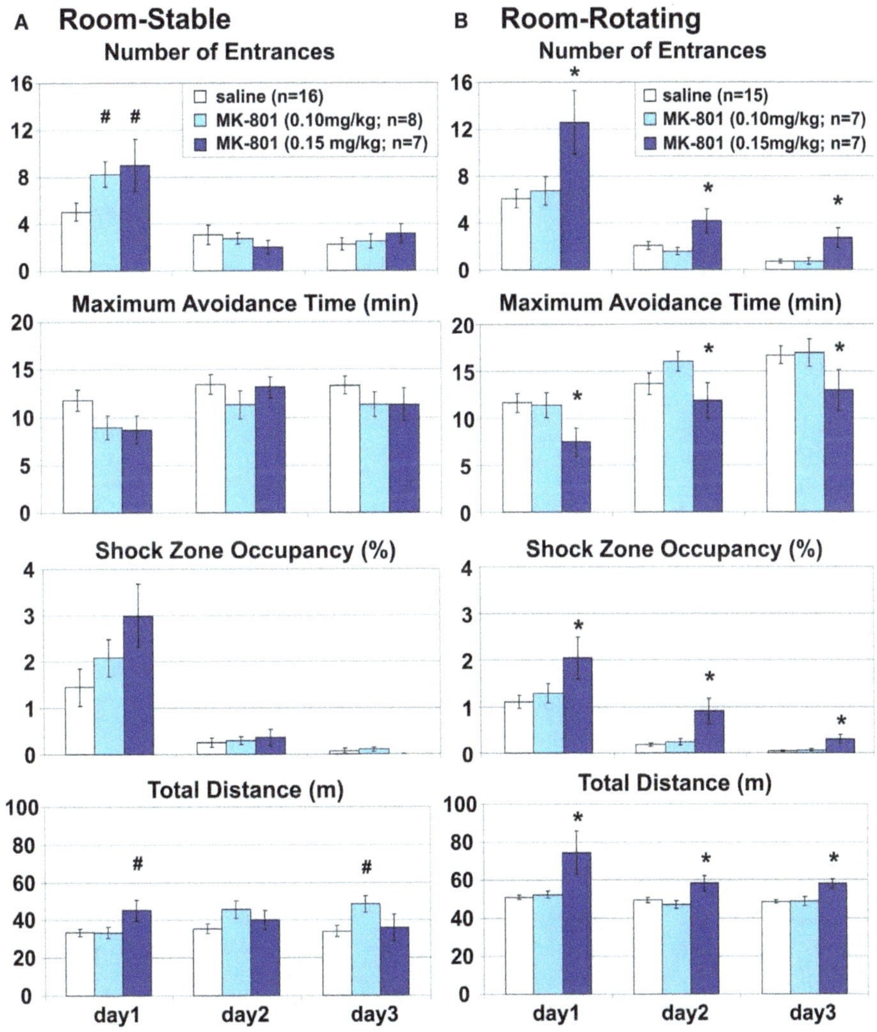

FIGURE 3 | Room-based place avoidance on a Stable and a Rotating arena. (A) Room-Stable place avoidance on a stationary dry arena with no demand for coordination of information from congruent spatial frames. Only a transient increase in the number of Entrances and a similar trend in the Shock Zone Occupancy were observed on day 1 on the Stable arena after either dose of MK-801. This effect was associated with transient hyperlocomotion after the high, but not the low dose of MK-801. **(B)** Room-Rotating Place Avoidance on a rotating dry arena with a high demand for coordination of information from the dissociated spatial frames. 0.15 mg/kg MK-801 persistently impaired all measures of avoidance and increased locomotion on the Rotating arena compared to the saline controls and 0.10 mg/kg MK-801. All rats improved their performance during training. *Significant effects of treatment; #significant effect of treatment × session interaction.

curve of control animals was relatively flat, especially in the MaxT parameter. To see if this was due to rapid learning on day 1, which was not captured in the between-session comparisons, we compared performance between the two halves of session 1. A two-way repeated measures ANOVA found a dramatic improvement during the session (E: $F_{1,28} = 55.4, p < 10^{-6}$; MaxT: $F_{1,28} = 33.1, p < 10^{-5}$; ED: $F_{1,28} = 12.2, p < 0.005$; pTime: $F_{1,28} = 46.2, p < 10^{-6}$).

ROOM-ROTATING: MK-801 (0.15 MG/KG) IMPAIRED PLACE AVOIDANCE IN DISSOCIATED SPATIAL FRAMES ON A ROTATING ARENA

Stationary room-defined PA on a continuously rotating dry arena (Carousel) was impaired when spatial reference frames were dissociated (**Figure 3B**). Cues from both the room and arena frames were available, but only the room cues predicted the shock while the arena cues were misleading and the coordination demand was high. All PA parameters were markedly impaired (E: $F_{2,26} = 10.4$, $p < 0.0005$; MaxT: $F_{2,26} = 5.76$, $p < 0.01$; pTime: $F_{2,26} = 11.5$, $p < 0.0005$; ED: $F_{2,26} = 4.26$, $p = 0.025$) and locomotion was increased (D: $F_{2,26} = 10.3, p > 0.001$) after the high ($E$: $p < 0.005$; MaxT: $p = 0.011$; ED: $p = 0.016$; pTime: $p < 0.001$; D: $p < 0.005$), but not the low dose of MK-801 (all $ps > 0.5$), compared to saline controls. An increased number of Entrances per unit Distance suggests that the PA deficit could not be attributed merely to hyperlocomotion (**Figure 6**; but see Discussion of this parameter in MK-801 Impaired Segregation of Discordant Spatial Information). All rats showed robust between-session learning (E: $F_{2,52} = 51.8$, $p < 10^{-6}$; MaxT: $F_{2,52} = 11.6$, $p < 10^{-4}$; TARG: $F_{2,52} = 56.8$, $p < 10^{-6}$; D: $F_{2,52} = 7.06, p < 0.005$; ED: $F_{2,52} = 57.9, p < 10^{-6}$). Marginally insignificant treatment × session interactions (E: $F_{4,52} = 2.32$, $p < 0.069$; D: $F_{4,52} = 2.54$, $p < 0.051$) reflected a trend toward hyperlocomotion and poorer avoidance after the higher dose of MK-801 specifically in session 1.

Comparison of the performance of control rats between Stable and Rotating arena found no effect of rotation on the avoidance (E: $F_{1,29} = 0.43, p > 0.5$; MaxT: $F_{1,29} = 1.39, p > 0.2$; pTime: $F_{1,29} = 0.82, p > 0.3$), but a highly significant effect on locomotion (D: $F_{1,29} = 37.3, p < 10^{-5}$). Since this effect could confound direct comparisons between different conditions, the effects of MK-801 were always compared to the respective vehicle controls in the same condition. Given the selectivity of the MK-801-induced PA deficit, we focused the following experiments on the effect of the high dose (0.15 mg/kg) on the rotating arena.

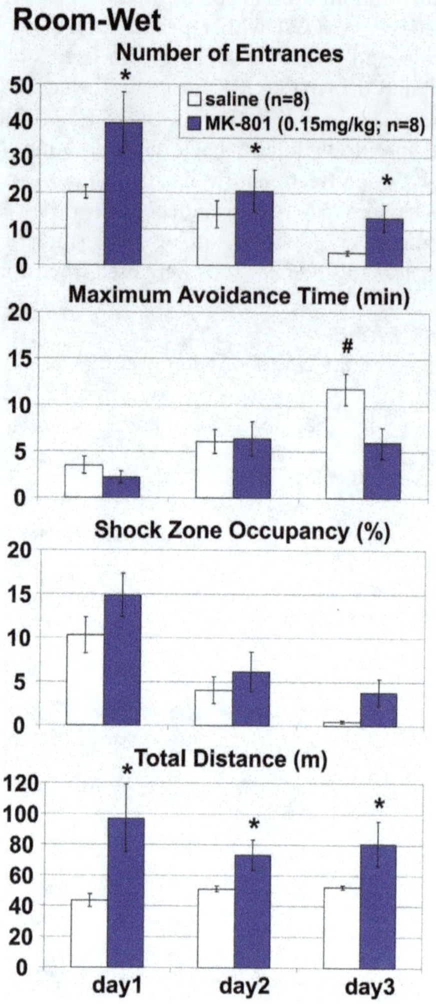

FIGURE 4 | Room-Wet place avoidance with rotating arena cues obscured by shallow water. The demand for coordination was reduced but not eliminated because arena-bound visual stimuli, path integration, and idiothetic information remained available. MK-801 (0.15 mg/kg) increased the number of Entrances, but the effect of treatment on other measures of avoidance did not reach significance. All rats improved their performance during training. *Significant effects of treatment; #significant effect of treatment × session interaction.

ROOM-WET: MK-801(0.15 MG/KG) IMPAIRED PLACE AVOIDANCE ON A ROTATING ARENA WITH LIMITED ACCESS TO IRRELEVANT ARENA CUES

Stationary room-defined PA in dissociated spatial frames was impaired when the salience of the rotating arena cues was attenuated by shallow water (**Figure 4**). Misleading substratal cues on the rotating arena surface were obscured, but arena-bound visual stimuli, path integration, and idiothesis were not removed and could interfere with the avoidance. The coordination demand was reduced, but not eliminated. MK-801 increased the number of Entrances (E: $F_{1,14} = 7.95$, $p = 0.014$) but not the number of Entrances per unit Distance (ED: $F_{1,14} = 1.25, p > 0.2$; **Figure 6**), indicating that this effect could be related to the observed hyperlocomotion (D: $F_{1,14} = 11.4$, $p < 0.005$). Other parameters were not significantly affected by MK-801 ($ps > 0.1$). Control rats also reached longer Maximum Avoidance Time on day 3. Again, robust learning was observed in all rats during the training (E: $F_{2,28} = 10.9$, $p < 0.0005$; MaxT: $F_{2,28} = 16.2$, $p < 10^{-4}$; pTime: $F_{2,28} = 30.9, p < 10^{-6}$; ED: $F_{2,28} = 32.0, p < 10^{-6}$). A significant treatment × day interaction on MaxT ($F_{2,28} = 4.61$, $p < 0.019$) reflected better performance by control rats on day 3 ($p < 0.05$).

ARENA-DARK: MK-801 (0.15 MG/KG) SPARED PLACE AVOIDANCE WITHOUT IRRELEVANT ROOM CUES ON AN ARENA ROTATING IN DARKNESS

While complete removal of arena frame information is difficult (but see Stuchlík et al., 2001), eliminating room-based, predominantly visual cues is very simple. Therefore, we compared Arena-based PA on a dry rotating arena with or without access to irrelevant, misleading visual stimuli in light or darkness, respectively. Avoidance of a rotating arena-defined place was not affected by MK-801 when irrelevant room cues were hidden by darkness and the coordination demand was low (**Figure 5A**). MK-801 caused a transient hyperlocomotion (D: $F_{2,20} = 4.37$, $p = 0.027$) on day 1 ($p < 0.01$), but did not affect any PA parameter. All rats showed robust learning during training (E: $F_{2,20} = 17.9$, $p < 10^{-4}$; MaxT: $F_{2,20} = 3.68$, $p = 0.043$; pTime: $F_{2,20} = 4.85$, $p = 0.019$; D: $F_{2,20} = 8.93$, $p < 0.005$; ED: $F_{2,20} = 32.7$, $p < 10^{-5}$).

ARENA-LIGHT: MK-801 (0.15 MG/KG) IMPAIRED PLACE AVOIDANCE IN DISSOCIATED SPATIAL FRAMES ON AN ARENA ROTATING IN THE LIGHT

Avoidance of an arena-defined place on a rotating arena in the light was severely impaired when irrelevant room cues were available and the coordination demand was high (**Figure 5B**). MK-801 impaired all PA parameters (E: $F_{1,14} = 10.6$, $p < 0.01$; MaxT: $F_{1,14} = 5.28$, $p = 0.037$; pTime: $F_{1,14} = 12.4$, $p < 0.005$; ED: $F_{1,14} = 5.34$, $p > 0.05$) and increased locomotion (D: $F_{1,14} = 11.8$, $p < 0.005$). A significant effect of MK-801 on the number of Entrances per unit Distance shows hyperlocomotion is an unlikely explanation of the PA deficit (**Figure 6**; but see Discussion of this parameter in MK-801 Impaired Segregation of Discordant Spatial Information). All rats improved performance during training (E: $F_{2,28} = 3.45$, $p = 0.046$; MaxT: $F_{2,28} = 3.88$, $p = 0.033$; pTime: $F_{2,28} = 5.78$, $p < 0.01$; ED: $F_{2,28} = 11.0$, $p < 0.0005$).

EXTENDED ROOM-ROTATING TRAINING: PLACE AVOIDANCE IS IMPAIRED AFTER SWITCHING TO OR FROM MK-801 (0.15 MG/KG)

Rats in both MK15/sal and sal/MK15 groups were impaired relative to control animals (sal/MK10). A two-way ANOVA with

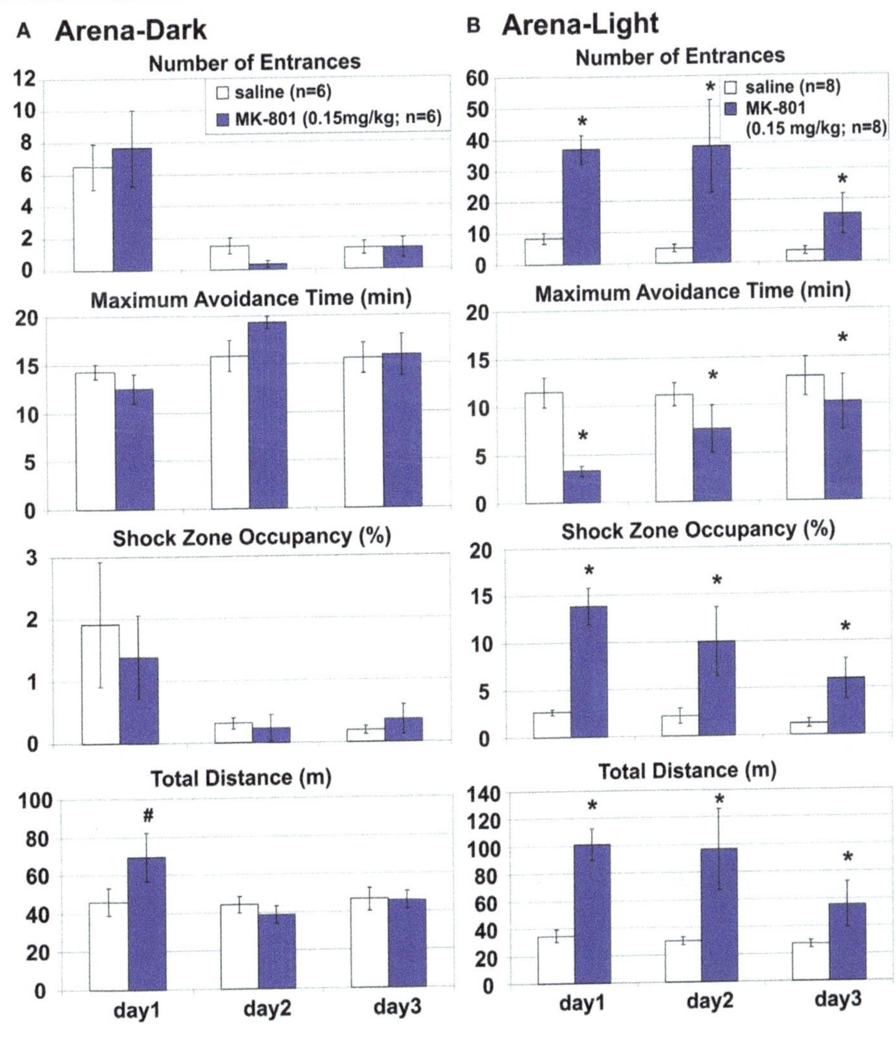

FIGURE 5 | Arena-based place avoidance on a rotating arena in Darkness and in Light. (A) Arena-Dark place avoidance posed no demand for coordination because the irrelevant room stimuli were hidden by darkness. MK-801 transiently increased locomotion in Darkness on day 1. **(B)** Arena-Light place avoidance with high demand for coordination due to interference from irrelevant room cues In contrast to darkness, MK-801 markedly and persistently impaired all place avoidance measures in Light. All rats improved their performance during training. *Significant effects of treatment; #significant effect of treatment × session interaction.

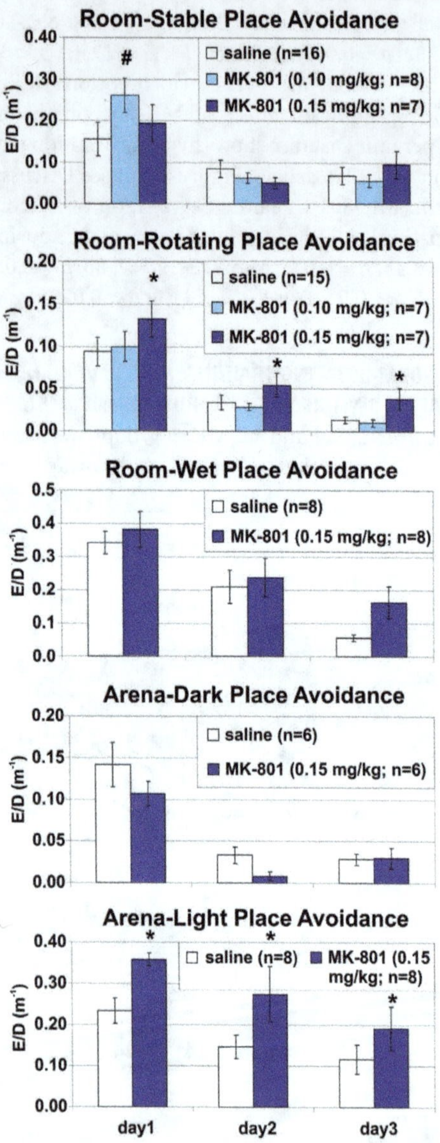

FIGURE 6 | Place avoidance normalized by locomotion in different versions of the place avoidance task. MK-801 (0.15 mg/kg) increased the number of entrances per unit distance (ED) in the Room-Rotating and Arena-Light conditions, suggesting that the place avoidance deficit was not due to hyperlocomotion. *Significant effects of treatment; #significant effect of treatment × session interaction.

repeated measures on the three extra days found a significant main effects of groups on all measures (*E*: $F_{2,18} = 7.48$, $p < 0.005$; MaxT: $F_{2,18} = 7.24$, $p < 0.005$; pTime: $F_{2,18} = 4.05$, $p = 0.035$; *D*: $F_{2,18} = 9.09$, $p < 0.005$; ED: $F_{2,18} = 10.0$, $p < 0.005$). *Post hoc* tests showed that rats in the sal/MK10 group avoided more than rats in MK15/sal (*E*: $p < 0.01$; MaxT: $p < 0.01$; pTime: $p = 0.039$; ED: $p = 0.001$) and sal/MK15 (*E*: $p = 0.014$; MaxT: $p < 0.01$; pTime: $p = 0.044$) groups. Locomotion was increased in the sal/MK15 group (*D*: ps < 0.005). Significant effects of days (*E*: $F_{2,36} = 5.71$, $p < 0.01$; pTime: $F_{2,36} = 5.17$, $p = 0.011$; ED: $F_{2,36} = 5.15$, $p = 0.011$) reflect improved performance on days 5 and 6 and group × day interaction (MaxT: $F_{4,36} = 2.86$, $p = 0.037$; ED: $F_{4,36} = 2.93$, $p = 0.034$) show markedly worse performance in the MK15/saline group on day 4. The *post hoc* tests showed that ED was increased compared to other days and groups (all ps < 0.005) and MaxT was shorter than on day 2 and 3 of saline/MK15 and all days in the controls (sal/MK10; all *ps* < 0.05). A similar pattern was observed for the marginal interaction on the number of Entrances ($F_{4,36} = 2.29$, $p = 0.078$), suggesting that the group effect for MK15/sal rats may be driven by impaired performance after the switch on day 4. In contrast, rats initially trained with saline appeared to display a less dramatic, but more sustained deficit after switching to 0.15 mg/kg MK-801 (sal/MK15; **Figure 7**).

To see if this is indeed the case, we compared their performance to controls selectively on days 5 and 6. The ANOVA (sal/MK15 vs. sal/MK10) found a significant group effect on pTime ($F_{1,12} = 7.44$, $p = 0.018$) and marginal effects on Entrances ($F_{1,12} = 4.23$, $p = 0.062$) and MaxT ($F_{1,12} = 4.72$, $p = 0.051$). No such effects were found for the MK15/sal rats (all *ps* > 0.26) suggesting that in contrast to the MK15/sal group, the effect of group on the 3-day performance was not driven solely by impairment on day 4 in the sal/MK15 group. To examine the immediate effect of MK-801 on well-learned PA within-subject, we compared performance on days 3 and 4 with paired *t*-tests. The analysis yielded only a marginally insignificant difference for the sal/MK15 group (E: $p = 0.082$; pTime: $p = 0.064$) and no difference in the MK15/sal group (all $p > 0.25$) and controls (sal/MK10; all $p > 0.59$). This result was puzzling given the significant difference between the sal/MK15 and the controls (sal/MK10) revealed by the ANOVA on days 4–6 of the extended training. We examined individual performance (**Figure 8**) to see if excessive variance could explain the lack of effect between days 3 and 4. Avoidance deteriorated and locomotion increased after switching to 0.15 mg/kg MK-801 in all rats except one (#7), which improved avoidance with no change in locomotion. This rat made one error on day 3 and none on day 4 resembling behavior of control rats (sal-to-MK10), which only made error(s) in one session, but never in both (**Figure 9**). Without this outlier (with respect to the general effect of 0.15 mg/kg MK-801), the *t*-tests were significant for all avoidance parameters in the sal/MK15 group (E: $p = 0.038$; MaxT: $p < 0.01$; pTime: $p = 0.029$; E/D: $p = 0.013$; D: $p = 0.052$). In addition, disproportional impairment in rat #6 represents another major source of variance as bringing the values closer to the group means restored significances for E and pTime. Combined, these two manipulations brought the *t*-tests on E and pTime to $p < 0.005$.

MK-801 REDUCED IEG EXPRESSION IN THE HIPPOCAMPUS

The effects of MK-801 on IEG expression in CA1 are illustrated in **Figure 10** and the IEG expression data analysis is summarized in **Figure 11**.

The three-way ANOVA found significant main effects of treatment ($F_{2,33} = 10.7$, $p < 0.0005$), behavior ($F_{2,33} = 12.1$, $p < 0.0005$), and session ($F_{1,33} = 21.7$, $p < 10^{-4}$), but no interaction (**Figures 11A,B**). *Post hoc* tests showed that both doses of MK-801 substantially reduced the IEG expression (*ps* < 0.001), that behavioral experience (A/A, A/B) dramatically increased the

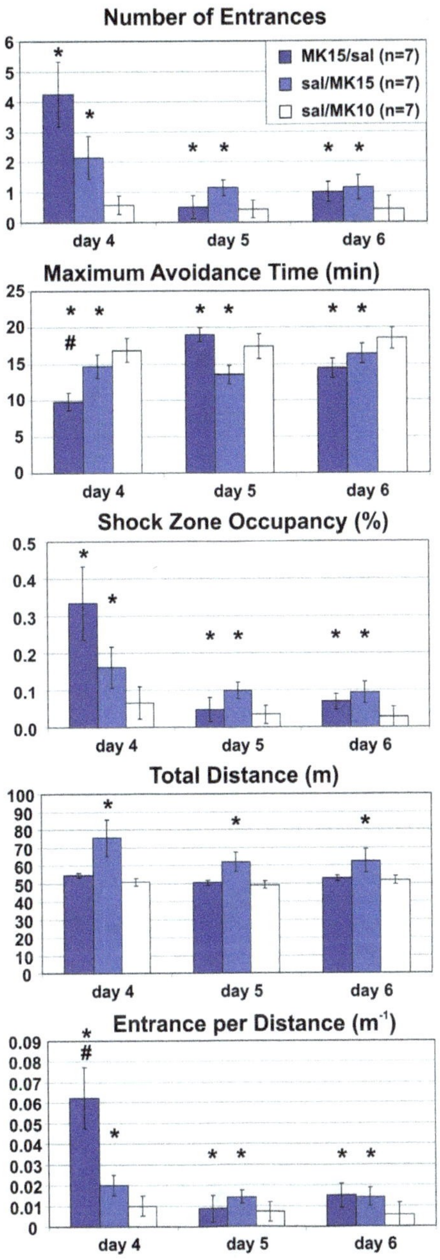

FIGURE 7 | **Room-Rotating place avoidance after reversed injections.** Rats trained with MK-801 (0.15 mg/kg) on days 1–3 received saline on days 4–6 (MK15/sal) and rats initially trained with saline received MK-801 at 0.15 mg/kg (sal/MK15) or 0.10 mg/kg (sal/MK10). Rats in the sal/MK10 group avoided better than the other rats. Locomotion was increased in the sal/MK15 group. Switching from MK-801 to saline caused a marked but transient place avoidance deficit on day 4, which disappeared on the next day (MK/sal). Switching from saline to MK-801 (0.15 mg/kg) caused a less dramatic, but more persistent place avoidance deficit. Significant effects of treatment are marked with asterisk (*) and a significant effect of treatment × session interaction is marked with number sign (#).

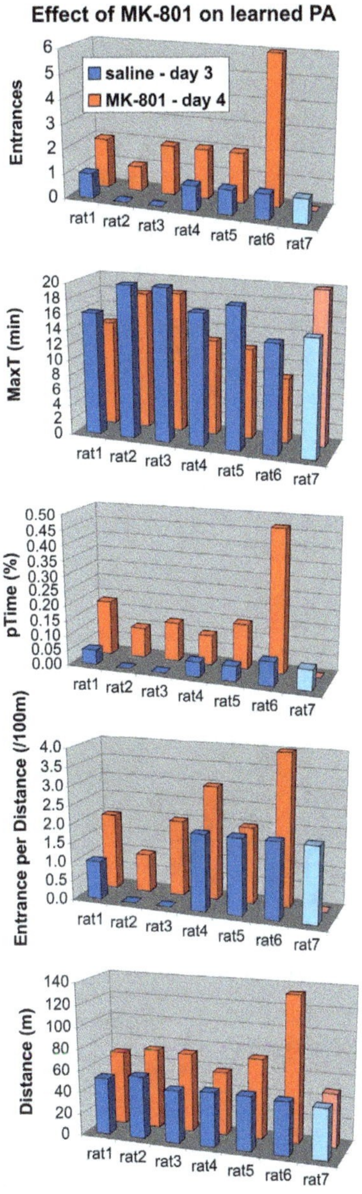

FIGURE 8 | **Effect of MK-801 (0.15 mg/kg) on well-trained avoidance.** MK-801 impaired avoidance and increased locomotion in all animals (sal/MK15) except rat 7. Rat 6 deteriorated approximately three times as much as other rats (except MaxT).

IEG expression compared to CC ($ps < 0.0005$), and that the IEG expression in session 2 was lower than in session 1 ($ps < 0.0005$). This last effect appeared to be driven largely by saline and 0.10 mg/kg MK-801 treatments in behaving animals (A/A and A/B) as opposed to 0.15 mg/kg MK-801 treatment and CC, but none of the interactions reached significance. To see if it could be due to large heterogeneity of the sample, we analyzed the expression separately in the behaving and CC animals.

MK-801 (0.15 MG/KG) PREVENTED HABITUATION OF THE IEG EXPRESSION RESPONSE

To examine the effect of MK-801 specifically on the behaviorally induced IEG expression, we focused the analysis on animals, which explored environments A/A and A/B during the test sessions. A three-way ANOVA found significant main effects of treatment ($F_{2,24} = 9.48$, $p < 0.001$) and session ($F_{1,24} = 25.4$, $p < 10^{-4}$), and a significant treatment × session interaction ($F_{2,24} = 4.35$, $p = 0.024$), but no effect of behavior ($F_{1,24} = 0.36$, $p > 0.5$). *Post hoc* tests showed that the IEG expression decreased after both doses of MK-801 (*ps* < 0.005) and that it was significantly lower in the second session than in the first in rats treated with saline ($p < 0.0005$) and 0.10 mg/kg ($p = 0.025$), but not 0.15 mg/kg MK-801 ($p > 0.6$). A separate two-way ANOVA on the IEG expression in CC animals found a significant effect of treatment ($F_{2,9} = 21.3$, $p < 0.0005$), but no effect of session, and no interaction. *Post hoc* tests showed that both doses of MK-801 (*ps* < 0.001) reduced IEG expression in CC.

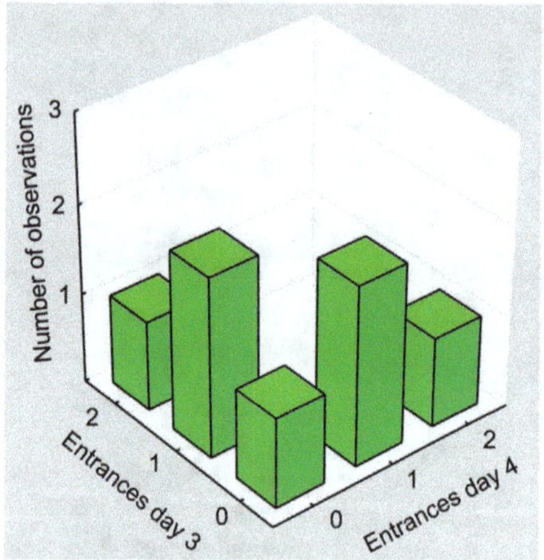

FIGURE 9 | Behavioral pattern in control animals (sal/MK10). A bivariate histogram for the number of Entrances on days 3 and 4. No rat entered the shock zone in both sessions. One entrance in one of the sessions was the most typical performance in the control group.

MK-801 (0.15 MG/KG) INCREASED SIMILARITY BETWEEN UNRELATED CA1 ENSEMBLES

To examine the effect of MK-801 treatment specifically on differences in CA1 ensemble similarity between A/A and A/B conditions,

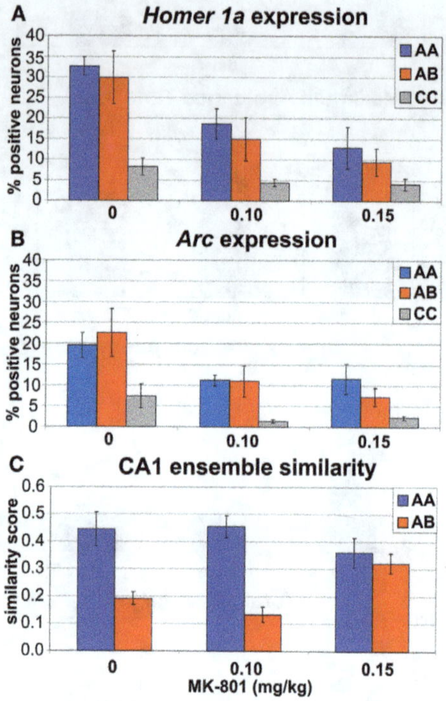

FIGURE 11 | Immediate-early gene imaging data summary. **(A,B)** both doses of MK-801 reduced expression of IEGs *Homer1a* **(A)** and *Arc* **(B)** in CA1 neurons. **(C)** Higher dose of MK-801 (0.15 mg/kg) increased similarity between CA1 ensembles activated in different environments **(A,B)** and eliminated the contextual specificity of the IEG expression observed after saline and 0.10 mg/kg MK-801.

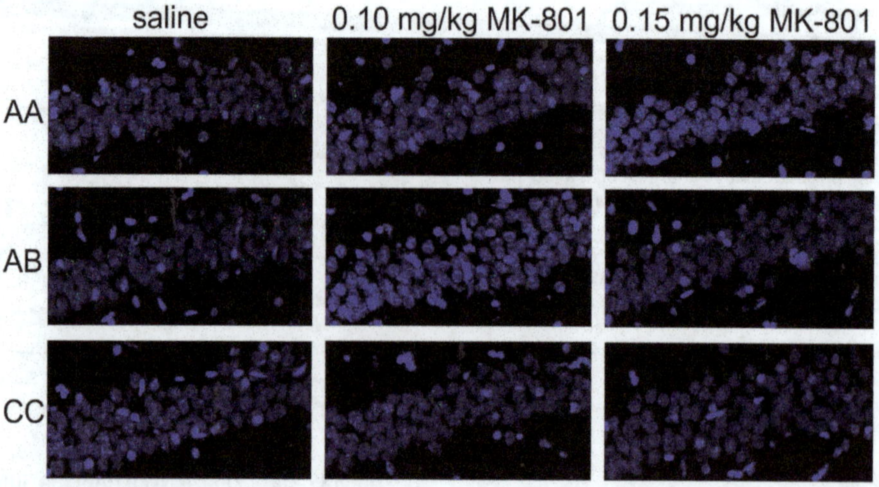

FIGURE 10 | Immediate-early gene expression in CA1. Representative images showing expression of *Homer 1a* (green) and *Arc/Arg3.1* (red) triggered in the CA1 region of the hippocampus by exploration of the same (AA) or two different environments (AB) after an injection of saline or MK-801 (0.10 and 0.15 mg/kg).

we analyzed similarity scores between CA1 ensembles expressing IEGs during sessions 1 and 2. A two-way ANOVA found a significant main effect of behavior ($F_{1,24} = 34.1$, $p < 10^{-4}$) and a significant treatment × behavior interaction ($F_{2,24} = 5.96, p < 0.01$), but no significant main effect of treatment ($F_{2,24} = 0.59, p > 0.5$). *Post hoc* tests showed that the similarity was lower in A/B than in A/A condition after saline ($p < 0.005$) and 0.10 mg/kg MK-801 ($p < 0.0005$). In contrast, after 0.15 mg/kg MK-801, similarity in A/B was equivalent to A/A ($p > 0.5$) and significantly higher than in A/B condition after saline ($p = 0.013$) or 0.10 mg/kg MK-801 ($p = 0.042$; **Figure 11C**).

DISCUSSION

MK-801 IMPAIRED SEGREGATION OF DISCORDANT SPATIAL INFORMATION

MK-801 (0.15 mg/kg) impaired PA when irrelevant information was present (Room-Rotating and Arena-Light), but not when it was absent (Room-Stable or Arena-Dark). These PA versions differed in their demand for segregation of relevant and irrelevant spatial information, but not in mnemonic or motivational demands, demonstrating that general learning impairment, selective impairment of either allothetic or idiothetic (egocentric) navigation, or MK-801-induced alterations in motivation or shock sensitivity cannot explain the PA deficit. Partial PA deficit was also observed when cues on the arena surface (such as scent marks, urine, or droppings) were obscured by shallow water. Note that misleading, Arena-bound cues, related to idiothesis and path integration were not affected by the water and could interfere with the Room-based avoidance. Poorer avoidance on the wet arena is likely due to the water reduced impedance between a rat and the grounded arena and alleviated perception of shock in the constant-current circuit. Indeed, despite the shock intensity was often set to the maximum of 0.7 mA, the control rats made many more errors and received many more shocks (~60) than in any dry arena version (10–15) on PA day 1. By day 3, however, the controls' avoidance matched other versions (entrances: 3.5 vs. 0.73–3.625; shocks: 4.125 vs. 0.73–8.0). Locomotion was slightly but consistently lower on the wet arena (~30 compared to 40 m on dry arena) during foraging before the first injection (version: $F_{1,36} = 21.2$, $p < 10^{-4}$). MK-801 increased locomotion on foraging day 4 (treatment: $F_{1,34} = 11.7$, $p < 0.005$), particularly on the wet arena (~80 vs. 45 m; interaction $F_{1,34} = 4.9$, $p < 0.05$). During avoidance, shallow water did not affect the locomotion of control rats, but accentuated MK-801-induced hyperlocomotion. The controls covered, on average, 43–52 m on the wet, compared to ~50 m on the dry rotating arena. MK-801 (0.15 mg/kg) increased that to 80–97 m on the wet and 58–74 m on the dry rotating arena (Room-Rotating; **Figures 3** and **4**). In agreement with previous reports (Stuchlík et al., 2004; Valeš et al., 2006), the low dose of MK-801 (0.10 mg/kg) had a little effect on the PA. Rotation of the arena itself did not affect the PA in control rats, but it substantially facilitated locomotion, presumably by continuously bringing rats toward the Shock zone. This pro-locomotory drive was absent on the stable arena. Hyperlocomotion invariably accompanied the PA deficit, but it was absent when PA was unaffected. Different locomotory demands could explain differences in locomotion and avoidance between the Stable and Rotating arena, but not between Light and Darkness. Furthermore, MK-801 impaired the number of Entrances per unit Distance, suggesting that hyperlocomotion does not suffice to explain the PA deficit (**Figure 6**). However, it should be noted that this effect was not significant after Bonferroni ($\alpha = 0.0167$) or Šidák correction ($\alpha = 0.0170$) for multiple comparisons in either the Room-Rotating ($F_{2,26} = 4.26$, $p = 0.025$) or the Arena-Light version ($F_{1,14} = 5.34$, $p = 0.037$). On the other hand, both comparisons proved significant using Tukey's HSD test ($p = 0.029$ and $p = 0.037$, respectively) as a weak control of Type I error connected with repeated measures. Together, the dependence of the MK-801-induced hyperlocomotion on the PA deficit and the effect of MK-801 on ED suggest that, rather than causing the PA deficit, the accompanying hyperlocomotion results from an inability to efficiently organize spatial behavior in dissociated reference frames.

Well-learned PA was impaired when MK-801 (0.15 mg/kg) was injected instead of saline during the extended training. The t-test analysis fell short of significance, but this shortcoming was partly due to too much impairment rather than too little and partly due to a single animal, which displayed neither deteriorated avoidance nor increased locomotion after switching to 0.15 mg/kg MK-801 and resembled behavioral pattern observed in controls. Given these were the main sources of variance responsible for the lack of significance in the primary t-test analysis, we conclude that the MK-801-induced PA deficit was not selective to learning. In summary, our behavioral data provide compelling evidence that 0.15 mg/kg MK-801 disrupted segregation of discordant spatial information into coherent representations on the Carousel.

That is not to imply that cognitive coordination is the only function affected by MK-801. Low doses of up to 0.10 mg/kg MK-801 impaired cognitive performance of Wistar rats without causing gross sensorimotor or motivational disturbances in a variety of behavioral tasks (van der Staay et al., 2011). The lack of effect of the low dose in this study may be due to higher sensitivity of Wistar rats to the effects of MK-801 (Valeš et al., 2006) or due to lower sensitivity of the PA task compared to spatial water maze (WM) (Stuchlík et al., 2004). MK-801 also induced social withdrawal in a model of negative symptoms of schizophrenia (Rung et al., 2005) and impaired visuospatial working memory (Zemanova et al., 2013) and reversal learning on the Carousel (Lobellova et al., 2013). Importantly, MK-801 also slightly reduced sensitivity to electric shock (van der Staay et al., 2011); therefore, we adjusted the shock intensity individually for each rat based on behavioral markers (escape response) to enhance comparability between the groups.

COGNITIVE COORDINATION IN THE HIPPOCAMPUS

The notion that the PA on the Carousel depends on cognitive coordination of room and arena cues is based on several observations. First, PA acquired on a stationary arena can later be expressed and extinguished separately in the arena frame in darkness, and in the room frame on a rotating arena in light (Bureš et al., 1997; Fenton et al., 1998). Second, hippocampal place cells represent locations in both room and arena frames dissociated by rotation (Zinyuk et al., 2000; Fenton et al., 2010; Kelemen and Fenton, 2010). Third, hippocampal ensemble activity rapidly switches between multiple representations of the same space on a rotating arena (Kelemen and Fenton, 2013) and during a "teleportation" task where two sets of cues are alternated within a single physical environment (Ježek et al., 2011). Fourth, injection of TTX into one hippocampus prevented the PA when room and arena frames were dissociated by rotation and misleading cues were present, but not when they were absent (Wesierska et al., 2005). When cues on the arena surface were obscured by shallow water, rats could perform the previously acquired PA, but new PA learning was not possible after the TTX injection (Kubik and Fenton, 2005). In contrast, retrieval of an existing memory trace was impaired but new spatial learning was spared in the WM after partial hippocampal inactivation (Fenton and Bureš, 1993; Moser and Moser, 1998) suggesting that WM and PA engage distinct hippocampal functions, spatial representation, and segregation, respectively (Kubik and Fenton, 2005). Specifically, whereas locating a small platform (1/330 area) in a large WM requires precise spatial representation, a relatively coarse spatial representation may be sufficient to support avoidance of a large (1/6 area) place on the rotating arena, provided that dissociated room- and arena-frame information can be segregated into coherent subsets. These findings demonstrated that multiple representations of the same space are coordinated within hippocampal neural activity.

IEG IMAGING OF HIPPOCAMPAL ENSEMBLE SIMILARITY

In agreement with previous reports (Guzowski et al., 1999; Vazdarjanova and Guzowski, 2004), more similar CA1 ensembles expressed the IEGs in the same environment (A/A) than in different environments (A/B) in rats injected with saline or the low dose of MK-801 (0.10 mg/kg). This contextual specificity was eliminated after the high dose of MK-801 (0.15 mg/kg), which also impaired cognitive coordination on the Carousel. Specifically, the ensemble similarity was increased in A/B, but not in A/A. Decreased IEG expression after either dose of MK-801 could be due to inhibition of NMDA receptors on pyramidal neurons and their role in inducing IEG expression and synaptic plasticity (Link et al., 1995; Steward and Worley, 2001; Czerniawski et al., 2011). On the other hand, the loss of contextual specificity was only observed after the high dose and it may be more closely related to the psychotomimetic effect of MK-801, presumably via its effect on NMDARs on inhibitory interneurons (Grunze et al., 1996; Li et al., 2002). *Arc* expression can be induced in hippocampal CA3 neurons rapidly enough to support one-trial memory formation. The expression is abolished by inactivation of medial septum known to disrupt hippocampal plasticity and learning (Miyashita et al., 2009). Interfering with *Arc* expression impairs maintenance of synaptic plasticity and memory consolidation (Guzowski et al., 2000; Plath et al., 2006), suggesting that *Arc* expression marks plasticity-inducing neural activity. Although the effects of systemic MK-801 are definitely not limited to the hippocampus, our IEG imaging data match the prediction of the Hypersynchrony theory and suggest that MK-801 induced coactivity and "co-plasticity" between hippocampal ensembles, which were previously not related. This mechanism could lead to hyperassociation observed in psychosis (Miller, 1989).

HYPERSYNCHRONY AND COGNITIVE DISORGANIZATION

The Hypersynchrony theory posits that behavioral cognitive coordination depends on selective activation of relevant neural representations and suppression of the irrelevant ones (neural coordination). Increasing coactivity between neurons that would normally not fire together impairs neural coordination and causes psychotic disorganization (Fenton, 2009). Several observations support this hypothesis. First, TTX injection into one hippocampus produced transient disinhibition in the uninjected hippocampus and increased coactivity between pairs of CA1 neurons, which did not fire together before the injection, whereas coactivity between previously coactive neurons was not affected (Olypher et al., 2006). This effect could be due to disrupted feed-forward inhibition mediated by the commissural projection (Buzsáki and Eidelberg, 1981). Second, impaired inhibition could also be responsible for the effects of NMDAr antagonists. Fast-spiking inhibitory interneurons display disproportionately higher sensitivity to NMDAr antagonists (Grunze et al., 1996; Li et al., 2002), which cause a disinhibition of pyramidal neurons (Breier et al., 1997; Vollenweider et al., 1997; Jackson et al., 2004; Lisman et al., 2008), increase interference between memories (Chrobak et al., 2008), and decrease cognitive flexibility (Nikiforuk and Popik, 2012). Third, cognitive coordination on the Carousel was disrupted and coactivity between hippocampal pyramidal neurons was increased after 5 mg/kg, but not 3 mg/kg, phencyclidine (PCP) another non-competitive NMDAr antagonist (Fenton et al., 2006). Fourth, PA on the Carousel and accompanying interhippocampal synchrony are also disrupted in a neurodevelopmental model of schizophrenia by neonatal lesions of the ventral hippocampus (Lee et al., 2012).

HYPERASSOCIATION IN SCHIZOPHRENIA

Alterations in the hippocampus (Weinberger, 1999; Harrison, 2004), and hippocampus-dependent memory deficits are typical for schizophrenia (Weiss et al., 2003; Boyer et al., 2007; Ragland et al., 2007; Ranganath et al., 2008; Tamminga et al., 2010). Aberrant inhibitory neurotransmission and loss of parvalbumin (PV)-positive interneurons is found in the hippocampus and the dorsolateral prefrontal cortex (Lewis et al., 2005; Benes et al., 2007; Adell et al., 2012). Reduced PV expression was observed in an animal model by repeated (Braun et al., 2007) or acute administration of MK-801 (Romón et al., 2011). Schizophrenia-like phenotype emerged in post-adolescent mice with a genetic ablation of the NMDA receptor function predominantly in PV+ cortical and hippocampal GABAergic interneurons during early postnatal development (Belforte et al., 2010). Reduced neurotransmission along the mossy fiber pathway from the dentate gyrus (DG) to areas CA3 and CA4 of the hippocampus emerge as a key pathophysiology in schizophrenia (Kerwin et al., 1990; Nowakowski et al., 2002; Kolomeets et al., 2005, 2007; Yamasaki et al., 2008; Kobayashi, 2009; Tamminga et al., 2012). Given the role of the DG in pattern separation (PS; Gilbert et al., 2001; Leutgeb et al., 2007; McHugh et al., 2007; Bakker et al., 2008), reduced DG output could disrupt the dynamic balance between PS and pattern completion (PC) in CA3 (Guzowski et al., 2004) and facilitate cross-linking between hippocampal representations of unrelated events. A hyperassociative hippocampal memory system can give rise to inappropriate associations, distorted perception, irrational expectations, and even hallucinations (Behrendt, 2010). In agreement with this perspective, patients with schizophrenia display excessive associations (Miller, 1989; Wentura et al., 2008; Manschreck et al., 2012), increased interference (Westerhausen et al., 2011), reduced cognitive flexibility (Elliott et al., 1998), and autonoetic awareness (Danion et al., 1999), lack of semantic specificity (Tüscher et al., 2005), difficulties to represent expected reward value (Gold et al., 2012), and deficits in emotional discrimination (Schneider et al., 2006).

CONCLUSION

Cognitive dysfunction precedes the manifestation of psychotic symptoms from early childhood (Reichenberg et al., 2010; Sørensen et al., 2010) and cognitive performance is the strongest predictor of the functional outcome in schizophrenia (Green, 1996; Green and Nuechterlein, 1999; Green et al., 2004; Bowie et al., 2006; Keefe et al., 2006; Rosenheck et al., 2006). However, cognitive benefits of available antipsychotics remain rather limited (Harvey and Keefe, 2001; Mishara and Goldberg, 2004; Hill et al., 2010). Cognitive disorganization has been proposed as a core cognitive deficit in schizophrenia (Phillips and Silverstein, 2003). The present data demonstrate that systemic MK-801 impairs cognitive coordination on the Carousel and increases similarity between unrelated hippocampal ensemble representations. In addition, it suggests that increased coactivity in previously unrelated neurons may translate into synaptic plasticity and result in hyperassociative psychotic memories. These findings support the Hypersynchrony theory, validate the PA on the Carousel as test of psychosis-related cognitive disorganization, and demonstrate that the concept of cognitive coordination in schizophrenia can be straightforwardly targeted in an animal model.

ACKNOWLEDGMENTS

This study was supported by GACR grant P303/10/P191, Marie Curie Reintegration grant PIR06-GA/2009-256581 from the EU, and by institutional funding to the Institute of Physiology RVO: 67985823. The authors thank to Dr. J. F. Guzowski for kindly providing the DNA constructs for riboprobe synthesis, B. Stuchlíková for arduous FISH image data analysis, A. J. Schiffman for developing the ImageJ macro for the analysis, and Dr. E. Kelemen, Dr. A. Pevzner, and two anonymous reviewers for valuable comments on earlier versions of the manuscript.

REFERENCES

Adell, A., Jiménez-Sánchez, L., López-Gil, X., and Romón, T. (2012). Is the acute NMDA receptor hypofunction a valid model of schizophrenia? *Schizophr. Bull.* 38, 9–14. doi:10.1093/schbul/sbr133

Bakker, A., Kirwan, C. B., Miller, M., and Stark, C. E. L. (2008). Pattern separation in the human hippocampal CA3and dentate gyrus. *Science* 319, 1640–1642. doi:10.1126/science.1152882

Barch, D. M. (2005). The cognitive neuroscience of schizophrenia. *Annu. Rev. Clin. Psychol.* 1, 321–353. doi:10.1146/annurev.clinpsy.1.102803.143959

Behrendt, R. P. (2010). Contribution of hippocampal region CA3 to consciousness and schizophrenic hallucinations. *Neurosci. Biobehav. Rev.* 34, 1121–1136. doi:10.1016/j.neubiorev.2009.12.009

Belforte, J. E., Zsiros, V., Sklar, E. R., Jiang, Z., Yu, G., Li, Y., et al. (2010). Postnatal NMDA receptor ablation in corticolimbic interneurons confers schizophrenia-like phenotypes. *Nat. Neurosci.* 13, 76–83. doi:10.1038/nn.2447

Benes, F. M., Lim, B., Matzilevich, D., Walsh, J. P., Subburaju, S., and Minns, M. (2007). Regulation of the GABA cell phenotype in hippocampus of schizophrenics and bipolars hippocampal GABA alterations in schizophrenia. *Proc. Natl. Acad. Sci. U.S.A.* 104, 10164–10169. doi:10.1073/pnas.0703806104

Bowie, C. R., Reichenberg, A., Patterson, T. L., Heaton, R. K., and Harvey, P. D. (2006). Determinants of real-world functional performance in schizophrenia subjects: correlations with cognition, functional capacity, and symptoms. *Am. J. Psychiatry* 163, 418–425. doi:10.1176/appi.ajp.163.3.418

Boyer, P., Phillips, J. L., Rousseau, F. L., and Ilitvitsky, S. (2007). Hippocampal abnormalities and memory deficits: new evidence of a strong pathophysiological link in schizophrenia. *Brain Res. Rev.* 54, 92–112. doi:10.1016/j.brainresrev.2006.12.008

Braun, I., Genius, J., Grunze, H., Bender, A., Möller, H. J., and Rujescu, D. (2007). Alterations of hippocampal and prefrontal GABAergic interneurons in an animal model of psychosis induced by NMDA receptor antagonism. *Schizophr. Res.* 97, 254–263. doi:10.1016/j.schres.2007.05.005

Breier, A., Malhotra, A. K., Pinals, D. A., Weisenfeld, N. I., and Pickar, D. (1997). Association of ketamine-induced psychosis with focal activation of the prefrontal cortex in healthy volunteers. *Am. J. Psychiatry* 154, 805–811.

Bubeníková-Valešová, V., Horacek, J., Vrajova, M., and Höschl, C. (2008a). Models of schizophrenia in humans and animals based on inhibition of NMDA receptors. *Neurosci. Biobehav. Rev.* 32, 1014–1023. doi:10.1016/j.neubiorev.2008.03.012

Bubeníková-Valešová, V., Stuchlík, A., Svoboda, J., Bureš, J., and Valeš, K. (2008b). Risperidone and ritanserin but not haloperidol block effect of dizocilpine on the active allothetic place avoidance task. *Proc. Natl. Acad. Sci. U.S.A.* 105, 1061–1066. doi:10.1073/pnas.0711273105

Bureš, J., Fenton, A. A., Kaminsky, Y., Rossier, J., Sacchetti, B., and Zinyuk, L. (1997). Dissociation of exteroceptive and idiothetic orientation cues: effect on hippocampal place cells and place navigation. *Philos. Trans. R. Soc. Lond. B Biol. Sci.* 352, 1515–1524. doi:10.1098/rstb.1997.0138

Buzsáki, G., and Eidelberg, E. (1981). Commissural projection to the dentate gyrus of the rat: evidence for feed-forward inhibition. *Brain Res.* 230, 346–350. doi:10.1016/0006-8993(81)90413-3

Christian, G. D. (2003). *Analytical Chemistry*, 6th Edn. New York: Wiley.

Chrobak, J. J., Hinman, J. R., and Sabolek, H. R. (2008). Revealing past memories: proactive interference and ketamine-induced memory deficits. *J. Neurosci.* 28, 4512–4520. doi:10.1523/JNEUROSCI.0742-07.2008

Cimadevilla, J. M., Wesierska, M., Fenton, A. A., and Bureš, J. (2001). Inactivating one hippocampus impairs avoidance of a stable room-defined place during dissociation of arena cues from room cues by rotation of the arena. *Proc. Natl. Acad. Sci. U.S.A.* 98, 3531–3536. doi:10.1073/pnas.051628398

Czerniawski, J., Ree, F., Chia, C., Ramamoorthi, K., Kumata, Y., and Otto, T. A. (2011). The importance of having Arc: expression of the immediate-early gene Arc is required for hippocampus-dependent fear conditioning and blocked by NMDA receptor antagonism. *J. Neurosci.* 31, 11200–11207. doi:10.1523/JNEUROSCI.2211-11.2011

Danion, J. M., Rizzo, L., and Bruant, A. (1999). Functional mechanisms underlying impaired recognition memory and conscious awareness in patients with schizophrenia. *Arch. Gen. Psychiatry* 56, 639–644. doi:10.1001/archpsyc.56.7.639

Deutsch, S. I., Rosse, R. B., Billingslea, E. N., Bellack, A. S., and Mastropaolo, J. (2002). Topiramate antagonizes MK-801 in an animal model of schizophrenia. *Eur. J. Pharmacol.* 449, 121–125. doi:10.1016/S0014-2999(02)02041-1

Ellenbroek, B. A., and Cools, A. R. (1990). Animal models with construct validity for schizophrenia. *Behav. Pharmacol.* 1, 469–490. doi:10.1097/00008877-199000160-00001

Elliott, R., McKenna, P. J., Robbins, T. W., and Sahakian, B. J. (1998). Specific neuropsychological deficits in schizophrenic patients with preserved intellectual function. *Cogn. Neuropsychiatry* 3, 45–70. doi:10.1080/135468098396242

Fenton, A. A. (2009). "Neural coordination and psychotic disorganization," in *Information Processing by Neuronal Populations*, eds C. Holscher and M. H. Munk (London: Cambridge University Press), 387–408.

Fenton, A. A., and Bureš, J. (1993). Place navigation in rats with unilateral TTX inactivation of the dorsal hippocampus: place but not procedural learning can be lateralised to one hippocampus. *Behav. Neurosci.* 107, 552–564. doi:10.1037/0735-7044.107.4.552

Fenton, A. A., Kenney, J., and Kao, H.-Y. (2006). Phencyclidine impairs cognition if and only if it co-activates initially independently active neurons. *Soc. Biol. Psychiatry* 59, 85S.

Fenton, A. A., Lytton, W. W., Barry, J. M., Lenck-Santini, P. P., Zinyuk, L. E., Kubík, S., et al. (2010). Attention-like modulation of hippocampus place cell discharge. *J. Neurosci.* 30, 4613–4625. doi:10.1523/JNEUROSCI.5576-09.2010

Fenton, A. A., Wesierska, M., Kaminsky, Y., and Bureš, J. (1998). Both here and there: simultaneous expression of autonomous spatial memories in rats. *Proc. Natl. Acad. Sci. U.S.A.* 95, 11493–11498. doi:10.1073/pnas.95.19.11493

Gilbert, P. E., Kesner, R. P., and Lee, I. (2001). Dissociating hippocampal subregions: double dissociation between dentate gyrus and CA1. *Hippocampus* 11, 626–636. doi:10.1002/hipo.1077

Gold, J. M., Waltz, J. A., Matveeva, T. M., Kasanova, Z., Strauss, G. P., Herbener, E. S., et al. (2012). Negative symptoms and the failure to represent the expected reward value of actions: behavioral and computational modeling evidence. *Arch. Gen. Psychiatry* 69, 129–138. doi:10.1001/archgenpsychiatry.2011.1269

Green, M. F. (1996). What are the functional consequences of neurocognitive deficits in schizophrenia? *Am. J. Psychiatry* 153, 321–330.

Green, M. F., Kern, R. S., and Heaton, R. K. (2004). Longitudinal studies of cognition and functional outcome in schizophrenia: implications for MATRICS. *Schizophr. Res.* 72, 41–51. doi:10.1016/j.schres.2004.09.009

Green, M. F., and Nuechterlein, K. H. (1999). Should schizophrenia be treated as a neurocognitive disorder? *Schizhopr. Bull.* 25, 309–319. doi:10.1093/oxfordjournals.schbul.a033380

Grunze, H. C., Rainnie, D. G., Hasselmo, M. E., Barkai, E., Hearn, E. F., McCarley, R. W., et al. (1996). NMDA-dependent modulation of CA1 local circuit inhibition. *J. Neurosci.* 16, 2034–2043.

Guzowski, J. F., Knierim, J. J., and Moser, E. I. (2004). Ensemble dynamics of hippocampal regions CA1 and CA3. *Neuron* 44, 581–584. doi:10.1016/j.neuron.2004.11.003

Guzowski, J. F., Lyford, G. L., Stevenson, G. D., Houston, F. P., McGaugh, J. L., Worley, P. F., et al. (2000). Inhibition of activity-dependent arc protein expression in the rat hippocampus impairs the maintenance of long-term potentiation and the consolidation of long-term memory. *J. Neurosci.* 20, 3993–4001.

Guzowski, J. F., McNaughton, B. L., Barnes, C. A., and Worley, P. F. (1999). Environment-specific expression of the immediate-early gene *Arc* in hippocampal neuronal ensembles. *Nat. Neurosci.* 2, 1120–1124. doi:10.1038/16046

Harrison, P. J. (2004). The hippocampus in schizophrenia: a review of the neuropathological evidence and its pathophysiological implications. *Psychopharmacology (Berl.)* 174, 151–162. doi:10.1007/s00213-003-1761-y

Harvey, P. D., and Keefe, R. S. (2001). Studies of cognitive change in patients with schizophrenia following novel antipsychotic treatment. *Am. J. Psychiatry* 158, 176–184. doi:10.1176/appi.ajp.158.2.176

Hemsley, D. R. (2005). The schizophrenic experience: taken out of context? *Schizhopr. Bull.* 31, 43–53. doi:10.1093/schbul/sbi003

Hill, S. K., Bishop, J. R., Palumbo, D., and Sweeney, J. A. (2010). Effect of second-generation antipsychotics on cognition: current issues and future challenges. *Expert Rev. Neurother.* 10, 43–57. doi:10.1586/ern.09.143

Jackson, M. E., Homayoun, H., and Moghaddam, B. (2004). NMDA receptor hypofunction produces concomitant firing rate potentiation and burst activity reduction in the prefrontal cortex. *Proc. Natl. Acad. Sci. U.S.A.* 101, 8467–8472. doi:10.1073/pnas.0308455101

Ježek, K., Henriksen, E. J., Treves, A., Moser, E. I., and Moser, M.-B. (2011). Theta-paced flickering between place-cell maps in the hippocampus. *Nature* 478, 246–249. doi:10.1038/nature10439

Keefe, R. S. E., Poe, M., Walker, T. M., Kang, J. W., and Harvey, P. D. (2006). The Schizophrenia Cognition Rating Scale: an interview-based assessment and its relationship to cognition, real-world functioning, and functional capacity. *Am. J. Psychiatry* 163, 426–432. doi:10.1176/appi.ajp.163.3.426

Kelemen, E., and Fenton, A. A. (2010). Dynamic grouping of hippocampal neural activity during cognitive control of two spatial frames. *PLoS Biol.* 8:e1000403. doi:10.1371/journal.pbio.1000403

Kelemen, E., and Fenton, A. A. (2013). Key features of human episodic recollection in the cross-episode retrieval of rat hippocampus representations of space. *PLoS Biol.* 11:e1001607. doi:10.1371/journal.pbio.1001607

Kerwin, R., Patel, S., and Meldrum, B. (1990). Quantitative autoradiographic analysis of glutamate binding sites in the hippocampal formation in normal and schizophrenic brain post mortem. *Neuroscience* 39, 25–32. doi:10.1016/0306-4522(90)90219-T

Kobayashi, K. (2009). Targeting the hippocampal mossy fiber synapse for the treatment of psychiatric disorders. *Mol. Neurobiol.* 39, 24–36. doi:10.1007/s12035-008-8049-5

Kolomeets, N. S., Orlovskaya, D. D., Rachmanova, V. I., and Uranova, N. A. (2005). Ultrastructural alterations in hippocampal mossy fiber synapses in schizophrenia: a postmortem morphometric study. *Synapse* 57, 47–55. doi:10.1002/syn.20153

Kolomeets, N. S., Orlovskaya, D. D., and Uranova, N. A. (2007). Decreased numerical density of CA3 hippocampal mossy fiber synapses in schizophrenia. *Synapse* 61, 615–621. doi:10.1002/syn.20405

Kubik, Š, and Fenton, A. A. (2005). Behavioral evidence that segregation and representation are dissociable hippocampal functions. *J. Neurosci.* 25, 9205–9212. doi:10.1523/JNEUROSCI.1707-05.2005

Kubik, Š, Miyashita, T., and Guzowski, J. F. (2007). Using immediate-early genes to map hippocampal subregional functions. *Learn. Mem.* 14, 758–770. doi:10.1101/lm.698107

Kubik, Š, Miyashita, T., Kubik-Zahorodna, A., and Guzowski, J. F. (2012). Loss of activity-dependent *Arc* gene expression in the retrosplenial cortex after hippocampal inactivation: interaction in a higher-order memory circuit. *Neurobiol. Learn. Mem.* 97, 124–131. doi:10.1016/j.nlm.2011.10.004

Ledoux, A. A., Phillips, J. L., Labelle, A., Smith, A., Bohbot, V. D., and Boyer, P. (2013). Decreased fMRI activity in the hippocampus of patients with schizophrenia compared to healthy control participants, tested on a wayfinding task in a virtual town. *Psychiatry Res.* 211, 47–56. doi:10.1016/j.pscychresns.2012.10.005

Lee, H., Dvorak, D., Kao, H.-Y., Duffy, A. M., Scharfman, H. E., and Fenton, A. A. (2012). Early cognitive experience prevents adult deficits in a neurodevelopmental schizophrenia model. *Neuron* 75, 714–724. doi:10.1016/j.neuron.2012.06.016

Lee, I., Yoganarasimha, D., Rao, G., and Knierim, J. J. (2004). Comparison of population coherence of place cells in hippocampal subfields CA1 and CA3. *Nature* 430, 456–459. doi:10.1038/nature02739

Leutgeb, J. K., Leutgeb, S., Moser, M. B., and Moser, E. I. (2007). Pattern separation in the dentate gyrus and CA3 of the hippocampus. *Science* 315, 961–966. doi:10.1126/science.1135801

Leutgeb, S., Leutgeb, J. K., Treves, A., Moser, M.-B., and Moser, E. I. (2004). Distinct ensemble codes in hippocampal areas CA3 and CA1. *Science* 305, 1295–1298. doi:10.1126/science.1100265

Lewis, D. A., Hashimoto, T., and Volk, D. W. (2005). Cortical inhibitory neurons and schizophrenia. *Nat. Rev. Neurosci.* 6, 312–324. doi:10.1038/nrn1648

Li, Q., Clark, S., Lewis, D. V., and Wilson, W. A. (2002). NMDA receptor antagonists disinhibit rat posterior cingulate and retrosplenial cortices: a potential mechanism of neurotoxicity. *J. Neurosci.* 22, 3070–3080.

Link, W., Konietzko, U., Kauselmann, G., Krug, M., Schwanke, B., Frey, U., et al. (1995). Somatodendritic expression of an immediate early gene is regulated by synaptic activity. *Proc. Natl. Acad. Sci. U.S.A.* 92, 5734–5738. doi:10.1073/pnas.92.12.5734

Lisman, J. E., Coyle, J. T., Green, R. W., Javitt, D. C., Benes, F. M., Heckers, S., et al. (2008). Circuit-based framework for understanding neurotransmitter and risk gene interactions in schizophrenia. *Trends Neurosci.* 31, 234–242. doi:10.1016/j.tins.2008.02.005

Lobellova, V., Entlerova, M., Svojanovska, B., Hatalova, H., Prokopova, I., Petrasek, T., et al. (2013). Two learning tasks provide evidence for disrupted behavioural flexibility in an animal model of schizophrenia-like behaviour induced by acute MK-801: a dose-response study. *Behav. Brain Res.* 246, 55–62. doi:10.1016/j.bbr.2013.03.006

Lyford, G. L., Yamagata, K., Kaufmann, W. E., Barnes, C. A., Sanders, L. K., Copeland, N. G., et al. (1995). Arc, a growth factor and activity-regulated gene, encodes a novel cytoskeleton-associated protein that is enriched in neuronal dendrites. *Neuron* 14, 433–445. doi:10.1016/0896-6273(95)90299-6

Manschreck, T. C., Merrill, A. M., Jabbar, G., Chun, J., and Delisi, L. E. (2012). Frequency of normative word associations in the speech of individuals at familial high-risk for schizophrenia. *Schizophr. Res.* 140, 99–103. doi:10.1016/j.schres.2012.06.034

Martin, P., Waters, N., Waters, S., Carlsson, A., and Carlsson, M. L. (1997). MK-801-induced hyperlocomotion: differential effects of M100907, SDZ PSD 958 and raclopride. *Eur. J. Pharmacol.* 335, 107–116. doi:10.1016/S0014-2999(97)01188-6

McHugh, T. J., Jones, M. W., Quinn, J. J., Balthasar, N., Coppari, R., Elmquist, J. K., et al. (2007). Dentate gyrus NMDA receptors mediate rapid pattern separation in the hippocampal network. *Science* 317, 94–99. doi:10.1126/science.1140263

Miller, R. (1989). Hyperactivity of associations in psychosis. *Aust. N. Z. J. Psychiatry* 23, 241–248. doi:10.3109/00048678909062141

Mishara, A. L., and Goldberg, T. E. (2004). A meta-analysis and critical review of the effects of conventional neuroleptic treatment on cognition in schizophrenia: opening a closed book. *Biol. Psychiatry* 55, 1013–1022. doi:10.1016/j.biopsych.2004.01.027

Miyashita, T., Kubík, Š, Haghighi, N., Steward, O., and Guzowski, J. F. (2009). Rapid activation of plasticity-associated gene transcription in hippocampal neurons provides a mechanism for encoding of one-trial experience. *J. Neurosci.* 29, 898–906. doi:10.1523/JNEUROSCI.4588-08.2009

Moscovitch, M., Nadel, L., Winocur, G., Gilboa, A., and Rosenbaum, R. S. (2006). The cognitive neuroscience of remote episodic, semantic and spatial memory. *Curr. Opin. Neurobiol.* 16, 179–190. doi:10.1016/j.conb.2006.03.013

Moser, E. I., and Moser, M. B. (1998). Distributed encoding and retrieval of spatial memory in the hippocampus. *J. Neurosci.* 18, 7535–7542.

Newcomer, J. W., and Krystal, J. H. (2001). NMDA receptor regulation of memory and behavior in humans. *Hippocampus* 11, 529–542. doi:10.1002/hipo.1069

Nikiforuk, A., and Popik, P. (2012). Effects of quetiapine and sertindole on subchronic ketamine-induced deficits in attentional set-shifting in rats. *Psychopharmacology (Berl.)* 220, 65–74. doi:10.1007/s00213-011-2487-x

Nowakowski, C., Kaufmann, W. A., Adlassnig, C., Maier, H., Salimi, K., Jellinger, K. A., et al. (2002). Reduction of chromogranin B-like immunoreactivity in distinct subregions of the hippocampus from individuals with schizophrenia. *Schizophr. Res.* 58, 43–53. doi:10.1016/S0920-9964(01)00389-9

Olypher, A. V., Klement, D., and Fenton, A. A. (2006). Cognitive disorganization in hippocampus: physiological model of the disorganization in psychosis. *J. Neurosci.* 26, 158–168. doi:10.1523/JNEUROSCI.2064-05.2006

Phillips, W. A., and Silverstein, S. M. (2003). Convergence of biological and psychological perspectives on cognitive coordination in schizophrenia. *Behav. Brain Sci.* 26, 65–82. doi:10.1017/S0140525X03000025

Plath, N., Ohana, O., Dammermann, B., Errington, M. L., Schmitz, D., Gross, C., et al. (2006). *Arc/Arg3.1* is essential for the consolidation of synaptic plasticity and memories. *Neuron* 52, 437–444. doi:10.1016/j.neuron.2006.08.024

Powel, S. B., and Geyer, M. A. (2007). Overview of animal models of schizophrenia. *Curr. Protoc. Neurosci.* 39, 9.24.1–9.24.20. doi:10.1002/0471142301.ns0924s39

Ragland, J. D., Yoon, J., Minzenberg, M. J., and Carter, C. S. (2007). Neuroimaging of cognitive disability in schizophrenia: search for a pathophysiological mechanism. *Int. Rev. Psychiatry* 19, 417–427. doi:10.1080/09540260701486365

Ranganath, C., Minzenberg, M. J., and Ragland, J. D. (2008). The cognitive neuroscience of memory function and dysfunction in schizophrenia. *Biol. Psychiatry* 64, 18–25. doi:10.1016/j.biopsych.2008.04.011

Reichenberg, A., Caspi, A., Harrington, H., Houts, R., Keefe, R. S. E., Murray, R. M., et al. (2010). Static and dynamic cognitive deficits in childhood preceding adult schizophrenia: a 30-year study. *Am. J. Psychiatry* 167, 160–169. doi:10.1176/appi.ajp.2009.09040574

Romón, T., Mengod, G., and Adell, A. (2011). Expression of parvalbumin and glutamic acid decarboxylase-67 after acute administration of MK-801. Implications for the NMDA hypofunction model of schizophrenia. *Psychopharmacology (Berl.)* 217, 231–238. doi:10.1007/s00213-011-2268-6

Rorabacher, D. B. (1991). Statistical treatment for rejection of deviant values: critical values of Dixon's "Q" parameter and related subrange ratios at the 95% confidence level. *Anal. Chem.* 63, 139–146. doi:10.1021/ac00002a010

Rosenheck, R., CATIE Study Investigators Group, Leslie, D., Keefe, R., McEvoy, J., Swartz, M., et al. (2006). Barriers to employment for people with schizophrenia. *Am. J. Psychiatry* 163, 411–417. doi:10.1176/appi.ajp.163.3.411

Rung, J. P., Carlsson, A., Rydén Markinhuhta, K., and Carlsson, M. L. (2005). (+)-MK-801 induced social withdrawal in rats; a model for negative symptoms of schizophrenia. *Prog. Neuropsychopharmacol. Biol. Psychiatry* 29, 827–832. doi:10.1016/j.pnpbp.2005.03.004

Schneider, F., Gur, R. C., Koch, K., Backes, V., Amunts, K., Shah, N. J., et al. (2006). Impairment in the specificity of emotion processing in schizophrenia. *Am. J. Psychiatry* 163, 442–447. doi:10.1176/appi.ajp.163.3.442

Silverstein, S. M., Kovacs, I., Corry, R., and Valone, C. (2000). Perceptual organization, the disorganization syndrome, and context processing in chronic schizophrenia. *Schizophr. Res.* 43, 11–20. doi:10.1016/S0920-9964(99)00180-2

Sørensen, H. J., Mortensen, E. L., Schiffman, J., Reinisch, J. M., Maeda, J., and Mednick, S. A. (2010). Early developmental milestones and risk of schizophrenia: a 45-year follow-up of the Copenhagen Perinatal Cohort. *Schizophr. Res.* 118, 41–47. doi:10.1016/j.schres.2010.01.029

Steward, O., and Worley, P. F. (2001). Selective targeting of newly synthesized Arc mRNA to active synapses requires NMDA receptor activation. *Neuron* 30, 227–240. doi:10.1016/S0896-6273(01)00275-6

Stuchlík, A., Fenton, A. A., and Bureš, J. (2001). Substratal idiothetic navigation of rats is impaired by removal or devaluation of extramaze and intramaze cues. *Proc. Natl. Acad. Sci. U.S.A.* 98, 3537–3542. doi:10.1073/pnas.051630498

Stuchlík, A., Rezácová, L., Valeš, K., Bubeníková, V., and Kubík, S. (2004). Application of a novel active allothetic place avoidance task (AAPA) in testing a pharmacological model of psychosis in rats: comparison with the Morris Water Maze. *Neurosci. Lett.* 366, 162–166. doi:10.1016/j.neulet.2004.05.037

Stuchlík, A., and Valeš, K. (2005). Systemic administration of MK-801, a non-competitive NMDA-receptor antagonist, elicits a behavioural deficit of rats in the active allothetic place avoidance (AAPA) task irrespectively of their intact spatial pretraining. *Behav. Brain Res.* 159, 163–171. doi:10.1016/j.bbr.2004.10.013

Tamminga, C. A., Southcott, S., Sacco, C., Wagner, A. D., and Ghose, S. (2012). Glutamate dysfunction in hippocampus: relevance of dentate gyrus and CA3 signaling. *Schizophr. Bull.* 38, 927–935. doi:10.1093/schbul/sbs062

Tamminga, C. A., Stan, A. D., and Wagner, A. D. (2010). The hippocampal formation in schizophrenia. *Am. J. Psychiatry* 167, 1178–1193. doi:10.1176/appi.ajp.2010.09081187

Tüscher, O., Silbersweig, D., Pan, H., Smith, T., Beutel, M., Zonana, J., et al. (2005). Processing of environmental sounds in schizophrenic patients: disordered recognition and lack of semantic specificity. *Schizophr. Res.* 73, 291–295. doi:10.1016/j.schres.2004.06.010

Uhlhaas, P. J., Silverstein, S. M., Phillips, W. A., and Lovell, P. G. (2004). Evidence for impaired visual context processing in schizotypy with thought disorder. *Schizophr. Res.* 68, 249–260. doi:10.1016/S0920-9964(03)00184-1

Valeš, K., Bubeníková-Valešová, V., Klement, D., and Stuchlík, A. (2006). Analysis of sensitivity to MK-801 treatment in a novel active allothetic place avoidance task and in the working memory version of the Morris water maze reveals differences between Long-Evans and Wistar rats. *Neurosci. Res.* 55, 383–388. doi:10.1016/j.neures.2006.04.007

van der Staay, F. J., Rutten, K., Erb, C., and Bloklande, A. (2011). Effects of the cognition impairer MK-801 on learning and memory in mice and rats. *Behav. Brain Res.* 220, 215–229. doi:10.1016/j.bbr.2011.01.052

Vazdarjanova, A., and Guzowski, J. F. (2004). Differences in hippocampal neuronal population responses to modifications of an environmental context: evidence for distinct, yet complementary, functions of CA3 and CA1 ensembles. *J. Neurosci.* 24, 6489–6496. doi:10.1523/JNEUROSCI.0350-04.2004

Vazdarjanova, A., McNaughton, B. L., Barnes, C. A., Worley, P. F., and Guzowski, J. F. (2002). Experience-dependent coincident expression of the effector immediate-early genes *Arc* and *Homer 1a* in hippocampal and neocortical neuronal networks. *J. Neurosci.* 22, 10067–10071.

Vollenweider, F. X., Leenders, K. L., Scharfetter, C., Antonini, A., Maguire, P., Missimer, J., et al. (1997). Metabolic hyperfrontality and psychopathology in the ketamine model of psychosis using positron emission tomography (PET) and [18F]fluorodeoxyglucose (FDG). *Eur. Neuropsychopharmacol.* 7, 9–24. doi:10.1016/S0924-977X(96)00039-9

Weinberger, D. R. (1999). Cell biology of the hippocampal formation in schizophrenia. *Biol. Psychiatry* 45, 395–402. doi:10.1016/S0006-3223(98)00331-X

Weiss, A. P., Schacter, D. L., Goff, D. C., Rauch, S. L., Alpert, N. M., Fischman, A. J., et al. (2003). Impaired hippocampal recruitment during normal modulation of memory performance in schizophrenia. *Biol. Psychiatry* 53, 48–55. doi:10.1016/S0006-3223(02)01541-X

Wentura, D., Moritz, S., and Frings, C. (2008). Further evidence for "hyper-priming" in thought-disordered schizophrenic patients using repeated masked category priming. *Schizophr. Res.* 102, 69–75. doi:10.1016/j.schres.2008.04.016

Wesierska, M., Dockery, C., and Fenton, A. A. (2005). Beyond memory, navigation and inhibition: behavioural evidence for hippocampus-dependent cognitive coordination in the rat. *J. Neurosci.* 25, 2413–2419. doi:10.1523/JNEUROSCI.3962-04.2005

Westerhausen, R., Kompus, K., and Hugdahl, K. (2011). Impaired cognitive inhibition in schizophrenia: a meta-analysis of the Stroop interference effect. *Schizophr. Res.* 133, 172–181. doi:10.1016/j.schres.2011.08.025

Yamasaki, N., Maekawa, M., Kobayashi, K., Kajii, Y., Maeda, J., Soma, M., et al. (2008). Alpha-CaMKII deficiency causes immature dentate gyrus, a novel candidate endophenotype of psychiatric disorders. *Mol. Brain* 1, 6. doi:10.1186/1756-6606-1-6

10

Reduced expression of Nogo-A leads to motivational deficits in rats

Thomas Enkel[1]*, Stefan M. Berger[1], Kai Schönig[1], Björn Tews[2] and Dusan Bartsch[1]

[1] *Department of Molecular Biology, Central Institute of Mental Health, Medical Faculty Mannheim, University of Heidelberg, Mannheim, Germany*
[2] *Schaller Research Group, Division of Molecular Mechanisms of Tumor Invasion, University of Heidelberg and German Cancer Research Center, Heidelberg, Germany*

Edited by:
Ales Stuchlik, Academy of Sciences of the Czech Republic, Czech Republic

Correspondence:
Thomas Enkel, Department Molecular Biology, Central Institute of Mental Health, Square J5, 68159 Mannheim, Germany
e-mail: thomas.enkel@zi-mannheim.de

Nogo-A is an important neurite growth-regulatory protein in the adult and developing nervous system. Mice lacking Nogo-A, or rats with neuronal Nogo-A deficiency, exhibit behavioral abnormalities such as impaired short-term memory, decreased pre-pulse inhibition, and behavioral inflexibility. In the current study, we extended the behavioral profile of the Nogo-A deficient rat line with respect to reward sensitivity and motivation, and determined the concentrations of the monoamines dopamine and serotonin in the prefrontal cortex (PFC), dorsal striatum (dSTR), and nucleus accumbens (NAcc). Using a limited access consumption task, we found similar intake of a sweet condensed milk solution following *ad libitum* or restricted feeding in wild-type and Nogo-A deficient rats, indicating normal reward sensitivity and translation of hunger into feeding behavior. When tested for motivation in a spontaneous progressive ratio task, Nogo-A deficient rats exhibited lower break points and tended to have lower "highest completed ratios." Further, under extinction conditions responding ceased substantially earlier in these rats. Finally, in the PFC we found increased tissue levels of serotonin, while dopamine was unaltered. Dopamine and serotonin levels were also unaltered in the dSTR and the NAcc. In summary, these results suggest a role for Nogo-A regulated processes in motivated behavior and related neurochemistry. The behavioral pattern observed resembles aspects of the negative symptomatology of schizophrenia.

Keywords: Nogo-A, reward sensitivity, anhedonia, motivation, avolition, schizophrenia, dopamine, serotonin

INTRODUCTION

Nogo-A is an important neurite growth-regulatory protein in the developing and adult nervous system (Schwab, 2010). While research originally focused on oligodendrocytic Nogo-A and its role in injury and repair of fiber tracts in the CNS, the fact that Nogo-A was found to be present also in neurons (Huber et al., 2002) has risen interest in its involvement in the generation of general behavior, as well. Indeed, in a wide-ranging analysis, Willi et al. (2009, 2010) could demonstrate behavioral alterations in Nogo-A knockout (Nogo-A$^{-/-}$) mice.

Recently, Nogo-A deficiency could be established in the rat species by using a transgenic, constitutively expressed artificial microRNA leading to a 50% reduction of Nogo-A levels in neurons (Tews et al., 2013). Similar to Nogo-A$^{-/-}$ mice, these Nogo-A deficient rats exhibited a variety of behavioral deficits, such as reduced pre-pulse inhibition of the acoustic startle response, behavioral inflexibility, and impairments in short-term memory. In addition, pronounced alterations in social behavior were found. Conducting basic research or preclinical studies in rats offer the advantage that, for example, they more readily learn difficult cognitive behavioral tasks and exhibit more complex social behaviors than mice (Poole and Fish, 1975; McNamara et al., 1996; Costantini and D'Amato, 2006; Cressant et al., 2007). Further, the rat Nogo-A knockdown model uses the well-characterized Sprague Dawley outbred strain and therefore offers increased translational value compared to inbred mice, which is particularly important when evaluating a possible role of neuronal growth regulation in psychiatric disorders (Tews et al., 2013). This latter point is of interest, as the behavioral and structural phenotypes of Nogo-A$^{-/-}$ mice and Nogo-A deficient rats make them potential tools to investigate the pathology of schizophrenia (SCZ; Kristofikova et al., 2013; Willi and Schwab, 2013).

Schizophrenia is a common and debilitating psychiatric disorder and believed to result from neurodevelopmental disturbances (Keshavan et al., 2008; Tandon et al., 2008; Lewis and Sweet, 2009). Interestingly, neuronal Nogo-A is highly expressed particularly during early neuronal development and down regulated later during adulthood in most regions, except the hippocampus, suggesting an important role in neuronal network formation (Huber et al., 2002; Kempf and Schwab, 2013; Mironova and Giger, 2013). In the current study, we aimed to investigate the consequences of Nogo-A deficiency with respect to two important aspects of the negative spectrum of SCZ symptoms, which have not yet been explored in rats nor in mice: *avolition*, a decrease in the motivation to take action and pursue goals, and *anhedonia*, the reduced ability to experience positive affect through reward (Tandon et al., 2009). The negative symptoms of SCZ have been particularly linked to genetic liability and neurodevelopmental disturbances (Dominguez et al., 2010). Further, it has been described before that interference with neuronal development by lesioning the neonatal brain can affect reward sensitivity (Le Pen et al., 2002) or motivated behavior (Schneider and Koch, 2005).

Motivational states in rats can be made accessible to quantification by the use of operant progressive ratio schedules introduced by Hodos and colleagues (Hodos, 1961; Hodos and Kalman, 1963). In this test, subjects need to exhibit progressively increasing effort (more lever pressing) to gain a stable amount of reward; the operant demand at which reward-related responding ceases is termed the "break point" and can serve as an index for reinforcer efficacy or a rat's motivational state (Barr and Phillips, 1998; Reilly, 1999; Mobini et al., 2000). In the Nogo-A deficient rat, we employed the spontaneous progressive ratio test (PR-Test) and additionally assessed operant responding under extinction conditions, i.e., when rewards were completely omitted. Reward sensitivity was investigated in a well-validated limited access consumption task for sweet rewards (Enkel et al., 2010; Schneider et al., 2010). Finally, to relate behavioral findings to underlying neurochemistry, we analyzed dopamine and serotonin (5-HT) content in brain regions associated with reward processing, namely nucleus accumbens (NAcc), dorsal striatum (dSTR), and prefrontal cortex (PFC).

MATERIALS AND METHODS

All experiments in this study were performed in accordance with national and international ethical guidelines, conducted in compliance with the German Animal Welfare Act and approved by the local authorities (Regierungspräsidium Karlsruhe, Germany).

SUBJECTS

Male, heterozygous Nogo-A deficient rats (Nogo-A KD rats) of the previously characterized and described transgenic line SD-Tg(CAG-RNAi:Nogo-A,EGFP)2ZI (Tews et al., 2013; L2 rats) and wild-type littermates (WT rats) were bred at the animal facilities of the Central Institute of Mental Health, Mannheim. At the beginning of the study they were 8 months old. They were housed in groups of three to four animals per cage under controlled conditions [22°C, 12 h light-dark cycle (lights-on at 7 a.m.), constant humidity]. Throughout the experiments, water was available *ad libitum* and food was restricted to 20 g/rat/day. Each rats' bodyweight was controlled continuously not to fall below 90% of free-feeding weight. Experiments were performed during the light phase between 09:00 and 12:00. Before the start of behavioral assessments, all rats were handled for 5 min daily on five consecutive days. For behavioral analysis, 18 rats were initially used but 1 rat from the WT group consumed neither the milk used as reward in the experiments nor any other food outside its home cage and it was therefore excluded from the study, resulting in the following group sizes: Nogo-A KD: $n = 9$; WT: $n = 8$. Group sizes in neurochemical experiments were: Nogo-A KD: $n = 15$; WT: $n = 9$; this cohort consisted of randomly chosen animals from the current study and age-matched animals used in a previous study (Tews et al., 2013).

CONSUMPTION TEST

Prior to the consumption test sessions, rats were given free access to the reward [a 25% solution of sweetened condensed milk (SCM), Milchmaedchen, Nestle Germany] in their home cage to reduce any neophagia. On the day preceding testing, rats were separated in small cages (type 3) for 1 h. Testing for SCM intake took place 24 h later in these cages. After 5 min of habituation, rats had access to a drinking bottle containing the SCM solution for 15 min. The amount of liquid consumed was recorded for each rat by weighing the bottle before and after 5 and 15 min of drinking time. Consume was calculated in relation to the individual body weight. The test was conducted twice, while rats were under the restricted feeding schedule (i.e., in hungry rats) and following overnight *ad libitum* feeding prior to the consumption test (i.e., in non-hungry rats).

OPERANT CONDITIONING PROCEDURES

All operant schedules were carried out in four identical rat operant training chambers (MedAssociates, Vermont, USA) controlled by a computer running MedPC-IV software and custom-made MedStat Notation code. During sessions, a fan provided constant background noise; sessions always started with illumination of the houselight, which remained on until the session was finished. On the first 2 days, rats received 30 min session of magazine training (levers retracted) in which the dispenser used to deliver 60 μl SCM was manually operated 10–15 times; at the end of the second session all rats reliably drank from the food trough. Magazine training was followed by acquisition of lever pressing under a continuous reinforcement schedule (fixed ratio 1). Each trial started with extension of the response lever. Pressing the lever resulted in its retraction and delivery of 60 μl of SCM; once a rat entered the food trough to consume the reward, the lever was extended for the next trial. Training continued with the so-called "lever access training," in which rats were required to nose poke into a newly installed response device on the opposite wall of the lever to initiate lever extension. All training sessions ended after 30 min or when 60 rewards had been earned (whatever occurred first). Once all rats showed stable trial initiation and responding, the PR-Test was performed. In a single session (fixed to 30 min duration) the operant demand was progressively increased such that the number of lever presses required to receive a reward was raised by one following each reward delivery (i.e., a dwell 1-step 1 sequence). Following measures were taken: (1) the ratio in which a first inactivity phase of 180 s occurred; this ratio was termed the "break point," (2) the highest completed ratio achieved within the 30-min session, (3) the latencies to respond on the lever after insertion (response latency), and (4) to consume the reward after delivery (consume latency). Note that after a break point had occurred, a rat was allowed to continue to press the lever for the whole 30 min duration of the session (i.e., the "highest completed ratio" achieved could be higher than or identical to the break point). One day after the PR-Test, lever pressing was tested in a single session under extinction conditions, i.e., all lever presses were unrewarded. To control for activity changes during this session an additional lever with no programed consequences was inserted into the chamber and the numbers of lever presses on both levers were recorded. Both levers were present throughout the session and therefore no nose poking was required.

NEUROCHEMISTRY

After decapitation under carbon dioxide anesthesia brains were removed, immediately frozen in isopentane, wrapped in aluminum foil, and stored at −80°. Using a cryotome (Leica, Nußloch,

Germany), 120 μm thick frontal sections were cut and brain tissue was dissected from the PFC (from +4.7 to +3.0 mm from Bregma; including medial and orbitofrontal parts), dSTR (from +2.2 to −1.7 mm from Bregma; caudate putamen), and NAcc (from +2.7 to +0.8 mm from Bregma, including NAcc core and shell subregions) using punching needles; respective brain regions were identified according to the Rat Brain Atlas by Paxinos and Watson (2007). Frozen tissue samples were collected in polypropylene tubes and stored at −80° until further processing.

For HPLC analysis samples were thawed, weighed, and immediately homogenized in an extraction solution (0.1 M perchloric acid, 1 mM EDTA) using a tissue homogenizer Mixer Mill (Qiagen, Hilden, Germany). Yielded solutions were subsequently centrifuged at 15000 × *g* for 10 min at 4°C. Cleared supernatants were analyzed by a HPLC system consisting of a Triathlon autosampler (Spark Holland B.V., Emmen, Netherlands), a Shimadzu LC-10 AD pump (Shimadzu Corporation, Kyoto, Japan), a 150 mm × 2.1 mm C18-Reprosil-AQ reverse phase column (3 μm particle size; Dr. Maisch HPLC GmbH, Ammerbuch, Germany) and a Decade II electrochemical detector (Antec Leyden, Zoeterwoude, Netherlands). The mobile phase was 50 mM sodium citrate, 2.4 mM sodium octyl sulfate, 0.1 mM EDTA, 10 mM NaCl, and 22% methanol at pH 4.0. The temperature applied on the system was 37°C. Tissue concentrations were determined by normalizing the quantified amounts of respective neurotransmitters and their metabolites to the corresponding weight of the individual tissue sample.

STATISTICS

Sweetened condensed milk intake was analyzed using a three-way repeated measure ANOVA with factors drinking time (5/15 min) × feeding status (restricted/*ad libitum*) × genotype (Nogo-A/WT) and *post hoc* paired *t*-Tests (two-tailed) where appropriate. For operant behavior, lever press activity during training sessions was analyzed as number of trials per minute due to varying session lengths; for the PR-Test, data were analyzed as completed ratios (for example, a ratio of "12" required 12 lever presses to be completed); under extinction, the exact number of lever presses made was taken for analysis. Behavioral parameters and neurotransmitter content were compared using two-tailed Student's *t*-test or, in cases of unequal variances, Welch's *t*-Test. Calculations were done with SPSS statistical software (Version 21, IBM Corporation). In all cases *p*-values of 5% or lower ($p \leq 0.05$) were accepted as statistically significant.

RESULTS

REWARD SENSITIVITY

No significant differences were found between the groups of rats regarding their bodyweight on the day before the first consumption test (Nogo-A KD: 632g ± 12; WT:648 g ± 16; $t_{15} = 0.79$, $p = 0.45$). **Figure 1** shows the amount of SCM consumed after 5 or 15 min access to the drinking bottle under each feeding status (restricted/*ad libitum*). There was no main effect of the factor genotype ($F_{1,15} = 0.85$, $p = 0.372$) and none of the other factors (feeding state or drinking time) interacted with genotype (all $p > 0.660$), indicating that Nogo-A KD rats consumed similar amounts compared to WT controls under each condition. Significant main effects were found for feeding state ($F_{1,15} = 158.78$, $p < 0.001$) and drinking time ($F_{1,15} = 457.37$, $p < 0.001$), and these two factors interacted significantly ($F_{1,15} = 113.71$, $p < 0.001$); further inspection of the data indicated that, after restricted feeding rats consumed more total SCM in 15 min ($t_{16} = 12.91$, $p < 0.001$) and they also consumed more SCM during the first 5 min of drinking time following restricted compared to *ad libitum* feeding ($t_{16} = 4.87$, $p < 0.001$).

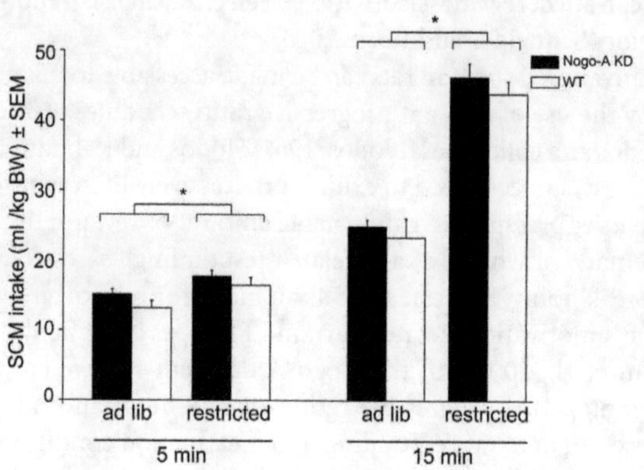

FIGURE 1 | Reward sensitivity in Nogo-A deficient rats. There were no differences in SCM intake between Nogo-A KD and WT rats under any feeding condition or at any time point. Restricted feeding prior to the consumption test resulted in higher SCM intake after 5 min ($p < 0.001$) and 15 min ($p < 0.001$). Data are expressed as means ± SEM. WT: $n = 8$, Nogo-A KD: $n = 9$. Asterisks (*) indicate statistically significant differences.

MOTIVATION

Acquisition of operant responding during the initial learning stage (days 1–5), and the performance during the "lever access" stage (days 6–8; nose poking required to access lever) was similar in both strains (**Figure 2A**). Explicitly, a planned comparison of the number of initiated trials during the last training session before the PR-Test (**Figure 2A**, day 8) confirmed that there was no statistically relevant difference between Nogo-A KD and WT rats (Nogo-A KD: 2.3 ± 0.3 trials/min, WT: 2.9 ± 0.2 trials/min; $t_{15} = 1.56$, $p = 0.139$). During the PR-Test (**Figure 2B**), Nogo-A KD rats exhibited a significantly lower break point (Nogo-A KD: 17 ± 2.8, WT: 24 ± 1.4; $t_{11.87} = 2.19$, $p = 0.049$) and, additionally, a tendency for a decreased "highest completed ratio" was found in Nogo-A KD rats (Nogo-A KD: 18 ± 2.6, WT: 24 ± 1.2; $t_{11.22} = 1.87$, $p = 0.088$). Further, response latencies were significantly increased in Nogo-A KD rats compared to WTs (Nogo-A KD: 6.7s ± 1.1, WT: 3.4 s ± 0.3; $t_{8.94} = 3.04$, $p = 0.014$), but consumption latencies were similar between groups (Nogo-A KD: 2.8 s ± 0.7, WT: 2.1 s ± 0.4; $t_{11.78} = 0.88$, $p = 0.398$; **Figure 2C**). Under the extinction schedule, i.e., when lever pressing was no longer rewarded, responding ceased earlier in Nogo-A KD rats than in WT rats (**Figure 2D**). While this was apparent for the previously rewarded lever (Nogo-A KD: 9.3 ± 1.5, WT: 17.3 ± 1.6; $t_{15} = 3.59$, $p = 0.003$), this was not the case for the alternatively available new lever (Nogo-A KD: 7.0 ± 2.1, WT: 9.4 ± 1.9; $t_{15} = 0.83$, $p = 0.419$) on which rats from both groups made less responses compared to the previously rewarded lever.

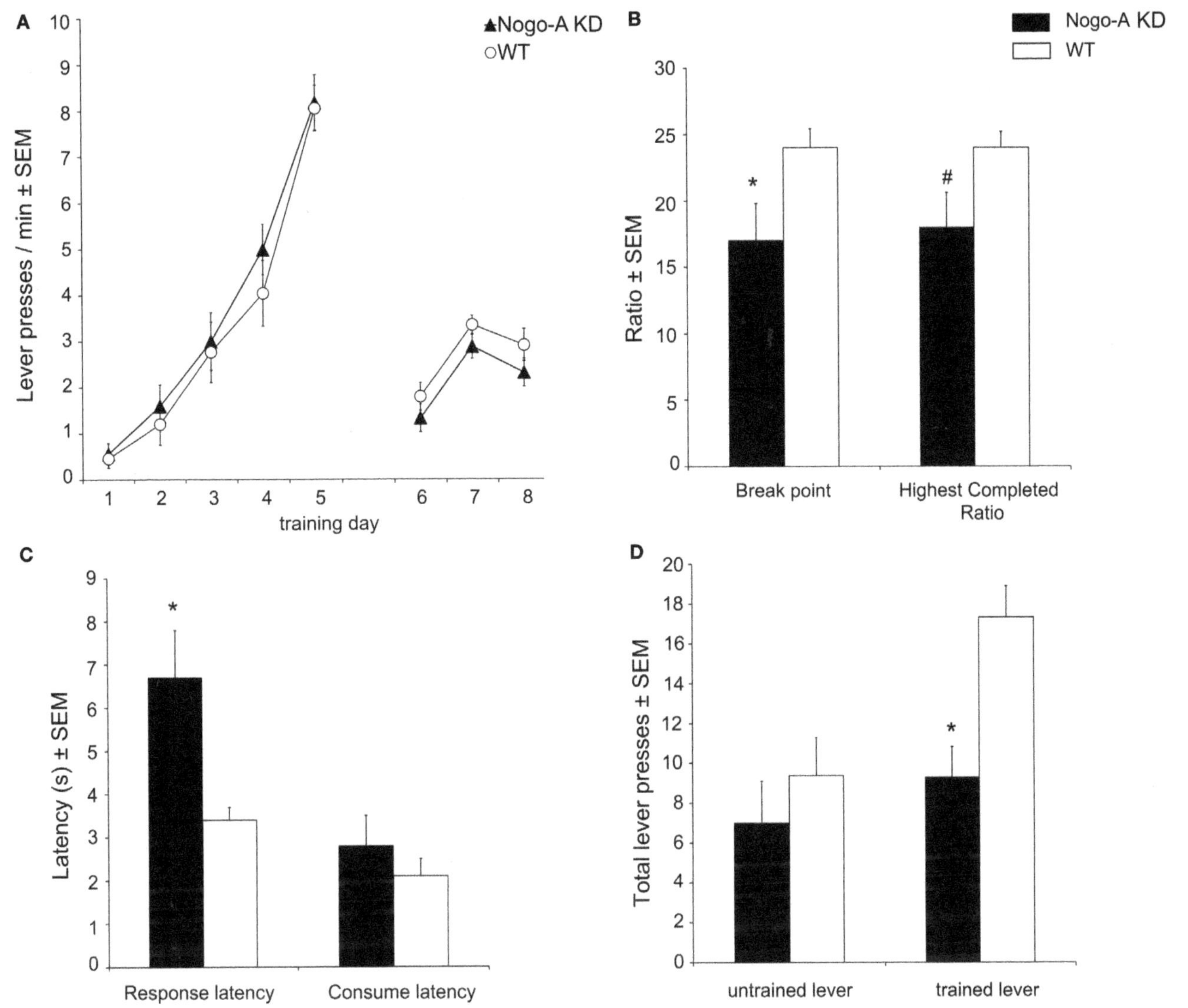

FIGURE 2 | Motivational behavior in Nogo-A deficient rats. **(A)** Nogo-A KD rats acquired operant responding similar to WT rats (days 1–5); additionally, there was no difference in baseline performance before the PR-Test (during days 6–8, when nose poking was required to get access to the lever). **(B)** In the PR-Test, Nogo-A KD rats had a significantly lower break point ($p = 0.049$) and tended to have a lower "highest completed ratio" ($p = 0.088$). **(C)** Response latency was increased in Nogo-A KD rats ($p = 0.014$) while the latency to consume the SCM was unaltered ($p = 0.398$). **(D)** Performance under extinction conditions. Nogo-A KD rats made significantly less lever presses than WT rats on the trained lever ($p = 0.003$). There was no difference for the untrained lever ($p = 0.419$). Data are expressed as means ± SEM. WT: $n = 8$, Nogo-A KD: $n = 9$. Asterisks (*) indicate statistically significant differences, the number sign (#) indicates a trend.

NEUROCHEMISTRY

Concentrations of monoamine neurotransmitters and their metabolites in tissue homogenates from PFC, dSTR, and NAcc of Nogo-A KD and WT rats are shown in **Table 1**. We found a highly significant 25% increase in 5-HT tissue levels in the PFC (WT:1.37 ± 0.07 pmol/mg, Nogo-A: 1.71 ± 0.08 pmol/mg; $t_{22} = 2.895$, $p = 0.008$) while the metabolite 5-Hydroxyindoleacetic acid (5-HIAA) was not altered. No further significant alterations of DA or its metabolites 3,4-dihydroxyphenylacetic acid (DOPAC) or homovanillic acid (HVA) or of 5-HT or its metabolite 5-HIAA were detected in any other brain region measured.

DISCUSSION

Deficiency of the Nogo-A protein, which is highly expressed during neurodevelopment (Huber et al., 2002), has been associated with a variety of behavioral abnormalities in adult rats (Tews et al., 2013). Here, we extended the behavioral profile of Nogo-A deficient rats with respect to reward sensitivity and motivation.

Consumption of a palatable SCM solution was taken as an indicator for reward sensitivity. This test has been shown to be sensitive to detect anhedonic states, for example, due to blockade of the opioid system (Schneider et al., 2010) or due to stress in an animal model of depression (Enkel et al., 2010). Intake after *ad libitum* pre-feeding with lab chow assumingly reflects mainly the hedonic

Table 1 | Brain tissue concentrations of monoamine neurotransmitters and their metabolites as well as monoamine turnover rates in WT and Nogo-A KD rats.

Region	Group	DA (pmol/mg)	DOPAC (pmol/mg)	HVA (pmol/mg)	DOPAC/DA	HVA/DA	5-HT (pmol/mg)	5-HIAA (pmol/mg)	5-HIAA/5-HT
PFC	WT	0.20 ± 0.03	0.15 ± 0.01	0.19 ± 0.03	0.81 ± 0.09	1.12 ± 0.35	1.37 ± 0.07	1.68 ± 0.27	1.27 ± 0.25
	Nogo-A	0.17 ± 0.02	0.13 ± 0.01	0.23 ± 0.02	1.25 ± 0.33	2.03 ± 0.50	1.72 ± 0.08**	1.63 ± 0.10	0.96 ± 0.06
dSTR	WT	45.88 ± 4.34	10.23 ± 1.04	2.50 ± 0.28	0.24 ± 0.03	0.06 ± 0.01	1.51 ± 0.21	2.40 ± 0.23	1.66 ± 0.11
	Nogo-A	43.27 ± 2.16	12.01 ± 1.16	2.83 ± 0.39	0.28 ± 0.072	0.06 ± 0.01	1.40 ± 0.11	2.34 ± 0.19	1.69 ± 0.07
NAcc	WT	15.36 ± 2.23	6.28 ± 1.21	1.56 ± 0.36	0.41 ± 0.06	0.10 ± 0.02	1.49 ± 0.26	2.03 ± 0.31	1.44 ± 0.21
	Nogo-A	14.46 ± 1.66	5.68 ± 0.56	1.37 ± 0.15	0.43 ± 0.04	0.10 ± 0.01	1.76 ± 0.21	2.25 ± 0.14	1.52 ± 0.20

5-HT levels were significantly increased in the PFC.
*Data are expressed as means ± SEM. **p = 0.008; WT: n = 9, Nogo-A: n = 15*

component of the reward, whereas intake after restricted feeding has an added component of hunger; indeed, when rats were hungry SCM intake was higher and more rapid. Nevertheless, under both conditions Nogo-A KD rats consumed similar amounts of SCM compared to WT and also the time pattern of consumption was similar, implying normal reward sensitivity and translation of hunger into feeding behavior. Our data therefore show that reduced levels of Nogo-A do not affect sensitivity to food rewards. Of course, anhedonia in other domains, e.g., for social reward, cannot be excluded.

Some studies interfering with neurodevelopmental processes have reported unaltered reward sensitivity, but found motivational deficits (Schneider and Koch, 2005). Correspondingly, Nogo-A KD rats exhibited pronounced motivational deficits under a progressive ratio schedule of operant responding. They had a lower break point, indicating that in these rats a "drop" in their motivation to engage in effortful lever pressing occurred earlier, i.e., at lower operant demands. Although some Nogo-A KD rats continued to press the lever after the break point had occurred, they were not willing to invest similar amounts of effort to obtain as much rewards as WT rats, as suggested by the tendency for a decreased "highest completed ratio." Importantly, inspection of the time courses of responding verified that the 30-min session duration did not pose time constraints on the animals; rather, animals from both groups were inactive during the last minutes of the session. After initiating a trial by nose poking, Nogo-A KD rats were slower to actually begin lever pressing but not to consume the reward once achieved, supporting the interpretation of a motivational deficit but normal reward sensitivity. Our results are not likely to be confounded by impaired learning, since WT and Nogo-A KD rats acquired lever pressing similarly and there were no baseline performance differences between groups prior to the PR-Test, or by decreased locomotor activity, since normal explorative behavior has been shown for Nogo-A KD rats (Tews et al., 2013).

From the current study, the functional origin of the motivational deficit cannot be definitely concluded. Our data allow excluding anhedonia as an explanation, given normal SCM consumption and normal consumption latencies in the PR-Test, but instead suggest disturbances in the instrumental phase of motivated behavior. The latter refers to several processes required to translate reward information into goal-directed behavior, such as "wanting," cost-benefit calculation and response initiation, which are more difficult to disentangle (Salamone and Correa, 2012). The fact that Nogo-A KD rats still initiated trials by nose poking to access the lever and performed lever pressing to a certain extent suggests normal response initiation. Further, this also suggests that the reward was still "wanted" and that a representation of the reward could be used to motivate them to start a new trial. But there are some hints that in Nogo-A KD rats either the representation of reward value itself or its use in cost/benefit calculations could indeed be altered. Interesting in this respect is a comparison of the performance in the PR-Test with the extinction session. In both groups, lever pressing ceased earlier under extinction conditions than in the PR-Test, but this effect was much stronger in Nogo-A KD rats. The main difference between these sessions is that during extinction any lever pressing is solely dependent on a representation of the reward (since no rewards can be physically experienced), while during the PR-Test the action-reward interval increases progressively and provides at least some hedonic experience (some rewards are delivered). Importantly, on the (never rewarded) control lever both groups made comparably few responses excluding overall lower activity in Nogo-A KD rats during extinction as an alternative explanation.

Our study also collected neurochemical data related to motivational processes. Although, our analysis of tissue monoamine levels under baseline conditions does not allow drawing substantial conclusions about direct functional relationships between altered monoaminergic activity and behavior, these data nevertheless provide some indirect information on the processes potentially contributing to the motivational deficit. Dopamine has been particularly linked to "wanting" and cost/benefit calculations (Salamone et al., 2007; Salamone and Correa, 2012) and the fact that we found no alterations in the dopaminergic transmitter system was surprising, but appears to be in line with our above discussed observation that Nogo-A KD rats were still wanting the reward. Of particular interest is therefore the highly significant increase in prefrontal 5-HT levels in Nogo-A KD rats. Increased brain serotonergic tone, due to deletion of the serotonin transporter or chronic 5-HT reuptake blockade, has been shown to decrease motivation for natural rewards in mice (Sanders et al., 2007). Particularly intriguing, increased serotonergic tone in the orbitofrontal areas of the PFC has been specifically associated with impaired ability to use the value of expected outcomes to guide behavior (Nonkes et al., 2010). This suggests that the motivational deficit in Nogo-A KD rats could indeed be a consequence of the observed alterations of 5-HT levels in the PFC. Brain microdialysis experiments monitoring transmitter release in the behaving rat could provide such correlative information. Alternatively, alterations in transmitter systems other than the dopaminergic or serotonergic systems could of course contribute to the motivational deficit. For example, the glutamatergic and GABAergic systems, which could not be measured in this study, have also been linked to motivational processes (Faure et al., 2010).

The findings of this study are of considerable interest given that reward-related disturbances are clinical features of many psychiatric disorders (Brown and Pluck, 2000), e.g., of the negative symptoms of SCZ which have been particularly linked to genetic liability and neurodevelopmental disturbances (Tandon et al., 2009; Dominguez et al., 2010). In our study Nogo-A KD rats did not show deficits in reward sensitivity; although anhedonia – which is defined as the decreased capacity to experience pleasure – has long been considered a symptom in SCZ, more recent research supports the idea that hedonic processing itself is indeed normal in patients but that cognitive deficits instead lead to negatively biased self-report about hedonic experience (Strauss and Gold, 2012). More important in this respect is that the motivational deficit in Nogo-A KD rats resembles avolition, which is defined as a lack in the motivation to pursue goals. Avolition is commonly seen in patients with SCZ and has always been considered a core negative symptom (Tandon et al., 2009; Messinger et al., 2011). Furthermore, an increase in serotonergic neurotransmission is suggested to be present in schizophrenic patients (Ngan et al., 2000; Dean, 2003). Our current results are therefore in line with earlier reports linking the behavioral phenotype of Nogo-A deficient rats (Tews et al., 2013), or of Nogo-A$^{-/-}$ mice (Willi et al., 2010), to a variety of schizophrenic symptoms.

The fact that the rats used in the current study and by Tews et al. (2013) were deficient of Nogo-A in neurons, but not in oligodendrocytes, allows an interesting comparison with earlier work in mice which bear the Nogo-A knockout in both cell types (Willi et al., 2010). Similar to these mice, Nogo-A KD rats exhibit behavioral deficits such as reduced pre-pulse inhibition of the acoustic startle response, behavioral inflexibility, impairments in short-term memory and impairments in management of reference frames (Tews et al., 2013; Petrasek et al., 2014). Additionally, they show the motivational deficits demonstrated in the current study. Given the cell-type specific temporal expression profile of Nogo-A, with high expression of Nogo-A in neurons mainly during early development and high expression in oligodendrocytes mainly in the postnatal nervous system, the behavioral deficits observed in the Nogo-A deficiency rat model and the Nogo-A$^{-/-}$ mouse model appear to be largely the consequences of disturbed brain developmental processes following Nogo-A deficiency particularly in neurons. Indeed, Nogo-A has been shown to be critically involved in early cortical development and neuronal maturation (Mingorance-Le Meur et al., 2007). This is intriguing since SCZ is considered to be a disorder of abnormal neurodevelopment (Lewis and Sweet, 2009). Notably, we found some clear differences between Nogo-A KD rats and Nogo-A$^{-/-}$ mice regarding alterations in neurotransmission: in contrast to rats, Nogo-A$^{-/-}$ mice had reduced tissue levels of DA and its metabolites DOPAC and HVA in the dSTR. Additionally, no reductions in tissue levels of 5-HT were found (Willi et al., 2010). Whether these differences to rats are related to the additional lack of oligodendrocytic Nogo-A in mice is unclear. Yet, since oligodendrocytic Nogo-A is crucial for myelination, which continues postnatally, ongoing perturbations in neuronal development might lead to the differential outcome in Nogo-A KD rats and Nogo-A$^{-/-}$ mice. Alternatively, in Nogo-A$^{-/-}$ mice compensatory upregulation of Nogo-B has been reported (Willi et al., 2010), an effect not present in Nogo-A deficient rats (Tews et al., 2013). More research is needed to determine possible differential contributions of neuronal or oligodendrocytic Nogo-A to the behavioral and neurochemical phenotypes observed. The Nogo-A deficiency rat model nevertheless provides a promising tool to complement the Nogo-A$^{-/-}$ mouse model to further elucidate the role of Nogo-A in neuropsychiatric disorders like SCZ.

AUTHOR CONTRIBUTIONS

Thomas Enkel, Kai Schönig, Björn Tews, and Dusan Bartsch initiated and designed the study; Thomas Enkel and Stefan M. Berger performed experiments; Thomas Enkel, Stefan M. Berger, Kai Schönig, Björn Tews, and Dusan Bartsch wrote the manuscript.

ACKNOWLEDGMENTS

The authors would like to thank Brigitte Pesold for excellent technical assistance with HPLC analysis. This work was funded by a National Bernstein Network for Computational Neuroscience grant and a HEALTH-F2-2007-201714 DEVANX (http://devanx.vitamib.com) grant.

REFERENCES

Barr, A. M., and Phillips, A. G. (1998). Chronic mild stress has no effect on responding by rats for sucrose under a progressive ratio schedule. *Physiol. Behav.* 64, 591–597. doi:10.1016/S0031-9384(98)00060-2

Brown, R. G., and Pluck, G. (2000). Negative symptoms: the "pathology" of motivation and goal-directed behaviour. *Trends Neurosci.* 23, 412–417. doi:10.1016/S0166-2236(00)01626-X

Costantini, F., and D'Amato, F. R. (2006). Ultrasonic vocalizations in rats and mice: social contexts and functions. *Acta Zool. Sin.* 52, 619–633.

Cressant, A., Besson, M., Suarez, S., Cormier, A., and Granon, S. (2007). Spatial learning in Long-Evans Hooded rats and C57BL/6J mice: different strategies for different performance. *Behav. Brain Res.* 177, 22–29. doi:10.1016/j.bbr.2006.11.010

Dean, B. (2003). The cortical serotonin2A receptor and the pathology of schizophrenia: a likely accomplice. *J. Neurochem.* 85, 1–13. doi:10.1046/j.1471-4159.2003.01693.x

Dominguez, M. D., Saka, M. C., Lieb, R., Wittchen, H. U., and van Os, J. (2010). Early expression of negative/disorganized symptoms predicting psychotic experiences and subsequent clinical psychosis: a 10-year study. *Am. J. Psychiatry* 167, 1075–1082. doi:10.1176/appi.ajp.2010.09060883

Enkel, T., Spanagel, R., Vollmayr, B., and Schneider, M. (2010). Stress triggers anhedonia in rats bred for learned helplessness. *Behav. Brain Res.* 209, 183–186. doi:10.1016/j.bbr.2010.01.042

Faure, A., Richard, J. M., and Berridge, K. C. (2010). Desire and dread from the nucleus accumbens: cortical glutamate and subcortical GABA differentially generate motivation and hedonic impact in the rat. *PLoS ONE* 5:e11223. doi:10.1371/journal.pone.0011223

Hodos, W. (1961). Progressive ratio as a measure of reward strength. *Science* 134, 943–944. doi:10.1126/science.134.3483.943

Hodos, W., and Kalman, G. (1963). Effects of increment size and reinforcer volume on progressive ratio performance. *J. Exp. Anal. Behav.* 6, 387–392. doi:10.1901/jeab.1963.6-387

Huber, A. B., Weinmann, O., Brosamle, C., Oertle, T., and Schwab, M. E. (2002). Patterns of Nogo mRNA and protein expression in the developing and adult rat and after CNS lesions. *J. Neurosci.* 22, 3553–3567.

Kempf, A., and Schwab, M. E. (2013). Nogo-A represses anatomical and synaptic plasticity in the central nervous system. *Physiology (Bethesda)* 28, 151–163. doi:10.1152/physiol.00052.2012

Keshavan, M. S., Tandon, R., Boutros, N. N., and Nasrallah, H. A. (2008). Schizophrenia, "just the facts": what we know in 2008 Part 3: neurobiology. *Schizophr. Res.* 106, 89–107. doi:10.1016/j.schres.2008.07.020

Kristofikova, Z., Vrajova, M., Sirova, J., Vales, K., Petrasek, T., Schonig, K., et al. (2013). N-Methyl-D-Aspartate receptor – nitric oxide synthase pathway in the cortex of Nogo-A-deficient rats in relation to brain laterality and schizophrenia. *Front. Behav. Neurosci.* 7:90. doi:10.3389/fnbeh.2013.00090

Le Pen, G., Gaudet, L., Mortas, P., Mory, R., and Moreau, J. L. (2002). Deficits in reward sensitivity in a neurodevelopmental rat model of schizophrenia. *Psychopharmacology (Berl.)* 161, 434–441. doi:10.1007/s00213-002-1092-4

Lewis, D. A., and Sweet, R. A. (2009). Schizophrenia from a neural circuitry perspective: advancing toward rational pharmacological therapies. *J. Clin. Invest.* 119, 706–716. doi:10.1172/JCI37335

McNamara, R. K., Namgung, U., and Routtenberg, A. (1996). Distinctions between hippocampus of mouse and rat: protein F1/GAP-43 gene expression, promoter activity, and spatial memory. *Brain Res. Mol. Brain Res.* 40, 177–187. doi:10.1016/0169-328X(96)00048-4

Messinger, J. W., Tremeau, F., Antonius, D., Mendelsohn, E., Prudent, V., Stanford, A. D., et al. (2011). Avolition and expressive deficits capture negative symptom phenomenology: implications for DSM-5 and schizophrenia research. *Clin. Psychol. Rev.* 31, 161–168. doi:10.1016/j.cpr.2010.09.002

Mingorance-Le Meur, A., Zheng, B., Soriano, E., and Del Rio, J. A. (2007). Involvement of the myelin-associated inhibitor Nogo-A in early cortical development and neuronal maturation. *Cereb. Cortex* 17, 2375–2386. doi:10.1093/cercor/bhl146

Mironova, Y. A., and Giger, R. J. (2013). Where no synapses go: gatekeepers of circuit remodeling and synaptic strength. *Trends Neurosci.* 36, 363–373. doi:10.1016/j.tins.2013.04.003

Mobini, S., Chiang, T. J., Ho, M. Y., Bradshaw, C. M., and Szabadi, E. (2000). Comparison of the effects of clozapine, haloperidol, chlorpromazine and D-amphetamine on performance on a time-constrained progressive ratio schedule and on locomotor behaviour in the rat. *Psychopharmacology (Berl)* 152, 47–54. doi:10.1007/s002130000486

Ngan, E. T., Yatham, L. N., Ruth, T. J., and Liddle, P. F. (2000). Decreased serotonin 2A receptor densities in neuroleptic-naive patients with schizophrenia: a PET study using [(18)F]setoperone. *Am. J. Psychiatry* 157, 1016–1018. doi:10.1176/appi.ajp.157.6.1016

Nonkes, L. J., Tomson, K., Maertin, A., Dederen, J., Maes, J. H., and Homberg, J. (2010). Orbitofrontal cortex and amygdalar over-activity is associated with an inability to use the value of expected outcomes to guide behaviour in serotonin transporter knockout rats. *Neurobiol. Learn. Mem.* 94, 65–72. doi:10.1016/j.nlm.2010.04.002

Petrasek, T., Prokopova, I., Bahnik, S., Schonig, K., Berger, S., Vales, K., et al. (2014). Nogo-A downregulation impairs place avoidance in the Carousel maze but not spatial memory in the Morris water maze. *Neurobiol. Learn. Mem.* 107, 42–49. doi:10.1016/j.nlm.2013.10.015

Poole, T. B., and Fish, J. (1975). An investigation of playful behaviour in Rattus norvegicus and *Mus musculus* (Mammalia). *J. Zool.* 175, 61–71. doi:10.1111/j.1469-7998.1975.tb01391.x

Reilly, S. (1999). Reinforcement value of gustatory stimuli determined by progressive ratio performance. *Pharmacol. Biochem. Behav.* 63, 301–311. doi:10.1016/S0091-3057(99)00009-X

Salamone, J. D., and Correa, M. (2012). The mysterious motivational functions of mesolimbic dopamine. *Neuron* 76, 470–485. doi:10.1016/j.neuron.2012.10.021

Salamone, J. D., Correa, M., Farrar, A., and Mingote, S. M. (2007). Effort-related functions of nucleus accumbens dopamine and associated forebrain circuits. *Psychopharmacology (Berl.)* 191, 461–482. doi:10.1007/s00213-006-0668-9

Sanders, A. C., Hussain, A. J., Hen, R., and Zhuang, X. (2007). Chronic blockade or constitutive deletion of the serotonin transporter reduces operant responding for food reward. *Neuropsychopharmacology* 32, 2321–2329. doi:10.1038/sj.npp.1301368

Schneider, M., Heise, V., and Spanagel, R. (2010). Differential involvement of the opioid receptor antagonist naloxone in motivational and hedonic aspects of reward. *Behav. Brain Res.* 208, 466–472. doi:10.1016/j.bbr.2009.12.013

Schneider, M., and Koch, M. (2005). Behavioral and morphological alterations following neonatal excitotoxic lesions of the medial prefrontal cortex in rats. *Exp. Neurol.* 195, 185–198. doi:10.1016/j.expneurol.2005.04.014

Schwab, M. E. (2010). Functions of Nogo proteins and their receptors in the nervous system. *Nat. Rev. Neurosci.* 11, 799–811. doi:10.1038/nrn2936

Strauss, G. P., and Gold, J. M. (2012). A new perspective on anhedonia in schizophrenia. *Am. J. Psychiatry* 169, 364–373. doi:10.1176/appi.ajp.2011.11030447

Tandon, R., Keshavan, M. S., and Nasrallah, H. A. (2008). Schizophrenia, "just the facts" what we know in 2008. 2. Epidemiology and etiology. *Schizophr. Res.* 102, 1–18. doi:10.1016/j.schres.2008.04.011

Tandon, R., Nasrallah, H. A., and Keshavan, M. S. (2009). Schizophrenia, "just the facts" 4. Clinical features and conceptualization. *Schizophr. Res.* 110, 1–23. doi:10.1016/j.schres.2009.03.005

Tews, B., Schonig, K., Arzt, M. E., Clementi, S., Rioult-Pedotti, M. S., Zemmar, A., et al. (2013). Synthetic microRNA-mediated downregulation of Nogo-A in transgenic rats reveals its role as regulator of synaptic plasticity and cognitive function. *Proc. Natl. Acad. Sci. U.S.A.* 110, 6583–6588. doi:10.1073/pnas.1217665110

Willi, R., Aloy, E. M., Yee, B. K., Feldon, J., and Schwab, M. E. (2009). Behavioral characterization of mice lacking the neurite outgrowth inhibitor Nogo-A. *Genes Brain Behav.* 8, 181–192. doi:10.1111/j.1601-183X.2008.00460.x

Willi, R., and Schwab, M. E. (2013). Nogo and Nogo receptor: relevance to schizophrenia? *Neurobiol. Dis.* 54, 150–157. doi:10.1016/j.nbd.2013.01.011

Willi, R., Weinmann, O., Winter, C., Klein, J., Sohr, R., Schnell, L., et al. (2010). Constitutive genetic deletion of the growth regulator Nogo-A induces schizophrenia-related endophenotypes. *J. Neurosci.* 30, 556–567. doi:10.1523/JNEUROSCI.4393-09.2010

11

Nogo-A-deficient transgenic rats show deficits in higher cognitive functions, decreased anxiety, and altered circadian activity patterns

Tomas Petrasek[1,2]*, Iva Prokopova[1], Martin Sladek[3], Kamila Weissova[3], Iveta Vojtechova[1], Stepan Bahnik[1,4], Anna Zemanova[1], Kai Schönig[5], Stefan Berger[5], Björn Tews[6,7,8], Dusan Bartsch[5], Martin E. Schwab[6,7], Alena Sumova[3] and Ales Stuchlik[1]*

[1] Department of Neurophysiology of Memory, Institute of Physiology, Academy of Sciences of the Czech Republic, Prague, Czech Republic
[2] First Faculty of Medicine, Charles University in Prague, Prague, Czech Republic
[3] Department of Neurohumoral Regulations, Institute of Physiology, Academy of Sciences of the Czech Republic, Prague, Czech Republic
[4] Social Psychology, Department of Psychology II, University of Würzburg, Würzburg, Germany
[5] Department of Molecular Biology, Central Institute of Mental Health, Mannheim, Germany
[6] Brain Research Institute, University of Zurich, Zurich, Switzerland
[7] Neurosciences, Department of Biology, Swiss Federal Institute of Technology Zurich, Zurich, Switzerland
[8] Division of Molecular Mechanisms of Tumor Invasion, German Cancer Research Center, Heidelberg, Germany

Edited by:
Tomiki Sumiyoshi, National Center of Neurology and Psychiatry, Japan

***Correspondence:**
Tomas Petrasek and Ales Stuchlik, Department of Neurophysiology of Memory, Institute of Physiology, Academy of Sciences of the Czech Republic, Videnska 1083, Prague 4 14220, Czech Republic
e-mail: disworlds@gmail.com; stuchlik@biomed.cas.cz

Decreased levels of Nogo-A-dependent signaling have been shown to affect behavior and cognitive functions. In Nogo-A knockout and knockdown laboratory rodents, behavioral alterations were observed, possibly corresponding with human neuropsychiatric diseases of neurodevelopmental origin, particularly schizophrenia. This study offers further insight into behavioral manifestations of Nogo-A knockdown in laboratory rats, focusing on spatial and non-spatial cognition, anxiety levels, circadian rhythmicity, and activity patterns. Demonstrated is an impairment of cognitive functions and behavioral flexibility in a spatial active avoidance task, while non-spatial memory in a step-through avoidance task was spared. No signs of anhedonia, typical for schizophrenic patients, were observed in the animals. Some measures indicated lower anxiety levels in the Nogo-A-deficient group. Circadian rhythmicity in locomotor activity was preserved in the Nogo-A knockout rats and their circadian period (tau) did not differ from controls. However, daily activity patterns were slightly altered in the knockdown animals. We conclude that a reduction of Nogo-A levels induces changes in CNS development, manifested as subtle alterations in cognitive functions, emotionality, and activity patterns.

Keywords: Nogo-A, AAPA, Carousel maze, passive avoidance, neophobia, anhedonia, circadian rhythmicity

INTRODUCTION

The protein Nogo-A, belonging to the Reticulon family of proteins, is an important member of the class of myelin-associated inhibitors of axonal growth. It is present principally in the oligodendrocytes, but is expressed by some neuron subpopulations as well. When exposed in the cellular membrane, the Nogo-A molecule acts via two principal receptors, Nogo-66 receptor (NgR) and paired immunoglobulin-like receptor B (PirB) (see Schwab, 2010 for review).

The Nogo-A is widely recognized for its relevance in various physiological and pathological processes. The protein was originally noted as an inhibitor blocking axonal regrowth and plasticity after CNS injuries (Chen et al., 2000; GrandPré et al., 2000; Schwab, 2004). Subsequently, the Nogo-A-dependent signaling has shown to be crucial in the development and migration of neurons (Mingorance et al., 2004; Mingorance-Le Meur et al., 2007) and glial cells (Pernet et al., 2008; Chong et al., 2012). In the adult brain, Nogo-A (especially the neuronal Nogo-A) contributes to the modulation of neuronal and synaptic plasticity (Akbik et al., 2012; Pernet and Schwab, 2012) and adult neurogenesis (Rolando et al., 2012).

It is therefore not surprising that the disruption of a Nogo signaling pathway in the developing brain has been suggested to play a role in neuropsychiatric diseases of neurodevelopmental origin, most notably schizophrenia and bipolar disorder (Willi and Schwab, 2013). This view is corroborated by a reported genetic linkage between chromosomal loci for the Nogo-A or its receptor and susceptibility to schizophrenia (Novak et al., 2002; Sinibaldi et al., 2004; Tan et al., 2005; Hsu et al., 2007; Budel et al., 2008; Voineskos, 2009; Jitoku et al., 2011). Schizophrenia is characterized by abnormal development and function of the hippocampus (Harrison, 2004). The hippocampus is a prime example of a structure exhibiting a high degree of neuronal and synaptic plasticity, as well as the neuronal expression of Nogo-A persisting well into adulthood. Therefore, it should be particularly liable to pathophysiological processes disrupting Nogo-A-dependent signaling, or corresponding experimental manipulations. The study was aimed to elucidate the behavioral effects of decreased Nogo-A expression on behavior, with a focus on hippocampal function and schizophrenia-like endophenotypes. We took advantage of a novel animal model, a Nogo-A knockdown rat exhibiting decreased expression of the Nogo-A protein in the brain tissue, most notably in neurons (Tews et al., 2013).

Apart from other places in the brain, Nogo-A has been found to be expressed in subsets of neurons of the retina (Huber et al., 2002; Wang et al., 2002; Hunt et al., 2003), which is a part of the internal time keeping circadian system (for review, see Meijer and Schwartz, 2003). Moreover, the function of the central circadian clock, located in the suprachiasmatic nuclei (SCN) of the hypothalamus, is modulated by neuronal connections with other brain areas including the hippocampus (Canteras and Swanson, 1992), and, vice versa, the circadian clock can affect hippocampal functions such as long-term memory formation (Stephan and Kovacevic, 1978; Tapp and Holloway, 1981). Therefore, we also focused on an analysis of basic circadian properties of the central clock in the SCN of Nogo-A knockdown rats, using daily rhythm in locomotor activity as a direct output of the clock.

We hypothesized that the animals should exhibit impairment in the active place avoidance task on the Carousel maze, which is highly sensitive in impairments of hippocampal function (Cimadevilla et al., 2001), and has been successfully employed in evaluation of animal models of schizophrenia (Stuchlik et al., 2004; Vales et al., 2006; Bubenikova-Valesova et al., 2008a). We also expect abnormal rhythmicity patterns resulting from changes in the circadian systems.

MATERIALS AND METHODS

TRANSGENIC MODEL

The transgenic rat model was prepared in the Central Institute of Mental Health (CIMH, Mannheim, Germany), in cooperation with Martin Schwab from the Brain Research Institute, University of Zurich and Department of Health Science and Technology, Swiss Federal Institute of Technology (ETH) Zurich, on the genetic background of the Sprague-Dawley rat. The particular transgenic line used in this study is designated as SD-Tg(CAG-RNAi: Nogo-A, EGFP)L2ZI, short L2; standing for line 2, and is of outbred genetic background. The parental subjects were obtained from Charles River, Germany.

The expression of Nogo-A was suppressed by means of the insertion of a genetic construct expressing a small interfering RNA, complementary to Nogo-A mRNA (targeting Nogo-A-specific exon 3 of *Rtn4*), binding to it with a high affinity and therefore preventing translation. Because the blockade is not total, the levels of neuronal Nogo-A were reduced to about 50% in the CNS as a whole, 30% in the cerebral cortex, and 60% in the hippocampus. Nogo-A levels in the oligodendrocytes were affected to a lesser extent relative to neurons (Tews et al., 2013).

The knockdown manifests itself on the cellular level by increased long-term potentiation, and leads to behavioral abnormalities as well (Tews et al., 2013). This resembles the schizophrenia-like behavior noted previously in knockout mice (Willi et al., 2010). Subtle cognitive deficit has been described in Petrasek et al. (2014). The distribution pattern of biochemical markers in the brains of the transgenic rats also paralleled some changes observed in human schizophrenic patients (Krištofiková et al., 2013).

ANIMALS

Male Nogo-A knockdown rats from two different litters and non-littermate, age-matched, and wild-type (WT) Sprague-Dawley controls obtained from the breeding colony of the CIMH, Mannheim, Germany, were used. After arrival at the Institute of Physiology, an appropriate acclimatization period (1 month) followed before the start of experimental procedures, and all the animals were accustomed to the experimenters during 1 week of daily handling. The rats were housed in groups of two or three in an air-conditioned animal room, with free access to food and water. The animals were kept on 12/12 light–dark cycle, and the experiments were performed during the light phase. The rats were 5 months old when the testing started (Carousel maze) and about 8 months old when sacrificed, their weights were between 540 and 750 g. For time schedule of the behavioral experiments, see **Table 1**.

The original group included nine Nogo-A knockdown and nine control animals, however, some individuals died before the completion of the experiments, therefore the group size was diminished in neophobia/anhedonia (eight Nogo-A knockdown rats and nine controls) and circadian rhythmicity tests (five Nogo-A knockdown rats and eight controls).

All animal experimentation complied with the Animal Protection Code of the Czech Republic and international guidelines including EU directives (2010/63/EC).

RNA ISOLATION AND REAL-TIME qRT-PCR

After completion of behavioral experiments, the rats were sacrificed by cervical dislocation, and hippocampal and cerebellar samples were removed and stored in RNA Later (Sigma, USA) at −80°C until processed. Total RNA was extracted by homogenization from the cerebellum, left and right hippocampus of five Nogo-A knockdown and eight control rats and subsequently purified using the RNeasy Mini kit (Qiagen, USA) according to the manufacturer's instructions. RNA concentrations were determined by spectrophotometry at 260 nm, and the RNA quality was assessed by electrophoresis on a 1.5% agarose gel. Moreover, the integrity of randomly selected samples of total RNA was tested using an Agilent 2100 Bioanalyzer (Agilent Technologies, USA).

The qRT-PCR method used to detect Nogo-A mRNA has been described previously (Sládek et al., 2007). Briefly, 1 μg of total RNA was reverse transcribed using the SuperScript VILO cDNA synthesis kit (Life Technologies, USA) with random primers. The resulting cDNAs were used as templates for qRT-PCR. Diluted cDNA was amplified on LightCycler 480 (Roche, Switzerland) using the Express SYBR GreenER qPCR SuperMix (Life Technologies, USA) and the corresponding primers for Nogo-A (forward 5′-CAG TGG ATG AGA CCC TTT TTG-3′, reverse 5′-GCT GCT CCA TCA AAT CCA TAA-3′) or GFP (forward 5′-CAA CAG CCA CAA CGT CTA TAT CAT-3′, reverse 5′-ATG TTG TGG CGG ATC TTG AAG-3′). Relative quantification was achieved using a standard curve and subsequently normalizing the gene expression to β2-microglobulin (B2M, forward 5′-TCT CAC TGA CCG GCC TGT ATG CTA TC-3′, reverse 5′-AAT GTG AGG CGG GTG GAA CTG TG-3′), which has been used as a housekeeping gene previously (Sládek et al., 2007). Its expression was stable throughout the day and did not vary among the analyzed tissues.

Table 1 | Time schedule of behavioral experiments.

Age (months)	5.3	5.5		5.7	5.9			6.1	6.3	6.5	6.7	6.9	7.1	7.3	7.5	7.7	7.9	7.9	8.0
Weeks	1	2		3	4			5	6	7	8	9	10	11	12	13	14	15	16
Task	Carousel maze				Step-through avoidance			Beam walking	Neophobia/ anhedonia			Circadian rhythmicity							Sacrifice
	Habituation	Acquisition	Retrieval	Reversal	Habituation	Acquisition	Test					12/12 LD cycle			Constant darkness				
Number of daily sessions	5	5	1	5	2	1	1	1	2			29			16				

PROTEIN ISOLATION AND WESTERN BLOT

Samples of the left hippocampus (50–100 mg) from five Nogo-A knockdown and three control animals were homogenized in 1 ml of CelLytic MT extraction reagent (Sigma, USA) according to the manufacturer's protocol. Protein concentration was determined by Bradford assay (Thermo Scientific, USA). All reagents for Western blot were purchased from Life Technologies, USA, unless stated otherwise. The hippocampal homogenate (21 μg of total protein) was mixed with a NuPAGE LDS Sample buffer and Sample reducing reagent, denatured at 70°C for 10 min, and separated with a protein ladder on a NuPAGE Tris–Acetate premade gel according to the manufacturer's instructions using a NuPAGE running buffer with an antioxidant. The protein was transferred by electro-blotting in a NuPAGE transfer buffer with 10% methanol onto a nitrocellulose membrane according to the manufacturer's instructions. The membrane was blocked in a Western Blocker solution (Sigma, USA) for 1 h and then incubated with a primary antibody against Nogo-A H300 (Santa Cruz, USA) diluted 1:2000 in a Western Blocker overnight at 4°C on a rocker. The membrane was then washed five times for 5 min in TBST (2.42 g Tris–HCl, 8 g NaCl, 1 ml Tween 20 in 1000 ml of redistilled water, pH 7.6) and incubated with a secondary anti-rabbit HRP-conjugated antibody (Promega, USA) diluted 1:40,000 in a Western Blocker at room temperature (RT) for 1 h on a rocker. The membrane was then washed 5× in TBST, incubated with a SuperSignal West Pico Chemiluminescent substrate (Pierce, USA), and immunoreactive bands were detected after 45-s exposure using a cooled camera system. The membrane was subsequently incubated for 30 min at 50°C in a stripping buffer (31.25 ml of 1 M Tris–HCl, 10 g SDS, 3.5 ml of 100 mM 2-Mercaptoethanol in 500 ml of redistilled water), washed 5× in TBST, blocked in a Western Blocker for 1 h, incubated with an anti-actin 20–33 antibody (Sigma, USA) 1:350 in a Western Blocker for 1 h at RT, washed 5× in TBST, incubated with a secondary anti-rabbit HRP-conjugated antibody (Promega, USA) diluted 1:20,000 in a Western Blocker at RT for 1 h, washed 5× in TBST, incubated with a West Pico substrate, and exposed for 3 s. Photographs of the blots were imported into ImageJ (NIH, USA) software, where the optical density of individual lanes of detected Nogo-A protein was quantified relative to the actin internal standard.

BEHAVIORAL TESTS

Carousel maze

The Carousel maze (for detailed description, see Stuchlik, 2007) consisted of a smooth featureless metallic circular arena (82 cm in diameter), enclosed by a 30-cm high transparent Plexiglas wall, and elevated 1 m above the floor of a 4 m × 5 m room containing an abundance of extra-maze cues. The behavior of the animals was recorded by a computer-based tracking system (Tracker, Biosignal Group, USA).

The active allothetic place avoidance (AAPA) task in the Carousel maze was employed, where the animals learned to avoid an unmarked sector, entrances into which were punished by mild electric shocks. The shock lasted 0.5 s, and was repeated after 1.5 s if the animal did not leave the sector. The intensity of current was individually adjusted for each rat to elicit escape reaction, ranging between 0.4 and 0.7 mA (50 Hz). There were no systematic differences in the shock levels between groups. The sector position was fixed in the reference frame of the room, so that the animals had to rely on extra-maze cues. Intra-maze cues (e.g., scent marks) were made unreliable by rotation of the arena, and the animals had to ignore these to solve the task. They also had to actively avoid the sector position, not to be transported there by movement of the arena.

The rats (tested at the age of 5–6 months) were trained during the light phase of the day, between 9:00 and 16:00 hours. Each daily session lasted for 20 min. The training consisted of three phases, each lasting 5 days: habituation (exploration of the whole apparatus without punishment), avoidance learning (acquisition), and training with a changed sector position (reversal). A single 5-min retrieval session (without shocks) was scheduled 24 h after the end of the acquisition phase, before onset of reversal training. No food deprivation or pellet chasing was involved.

To master this task, the animals need navigation skills and spatial memory to locate the to-be-avoided sector (which is directly imperceptible), as well as the ability to separate the landmarks into coherent representations and choose the relevant one. Separation of spatial frames has been suggested as an animal model of cognitive coordination (Wesierska et al., 2005), which is impaired in schizophrenic patients (Phillips and Silverstein, 2003), making the AAPA task very important in the study of animal models of schizophrenia.

This paradigm was similar, but simpler than the testing battery described in Petrasek et al. (2014), and was chosen for easier comparison with a large body of experimental results gained with the AAPA task.

Step-through avoidance

In this experiment, the same group of rats was used as in the Carousel maze experiment (7–8 months old during testing), with $n = 9$ for Nogo-A knockdown rats and $n = 9$ for controls. The step-through avoidance took place in an apparatus consisting of two compartments, one of which was open and brightly lit (1500 lx), while the second remained dark (<10 lx). Rats have a natural tendency to prefer the dark environment to the light, so they usually left the light compartment, where they were initially placed, and entered the dark half of the apparatus. After the entrance, the door between the compartments was always shut. The latency to step-through the door between compartments was recorded. During the two habituation trials, the entrance was neither rewarded nor punished. In the third, acquisition trial, however, a foot-shock (1.5 mA) was applied after entrance into the dark compartment. Individuals failing to enter the dark compartment altogether on this trial (lasting 5 min) were excluded from the experiment. After a 24-h delay, a testing session followed, during which the rats were exposed to the environment again. Increased latency to enter the dark compartment reflected memory from the previous experience.

Neophobia/anhedonia

The same group of rats was used in this experiment as in the previous ones, with $n = 8$ for Nogo-A knockdown rats and $n = 9$ for controls. Each rat, deprived of drinking water and food for 22 h, was put into a box containing two drinking bottles. One of them contained drinking water and the other was filled with saccharin solution (concentration 0.2%). After 60 min, the session was terminated and both bottles weighed to measure the amount of pure and sweetened water consumed. After this initial experience, the session was repeated after 24 h. The first session should elicit a conflict between preference for the sweet taste and the avoidance of the unfamiliar (neophobia), as the rats had never tasted saccharin before. In the second session, the rats were already familiar with the saccharin solution, and the amount consumed should reflect their taste preference. Failure to prefer the sweet taste could be taken as a sign of anhedonia, inability to enjoy a pleasant experience, observed in schizophrenia and depression (Pelizza and Ferrari, 2009) or in their animal models (Le Pen et al., 2002).

Beam walking test

The beam walking test was used to assess motor coordination of the same group of rats. The test requires a subject to cross a 2-m-long wooden beam that leads to a home-cage. Latency to reach the home-cage and number of slips and falls are measured to assess motor coordination. The results were already described in a different publication (Petrasek et al., 2014); therefore, we will not report them in detail in the present paper. Briefly, we did not find any difference between groups in any of the measured parameters.

MONITORING OF CIRCADIAN LOCOMOTOR ACTIVITY

Nogo-A knockdown and WT Sprague-Dawley rats were kept in a 12-h of light and 12 h of darkness cycle (LD12:12) with free access to food and water for 29 days and then in constant darkness (DD) for 16 days. The rats were monitored for spontaneous activity during the entire protocol. To monitor locomotor activity, rats of both genotypes were kept individually in cages equipped with infrared movement detectors that were attached above the center of the cage top. A circadian activity monitoring system (Dr. H. M. Cooper, INSERM, France) was used to measure activity every minute, and double-plotted actograms were generated to evaluate the activity. The resulting data were analyzed using the ClockLab toolbox (Actimetrics, USA).

MEASURED PARAMETERS AND STATISTICAL DESIGN

mRNA and protein levels

The differences in mRNA and protein levels between both rat genotypes were evaluated by a Student's t-test.

Carousel maze

The Carousel maze performance was evaluated using the track analysis program CM Manager 0.3.5 (Bahnik, 2013). Several behavioral measures were assessed. *Total distance* measured overall path traveled by a rat during a session, and was computed as a sum of linear distances between points selected every 1 s. Total distance can suggest deficits in locomotion or reveal rats that did not actively leave the to-be-avoided sector. *Maximum time avoided* was defined as the longest continuous time interval spent without an entrance into the to-be-avoided sector and was used as a measure of avoidance ability. *Mean distance from the center* of the arena was used as a measure of thigmotaxis. *Defecation* was assessed by counting the number of feces left on the arena floor after each session, serving as an additional measure of anxiety level. All these measures were used for analysis of performance during the acquisition and reversal phases. Furthermore, total distance, mean distance from the center, and defecation were used to assess locomotion, thigmotaxis, and anxiety during the habituation phase. Additionally, the *proportion of time spent in the opposite sector* was used to distinguish different behavioral strategies by assessing the time spent in the sector located 180° from the to-be-avoided sector. This measure was computed as a proportion of time spent in the opposite sector to the total time not spent in the to-be-avoided sector. We did not include time spent in the to-be-avoided sector in the denominator, otherwise the measure would be dependent on the avoidance ability. This measure was introduced for evaluating the reversal phase of the experiment, because the opposite sector during the reversal phase was in the same place as the to-be-avoided sector during the acquisition phase (the width of both sectors was the same, i.e., 60°). This measure was used to evaluate perseverance, which was observed in Nogo-A knockdown rats (and knockout mice) in some previous studies.

The parameters for acquisition and reversal phases were averaged across sessions before analysis. This was done because some values (approximately 0.6%) were missing for various reasons (e.g., tracking problems). Computing the averages enabled us to include all rats in the analysis. Before the averaging, we standardized values for each session. This was done because performance changed during subsequent days, and therefore the averages would be otherwise dependent on days when rats had missing values. To simplify comparison between phases, the averages were standardized again. Thus, we obtained one value for each rat for each of the two phases and every parameter. All parameters were then analyzed with mixed analysis of variance (ANOVA) with group (Nogo-A knockdown or control) as a between-subject factor and phase (acquisition and reversal) and as a within-subject factor. Since the mean value of all subjects for both phases was always zero due to the final standardization, the phase factor was included only to test for the interaction of group and phase factors (we used a similar analysis previously, Prokopova et al., 2012; Petrasek et al., 2014). Analyses for the habituation phase and for proportion of time spent in the opposite sector in the reversal phase were done in a similar manner, but the group comparisons were done with a Welch's t-test. Correlations between used parameters are displayed in **Table 2**.

As it is shown in the results, three rats from the control group exhibited prolonged periods of immobility during the testing sessions and were not able to learn avoidance of the to-be-avoided sector. Therefore, we describe two analyses – one included all subjects from both groups, and the other excluded the three rats that were not able to learn the avoidance along with three rats from Nogo-A knockdown group that had the worst performance as determined by mean maximum time avoided from both phases (exclusion of these subjects had to be done, otherwise a possible difference between groups could have been explained by a selective exclusion of subjects from control group). Because the performance of immobile rats is not related to their cognitive abilities in any way, we believe that the analysis with exclusion of those subjects may better reveal differences between the two groups. The exclusion was not necessary for the habituation phase because no avoidance was needed during this phase. Note that after the exclusion, it was no longer true that the means for both phases had to be equal to zero, however, the phase factor would assess only in which phase were the excluded subjects relatively better, and therefore it was of no interest and its analysis is not reported in the Section "Results."

Since values for three subjects were missing for retrieval phase and two other rats did not learn to avoid the to-be-avoided sector (as described above and in the Results), we did not perform any analysis for the retrieval phase. The number of subjects with valid values was low, and hence the low resulting statistical power would not enable us to find any effect other than extreme, which we did not expect.

All analyses were done with an R version 3.0.1 (R Core Team, 2013), which is also true for the step-through avoidance and neophobia/anhedonia tasks. Effect sizes are reported with generalized eta squared (Bakeman, 2005) or with a correlation coefficient.

Step-through avoidance

For the comparison of time it took subjects to move into the dark compartment during habituation and acquisition trials, we used a mixed ANOVA where group (Nogo-A knockdown or control) served as a between-subject factor and trial (two habituation trials and an acquisition trial were ordered and analyzed together) served as a within-subject factor. Polynomial contrasts were used for the trial factor. Because all but one subject remained in the light compartment during the entire testing session, the analysis was not deemed necessary for the testing session.

Neophobia/anhedonia

To compare the amount of saccharin consumed by both groups, we used a mixed ANOVA with group (Nogo-A knockdown or control) as a between-subject factor and session as a within-subject factor. Since the total amount of liquid consumed by both groups somewhat differed, we used a ratio of consumed saccharin solution to total amount of liquid consumed as a dependent variable.

Circadian rhythmicity

The differences in locomotor activity (i.e., the values of the total 24 h-activity and activity/rest ratio) between both rat genotypes were evaluated by a Student's t-test, while difference in period was analyzed by the Mann–Whitney test. The analysis was done in Prism 6 software (Graphpad, USA).

RESULTS

CONFIRMATION OF Nogo-A KNOCKDOWN GENOTYPE

The relative expression levels of Nogo-A were compared in the hippocampus and cerebellum of Nogo-A knockdown rats and Sprague-Dawley controls (**Figure 1**). In both tissues, the levels of Nogo-A mRNA were significantly reduced in the Nogo-A knockdown rats compared with controls [hippocampus $t(22) = 3.52$, $p = 0.002$, $r = 0.60$; cerebellum $t(10) = 2.90$, $p = 0.02$, $r = 0.68$; Student's t-test]. The reduction was by about $40.9 \pm 7.5\%$ (mean $\pm$ SEM) in the hippocampus and $43.6 \pm 17.5\%$ in the cerebellum. Apart from mRNA, protein levels were also compared in the hippocampus of the Nogo-A knockdown and WT rats (**Figure 1**). The Nogo-A protein levels were significantly reduced in Nogo-A knockdown compared with WT rats by about $22.1 \pm 5.5\%$ [$t(6) = 2.83$, $p = 0.03$, $r = 0.76$; Student's t-test].

CAROUSEL MAZE

Visual observation showed normal behavior during the habituation phase and rapid acquisition of the task in the majority of the rats. Three individuals from the control group, however, exhibited marked immobility during avoidance sessions. We assume that these animals adopted passive behavior (freezing) instead of an active approach (escape) as a reaction to the aversive nature of the task. Active locomotion is a basic prerequisite for the successful mastering of this task, therefore, the animals exhibiting freezing as the dominant strategy were excluded as "non-solvers" along with three other rats from the Nogo-A knockdown group for the reasons explained in the Section "Measured Parameters and Statistical Design." The visual observation was supported by values of the non-solvers for total distance parameter. We computed standardized averages of total distance for each rat for acquisition and reversal sessions as described in the Section "Measured Parameters and Statistical Design." We then averaged these values and standardized them again. The three rats displaying freezing behavior had z-scores for the resultant total distance parameter -2.7, -1.9, and -1.2 while all other rats had values in a range from -0.4 to 1.0 (values for total distance are shown in **Figure 2A**). Additionally, the freezing behavior can be seen in the subject's response

Table 2 | Correlations between measured parameters in the AAPA task.

	Maximum time avoided – acquisition	Maximum time avoided – reversal	Distance from center – habituation	Distance from center – acquisition	Distance from center – reversal	Total distance – habituation	Total distance – acquisition	Total distance – reversal	Defecation – habituation	Defecation – acquisition	Defecation – reversal	Time in opposite – reversal
Maximum time avoided – acquisition												
Maximum time avoided – reversal	0.32											
Distance from center – habituation	−0.50	−0.01										
Distance from center – acquisition	−0.62*	−0.11	0.54									
Distance from center – reversal	−0.68*	−0.31	0.57*	0.91**								
Total distance – habituation	0.36	0.38	−0.72*	−0.35	−0.52							
Total distance – acquisition	0.90*	0.51	−0.56	−0.66*	−0.67*	0.66*						
Total distance – reversal	0.79	0.80	−0.31	−0.17	−0.29	0.27	0.55					
Defecation – habituation	−0.03	−0.39	−0.17	0.03	−0.02	−0.18	−0.07	−0.60				
Defecation – acquisition	0.19	0.07	0.02	−0.26	−0.14	−0.40	0.07	0.09	0.16			
Defecation – reversal	0.12	−0.20	−0.20	−0.36	−0.12	0.06	0.41	−0.16	0.46	0.59*		
Time in opposite – reversal	0.67	0.79*	−0.35	−0.24	−0.37	0.58	0.75**	0.61*	−0.18	−0.11	0.00	

The table shows correlations between all parameters that were used for analysis of the AAPA task. Generally, there are large correlations between the same parameters during different phases. Additionally, total distance, maximum time avoided, and proportion of time spent in the opposite sector are positively correlated with each other and negatively with mean distance from the center. Defecation does not appear to be reliably correlated with any other measure. The correlations were computed for both groups separately and pooled thereafter. $^{*}p < 0.05$; $^{**}p < 0.01$.

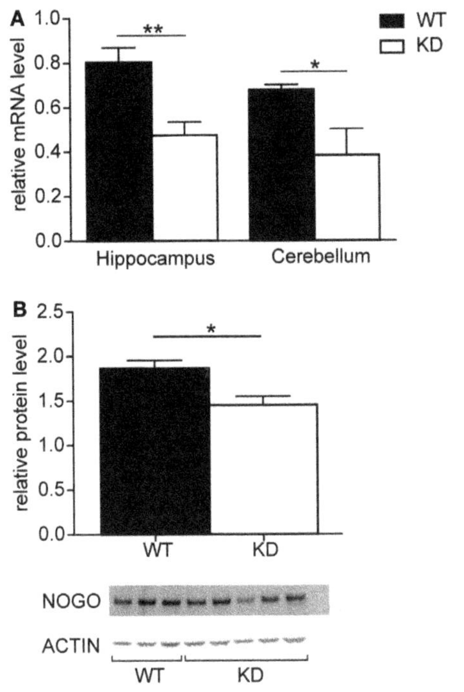

FIGURE 1 | Nogo-A mRNA and protein expression in Nogo-A knockdown rats (designated KD) and wild-type (WT) controls. **(A)** Relative levels of Nogo-A mRNA in the hippocampus ($n = 14$ for WT, $n = 10$ for KD) and cerebellum ($n = 7$ for WT, $n = 5$ for KD) of wild-type (black) and knockdown (white) animals. **(B)** Relative levels of Nogo-A protein in the hippocampus of wild-type (black) and knockdown (white) animals. The graph shows mean optical density of Nogo-A normalized to actin of three WT and five KD animals.

to obtaining a shock. We used the median absolute speed after shock to assess this response. This parameter is computed as a median of angular speed during 1 s following a shock. Since subjects can move outside of the sector both by moving with or against the direction of rotation of the arena, we used absolute speeds to assess whether administration of a shock elicited a response. While all other rats showed some active response (mean median absolute speed after shock higher than 8°/s), the three non-solvers displayed no such behavior (mean median absolute speed after shock lower than 2°/s).

Results for total distance from the habituation phase showed a significant difference between the two groups, $t(14.93) = 2.37$, $p = 0.03$, $r = 0.51$, with the control group having a lower total distance than the Nogo-A knockdown group. Additionally, there was a significant difference in the mean distance from the center, $t(13.15) = -3.99$, $p = 0.002$, $r = -0.71$. Nogo-A knockdown rats preferred positions closer to the center of arena than rats from the control group. Defecation was higher in the control group, but not significant, $t(13.51) = -1.76$, $p = 0.10$, $r = -0.40$.

The analysis of maximum time avoided (**Figure 3A**) for acquisition and reversal phases with all subjects included revealed no effect of group, $F(1, 16) < 1$, $p = 0.67$, $\eta^2_G = 0.01$, and no interaction between group and phase factors, $F(1, 16) = 1.41$, $p = 0.25$, $\eta^2_G = 0.02$. For total distance, we found a marginally significant effect of group, with the control group having lower total distance than the Nogo-A knockdown group, $F(1, 16) = 3.55$, $p = 0.08$, $\eta^2_G = 0.16$, and no interaction of group and phase factors, $F(1, 16) < 1$, $p = 0.85$, $\eta^2_G = 0.00$. For mean distance from the center, results revealed lower mean distance from the center in Nogo-A knockdown rats, $F(1, 16) = 26.79$, $p = 0.0001$, $\eta^2_G = 0.58$, and no interaction between group and phase factors, $F(1, 16) = 1.43$, $p = 0.25$, $\eta^2_G = 0.01$. Finally, analysis of defecation showed lower defecation in Nogo-A knockdown rats, $F(1, 16) = 10.04$, $p = 0.006$, $\eta^2_G = 0.32$, but no interaction between group and phase factors, $F(1, 16) < 1$, $p = 0.60$, $\eta^2_G = 0.00$.

Similar analysis for maximum time avoided with the three rats from each group excluded showed lower maximum time avoided in the Nogo-A knockdown group, $F(1, 10) = 17.19$, $p = 0.002$, $\eta^2_G = 0.27$, and no interaction between group and phase factors, $F(1, 10) = 1.07$, $p = 0.33$, $\eta^2_G = 0.08$. Analysis for total distance without the excluded subjects showed neither an effect of group, $F(1, 10) = 1.20$, $p = 0.30$, $\eta^2_G = 0.06$, nor an interaction between group and phase factors, $F(1, 10) = 1.78$, $p = 0.21$, $\eta^2_G = 0.08$. Without the excluded subjects, lower mean distance from the center was again observed for the Nogo-A knockdown group, $F(1, 10) = 24.13$, $p = 0.0006$, $\eta^2_G = 0.65$, while the interaction between group and phase factors was not significant, $F(1, 10) = 1.44$, $p = 0.26$, $\eta^2_G = 0.03$ (**Figure 2B**). Finally, analysis of defecation after the exclusion of rats again revealed lower defecation in Nogo-A knockdown rats, $F(1, 10) = 7.24$, $p = 0.02$, $\eta^2_G = 0.37$, and no interaction between group and phase factors, $F(1, 10) < 1$, $p = 0.81$, $\eta^2_G = 0.00$(**Figure 2C**).

Analysis of proportion of time in the opposite sector revealed no significant difference between groups when done both without, $t(10.40) = 1.40$, $p = 0.19$, $r = 0.33$, and with the exclusion, $t(6.70) = 1.89$, $p = 0.10$, $r = 0.51$. Surprisingly, in both cases, the proportion of time spent in the opposite sector was higher in the Nogo-A knockdown group, which is in contrast to the expectation of higher perseverance (**Figure 3B**). That the difference did not decrease after the exclusion of subjects shows that it was not caused only by the lower values of the rats displaying freezing behavior.

STEP-THROUGH AVOIDANCE

A mixed ANOVA for time required to move into the dark compartment showed a significant effect of group, $t(16) = 2.29$, $p = 0.04$, $r = 0.50$, marginally significant linear contrast for trial, $t(32) = -1.94$, $p = 0.06$, $r = -0.32$, and insignificant quadratic contrast for trial, $t(32) = 0.29$, $p = 0.78$, $r = 0.05$. The interaction between linear contrast for trial and group was significant, $t(32) = 2.37$, $p = 0.02$, $r = 0.38$, while the interaction between quadratic contrast for trial and group was not, $t(32) = -0.99$, $p = 0.33$, $r = -0.17$. To explore the interaction between linear contrast for trial and group, we conducted separate repeated measures ANOVAs for both groups. The analyses showed that whereas for the Nogo-A knockdown group the coefficient for linear contrast was positive, although insignificant, $t(16) = 1.46$, $p = 0.16$, $r = 0.34$, it was negative and marginally significant for control group, $t(16) = -1.88$, $p = 0.08$, $r = -0.42$. The interaction can be additionally explored with a separate Welch's t-tests for each trial. While there was no difference between groups for the first trial,

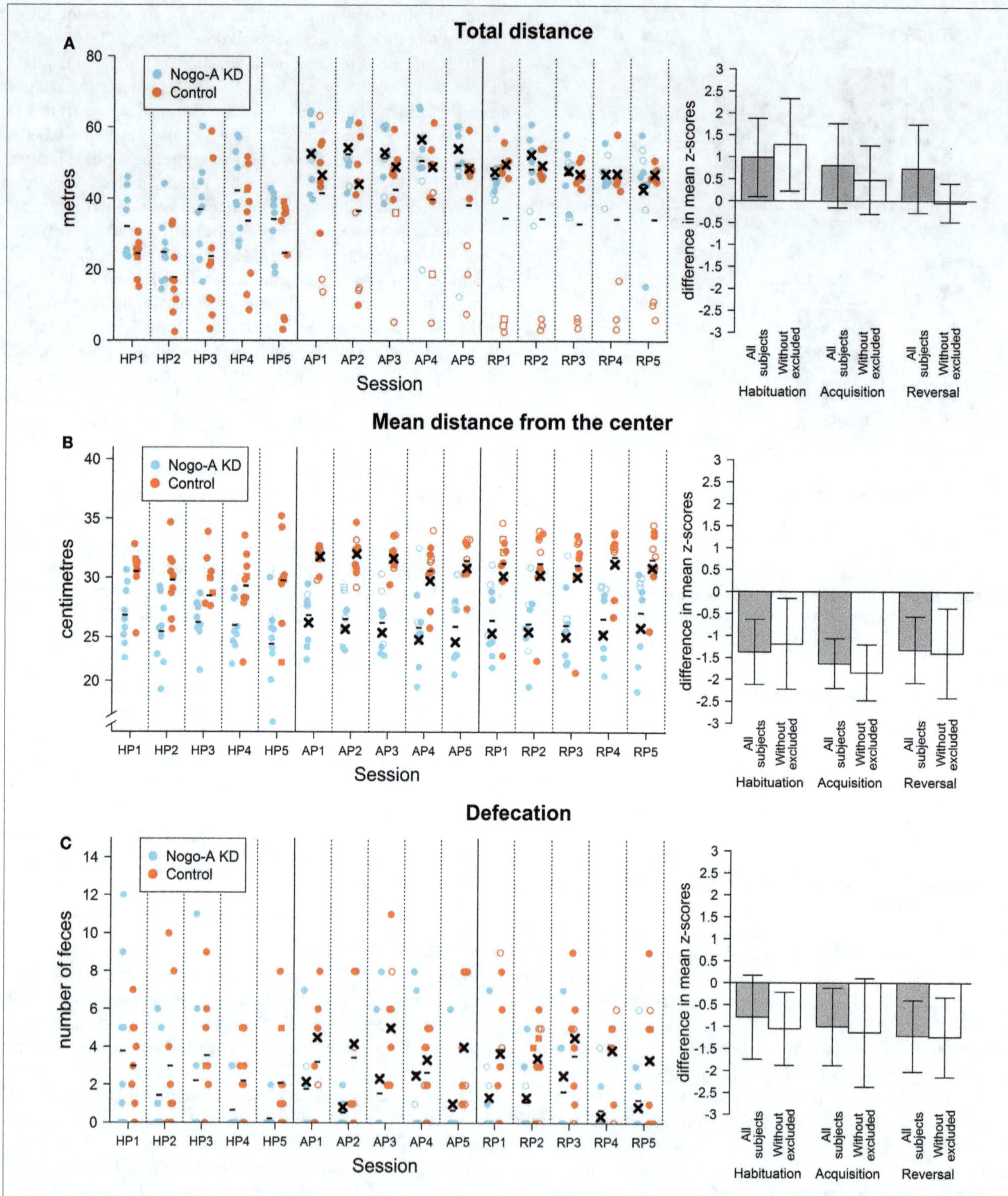

FIGURE 2 | Results of non-cognitive parameters in the AAPA task. The plots on the left show individual values for each rat during every session. The sessions are labeled by HP, habituation phase; AP, acquisition phase; RP, reversal phase. Missing values are indicated by square points. These values were imputed by the closest value from the same phase for a given subject. When the missing value was in the middle of the phase and values for both adjacent sessions were valid, the missing value was imputed by their average. Missing values were not imputed and used in the analysis described in the text. For the acquisition and reversal phases, empty points indicate values for subjects that were excluded from analysis (see text for details). Minus signs indicate mean group values for a given session computed from all subjects and crosses indicate mean values computed from values without the excluded subjects. The means are computed from values including the imputed. For the habituation phase, no subjects were excluded from the analyses; therefore, only mean values computed for all subjects in a group are *(Continued)*

FIGURE 2 | Continued
depicted. The bar plots on the right show differences between groups in the AAPA task for means of parameters averaged across sessions within a single phase. The differences are positive if Nogo-A knockdown group had higher values than control group. For every phase, both differences with and without excluded subjects are shown. Error bars show 95% confidence intervals of differences of means. Therefore, the error bars indicate whether there was a significant difference between groups for a given phase (which happens when the range within error bars does not include zero). However, they cannot be used for comparison between phases because they are not adjusted for dependency on the data. Furthermore, their use for comparison of the analyses with and without excluded subject is not meaningful as well. Even though the analysis of the habituation phase with the exclusion of subjects is not reported in text because the subjects could not show shock-induced freezing behavior during this phase, the differences with exclusion are depicted for this phase. **(A)** Results for total distance (left plot in meters). A difference between groups can be seen in all sessions in the habituation phase with Nogo-A knockdown rats displaying higher locomotion. The difference is still present during the subsequent phases, but only when values for all rats are compared. The difference in these phases is therefore mainly due to the rats in control group that did not actively avoid the to-be-avoided sector (i.e., rats depicted by empty points in the left plot). It can be seen that these rats generally moved <20 m during a session and they were even less active during the reversal phase. It can be observed that one of these rats moved in a degree comparable to other rats at the beginning of the acquisition phase but its locomotion hugely decreased in subsequent sessions. **(B)** Results for mean distance from the center (left plot in centimeters). A large difference between groups can be seen for mean distance from the center in all phases and sessions. Furthermore, the difference is not dependent on the exclusion of the subjects. Nogo-A knockdown rats tended to be present closer to the center of the arena than rats from control group. Note that the *y*-axis in the left plot does not start at zero. Arena diameter is 82 cm, therefore the maximum theoretically possible value of mean distance from the center is somewhat lower than 41 cm, which would correspond to being next to the margin of the arena during the entire session. **(C)** Results for defecation. Defecation was lower in Nogo-A knockdown rats in all three phases. However, the difference was not significant in the habituation phase. There appears to be little difference between the results of the analyses done with and without the excluded rats.

$t(15.13)=0.28, p=0.78, r=0.07$, the Nogo-A knockdown group had higher values in the second, $t(14.46)=2.15, p=0.05, r=0.47$, and third trials, $t(8.46)=3.44$, $p=0.008$, $r=0.65$ (**Figure 4**). Therefore, the results showed that time required to move into the dark compartment was the same during the first trial and then decreased for the control group. However, it slightly increased for the Nogo-A knockdown group, which caused a widening difference between both groups during the second and third trial. Both the experimental and control groups exhibited increased latency to enter the dark compartment during the testing session (after the foot-shock), demonstrating successful memory for the unpleasant experience. In fact, only one of the Nogo-A knockdown subjects moved into the dark compartment and none of the control subjects did.

NEOPHOBIA/ANHEDONIA

All animals behaved as expected during the testing sessions, i.e., tasted and drank the presented liquids. The rats drank slightly more liquid in the second session compared to the first one. For easier comparison, the ratio of consumed saccharine to total amount of liquid consumed was evaluated. We found no effect of group, $F(1, 15) < 1, p=0.60, \eta_G^2 = 0.01$, session, $F(1, 15)=2.71$, $p=0.12, \eta_G^2 = 0.08$, and no effect of interaction between group and session, $F(1, 15) < 1$, $p=0.55$, $\eta_G^2 = 0.01$, on ratio of consumed saccharine to total amount of liquid consumed (**Figure 5**).

CIRCADIAN LOCOMOTOR ACTIVITY

Spontaneous locomotor activity was monitored continuously in rats maintained under LD12:12 for 1 month and then released into DD for 16 days. The representative activity records (actograms) of one Nogo-A knockdown and one control rat are depicted in **Figure 6A**. Under LD12:12, the activity exhibited clear daily rhythm with increased levels during the dark phase and decreased levels during the light phase in both rat genotypes. The accumulated activity profiles measured under LD12:12 did not reveal significant differences between the Nogo-A knockdown and WT rats in the phasing or amplitude of the activity levels during the dark and light phases of the light/dark cycle (**Figure 6B**). Also, total activity (**Figure 6D**) and activity/rest ratio (**Figure 6E**) were not significantly different [$t(11)=0.39$, $p=0.70$, $r=0.12$ and $t(11)=1.42$, $p=0.18$, $r=0.39$, respectively] between both rat genotypes maintained under LD cycle. After releasing the rats into constant darkness, the behavioral activity maintained the circadian rhythm, which ran with an endogenous circadian period tau (**Figure 6A**). Comparison of the endogenous periods tau calculated from the periodograms (**Figure 6C**) revealed a marginally significant difference ($U=7$, $p=0.05$; Mann–Whitney test) between the Nogo-A knockdown (mean ± SD, 24.1 ± 0.1 h, $n=5$) and WT (24.2 ± 0.1 h, $n=8$) rats. Under DD, the total activity of the Nogo-A knockdown rats was significantly reduced [$t(11)=2.24$, $p=0.05$, $r=0.56$] (**Figure 6D**) and there was a trend toward increased activity/rest ratio compared with the controls (**Figure 6E**) [$t(11)=1.93$, $p=0.08$, $r=0.50$; Student's t-test]. Whereas the controls activity/rest ratio significantly dropped [$t(14)=4.64$, $p=0.0004$, $r=0.78$; Student's t-test] after releasing from LD12:12 into DD, in Nogo-A knockdown, the decline in the ratio was not significant [$t(8)=1.23$, $p=0.25$, $r=0.40$; Student's t-test].

DISCUSSION

Nogo-A KNOCKDOWN IS LINKED TO A COGNITIVE DEFICIT IN THE CAROUSEL MAZE

During the active place avoidance training in the Carousel maze, both groups of rats exhibited comparable locomotor activity, as measured by total distance (**Figure 2A**). The Nogo-A knockdown animals performed significantly worse as shown by the lower maximum time avoided. The impairment was slightly (but not significantly) more pronounced during reversal, when the sector position was changed and the animals had to adjust their behavior accordingly (**Figure 3A**). We might therefore assume that the Nogo-A knockdown rats were impaired in spatial learning and reference frames segregation *per se*, with a possible contribution of behavioral inflexibility. This finding closely parallels that of Petrasek et al. (2014), although the task used here is slightly different (in the present study, the task was purely aversive, without simultaneous foraging).

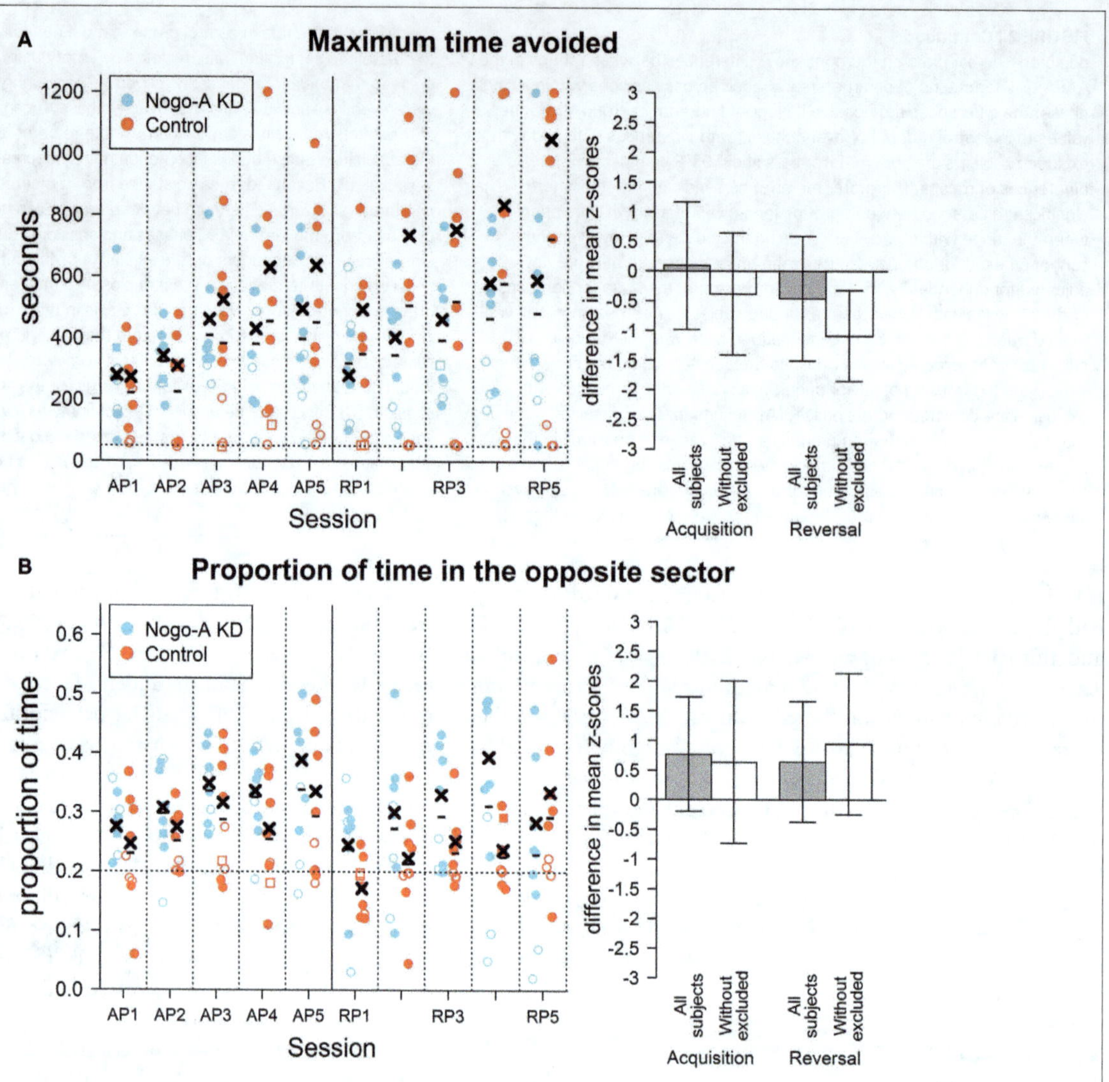

FIGURE 3 | Results of cognitive parameters in the AAPA task. The plots on the left show individual values for each rat during both sessions. The sessions are labeled by abbreviations: AP, acquisition phase; RP, reversal phase. Missing values are indicated by square points. Empty points indicate values for subjects that were excluded from analysis (see text for details). Minus signs indicate mean group values for a given session computed from all subjects and crosses indicate mean values computed from values without the excluded subjects. The bar plots on the right show differences between groups in the AAPA task for means of parameters averaged across sessions within a single phase. The differences are positive if Nogo-A knockdown group had higher values than control group. For both phases, both difference with and without excluded subjects is shown. Error bars show 95% confidence intervals of differences of means. See description of the **Figure 2** for further details. **(A)** Results for maximum time avoided (left plot in seconds). No difference between groups is visible when all subjects are compared. However, a significant difference can be seen when the comparison is done without the excluded rats. Note, especially, the large difference in means for the last few session of the reversal phase. The horizontal dotted line in the left plot represents 50 s, which corresponds to a time of maximum time avoided for a subject that is fully immobile. The excluded rats from control group do not usually show better avoidance ability than they would have if they did not move at all. Maximum possible value for maximum time avoided is 1200 s, which corresponds to no entrance to the to-be-avoided sector. **(B)** Results for proportion of time in the opposite sector. A slight, but not significant, increase in the proportion of time in the opposite sector can be seen in Nogo-A knockdown rats in all sessions with exception of the last one. The result is contrary to that expected based on previous research suggesting perseverance in Nogo-A knockdown animals. The horizontal dotted line in the left plot depicts a proportion that would be measured for totally immobile subjects. It can be seen that the three excluded rats from Nogo-A knockdown group have values close to this line. The acquisition phase was not included in analysis and is shown only for comparison.

Reversal learning in the active place avoidance has been recently suggested to tap mnemonic segregation (distinguishing the original learned response, now irrelevant, from the new and relevant), adding another dimension of pattern separation to the already present demand to separate spatial frames (Abdel Baki et al., 2009; Burghardt et al., 2012). It is therefore not surprising that very mild deficits became pronounced during this phase of training. Impairment of reversal learning in a spatial task (water *T*-maze) has been already described in Nogo knockdown mice (Willi et al., 2010) and rats (Tews et al., 2013) and attributed to perseveration. However, in the present study, the Nogo-A knockdown animals exhibited no signs of excessive perseveration, i.e., prolonged avoidance of

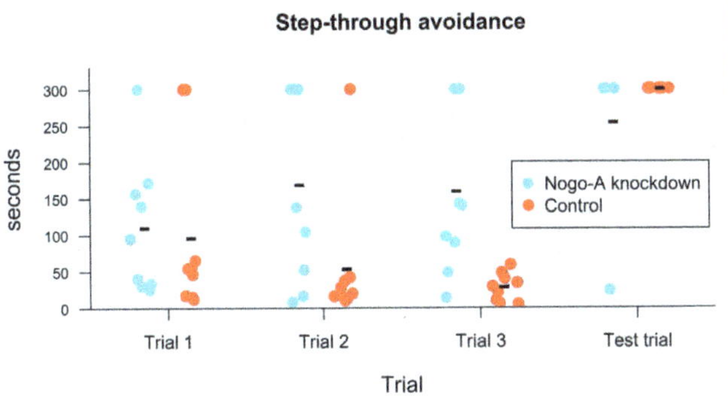

FIGURE 4 | Results of step-through avoidance in seconds. Individual points display values for each subject. Group mean is shown with a minus sign. While no difference is present in the first trial, in the subsequent two trials it took longer for Nogo-A knockdown rats to move into the dark compartment. All subjects with the exception of one remained in the light compartment during the entire test trial, i.e., after obtaining a shock in the dark compartment in the third trial (the three Nogo-A knockdown rats, which did not move into the dark compartment during the third trial were not given the test trial since they did not obtain the shock). Maximum possible duration of the trial was 300 s.

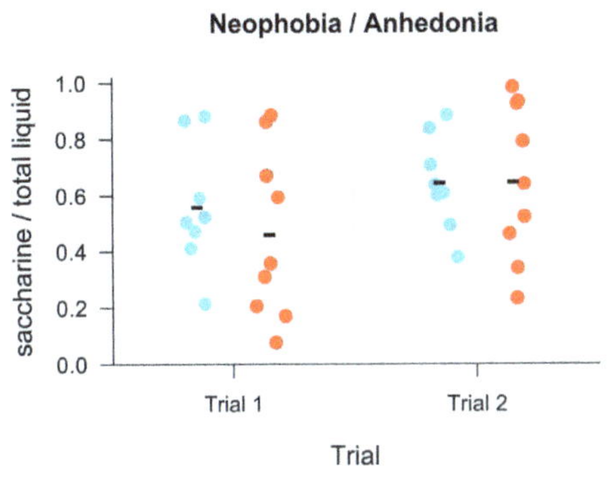

FIGURE 5 | Results of the neophobia/anhedonia task as a ratio of consumed saccharine to total consumed liquid. Individual points display values for each subject. Group mean is shown with a minus sign. No difference is seen between groups (blue – Nogo-A knockdown, red – control) in either trial.

the no-longer-punished sector. They actually spent *more* time in the former to-be-avoided sector during reversal phase, as shown in **Figure 3B**.

While our study focused on Nogo-A knockdown, there is a robust body of evidence connecting *facilitated* Nogo-A signaling with impairments of hippocampus-dependent cognitive functions. For example, mice over-expressing NgR show impairment of hippocampus-dependent long-term memory (Karlén et al., 2009). Increased levels of hippocampal Nogo-A showing strong positive correlation with cognitive decline in aged rats (VanGuilder et al., 2011, 2012) and cognitive impairments in a mouse model of Alzheimer's disease can be ameliorated by genetic deletion of Nogo-A (Masliah et al., 2010). The effects of decreased Nogo-A expression on the behavior of otherwise intact animals are less well explored. In several studies, no behavioral effects were reported after acute blockade of Nogo-A by antibodies in healthy mice (Lenzlinger et al., 2005; Marklund et al., 2007). The permanent absence of Nogo-A in knockout models seems to be more relevant from the neurodevelopmental viewpoint. In some studies, no behavioral effect of knockout has been noted in otherwise intact animals (Marklund et al., 2009; Masliah et al., 2010). In other cases, the deletion of the Nogo-A led to schizophrenia-related endophenotypes, as reported by Willi et al. (2010). The symptoms included disrupted sensorimotor gating and latent inhibition, perseverative behavior in reversal learning, and increased sensitivity to amphetamines. This discrepancy can be explained by differences in the behavioral paradigms employed, as the tasks used by Willi et al. (2010) were specifically chosen to search for schizophrenia-like behavior. Subtle cognitive deficits in Nogo-A knockdown rats have been confirmed by Tews et al. (2013) and our own previous work (Petrasek et al., 2014).

Nogo-A KNOCKDOWN DECREASES ANXIETY LEVELS

Some of the rats, especially from the control group, showed signs of excessive anxiety or fear during the testing, in some cases resulting in persistent freezing across multiple sessions ("non-solvers"). This behavior has been noted in healthy Sprague-Dawley rats in an active place avoidance task before (the "poor learners" in Carr et al., 2011). As immobile animals are incapable of solving the task, regardless of their cognitive abilities, such animals had to be removed from the analysis. In Nogo-A knockdown rats, passive behavior occurred rarely and never persisted across multiple sessions. Even after the exclusion of "non-solvers," control animals were apparently more anxious than the Nogo-A knockdown group, as revealed by more pronounced thigmotaxis and increased defecation during avoidance sessions (**Figures 2B,C**). The difference was apparently present even before introduction of the foot-shock, as the Nogo-A knockdown rats were less thigmotactic and more active than controls even during habituation sessions, when no aversive stimulus was present, except for the novel environment itself. The preferential occurrence of "non-solvers" in the control group was thus presumably linked to the higher anxiety levels, perhaps in a manner similar to learned helplessness. The strong difference in anxiety levels is somewhat surprising, as previous studies both in the rat model (Tews et al., 2013) and in knockout mice (Willi et al., 2009) did not show any difference in anxiety levels.

PASSIVE AVOIDANCE TASK REVEALS SPARED NON-SPATIAL MEMORY AND NORMAL HABITUATION TO A NOVEL TASTE

In the passive avoidance task, both the experimental and control groups exhibited increased latency to enter the dark compartment during the testing session (after the foot-shock), demonstrating successful memory for the unpleasant stimulus after 24 h. However, their behavior during the first three trials (i.e., without previous experience of the punishment) was different: while control animals entered the preferred dark environment with shorter and shorter latency in subsequent sessions, the Nogo-A knockdown rats exhibited similar or even increased latency with repeated experience, and some of them did not enter it at all (**Figure 4**). In the context of the Carousel maze results, we can assume that the Nogo-A knockdown rats were less anxious and therefore less motivated to seek shelter in the dark compartment.

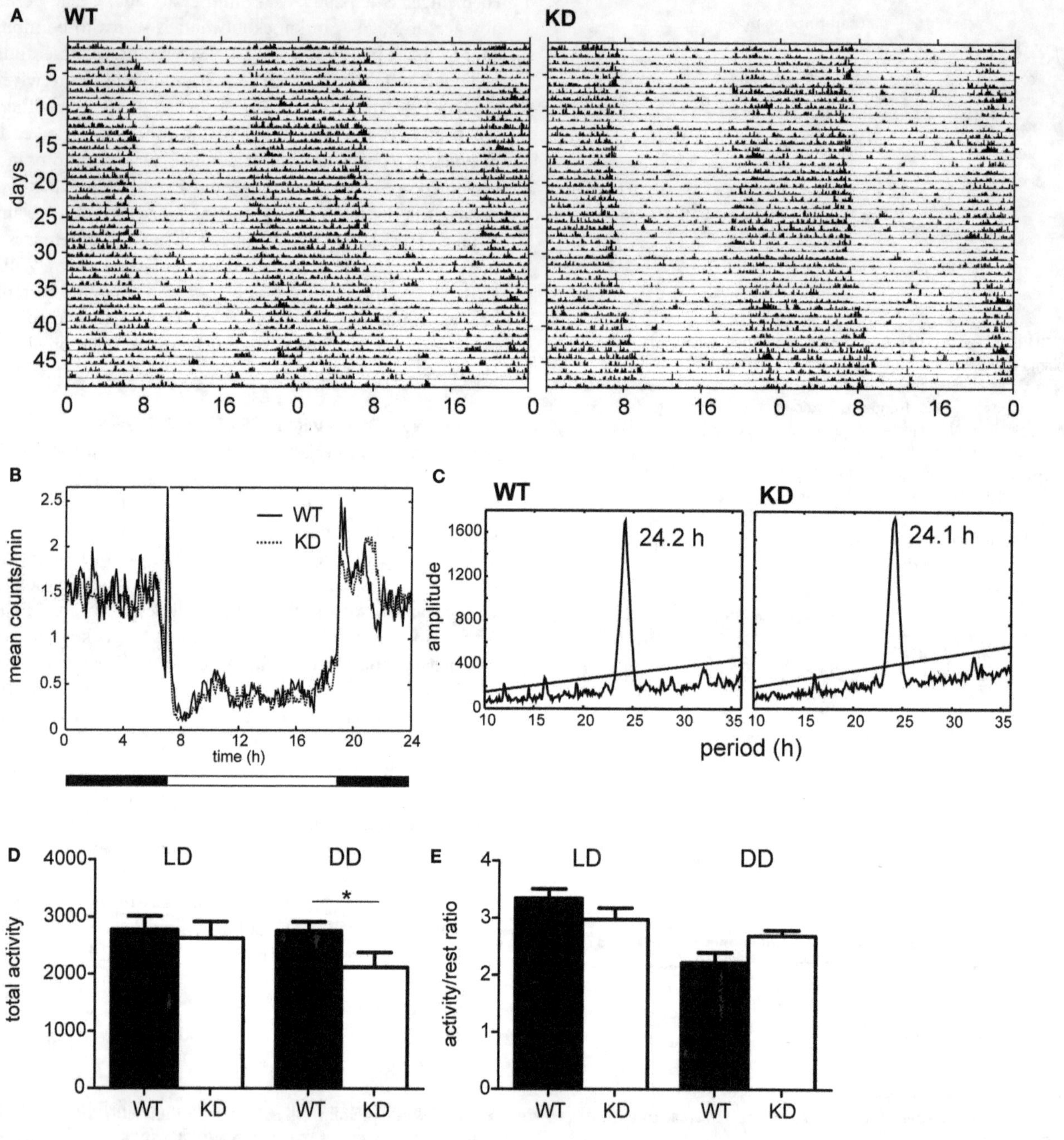

FIGURE 6 | Activity profiles of Nogo-A knockdown rats (designated KD) and wild-type (WT) controls. **(A)** Representative double-plotted actograms of locomotor activity of WT (left) and KD (right) rats maintained under a light–dark regime with 12 h of light and 12 h of darkness (LD12:12) for 29 days and subsequently under constant darkness (DD) for 16 days. **(B)** Cumulative locomotor activity profile of eight WT (solid line) and six KD (dashed line) rats kept under LD12:12. **(C)** Cumulative periodogram of eight WT (left) and six KD (right) rats kept under DD. **(D)** Total locomotor activity of eight WT (black) and six KD (white) rats kept under LD12:12 (left) or under DD (right). **(E)** Activity/rest ratio of eight WT (black) and six KD (white) rats kept under LD12:12 (left) or under DD (right).

The neophobia/anhedonia experiment revealed no difference in taste preferences between the groups (**Figure 5**).

CHANGES IN CIRCADIAN RHYTHMICITY

Nogo-A knockdown rats exhibited daily and circadian rhythms in locomotor activity. Therefore, the ability of the circadian clock to entrain to LD cycle and to drive the circadian rhythms was not affected by the reduction of Nogo-A mRNA and protein levels in retina and brain. Nevertheless, under constant dark conditions, the circadian rhythm in locomotor activity was better expressed in Nogo-A knockdown rats, because the ratio of their activity during the subjective night and subjective day was higher compared with the WT controls. The difference was not due to greater activity in the Nogo-A knockdown rats because their total activity in DD was rather reduced compared with controls. The difference was likely related to the endogenous state of the circadian clock in the SCN, which directly drives the activity rhythm in constant darkness, because the difference between both phenotypes was not apparent in LD conditions, when the activity was regulated by the circadian clock as well as directly suppressed by light via masking effect (**Figure 6**). Therefore, the data suggest that the partial developmental deficit in Nogo-A may modulate the clock function. It is, however, not known whether the modulation arises from changes of the clock property *per se* or from the fact that the input neural pathways from other brain areas may be modulated by the Nogo-A deficiency. Also, an impact of the genotype on the sensitivity of the locomotor activity to LD cycle cannot be completely ruled out because in mice with complete deletion of Nogo-A activity during the dark phase of the LD cycle was higher than in WT controls. The activity during the light phase was not different, which means that the activity/rest ratio in the Nogo-A knockout mice was increased even under LD cycle (Willi et al., 2009).

The aforementioned data suggest that the circadian clock in Nogo-A knockdown might function as a "stronger" circadian pacemaker than that of WT rats. As the robustness of the circadian clock in the SCN is highly dependent on the synaptic communication among the individual oscillators (Liu et al., 2007), the reduction of the neurite outgrowth inhibitor during development in Nogo-A knockdown rats might theoretically be beneficial for the clock function. However, this highly speculative conclusion would need to be verified in future experiments comparing the synaptic strength and amplitudes of clock gene and protein expression level profiles directly in the SCN between the Nogo-A knockdown and WT control rats.

CAVEATS

Because of the necessary exclusions, the number of animals used in this work was not large, raising concerns about power of the statistical tests used. However, in some measures, the difference between the two groups was large enough to be detected unambiguously.

Another caveat is that the Nogo-A knockdown group consisted of two litters. While we do not believe that this seriously affected the results, it should be taken into account in interpreting the results.

Nogo-A KNOCKDOWN AS A MODEL OF SCHIZOPHRENIA

In mouse and rat models, Nogo-A-deficient animals exhibit symptoms such as disrupted sensorimotor gating and latent inhibition, deficits of memory, cognitive flexibility, and social behavior (Willi et al., 2010; Tews et al., 2013; Petrasek et al., 2014, the present work), which are characteristic for schizophrenia models, and are considered analogous to cognitive and negative symptoms in humans (Bubenikova-Valesova et al., 2008b; Jones et al., 2011). As disruption of Nogo-A signaling may be relevant at least in some cases of human schizophrenia pathogenesis (Willi and Schwab, 2013), this model can exhibit construct validity as well.

Hyperlocomotion and stereotypic behavior are considered animal analogs to positive (psychotic) symptoms (Bubenikova-Valesova et al., 2008b). In the Nogo-A-deficient models, changes in locomotor behavior are rather subtle and reported only in some experimental settings, while stereotypies (e.g., stereotypic grooming) have not been observed. This might indicate that the Nogo-A knockout/knockdown induces alterations similar to negative and cognitive, but not positive schizophrenia symptoms. Differential expression of symptoms, often with some classes less pronounced or entirely missing, is rather typical for animal models of schizophrenia, as well as the disease itself in human patients. Preferential expression of negative and cognitive symptoms in an animal model might be even viewed as an advantage, as these classes are rather under-represented in the traditional models of the disease (Jones et al., 2011).

Our results from the present work and Petrasek et al. (2014) demonstrate mostly cognitive deficits specific for Carousel maze tasks requiring spatial frames segregation and cognitive flexibility, which is consistent with schizophrenia-like symptomatology, as can be demonstrated in comparison with similar studies using different models. Ample experimental data from the Carousel maze tests have been collected using pharmacological dizocilpine (MK-801) model of schizophrenia (Stuchlik et al., 2004; Vales et al., 2006; Bubenikova-Valesova et al., 2008a). Dizocilpine can disrupt Moris Water Maze performance even before Carousel maze performance (Stuchlik et al., 2004), unlike Nogo-A knockdown model, where Water Maze learning is intact (Petrasek et al., 2014). On the other hand, dizocilpine administration leads to deficits in spatial reversal learning (Lobellova et al., 2013), which is similar to Nogo-A deficiency.

Neurodevelopmental models of schizophrenia should be perhaps more comparable to the Nogo-A knockdown and knockout models than acute pharmacological treatments, but their influence on Carousel maze performance is less well studied. An exception is the neonatal ventral hippocampal lesion (NVHL) model (Lecourtier et al., 2012; Lee et al., 2012; Swerdlow et al., 2012). Lee et al. (2012) have found that the NVHL rats are impaired in the Carousel maze learning, and even more in reversal learning, which parallels our findings in Nogo-A knockdown rats.

We must note that there is no "ideal" animal model of schizophrenia. Etiology of schizophrenia is largely unknown (and probably multi-factorial), and all we can reasonably assess is the similarity of symptoms (face validity). Furthermore, there is no unambiguous biochemical, anatomical, pharmacological, or behavioral marker of schizophrenia that could be used to reliably validate proposed animal models (Lipska and Weinberger, 2000). From this perspective, Nogo-A-deficient transgenic animals constitute a novel candidate model of schizophrenia with proposed construct validity and good face validity at least for negative and cognitive symptoms.

SUMMARY

Results of the present study clearly demonstrate behavioral differences between the rats with decreased Nogo-A expression and WT Sprague-Dawley controls. We can conclude that the Nogo-A knockdown rats exhibited marked cognitive deficit in the Carousel maze. In spite of their reduced ability to avoid punishment, they seemed less anxious than their WT counterparts. Non-spatial long-term memory, assessed in the passive avoidance task, and neophobic reaction to a novel taste and preference of a sweet taste did not differ between groups. The period of circadian rhythms was not affected, but in constant darkness, the rhythm in locomotor activity was more pronounced in the Nogo-A knockdown animals.

When taken together with the biochemical assessment of key protein expression and laterality in the brain of the same transgenic rat line (Krištofiková et al., 2013), our results are mostly consistent with the proposed link between decreased Nogo-A levels and schizophrenia-like behavior in the rat, even though some of the results suggest that changes caused by Nogo-A knockdown are more complex than previously thought.

ACKNOWLEDGMENTS

This work was funded mainly by GAUK grant 365911 (awarded to Tomas Petrasek) and GACR 14-03627S (awarded to Ales Stuchlik). Additional support came from IGA MZ CR NT13386 and AVCR M200111204 awarded to Ales Stuchlik. Support for foreign partners was provided by grants from the German Ministry for Education and Research (BMBF, 01GQ1003B), National Bernstein Network for Computational Neuroscience, HEALTH-F2-2007-201714 DEVANX (awarded to Dusan Bartsch), and the Grant No. 31-122527/1 (awarded to Martin E. Schwab). The work of Stepan Bahnik was partly supported by the Deutsche Forschungsgemeinschaft (DFG-RTG 1253/2).

REFERENCES

Abdel Baki, S. G., Kao, H. Y., Kelemen, E., Fenton, A. A., and Bergold, P. J. (2009). A hierarchy of neurobehavioral tasks discriminates between mild and moderate brain injury in rats. *Brain Res.* 1280, 98–106. doi:10.1016/j.brainres.2009.05.034

Akbik, F., Cafferty, W. B., and Strittmatter, S. M. (2012). Myelin associated inhibitors: a link between injury-induced and experience-dependent plasticity. *Exp. Neurol.* 235, 43–52. doi:10.1016/j.expneurol.2011.06.006

Bahnik, S. (2013). *Carousel Maze Manager (Version 0.3.5) [Software].* Available at: https://github.com/bahniks/CM_Manager_0_3_5.

Bakeman, R. (2005). Recommended effect size statistics for repeated measures designs. *Behav. Res. Methods* 37, 379–384. doi:10.3758/BF03192707

Bubenikova-Valesova, V., Stuchlik, A., Svoboda, J., Bures, J., and Vales, K. (2008a). Risperidone and ritanserin but not haloperidol block effect of dizocilpine on the active allothetic place avoidance task. *Proc. Natl. Acad. Sci. U.S.A.* 105, 1061–1066. doi:10.1073/pnas.0711273105

Bubenikova-Valesova, V., Horacek, J., Vrajova, M., and Höschl, C. (2008b). Models of schizophrenia in humans and animals based on inhibition of NMDA receptors. *Neurosci. Biobehav. Rev.* 32, 1014–1023. doi:10.1016/j.neubiorev.2008.03.012

Budel, S., Padukkavidana, T., Liu, B. P., Feng, Z., Hu, F., Johnson, S., et al. (2008). Genetic variants of Nogo-66 receptor with possible association to schizophrenia block myelin inhibition of axon growth. *J. Neurosci.* 28, 13161–13172. doi:10.1523/JNEUROSCI.3828-08.2008

Burghardt, N. S., Park, E. H., Hen, R., and Fenton, A. A. (2012). Adult-born hippocampal neurons promote cognitive flexibility in mice. *Hippocampus* 22, 1795–1808. doi:10.1002/hipo.22013

Canteras, N. S., and Swanson, L. W. (1992). Projections of the ventral subiculum to the amygdala, septum, and hypothalamus: a PHAL anterograde tract-tracing study in the rat. *J. Comp. Neurol.* 324, 180–194. doi:10.1002/cne.903240204

Carr, Z. J., Torjman, M. C., Manu, K., Dy, G., and Goldberg, M. E. (2011). Spatial memory using active allothetic place avoidance in adult rats after isoflurane anesthesia: a potential model for postoperative cognitive dysfunction. *J. Neurosurg. Anesthesiol.* 23, 138–145. doi:10.1097/ANA.0b013e3182049f19

Chen, M. S., Huber, A. B., van der Haar, M. E., Frank, M., Schnell, L., Spillmann, A. A., et al. (2000). Nogo-A is a myelin-associated neurite outgrowth inhibitor and an antigen for monoclonal antibody IN-1. *Nature* 403, 434–439. doi:10.1038/35000219

Chong, S. Y. C., Rosenberg, S. S., Fancy, S. P. J., Zhao, C., Shen, Y.-A. A., Hahn, A. T., et al. (2012). Neurite outgrowth inhibitor Nogo-A establishes spatial segregation and extent of oligodendrocyte myelination. *Proc. Natl. Acad. Sci. U.S.A.* 109, 1299–1304. doi:10.1073/pnas.1113540109

Cimadevilla, J. M., Wesierska, M., Fenton, A. A., and Bures, J. (2001). Inactivating one hippocampus impairs avoidance of a stable room-defined place during dissociation of arena cues from room cues by rotation of the arena. *Proc. Natl. Acad. Sci. U.S.A.* 98, 3531–3536. doi:10.1073/pnas.051628398

GrandPré, T., Nakamura, F., Vartanian, T., and Strittmatter, S. M. (2000). Identification of the Nogo inhibitor of axon regeneration as a reticulon protein. *Nature* 403, 439–444. doi:10.1038/35000226

Harrison, P. J. (2004). The hippocampus in schizophrenia: a review of the neuropathological evidence and its pathophysiological implications. *Psychopharmacology (Berl.)* 174, 151–162. doi:10.1007/s00213-003-1761-y

Hsu, R., Woodroffe, A., Lai, W. S., Cook, M. N., Mukai, J., Dunning, J. P., et al. (2007). Nogo Receptor 1 (RTN4R) as a candidate gene for schizophrenia: analysis using human and mouse genetic approaches. *PLoS ONE* 2:1234. doi:10.1371/journal.pone.0001234

Huber, A. B., Weinmann, O., Brösamle, C., Oertle, T., and Schwab, M. E. (2002). Patterns of Nogo mRNA and protein expression in the developing and adult rat and after CNS lesions. *J. Neurosci.* 22, 3553–3567.

Hunt, D., Coffin, R. S., Prinjha, R. K., Campbell, G., and Anderson, P. N. (2003). Nogo-A expression in the intact and injured nervous system. *Mol. Cell. Neurosci.* 24, 1083–1102. doi:10.1016/j.mcn.2003.09.002

Jitoku, D., Hattori, E., Iwayama, Y., Yamada, K., Toyota, T., Kikuchi, M., et al. (2011). Association study of Nogo-related genes with schizophrenia in a Japanese case-control sample. *Am. J. Med. Genet. B Neuropsychiatr. Genet.* 156B, 581–592. doi:10.1002/ajmg.b.31199

Jones, C. A., Watson, D. J., and Fone, K. C. (2011). Animal models of schizophrenia. *Br. J. Pharmacol.* 164, 1162–1194. doi:10.1111/j.1476-5381.2011.01386.x

Karlén, A., Karlsson, T. E., Mattsson, A., Lundströmer, K., Codeluppi, S., Pham, T. M., et al. (2009). Nogo receptor 1 regulates formation of lasting memories. *Proc. Natl. Acad. Sci. U.S.A.* 106, 20476–20481. doi:10.1073/pnas.0905390106

Krištofiková, Z., Vrajová, M., Šírová, J., Valeš, K., Petrásek, T., Schönig, K., et al. (2013). N-methyl-D-aspartate receptor – nitric oxide synthase pathway in the cortex of Nogo-A-deficient rats in relation to brain laterality and schizophrenia. *Front. Behav. Neurosci.* 7:90. doi:10.3389/fnbeh.2013.00090

Le Pen, G., Gaudet, L., Mortas, P., Mory, R., and Moreau, J. L. (2002). Deficits in reward sensitivity in a neurodevelopmental rat model of schizophrenia. *Psychopharmacology (Berl.)* 161, 434–441. doi:10.1007/s00213-002-1092-4

Lecourtier, L., Antal, M. C., Cosquer, B., Schumacher, A., Samama, B., Angst, M. J., et al. (2012). Intact neurobehavioral development and dramatic impairments of procedural like memory following neonatal ventral hippocampal lesion in rats. *Neuroscience* 207, 110–123. doi:10.1016/j.neuroscience.2012.01.040

Lee, H., Dvorak, D., Kao, H. Y., Duffy, ÁM., Scharfman, H. E., and Fenton, A. A. (2012). Early cognitive experience prevents adult deficits in a neurodevelopmental schizophrenia model. *Neuron* 75, 714–724. doi:10.1016/j.neuron.2012.06.016

Lenzlinger, P. M., Shimizu, S., Marklund, N., Thompson, H. J., Schwab, M. E., Saatman, K. E., et al. (2005). Delayed inhibition of Nogo-A does not alter injury-induced axonal sprouting but enhances recovery of cognitive function following experimental traumatic brain injury in rats. *Neuroscience* 134, 1047–1056. doi:10.1016/j.neuroscience.2005.04.048

Lipska, B. K., and Weinberger, D. R. (2000). To model a psychiatric disorder in animals: schizophrenia as a reality test. *Neuropsychopharmacology* 23, 223–239. doi:10.1016/S0893-133X(00)00137-8

Liu, A. C., Welsh, D. K., Ko, C. H., Tran, H. G., Zhang, E. E., Priest, A. A., et al. (2007). Intercellular coupling confers robustness against mutations in the SCN circadian clock network. *Cell* 129, 605–616. doi:10.1016/j.cell.2007.02.047

Lobellova, V., Entlerova, M., Svojanovska, B., Hatalova, H., Prokopova, I., Petrasek, T., et al. (2013). Two learning tasks provide evidence for disrupted behavioural flexibility in an animal model of schizophrenia-like behaviour induced by acute MK-801: a dose-response study. *Behav. Brain Res.* 246, 55–62. doi:10.1016/j.bbr.2013.03.006

Marklund, N., Bareyre, F. M., Royo, N. C., Thompson, H. J., Mir, A. K., Grady, M. S., et al. (2007). Cognitive outcome following brain injury and treatment with an inhibitor of Nogo-A in association with an attenuated downregulation of hippocampal growth associated protein-43 expression. *J. Neurosurg.* 107, 844–853. doi:10.3171/JNS-07/10/0844

Marklund, N., Morales, D., Clausen, F., Hånell, A., Kiwanuka, O., Pitkänen, A., et al. (2009). Functional outcome is impaired following traumatic brain injury in aging Nogo-A/B-deficient mice. *Neuroscience* 163, 540–551. doi:10.1016/j.neuroscience.2009.06.042

Masliah, E., Xie, F., Dayan, S., Rockenstein, E., Mante, M., Adame, A., et al. (2010). Genetic deletion of Nogo/Rtn4 ameliorates behavioral and neuropathological outcomes in amyloid precursor protein transgenic mice. *Neuroscience* 169, 488–494. doi:10.1016/j.neuroscience.2010.04.045

Meijer, J. H., and Schwartz, W. J. (2003). In search of the pathways for light-induced pacemaker resetting in the suprachiasmatic nucleus. *J. Biol. Rhythms* 18, 235–249. doi:10.1177/0748730403018003006

Mingorance, A., Fontana, X., Solé, M., Burgaya, F., Ureña, J. M., Teng, F. Y., et al. (2004). Regulation of Nogo and Nogo receptor during the development of the entorhino-hippocampal pathway and after adult hippocampal lesions. *Mol. Cell. Neurosci.* 26, 34–49. doi:10.1016/j.mcn.2004.01.001

Mingorance-Le Meur, A., Zheng, B., Soriano, E., and del Río, J. A. (2007). Involvement of the myelin-associated inhibitor Nogo-A in early cortical development and neuronal maturation. *Cereb. Cortex* 17, 2375–2386. doi:10.1093/cercor/bhl146

Novak, G., Kim, D., Seeman, P., and Tallerico, T. (2002). Schizophrenia and Nogo: elevated mRNA in cortex, and high prevalence of a homozygous CAA insert. *Brain Res. Mol. Brain Res.* 107, 183–189. doi:10.1016/S0169-328X(02)00492-8

Pelizza, L., and Ferrari, A. (2009). Anhedonia in schizophrenia and major depression: state or trait? *Ann. Gen. Psychiatry* 8, 22. doi:10.1186/1744-859X-8-22

Pernet, V., Joly, S., Christ, F., Dimou, L., and Schwab, M. E. (2008). Nogo-A and myelin-associated glycoprotein differently regulate oligodendrocyte maturation and myelin formation. *J. Neurosci.* 28, 7435–7444. doi:10.1523/JNEUROSCI.0727-08.2008

Pernet, V., and Schwab, M. E. (2012). The role of Nogo-A in axonal plasticity, regrowth and repair. *Cell Tissue Res.* 349, 97–104. doi:10.1007/s00441-012-1432-6

Petrasek, T., Prokopova, I., Bahnik, S., Schonig, K., Berger, S., Vales, A., et al. (2014). Nogo-A downregulation impairs place avoidance in the Carousel maze but not spatial memory in the Morris water maze. *Neurobiol. Learn. Mem.* 107, 42–49. doi:10.1016/j.nlm.2013.10.015

Phillips, W. A., and Silverstein, S. M. (2003). Convergence of biological and psychological perspectives on cognitive coordination in schizophrenia. *Behav. Brain Sci.* 26, 65–82. doi:10.1017/S0140525X03000025

Prokopova, I., Bahnik, S., Doulames, V., Vales, K., Petrasek, T., Svoboda, J., et al. (2012). Synergistic effects of dopamine D2-like receptor antagonist sulpiride and beta-blocker propranolol on learning in the Carousel maze, a dry-land spatial navigation task. *Pharmacol. Biochem. Behav.* 102, 151–156. doi:10.1016/j.pbb.2012.04.003

R Core Team. (2013). *R: A Language and Environment for Statistical Computing.* Vienna: R Foundation for Statistical Computing.

Rolando, C., Parolisi, R., Boda, E., Schwab, M. E., Rossi, F., and Buffo, A. (2012). Distinct roles of Nogo-A and Nogo receptor 1 in the homeostatic regulation of adult neural stem cell function and neuroblast migration. *J. Neurosci.* 32, 17788–17799. doi:10.1523/JNEUROSCI.3142-12.2012

Schwab, M. E. (2004). Nogo and axon regeneration. *Curr. Opin. Neurobiol.* 14, 118–124. doi:10.1016/j.conb.2004.01.004

Schwab, M. E. (2010). Functions of Nogo proteins and their receptors in the nervous system. *Nat. Rev. Neurosci.* 11, 799–811. doi:10.1038/nrn2936

Sinibaldi, L., De Luca, A., Bellacchio, E., Conti, E., Pasini, A., Paloscia, C., et al. (2004). Mutations of the Nogo-66 receptor (RTN4R) gene in schizophrenia. *Hum. Mutat.* 24, 534–535. doi:10.1002/humu.9292

Sládek, M., Jindráková, Z., Bendová, Z., and Sumová, A. (2007). Postnatal ontogenesis of the circadian clock within the rat liver. *Am. J. Physiol. Regul. Integr. Comp. Physiol.* 292, R1224–R1229. doi:10.1152/ajpregu.00184.2006

Stephan, F. K., and Kovacevic, N. S. (1978). Multiple retention deficit in passive avoidance in rats is eliminated by suprachiasmatic lesions. *Behav. Biol.* 22, 456–462. doi:10.1016/S0091-6773(78)92565-8

Stuchlik, A. (2007). Further study of the effects of dopaminergic D1 drugs on place avoidance behavior using pretraining: some negative evidence. *Behav. Brain Res.* 178, 47–52. doi:10.1016/j.bbr.2006.11.046

Stuchlik, A., Rezacova, L., Vales, K., Bubenikova, V., and Kubik, S. (2004). Application of a novel Active Allothetic Place Avoidance task (AAPA) in testing a pharmacological model of psychosis in rats: comparison with the Morris Water Maze. *Neurosci. Lett.* 366, 162–166. doi:10.1016/j.neulet.2004.05.037

Swerdlow, N. R., Light, G. A., Breier, M. R., Shoemaker, J. M., Saint Marie, R. L., Neary, A. C., et al. (2012). Sensory and sensorimotor gating deficits after neonatal ventral hippocampal lesions in rats. *Dev. Neurosci.* 34, 240–249. doi:10.1159/000336841

Tan, E. C., Chong, S. A., Wang, H., Chew-Ping Lim, E., and Teo, Y. Y. (2005). Gender-specific association of insertion/deletion polymorphisms in the nogo gene and chronic schizophrenia. *Brain Res. Mol. Brain Res.* 139, 212–216. doi:10.1016/j.molbrainres.2005.05.010

Tapp, W. N., and Holloway, F. A. (1981). Phase shifting circadian rhythms produces retrograde amnesia. *Science* 211, 1056–1058. doi:10.1126/science.7193351

Tews, B., Schönig, K., Arzt, M. E., Clementi, S., Rioult-Pedotti, M. S., Zemmar, A., et al. (2013). Synthetic miRNA-mediated downregulation of Nogo-A in transgenic rats reveals its role as regulator of plasticity, learning and memory. *Proc. Natl. Acad. Sci. U.S.A.* 110, 6583–6588. doi:10.1073/pnas.1217665110

Vales, K., Bubenikova-Valesova, V., Klement, D., and Stuchlik, A. (2006). Analysis of sensitivity to MK-801 treatment in a novel active allothetic place avoidance task and in the working memory version of the Morris water maze reveals differences between Long-Evans and Wistar rats. *Neurosci. Res.* 55, 383–388. doi:10.1016/j.neures.2006.04.007

VanGuilder, H. D., Bixler, G. V., Sonntag, W. E., and Freeman, W. M. (2012). Hippocampal expression of myelin-associated inhibitors is induced with age-related cognitive decline and correlates with deficits of spatial learning and memory. *J. Neurochem.* 121, 77–98. doi:10.1111/j.1471-4159.2012.07671.x

VanGuilder, H. D., Farley, J. A., Yan, H., Van Kirk, C. A., Mitschelen, M., Sonntag, W. E., et al. (2011). Hippocampal dysregulation of synaptic plasticity-associated proteins with age-related cognitive decline. *Neurobiol. Dis.* 43, 201–212. doi:10.1016/j.nbd.2011.03.012

Voineskos, A. N. (2009). Converging evidence for the Nogo-66 receptor gene in schizophrenia. *J. Neurosci.* 29, 5045–5047. doi:10.1523/JNEUROSCI.0477-09.2009

Wang, K. C., Koprivica, V., Kim, J. A., Sivasankaran, R., Guo, Y., Neve, R. L., et al. (2002). Oligodendrocyte-myelin glycoprotein is a Nogo receptor ligand that inhibits neurite outgrowth. *Nature* 417, 941–944. doi:10.1038/nature00867

Wesierska, M., Dockery, C., and Fenton, A. A. (2005). Beyond memory, navigation, and inhibition: behavioral evidence for hippocampus-dependent cognitive coordination in the rat. *J. Neurosci.* 25, 2413–2419. doi:10.1523/JNEUROSCI.3962-04.2005

Willi, R., Aloy, E. M., Yee, B. K., Feldon, J., and Schwab, M. E. (2009). Behavioral characterization of mice lacking the neurite outgrowth inhibitor Nogo-A. *Genes Brain Behav.* 8, 181–192. doi:10.1111/j.1601-183X.2008.00460.x

Willi, R., and Schwab, M. E. (2013). Nogo and Nogo receptor: relevance to schizophrenia? *Neurobiol. Dis.* 54, 150–157. doi:10.1016/j.nbd.2013.01.011

12

Low-dose memantine-induced working memory improvement in the allothetic place avoidance alternation task (APAAT) in young adult male rats

Malgorzata J. Wesierska[1]*, Weronika Duda[1] and Colleen A. Dockery[1,2]

[1] *Laboratory of Neuropsychology, Department of Neurophysiology, Nencki Institute of Experimental Biology, Polish Academy of Sciences, Warsaw, Poland*
[2] *Faculty of Life Sciences, Albstadt-Sigmaringen University of Applied Sciences, Sigmaringen, Germany*

Edited by:
Ales Stuchlik, Institute of Physiology Academy of Sciences of the Czech Republic, Czech Republic

****Correspondence:***
Malgorzata J. Wesierska, Laboratory of Neuropsychology, Department of Neurophysiology, Nencki Institute of Experimental Biology, Polish Academy of Sciences, 3 Pasteur Street, 02-093 Warsaw, Poland
e-mail: m.wesierska@nencki.gov.pl

N-methyl-D-aspartate receptors (NMDAR) are involved in neuronal plasticity. To assess their role simultaneously in spatial working memory and non-cognitive learning, we used NMDAR antagonists and the Allothetic Place Avoidance Alternation Task (APAAT). In this test rats should avoid entering a place where shocks were presented on a rotating arena which requires cognitive coordination for the segregation of stimuli. The experiment took place 30 min after intraperitoneal injection of memantine (5, 10, 20 mg/kg b.w.: MemL, MemM, MemH, respectively) and (+)MK-801 (0.1, 0.2, 0.3 mg/kg b.w.: MK-801L, MK-801M, MK-801H, respectively). Rats from the control group were intact or injected with saline (0.2 ml/kg). Over three consecutive days the rats underwent habituation, two avoidance training intervals with shocks, and a retrieval test. The shock sector was alternated daily. The after-effects of the agents were tested on Day 21. Rats treated with low dose memantine presented a longer maximum time avoided and fewer entrances than the MemH, MK-801M, MK-801H and Control rats. The shocks per entrances ratio, used as an index of cognitive skill learning, showed skill improvement after D1, except for rats treated by high doses of the agents. The activity levels, indicated by the distance walked, were higher for the groups treated with high doses of the agents. On D21 the MK801H rats performed the memory task better than the MemH rats, whereas the rats' activity depended on condition, not on the group factor. These results suggest that in naïve rats mild NMDAR blockade by low-dose memantine improves working memory related to a highly challenging task.

Keywords: working memory, cognitive skill learning, locomotor activity, MK-801, memantine, Allothetic Place Avoidance Alternation Task (APAAT)

RESEARCH HIGHLIGHTS

Improvement of working memory was induced by low dose memantine;

The negative effects of high doses on cognitive function were diminished after a long break post-MK-801 administration, but not post-memantine.

The APAAT is a useful behavioral tool to study the effects of pharmacological treatments on both non-cognitive functions and the cognitive functions, learning, memory and executive functions.

INTRODUCTION

Working memory is fundamental for sustaining successful daily activity in humans and animals. The brain areas involved in working memory include the prefrontal cortex, hippocampus and subcortical areas (Goldman-Rakic, 1995; Westerberg and Klingberg, 2007; Heuer and Bachevalier, 2012). The prelimbic and medial orbital cortices are part of the rat homologs of the human prefrontal cortex, which receive hippocampal projections from the ventral CA1 of the Ammon's horn and subiculum (Jay and Witter, 1991). A functional hippocampal-prefrontal network has been documented in the rat brain (Schwarz et al., 2013) and was found to be engaged in the rapid acquisition and short-term maintenance of spatial information (Burette et al., 2000). The prelimbic cortex is reciprocally connected with the rest of the prefrontal cortex (Jay and Witter, 1991); hence this area is capable of functionally integrating contributions from the hippocampus and prefrontal cortex, which further validate their participation in spatial working memory.

In human working memory function, temporary storage of current information occurs simultaneously along with the execution of higher cognitive function and skill performance (Baddeley, 1992; Repovs and Baddeley, 2006). It involves a multi-component system of short-term and long-term memory, which is distinguished by low and high capacities for information retention (Cowan, 2008). Animal models of working memory have utilized delayed alternation, the radial maze test, the water maze and the place avoidance test for their assessment (Dudchenko, 2004). The latter of these tasks, the place avoidance test with alternation of the target sector, involves a new set of spatial information about the task but does not require prior skill pretraining, which permits demonstration of skill improvement across time through training (Dockery and Wesierska, 2010).

It has been proven, that repetitive working memory training of a spatial task promotes improvement in the general learning performance and cognitive abilities (Klingberg, 2010). This improvement is known as cognitive skill learning (CSL), and just as for working memory in humans, it is domain-specific (e.g., visual-spatial or phonological information), and results in task-relevant improvements in terms of storage and assessment (Olesen et al., 2004; Lee et al., 2007). During CSL, such as evoked by exposure to novel task conditions, various learning mechanisms are involved including both declarative knowledge and procedural form (Anderson et al., 1997). CSL requires associative memory processes and intact fronto-striatal circuitry (Poldrack et al., 1999), in addition to normal activity in the dorsolateral prefrontal cortex (DLPFC) and the hippocampus (Cerella et al., 2006). Furthermore, there is a relationship between spatial working memory performance and motor skill learning, whereby spatial working memory, particularly in early learning, is predictive of the rate of motor learning in humans (specifically sensorimotor adaptation) with significant neural overlap between the two involving activation in the right DLPFC (Seidler et al., 2012).

CSL related to working memory in rodents has not, however, been shown to have an effect on the exploratory tendencies or other non-specific behavioral consequences of exposure to environments outside of the home cage (Light et al., 2010). Beyond the impact of training on CSL, improvement of working memory has been found as an immediate and latent effect of cathodal and anodal transcranial direct current brain stimulation (tDCS) when paired with training in humans (Dockery et al., 2009). The benefits of tDCS on spatial working memory and CSL in a rat model have furthermore been demonstrated in the place avoidance alternation task (Dockery et al., 2011). Interestingly, recent evidence suggests that anodal tDCS results in a reduction of GABA concentration, while cathodal stimulation decreases glutamate concentrations, in correlation with reduced GABA levels, as measured by magnetic resonance spectroscopy in the sensorimotor cortex (Stagg et al., 2009). It has been proposed that the cumulative benefits on working memory may result from homeostatic effects of tDCS through its interaction with mediators of neuronal function and plasticity in rats and humans (Dockery, 2013).

Activation of N-Methyl-D-aspartate (NMDA) receptors by glutamate is critical for long-term potentiation (LTP) and long term depression (LTD). They comprise a form of experience–dependent change in synaptic efficacy which is accepted as a cellular analog of learning, long-term memory storage (Lynch, 2004; Pastalkova et al., 2006), working memory and cognitive function (Timofeeva and Levin, 2011; Wang et al., 2013). Over expression of glutamate excitation involves increased intracellular Ca^{2+} and Na^{+} ions which generate excitotoxic effects. These effects are responsible for triggering neurodegeneration in many neurological diseases and disorders such as: AD, stroke, status epilepticus and head trauma. Impairment of working memory is a symptom of cognitive dysfunction which occurs with ageing, brain trauma, and neuropsychiatric diseases such as depression, Alzheimer's disease (AD) or schizophrenia (Elvevåg et al., 2000).

By studying the effect of NMDAR blockade on cognitive and non-cognitive processes, the role of NMDA receptors in the hippocampus, involved in working memory encoding and retrieval (Yoshihara and Ichitani, 2004), and their role in the prefrontal cortex, subserving persistent neuronal firing in the absence of sensory stimulation (Wang et al., 2013), can be further elucidated. Loss of the NMDA receptor NR1 subunit in the granule cells of the dentate gyrus impaired spatial memory (Niewoehner et al., 2007), and NMDA receptor deletion has been shown to both restrict CA3 pyramidal cells (Nakazawa et al., 2003) and affect spatial working memory. Moreover, blockade of NMDARs in the different subregions of the hippocampus has been found to affect different stages of spatial working memory (Lee and Kesner, 2002).

The NMDAR is a complex comprised of several heterogeneous subunits, which contains binding sites for the different modes of action of non-competitive antagonists such as (+)MK-801 (commercial name: Dizocilpine) or memantine (Paoletti et al., 2013). MK-801 acts without subunit selectivity and, with a long dwell-time in the ion channel, results in a slow off-rate and high affinity to NMDAR (Wong et al., 1986; Chen and Lipton, 2006). Memantine acts via a shorter dwell-time (faster off-rate), lower affinity and higher voltage dependence (Parsons et al., 1995; Chen and Lipton, 2006). It blocks excessive NMDA receptor activity without impairing normal activity, which is a feature of uncompetitive antagonists. Blockade of NMDA receptors by memantine and MK-801 has been proposed as a therapeutic intervention for neuroprotection in neurodegenerative diseases such as Alzheimer and Parkinson's Disease or stroke (Zajaczkowski et al., 1996; Danysz et al., 1997). However, the different properties of the two agents in regard to NMDARs influence the differential effects on cognitive and non-cognitive behavior.

NMDAR activity relates to normal and abnormal function of the nervous system via their excitatory activity (Chen and Lipton, 2006), whereby the levels of transmission represent a continuum with polarities between excessive and inadequate transmission. The critical aspect then in achieving therapeutic efficacy to ameliorate neurological diseases and psychiatric disorders, is through the capacity to register the current state of the NMDAR activity on this continuum and apply appropriate dosing of NMDAR antagonism to achieve health and reinstate proper function. MK-801 application in animal studies was found to impair food consumption, and disturb mobility (locomotor activity) and psychogenic activity (stereotypic activity and ataxia) (Mondadori et al., 1989; Whishaw and Auer, 1989), in addition to psychotic dysfunction in rats (Manahan-Vaughan et al., 2008). In healthy humans, MK-801 administration has been associated with hallucinations, delusions and affective blunting. Memantine in high doses has also been found to disturb motor function and spontaneous responses such as rearing (Creeley et al., 2006). However, in contrast to MK-801, for memantine the distinction between doses which produced undesirable side effects and those which elicit promising therapeutic effects are clearly distinguishable (Morè et al., 2008). A pharmacological study showed that injection of 5 mg/kg of memantine resulted in plasma concentrations in a therapeutic range (about 1.0 umol/l), which is safe and does not cause learning and memory impairment. Whereas higher doses of memantine (10 mg/kg) were found to produce plasma level concentrations that were fivefold higher than those which mediated therapeutic effects in patients requiring treatment (Zoladz et al., 2006).

The effects of MK-801 and memantine have been studied in relation to cognitive function in animal models of long- and short-term memory, but have rarely been tested in working memory paradigms. The effects on memory have been shown to be dose- and time-dependent. When applied 30 min before the experiment both memantine (in 0.5 or 1.0 mg/kg doses) and MK-801 (in 0.025 or 0.05 mg/kg doses) preserved intact working memory performance in a delayed match–to–position task (Smith et al., 2011). Whereas memantine in 5 mg/kg or MK-801 in801 in 0.1 mg/kg doses impaired working memory in the same test. The low and high doses of MK-801 (0.25, 0.5, 1.0, 4.0 mg/kg) made working memory worse in the water maze test shortly after injections (from 3h to 1 day post-treatment), but not on the third or the fourth post-treatment day (Whishaw and Auer, 1989). In the radial maze, working memory was intact in rats with high doses of memantine (20 mg/kg per day) and MK-801 (0.312 mg/kg per day) applied as a chronic infusion during the experiment (Zajaczkowski et al., 1996) or post-administration of a 5 mg/kg dose of MK-801 and high doses of memantine (20 and 40 mg/kg) with a long delay (8 days) (Zajaczkowski et al., 2000). Also acute application of moderate doses of memantine (2.5, 5.0, 10.0 mg/kg) preserved short-term memory in the radial water maze test (Zoladz et al., 2006). After a high dose of memantine (20 mg/kg) a slight improvement in working memory was observed at the onset of training in the radial maze (Zajaczkowski et al., 2000).

The experimental results collectively suggest palliative effects of memantine in low doses with mixed results for MK-801. As a consequence of such experimental results, memantine received authorization as a treatment for AD in 2002 in the EU and in 2003 in the USA (Parsons et al., 2007). In contrast, MK-801 dose-dependently induced mobility disturbances and long-lasting spatial memory impairment (Zajaczkowski et al., 1996), which mimics symptoms of schizophrenia. Therefore, application of MK-801 has been proposed as an animal model of schizophrenia using the active allothetic place avoidance method (Vales et al., 2010).

In active place avoidance tasks, a freely walking rat must remember and avoid an unmarked place on an elevated arena where foot-shocks are administered. When associated with a rotating arena in light, this place, or "to-be-avoided sector," is oriented according to room frame coordinates in which place avoidance demands segregation of relevant extramaze room stimuli from irrelevant intramaze arena stimuli. To achieve accurate memory performance in the active place avoidance task, segregation of relevant from irrelevant arena frame stimuli is required, a process which engages cognitive coordination (Wesierska et al., 2005). The inability to segregate stimuli has been proposed as a disturbance in cognitive coordination which is found in patients with schizophrenia (Phillips and Silverstein, 2003).

In order to specifically test working memory and CSL, a variant of the active place avoidance, the Allothetic Place Avoidance Alternation Task (APAAT), has been developed (Dockery and Wesierska, 2010). Due to the alternation aspect of the APAAT task, in which the to-be-avoided sector is alternated daily, new information is needed for each session in order for rats to perform place avoidance correctly. As training progresses, simultaneously the memory load also increases, as rats are obliged to continually update the location of the to be-avoided sector since its location changes for each day. To date a dose-response relationship concerning the effects of NMDAR blockade on APAAT performance has not been established. By determining the dose-response curve in this task, the possible remedial effects of the relevant drugs could be clarified. The aim of the presented study was to compare the cognitive and non-cognitive processes during, immediately after, and following a long delay post-drug administration of a range of doses of memantine and MK-801 in this task. Thereby, the APAAT allowed for simultaneous examination of spatial working memory capacity and the efficiency of CSL, in addition to locomotor activity as a non-cognitive process. Such comparisons have never been previously conducted.

MATERIALS AND METHODS

ANIMALS

Eighty-one naïve adult (3.5-month-old) male Long Evans rats, weighing 270–360 g, were obtained from the breeding colony of the Nencki Institute of Experimental Biology, Polish Academy of Science, Warsaw, Poland. They were accommodated in transparent plastic home cages, four per cage, under standard conditions (a constant temperature of 22°C, 12:12 light/dark cycle, humidity at 23%). Water and food were available in the cages *ad-libitum*. The animals were handled for four days prior to the onset of the experiment. All manipulations were done according to the European Community Directive for the ethical use of experimental animals and the Polish Communities Council for the care and use of laboratory animals.

DRUG TREATMENT

Memantine—(3, 5-Dimethyl-1-adamantanamine hydrochloride, 3,5-Dimethylamantadine hydrochloride; Sigma Aldrich) was dissolved in saline (5, 10, 20 mg/ml) and injected intraperitoneally (5, 10, 20 mg/kg b.w.). (+)MK-801–((5S,10R)-(+)-5-Methyl-10,11-dihydro-5H-dibenzo[a,d]cyclohepten-5,10-imine hydrogen maleate, Dizocilpine hydrogen maleate; Sigma Aldrich) was dissolved in saline solution (0.1, 0.2, 0.3 mg/ml) and injected intraperitoneally (0.1, 0.2, 0.3 mg/kg b.w.). For both drug treatments, the animals received the same volume of liquid per kg of body weight which was applied 30 min before the training sessions on Days 1, 2, and 3.

APPARATUS

The active allothetic place avoidance apparatus was previously described in detail (Wesierska et al., 2009). Briefly, the apparatus consisted of an 80-cm-diameter, rotating (1 rpm) platform or "arena" made of aluminum. It was elevated (80 cm), and located in a room with dim light and explicit visual landmarks (pictures, lamp, furniture). Rats wore a latex harness on their back upon which an infrared light-emitting diode (LED) was fixed. The second LED was attached to the periphery of the arena. The infrared TV camera was connected to a computer system which allowed for monitoring the position of the rat. Rats were pierced between the shoulders with a subcutaneous connector (surgical needle) which provided an anchor for a mini-alligator clip that was connected by a cable to the shock box. Every time the rat entered the to-be-avoided sector (60°) a mild, constant current foot-shock was delivered through the connector placed on the rat's back. The shock was repeated every 1.5 s until the rat escaped from the shock sector. The data were collected and analyzed by the place avoidance system (Bio-Signal Group, Brooklyn, New York).

EXPERIMENTAL GROUPS

Rats ($n = 81$) were randomly divided into eight groups. The Control group of rats consisted of intact animals ($n = 12$) and rats treated with saline ($n = 11$; 1 ml/kg b.w.). The memantine group was divided into three subgroups according to the dosage: a low (MemL) 5 mg/kg ($n = 12$), medium (MemM) 10 mg/kg ($n = 12$) and high (MemH) 20 mg/kg ($n = 10$) dosage group. Likewise, the dizocilpine ((+)-MK-801) group of rats was divided into three subgroups: a low (MK-801L) 0.1 mg/kg ($n = 8$), medium (MK-801M) 0.2 mg/kg ($n = 8$) and high (MK-801H) 0.3 mg/kg ($n = 8$) dosage group (**Table 1**).

BEHAVIORAL PROCEDURES

The experiment was divided into two stages. The first stage consisted of Days 1, 2, and 3 (D1, D2, D3), during which rats were injected with drugs and underwent training and testing sessions on the rotating arena. The second stage consisted of a single session, Day 21 (D21), which served as a follow-up to test the long-term influence of prior memantine and MK-801 injections paired with training on performance in the APAAT. On D21 rats were not injected before the behavioral session, however, the behavioral conditions were the same as for the first stage.

The experiment started on Day 0 which served as the habituation during which the rats were placed on the rotating arena for 5 min without an active shock sector. The next days (D1, D2, and D3) were training days during which the rats were injected intraperitoneally 30 min before the avoidance training began. Each behavioral session began with habituation (ha) on the rotating arena with an inactive shock sector. After 5 min of habituation the to-be-avoided sector was activated. The rats which were able to avoid the sector consistently for at least 90 s. completed the two training intervals after 10 min (5 min for tr1 and 5 min for tr2) and were removed from the arena. If a rat did not reach this criterion before the end of the 10 min, they underwent an additional 5 min of training. Those rats then underwent a 5 min delay period in a cage in an adjacent room. Afterwards, they were returned to the rotating arena for the 5 min retrieval test (ts). During the test the original shock sector was inactivated. The to-be-avoided sector was defined by room frame coordinates and was changed each day according to the following order: D1–Northwest, D2–Northeast, D3–Southwest, D21–Southeast.

MEASURES

The independent variables taken to describe cognitive working memory processes included the number of entrances into the shock sector (ENTR), the maximum time spent avoiding the shock sector (s) (Tmax) and the number of shocks per entrance (SH/ENTR). For habituation and the retrieval test, the shock was inactivated, however, the program still registered undelivered number of shocks related to the rat's presence in the to-be-avoided sector. This provided an index of "untrained behavior." During training, a high SH/ENTR ratio expresses poor CSL. Non-cognitive functions were assessed by locomotor activity by the total path length (distance) (m) and linearity (Lin). The latter was calculated as the average ratio of linear distance during each two-second time bin divided by the sum of the path distance determined by each 20 ms epoch.

DATA ANALYSIS

Based on the above measures for D1–3, analysis of the across session effects on performance was performed by a three-way ANOVA (group (MemL, MemM, MemH, MK-801L, MK-801M, MK-801H, CONTR) × day (D1, D2, D3) × condition (ha, tr1, tr2, ts): 7 × 3 × 4; with repeated measures on the last factors) followed by a Tukey HSD multiple comparison *post-hoc* test. On D21, a two-way ANOVA (group (MemL, MemM, MemH, MK-801L, MK-801M, MK-801H, CONTR) x condition (ha, tr1, tr2, ts): 7 × 4; with repeated measures on the last two factors) was performed with a Tukey HSD test for multiple comparisons. Significance was accepted at a level of $P < 0.05$. The statistical analysis was performed with STATISTICA 7.1. Group averages and ±s.e.m. values are reported.

RESULTS

DOSE-RELATED EFFECTS OF MEMANTINE AND MK-801 ADMINISTRATION ON WORKING MEMORY TRAINING (DAYS 1–3) EVALUATED BY THE NUMBER OF ENTRANCES INTO AND MAXIMUM TIME SPENT AVOIDING THE SHOCK SECTOR. HIGH DOSES OF BOTH AGENTS IMPAIRED WORKING MEMORY, WHILE LOW DOSES HELPED MAINTAIN OR EVEN IMPROVE (MEMANTINE) IT

Working memory performance expressed as the number of entrances (ENTR) into the shock sector changed according to the agents used and their doses [$F_{(6,\ 74)} = 29.068$; $P < 1 \times 10^{-16}$; MemH, MK-801H > CONTR, MK-801L, MK-801M, MemL, MemM], across days [$F_{(2,\ 148)} = 5.42$; $P < 0.005$; D1, D2 > D3] and for the different conditions within a session [$F_{(3,\ 222)} = 74.70$; $P < 0.000001$; tr2 < ts < tr1 < ha] (**Figure 1A**). Working memory was worse (more entrances) after the high doses of both agents ($P < 0.0001$). Rats performed better on D3 than on D1, and D2 ($P < 0.001$). Although during the test condition rats had more entrances than during tr2, it was significantly less than in tr1 and ha ($P < 0.0008$). The *post-hoc* evaluation of the group by day interaction [$F_{(12,\ 148)} = 6.27$; $P < 6.7 \times 10^{-8}$] confirmed that rats from the MemL, MK-801L, and CONTR groups showed a lower number of ENTR across the consecutive days. Their performance was better (fewer entrances) than in the rats with MemH on D2 and D3, and MK-801H on D1 and D2 ($P < 0.001$). The *post-hoc* test for the group by condition interaction [$F_{(18,\ 222)} = 3.26$; $P < 1.8 \times 10^{-4}$] showed that avoidance during tr2 was better than in the other conditions for the MemL, MK-801L, and CONTR groups ($P < 0.01$). In contrast, the number of ENTR for MemH and MK-801H was at a similar level for all the session conditions and was worse (more entrances) than in the other groups ($P < 0.001$). On D3 the number of ENTR

Table 1 | Description of experimental groups.

Group / Dosage	Memantine			(+)MK-801(Dizocilpine)			Control
	MemL	MemM	MemH	MK-801L	MK-801M	MK-801H	Saline $n = 11$ (1 ml/kg)
mg/kg b.w.	5	10	20	0.1	0.2	0.3	
#Rat's per group	$n = 12$	$n = 12$	$n = 10$	$n = 8$	$n = 8$	$n = 8$	Intact $n = 12$
							Σ $n = 23$

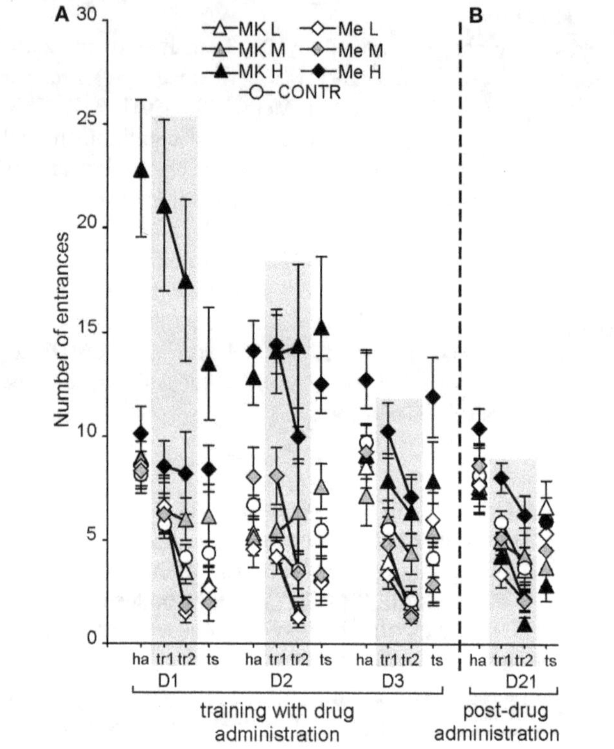

FIGURE 1 | The high dose of memantine and MK-801 (MemH and MK-801H, respectively), in contrast to the low doses, impaired working memory performance in the allothetic place avoidance alternation task as shown by a high number of entrances for D1–3 (A). This effect was absent for the long-term follow-up when no drug was administered (D21), however, rats previously treated with MemH performed worse than those previously treated with MK-801H **(B)**. The values are presented as the average number of entrances (±s.e.m.) for groups, across all days and for all conditions. The values are presented as the grand average (±s.e.m.) according to group, day and condition. Memantine doses: low MemL–5 mg/kg, medium MemM–10 mg/kg and high MemH–20 mg/kg. (+)MK-801 doses: low MK-801L–0.1 mg/kg, medium MK-801M–0.2 mg/kg and high MK-801H–0.3 mg/kg. The shaded columns represent the conditions during which shock was activated.

during tr2 was lower than for the other session conditions for all days as shown by a *post-hoc* for the day by condition interaction [$F_{(6, 444)} = 10.69$; $P < 4 \times 10^{-10}$; *post-hoc* test; $P < 0.0004$].

In the APAAT, the maximum time avoided (Tmax) is used to represent working memory performance. It differed depending on the group [$F_{(6, 74)} = 18.70$; $P < 4 \times 10^{-12}$; MemL > CONTR, MemH,MK-801H, MK-801M] and condition [$F_{(3, 222)} = 83.39$; $P < 0.00000$; tr2 > ts > tr1 > ha], whereas there was no significant effect of days (**Figure 2A**). The *post-hoc* test confirmed that rats treated with MemL avoided better (a higher Tmax) than the CONTR ($P < 0.02$), MemH, MK-801M, and MK-801H ($P < 0.001$; $P < 0.0001$) groups. No differences were found between the MemL and MK-801L, or between the MK-801L and control rats. The rats treated with MemH or MK-801H performed worse than the rats from the other groups. For condition, the shock sector was avoided with a longer Tmax during tr2 than during the other conditions (*post-hoc*; $P < 0.002$). Although the Tmax during the retrieval test (shock inactivated) was shorter than during tr2 (*post-hoc* test; $P < 0.0008$), it was longer than the Tmax during tr1 and ha (*post-hoc* test; $P < 7 \times 10^{-6}$). The *post-hoc* for the group by condition interaction [$F_{(18, 222)} = 4.86$; $P < 3 \times 10^{-8}$] showed that the Tmax during tr2 was shorter for the control than for MemL ($P < 0.02$), MemH and MK-801H ($P < 0.0001$) groups, and similar as that for the MK-801L, MK-801M, and MemM groups. The rats treated by high memantine or MK-801 presented a low Tmax for all conditions. The *post-hoc* for the day by condition interaction [$F_{(6, 444)} = 5.59$; $P < 1 \times 10^{-4}$; $P < 0.02$] showed that the Tmax was similar for tr2 across all days. The Tmax was higher for tr2 than for tr1, ha (D1-3) and ts (except for on D1).

DOSE-RELATED EFFECTS OF MEMANTINE AND MK-801 ADMINISTRATION ON COGNITIVE SKILL LEARNING (DAYS 1–3) EVALUATED AS THE SHOCKS PER ENTRANCE RATIO (SH/ENTR). RAPID ACQUISITION OF COGNITIVE SKILL LEARNING (WITHIN THE FIRST SESSION) OCCURRED AND WAS MAINTAINED OVER THE LONG-TERM (BETWEEN SESSIONS) AFTER TREATMENT WITH LOW DOSAGES OF BOTH OF THE NMDAR ANTAGONISTS

CSL was expressed as the shock per entrances ratio (SH/ENTR). It was dependent on condition [$F_{(3, 222)} = 77.48$; $P < 0.0000$)(ha > tr1, ts > tr2], but not day [$F_{(2, 148)} = 0.83$; $P = 0.43$] (**Figure 3A**). Although the main effect of treatment [$F_{(6, 74)} = 2.91$; $P < 0.013$] was significant, the *post-hoc* did not show a significant difference between groups. The SH/ENTR ratio was the highest during habituation ($P < 6 \times 10^{-5}$) and the lowest during tr2 ($P < 7 \times 10^{-4}$). The *post-hoc* test for the group by day interaction [$F_{(12, 148)} = 2.22$; $P < 0.013$] showed that the SH/ENTR ratio was similar for all groups on D1 and D2. On D3 the ratio for MemH was lower than that for MK-801M only ($P < 0.001$).

The *post-hoc* evaluation of the group by condition interaction [$F_{(18, 222)} = 5.35$; $P < 2 \times 10^{-9}$; $P < 0.01$] confirmed that during tr1 the SH/ENTR ratio was lower than during ha for the CONTR, MK-801L and MemL groups ($P < 0.01$), whereas rats

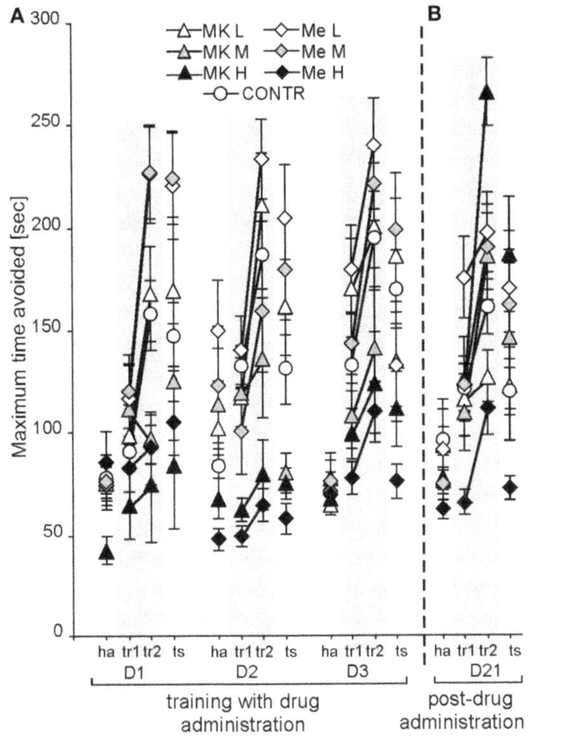

FIGURE 2 | The benefit of low-dose memantine on working memory performance was evidenced by a longer maximum time avoided (Tmax) in comparison to the control, MemH and MK-801H rats ($P < 0.02$; $P < 0.0001$; $P < 0.0001$, respectively) (A). Without any drug administration (D21) working memory performance was similar for all groups, but post-treatment MemH rats were worse than post-MK-801H **(B)**. The values are presented as the average Tmax (±s.e.m.) for groups across days and for all conditions. Other figure elements are the same as in **Figure 1**.

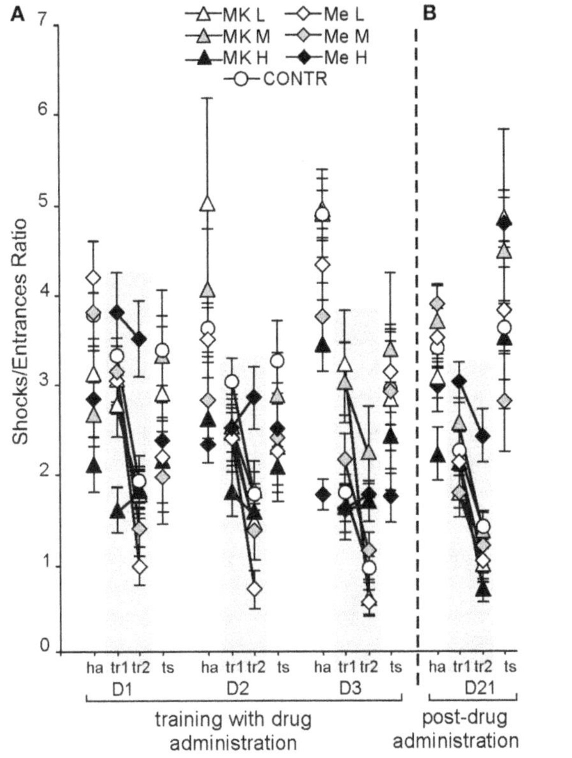

FIGURE 3 | Cognitive skill learning in the allothetic place avoidance alternation task was calculated as the ratio of shocks per entrances (SH/ENTR) into the shock sector which developed according to day and condition (A). On D1 the ratios for ha and tr1 were similar, whereas for D2 and D3 it decreased for tr1 in comparison to ha. Without any drug administration (D21), all rats presented similar skill levels in which performance was dependent on condition **(B)**. The values are presented as the grand average (±s.e.m.) according to group, day and condition. Other figure elements are the same as in **Figure 1**.

treated with middle or high doses of MK-801 and memantine presented similar ratios during ha and tr1. Rats from the high MK-801 and memantine groups presented similar ratios across all conditions. The *post-hoc* evaluation for the day by condition interaction [$F_{(6, 444)} = 6.27$; $P < 2 \times 10^{-5}$] showed that the ratios for ha and tr1 on D1 were similar, whereas on the next days the ratio for tr1 decreased compared to ha ($P < 0.0003$).

DOSE-RELATED EFFECTS OF MEMANTINE AND MK-801 ADMINISTRATION ON NON-COGNITIVE FUNCTIONS EXPRESSED BY THE DISTANCE WALKED BY RATS AND THE LINEARITY (STRAIGHTNESS), OF THE RAT'S PATH. THE HIGH DOSE OF MK-801 WAS ASSOCIATED WITH HYPERACTIVITY, BUT DID NOT AFFECT LINEARITY

The distance walked by rats was dependent on treatment and condition as confirmed by a significant effect of group [$F_{(6, 72)} = 21.01$; $P < 4 \times 10^{-13}$; MK-801H > all other groups] and condition [$F_{(3, 216)} = 4.69$; $P < 0.003$; tr2 > ha, tr1, ts], whereas an effect of day was not significant [$F_{(2, 144)} = 2.34$; $P = 0.099$] (**Figure 4A**). The *post-hoc* test for groups showed that the MK-801H rats walked more than the other rats ($P < 0.0001$; $P < 0.05$ for MemH). The rats from the CONTR group walked a shorter distance than the rats treated by high doses of memantine and MK-801. The *post-hoc* test for condition confirmed a longer distance for tr2 than for the other conditions ($P < 0.004$). Rats presented a similar distance during tr1, ha, and ts. The *post-hoc* evaluation of the group by day interaction [$F_{(12, 144)} = 8.81$; $P < 1.7 \times 10^{-11}$] confirmed that the MK-801H rats walked a similarly long distance every day, which was similar to that of the MemH rats on D3 ($P < 1.7 \times 10^{-5}$). Rats treated with MK-801H walked a long distance for all conditions [group by condition interaction $F_{(18, 216)} = 5.08$; $P < 1.2 \times 10^{-8}$; $P < 0.001$]. The *post-hoc* evaluation of the day by condition interaction [$F_{(6, 432)} = 7.19$; $P < 2.5 \times 10^{-6}$] confirmed a shorter path during habituation on D2 and D3 than for the other conditions ($P < 0.01$). No differences were found between tr1 and tr2 for all days.

Linearity, which represents the straightness of a rat's path in the arena according to a 20 ms sampling rate, changed dependent on treatment [$F_{(6, 72)} = 16.22$; $P < 10 \times 10^{-10}$; Control, low and MK-801M and MemM < MK-801H and MemH] and condition [$F_{(3, 216)} = 2.78$; $P < 0.04$; tr1 > ha] (**Figure 5A**). Rats from the high MK-801 and memantine groups walked straighter than the other rats (a high linearity value) ($P < 0.002$). Rats walked

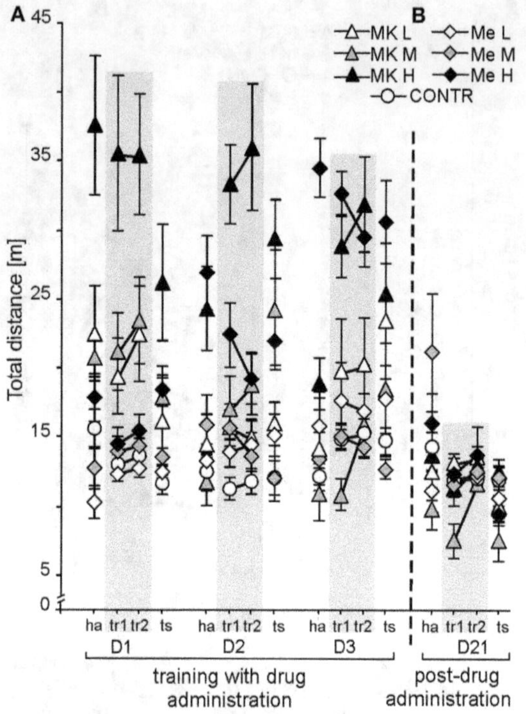

FIGURE 4 | Non-cognitive function was represented by the activity levels measured by the distance [m] walked in the allothetic place avoidance alternation task. After the high dose of MK-801 (MK-801H) the activity level was high across all days (D1-3), while it was only high for D3 following the high memantine dose (MemH) **(A)**. Without any drug administration (Day 21), hyperlocomotion in MK-801H rats post-treatment ceased and locomotion returned to a similar level as in other post-treated rats **(B)**. The values are presented as the grand average (±s.e.m.) according to group, day and condition. Other figure elements are the same as in **Figure 1**.

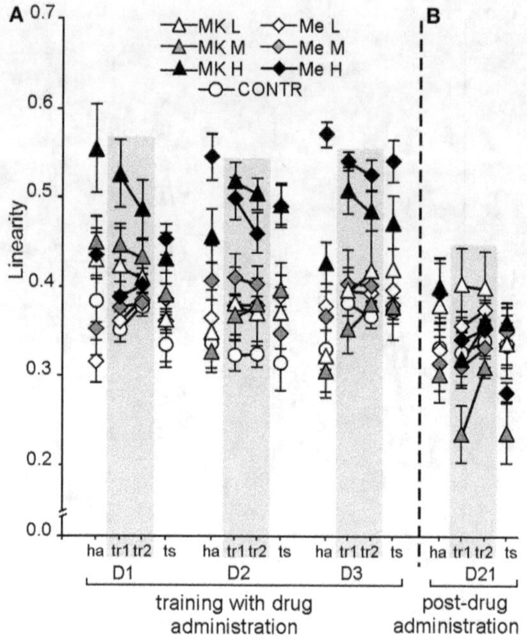

FIGURE 5 | The linearity of the path on the arena in the allothetic place avoidance task was straighter for the MK-801H rats across days (D1–3), and on D2 and D3 for the MemH rats (A). On D21, the linearity was dependent on condition **(B)**. The values are presented as the grand average (±s.e.m.) according to group, day and condition for rats treated with different doses of memantine or MK-801. Other figure elements are the same as in **Figure 1**.

straighter during tr1 than during ha and ts ($P < 0.03$), with no differences found between tr2 and the other conditions. The *post-hoc* evaluation of the group by day interaction [$F_{(12,\ 144)} = 5.54$; $P < 9 \times 10^{-7}$] showed that MK-801H rats presented a similar linearity value across days, which was similar to MemH except for on D1, but was higher than in the other groups of rats (*post-hoc* test; $P < 0.001$). The *post-hoc* evaluation of the group by condition interaction [$F_{(18,\ 216)} = 1.91$; $P < 0.016$] confirmed that the MK-801H and MemH rats had a similar linearity across conditions, which was higher than in the other groups independent of condition ($P < 0.0001$). The linearity values during ha and tr1on D1 and D2 were similar, which were lower than during tr1, tr2, and ts on D3 (*post-hoc*; $P < 0.01$) for the day by condition interaction [$F_{(6,\ 432)} = 4.941$; $P < 6 \times 10^{-4}$].

LONG-TERM EFFECTS (D21) ON WORKING MEMORY WITHOUT DRUG ADMINISTRATION

Proper functioning of working memory post-drug administration and early training (D21) was evidenced by a low number of entrances with a long maximum time avoided and via demonstration of the effective skill to avoid the new to-be-avoided sector.

Working memory performance in control rats and rats after memantine or MK-801 administration was assessed on D21 according to the number of entrances. A significant effect was confirmed for group [$F_{(6,\ 74)} = 3.98$; $P < 0.002$] and condition [$F_{(3,\ 222)} = 34.501$; $P < 2 \times 10^{-18}$] (**Figure 1B**). The *post-hoc* for group confirmed that MK-801H rats (no drug administered) performed better than MemH rats ($P < 0.002$), but the difference between the control and other treatment groups was not significant. The number of ENTR during tr2 was lower than during the other conditions (ha > tr2 < tr1, ts; $P < 0.001$).

The maximum time avoided showed significant effects of group [$F_{(6,\ 74)} = 6.37$; $P < 1,9 \times 10^{-4}$] and condition [$F_{(3,\ 222)} = 37.47$; $P < 1,2 \times 10^{-18}$], and a group by condition interaction [$F_{(18,\ 222)} = 1.80$; $P < 0.03$] (**Figure 2B**). Although the MK-801H rats presented a longer maximum avoidance time than the MK-801L, MK-801M and MemH rats ($P < 0.04$), it was similar to that for the control rats. The Tmax was longer during tr2 than during the tr1, ts and ha conditions ($P < 0.0001$), but no difference was found between tr1 and ts. The *post-hoc* test for the group by condition interaction confirmed that during tr2 the rats from the MK-801H group had a longer Tmax than the rats from the MK-801L, MemH and CONTR groups ($P < 0.03$). The MemH rats presented a shorter Tmax across all conditions.

The SH/ENTR ratio on D21 showed significant effects for condition [$F_{(3,\ 222)} = 74.04$; $P < 0.00001$] and for the group by condition interaction [$F_{(18,\ 222)} = 2.06$; $P < 0.008$]. There was a low ratio during tr2 and a high ratio during the ts compared to during tr1 and ha (*post-hoc* test; $P < 0.0002$). The ratio during tr1 was lower than during ha and the ts (*post-hoc* test; $P < 1 \times 10^{-7}$). The *post-hoc* test for the interaction showed similar SH/ENTR values during tr2 across groups (**Figure 3B**).

LONG-TERM EFFECTS (D21) ON NON-COGNITIVE FUNCTION WITHOUT DRUG ADMINISTRATION

On D21 the locomotor activity was dependent on condition [$F_{(3, 219)} = 9.66$; $P < 5 \times 10^{-5}$] and showed a group by condition interaction [$F_{(18, 219)} = 2.41$; $P < 0.0015$] (**Figure 4B**). All rats walked more during habituation and tr2 than during tr1 and ts ($P < 0.0001$). The *post-hoc* for the group by condition interaction confirmed that during habituation rats previously treated by MemM walked a longer distance than the other rats, except for the rats previously treated with MemH ($P < 0.001$). Furthermore, on D21 linearity was dependent on condition [$F_{(3, 216)} = 3.62$; $P < 0.01$] (**Figure 5B**). All rats walked a straighter path (higher linearity values) during tr2 than the ts ($P < 0.04$), while the values were equivalent during tr1 and the ts.

DISCUSSION

The presented study focused on comparisons of on-going cognitive and non-cognitive processes in the spatial working memory test, the APAAT task, using a wide range of doses of memantine and MK-801. We have shown that a low dose of memantine was associated with a short-lasting improvement in spatial working memory in comparison to the controls. Such an effect was not observed after application of a low dose of MK-801. However, at the low dose no differences in working memory were found between the two drug groups. CSL developed during the first training interval for groups with low doses of the agents. In contrast, high doses of the agents impaired working memory, negatively affected CSL and involved hyperactivity. In the same rats the after-effects of both agents were studied on D21 in the APAAT without drug application. Although all rats performed well in the working memory task and both maintained and updated their skill appropriately according to the novel sector location and the established session conditions, the MK-801H group avoided better during training 2 than the control, MK-801L and MemH groups. In contrast, the non-cognitive indices of locomotor activity (path length and linearity) showed dependence on the training conditions only.

In our working memory variant of the place avoidance test, in order to achieve accurate daily place avoidance, both stimuli segregation and short-term memory was required. The latter being necessary for the formation of new representations of the novel location of the shock sector. Memory acquisition occurred during tr1 and tr2, when the shock was presented, and was tested during the retrieval test (shock inactivated), which started 5 min after the end of tr2. With exposure to these conditions, intact rats improved place avoidance throughout the training sessions, when shocks were presented, and they generally continued to avoid even when the shock was inactivated during the retrieval test (Dockery and Wesierska, 2010). This variant differed from a previously presented working memory variant of place avoidance, wherein the location of the shock sector was alternated from day to day but the daily session did not include a habituation condition (5 min ha before avoidance training in our procedure) and consisted of only a single training interval (Cimadevilla et al., 2000). In such trials, comparison of working memory and CSL within a session was not possible as within a session the two abilities were mutually exclusive. This is due to the fact that in non-alternative variant of place avoidance the rats are always confronted with the same shock-sector location, meaning that they only have to learn the place it occurs in the room-frame coordinates itself. It does not necessitate, however, the application of the rule of how to avoid a to-be-a-frame (in any location), as is required in the alternative variant.

When taking into consideration the three components which comprise the working memory system in animals: goal maintenance, interference control, and memory capacity (Dudchenko et al., 2012), the working memory variant of active place avoidance used in this study seems to be a very useful tool to control the relation between these components. Furthermore, it offers the possibility to test non-cognitive behavior in intact and pharmacologically treated animals. To break down the components according to the APAA task conditions, the place avoidance during tr1, tr2 can be related to goal maintenance, as the rats must use the representation of the shock sector in order to avoid, for a long period of time, entering the actual place where shocks could be delivered. Moreover, interference control also relates to formation of a new representation, which occurs in the consequent session (e.g., from D1 to D2). Thus, interference control would be responsible for proper avoidance in each consecutive session. Better place avoidance performance in tr2 compared to tr1 depends on more effective on-going memory and, in this way, could be related to memory capacity. All components, maintenance, interference control and memory capacity were impaired under NMDARs blockade by high doses, in contrast to low and middle doses of the antagonists, memantine and MK-801. Hence, although the APAAT currently has no complementary human setup, it has been shown to be a useful tool to study the relation between components of working memory and the underlying mechanisms which control this system.

Working or short-term memory has been previously monitored by other authors/research groups in several animal models of spatial working memory under different doses of memantine or MK-801 with the primary aim to utilize these NMDAR antagonists as therapeutic treatment against excitotoxicity in neurodegenerative diseases (see Ref. in Introduction). In the presented study, acute application of memantine in a dose of 5 mg/kg preserved or even facilitated spatial working memory functioning in the APAAT. Similar to the control rats, this therapeutic dose resulted in a low number of entrances during the training and test conditions and also involved short-lasting enhancement of memory in tr 2, which manifested as a significantly longer maximum time avoided. For comparisons low doses of memantine (0.3; 0.56 mg/kg), but not a higher dose (1.0 mg/kg), enhanced spatial memory after a 18 h delay in the radial maze task, whereas higher doses (3 and 10 mg/kg) totally abolished choice accuracy in the same test (Wise and Lichtman, 2007). In contrast, enhancement of long-term memory was found after a 24 h delay in the radial arm water maze for the 5 and 7.5 mg/kg, but not the 2.5

and 3.75 mg/kg doses. In the same test the same doses had no effect on short–term memory acquisition and retention which was tested after a 15 min delay (Zoladz et al., 2006). Daily continuous infusion of 20 mg/kg memantine by minipumps did not impair working memory in the radial maze (Zajaczkowski et al., 1996). Contradictory to this data, acute memantine application at a high dose (20 mg/kg) negatively affected working memory in our experimental conditions, which manifested as a higher number of entrances with a short maximum time avoided across days.

Discrepancy in the obtained results, as reflected by the data reported here from various behavioral procedures (dry vs. water maze; appetitive vs. aversive conditions), are the result of differences in the memantine plasma concentration during the experimental session, which are dependent on the dose and means of administration (Zoladz et al., 2006).

In view of the similarities and differences between memantine and MK-801, an effect of the latter drug was also studied in terms of memory functioning. Unlike low dose memantine, the low dose of MK-801 (0.1 mg/kg) had no effect on working memory enhancement. However, alike memantine, the high dose of MK-801 (0.3 mg/kg) abolished working memory across the training and test conditions. These results are consistent with recently published data from the Stuchlik Laboratory (Zemanova et al., 2013) which revealed memory impairment in the APAAT after MK-801 in doses of 0.12 and 0.15 mg/kg in naive rats but not in pre-trained rats. Moreover, in the active place avoidance task, MK-801 in the 0.2, but not the 0.15 mg/kg impaired reacquisition of avoidance in the training conditions, whereas both doses impaired place avoidance performance in a new environment (Stuchlík and Vales, 2005). Our experiment was conducted on naive rats in the same environment with doses lower (0.1 mg/kg) and higher (0.3 mg/kg) than those in the previous studies which further supports the reliability of our results. Effect of MK-801 on working memory depending on the dose also in other tests on spatial memory. In the radial maze task working memory was preserved with the 0.05, 0.01, mg/kg 0.08 and 0.1 mg/kg doses and impaired with 0.12, 0.15 or 0.2 mg/kg of MK-801 (Wozniak et al., 1990; White and Best, 1998; Kretschmer and Fink, 1999). However, acquisition of working memory itself and in a new environment in the radial maze was impaired after a 0.0625 mg/kg dose of MK-801 (Shapiro and O'Connor, 1992). Chronic application of MK-801 at a 0.312 mg/kg daily dose by minipumps not impaired working memory in the radial maze test (Zajaczkowski et al., 1996). Contrary to dry radial maze test a single application of MK-801 at the 0.25, 0.5, 2, and 4 mg/kg doses impaired spatial working memory in the water maze on day 1 but this effect disappeared on day 4 (Whishaw and Auer, 1989). It has also been shown that the effect of different doses of MK-801 on spatial memory performance and locomotor activity depend on the experimental procedure, e.g., the water maze test seems to be more sensitive to MK-801 than the dry open field test (Wegener et al., 2011).

To summarize, MK-801 in low doses (0.05 mg/kg, 0.08 mg/kg), was found to have no effect on working memory in naive rats (Wozniak et al., 1990; Kretschmer and Fink, 1999), whereas pre-training in the working memory task preserved memory function even with the higher dose of MK-801 (0.12 or 0.15 mg/kg) (Zemanova et al., 2013). Thus, taking into account the cited literature, we believe that the 0.1 mg/kg dose of (+)MK-801 is sufficiently low, and that lowering it would likely produce negligible effects on working memory in our APAAT.

The shocks/entrance ratio was a useful tool to measure CSL, by which a high ratio expressed poor learning. During habituation, when shock was never applied, the SH/ENTR ratio expresses a "dummy" ratio. Here it was at a similarly high level for all rats, thus confirming that drugs application and the experimental conditions, such as the arena rotation, which was the same for all rats, did not change the rats' spontaneous activity. On D1 the value of the SH/ENTR ratio in all groups was similar for ha and tr1. On this day the task rules were acquired. For D2-3 in all groups, except the high dose groups, the SH/ENTR ratio was lower during tr2 than during tr1 and ha. It means that the rats with low and mild doses of both drugs successfully acquired the task rules. However, on D2-3, it was only for the rats under high doses of both agents that the ratio during tr1 and tr2 was similar with no improvement. That means that high doses of those agents suppressed CSL.

This is in concert with proper performance of working memory and flexible cognitive skill acquisition after low doses of the agents, and consequently memory impairment and disturbed CSL after the high doses related to the within session conditions and an across session learning effect. In spite of a high number of entrances after high doses of memantine and MK-801, the SH/ENTR ratio was at a similar level across session conditions which was similar to other groups (a non-significant group effect). This suggests that high doses of both agents did not disturb the ability to quickly recognize the shock sector and minimize the shocks by escaping, thereby reducing the total number of shocks obtained per entrance even while the number of entrances itself may have been high. Such an effective escape reaction could be due to the higher locomotor activity after high MK-801 across days and high memantine on D3. The different results for working memory performance and CSL could be explained by the heterogeneous nature of the components which belong to the working memory system (Baddeley, 1992; Dudchenko et al., 2000).

Measures of non-cognitive behavior were indexed by the activity characteristics: path length, and linearity. The path length was longer with the high dose of MK-801 independent of day and session condition. Contrary to the high dose of MK-801, hyperactivity related to the high dose of memantine developed throughout the training sessions. Independent of the doses of both agents, all rats walked more during tr 2 than in the other conditions. This result was in opposite to the findings presented by Zemanova et al. (2013), who showed that dose and day but not condition affect the impact of MK-801 on total distance. In training which focused on a stable shock sector location on arena, locomotor activity also increased with the 0.2 mg/kg, but not the 0.15 or 0.1 mg/kg of MK-801 (Stuchlík and Vales, 2005; Vales et al., 2010). In a swimming task the locomotor activity was dose-dependent and time dependent, in which it was impaired 3 h after MK-801 treatment in the doses: 0.25, 0.5, 1.0, 2.0, and 4.0 mg/kg. This was relevant for four of the consecutive post–treatment days, but not for the fifth day (Whishaw and Auer, 1989). Moreover, MK-801 in the 10 mg/kg dose resulted in catalepsy and doses higher than 10 mg/kg were found to be lethal (Whishaw and Auer, 1989). Memantine in a high dose (20 mg/kg) was reported to produce strong motor disturbance in females rats, which was expressed as hypoactivity 10 min after application and progressed to hyperactivity 90 min after drug administration (Creeley et al., 2006). The male rats in our experiments also presented higher locomotor activity after 20 mg/kg memantine but they were able to solve the APAAT task.

Linearity is a unique measure of motor activity that according to our knowledge is currently only calculated using the place avoidance method. Here, a high linearity score (a straighter path) was observed in high dose MK-801 group, which also showed a significantly longer walk distance compared to other groups. Both a long path length and high linearity were noted in rats from the high dose memantine group on all days of training except the first one.

The after-effect of memantine and MK-801 treatment on cognitive and non-cognitive functions was tested with a new shock sector location on D21, 18 days from the last exposure to the agents. Because this period was over the half-life time for memantine and MK-801 (Morè et al., 2008; Wegener et al., 2011) proper place avoidance by rats from all groups was expected without side effects. The results confirmed a lack of differences in working memory performance between the control rats and the rats previously treated with either low or high doses of the agents. This is in accordance with results in which a high dose of MK-801 (5 mg/kg) and memantine (20 or 40 mg/kg) administered intraperitoneally 8 days before training in the radial maze did not affect acquisition of spatial working memory (Zajaczkowski et al., 2000). However, detailed analysis of working memory performance across session conditions shows that during tr2, rats previously treated with the high MK-801 presented a lower number of entrances with a longer maximum time avoided than the groups previously treated with the high memantine dose, low MK-801 dose and the control rats. All rats on D21 showed a similar level of performance for cognitive skill retention/learning. The results primarily show an effect of the session condition in which locomotor activity and linearity was better (short distance, with a low level of linearity) for all groups of rats during the last 5 min of place avoidance training (tr2) than in the other conditions.

CONCLUSION

We found that, independent of dose, memantine and MK-80 have different effects on cognitive and non-cognitive functions. Furthermore, dose-dependent effects were found in which memantine in a low dose involved short-lasting improvement in spatial working memory. MK-801 in a low dose, which was found to produce schizophrenia-like symptoms in an animal model, supported working memory performance at the level of the control rats. Both agents in low doses had no effect on non-cognitive functions.

Severe impairment of working memory and disturbance in locomotor activity were produced by the high dose of MK-801 already on the first training session, whereas similar effects with the high dose of memantine developed over time. Differential results for the intra- and across session effects were found for the cognitive processes, working memory and CSL, which confirms that these components reflect the heterogeneous nature of the working memory system. No delayed (long-term) effects of previous drug treatment, except for high dose of memantine, on either cognitive or non-cognitive functions were observed. After a long break without memantine and MK-801 treatment performance was associated with proper working memory and locomotor activity comparable to that of controls. Interestingly, the high dose of MK-801 resulted in improved cognitive performance 18 days after the last drug administration.

The APAAT method offers a valuable and unique behavioral tool to simultaneously compare cognitive and non-cognitive functions under pharmacological intervention. In this study specifically NMDAr blockade, which can help develop concrete models for the therapeutic treatment of neurodegenerative disorders and diseases related to excitotoxicity, was employed. This expands the value of the APAAT beyond its capacity to measure working memory and CSL (Dockery and Wesierska, 2010).

AUTHORS CONTRIBUTIONS

Malgorzata J. Wesierska and Colleen A. Dockery designed the research; Malgorzata J. Wesierska, Colleen A. Dockery, equally contributed to ca. 60% of experimentation; Weronika Duda performed ca. 40% of the experiments; Malgorzata J. Wesierska analyzed and interpreted the data and prepared the manuscript; Colleen A. Dockery also prepared the manuscript and was responsible for corrections of the English.

ACKNOWLEDGMENTS

The authors thank J. Sadowska and W. Borkowski for their substantial technical assistance. Supported by grant MNiSW, NCN, 8165/B/P01/2011/40.

REFERENCES

Anderson, J. R., Fincham, J. M., and Douglass, S. (1997). The role of examples and rules in the acquisition of a cognitive skill. *J. Exp. Psychol. Learn. Mem. Cogn.* 23, 932–945. doi: 10.1037/0278-7393.23.4.932

Baddeley, A. (1992).Working memory. Science 255, 556–559. doi: 10.1126/science.1736359

Burette, F., Jay, T., and Laroche, S. (2000). Synaptic depression of the hippocampal to prefrontal cortex pathway during a spatial working memory task. *Cur. Psychol. Lett.* 1, 9–23.

Chen, H.S., and Lipton, S.A. (2006). The chemical biology of clinically tolerated NMDA receptor antagonists. J. Neurochem. 97, 1611–1626. doi: 10.1111/j.1471-4159.2006.03991.x

Cerella, J., Onyper, S. V., and Hoyer, W. J. (2006). The associative-memory basis of cognitive skill learning: adult age differences. *Psychol. Aging* 21, 483–498. doi: 10.1037/0882-7974.21.3.483

Cimadevilla, J. M., Kaminsky, Y., Fenton, A., and Bures, J. (2000). Passive and active place avoidance as a tool of spatial memory research in rats. *J. Neurosci. Methods* 102, 155–164. doi: 10.1016/S0165-0270(00)00288-0

Cowan, N. (2008). What are the differences between long-term, short-term, and working memory? *Prog. Brain Res.* 169, 323–338. doi: 10.1016/S0079-6123(07)00020-9

Creeley, C., Wozniak, D. F., Labruyere, J., Taylor, G. T., and Olney, J. W. (2006). Low doses of memantine disrupt memory in adult rats. *J. Neurosci.* 26, 3923–3932. doi: 10.1523/JNEUROSCI.4883-05.2006

Danysz, W., Parsons, C. G., Kornhuber, J., Schmidt, W. J., and Quack, G. (1997). Aminoadamantanes as NMDA receptor antagonists and antiparkinsonian agents–preclinical studies. Neurosci. Biobehav. Rev. 21, 455–468. doi: 10.1016/S0149-7634(96)00037-1

Dockery, C. A. (2013). "The human experiment: how we won't win the rat race. what can we learn from brain stimulation in humans and rats about enhancing the functional neurobiology of higher cognitive functions?," in *Cognitive Enhancement. An Interdisciplinary Perspective Series (Trends in Augmentation of Human Performance)*, eds E. Hilde and A. G. Franke (Dordrecht: Springer), 73–91.

Dockery, C. A., Hueckel-Weng, R., Birbaumer, N., and Plewnia, C. (2009). Enhancement of planning ability by transcranial direct current stimulation. *J. Neurosci.* 29, 7271–7277. doi: 10.1523/JNEUROSCI.0065-09.2009

Dockery, C. A., Liebetanz, D., Birbaumer, N., Malinowska, M., and Wesierska, M. J. (2011). Cumulative benefits of frontal transcranial direct current stimulation on visuospatial working memory training and skill learning in rats. *Neurobiol. Learn. Mem.* 96, 452–460. doi: 10.1016/j.nlm.2011.06.018

Dockery, C. A., and Wesierska, M. J. (2010). A spatial paradigm, the allothetic place avoidance alternation task, for testing visuospatial working memory and skill learning in rats. *J. Neurosci. Methods* 191, 215–221. doi: 10.1016/j.jneumeth.2010.06.029

Dudchenko, P. A. (2004). An overview of the tasks used to test working memory in rodents. Neurosci. Biobehav. Rev. 28, 699–709. doi: 10.1016/j.neubiorev.2004.09.002

Dudchenko, P. A., Talpos, J., Young, J., and Baxter, M. G. (2012). Animal models of working memory: a review of tasks that might be used in screening drug treatments for the memory impairments found in schizophrenia. *Neurosci. Biobehav. Rev.* 37, 2111–2124. doi: 10.1016/j.neubiorev.2012.03.003

Dudchenko, P. A., Wood, E. R., and Eichenbaum, H. (2000). Neurotoxic hippocampal lesions have no effect on odor span and little effect on odor recognition memory but produce significant impairments on spatial span, recognition, and alternation. *J. Neurosci.* 20, 2964–2977.

Elvevåg, B., Weinberger, D. R., Suter, J. C., and Goldberg, T. E. (2000). Continuous performance test and schizophrenia: a test of stimulus-response compatibility, working memory, response readiness, or none of the above? *Am. J. Psychiatry* 157, 772–780. doi: 10.1176/appi.ajp.157.5.772

Goldman-Rakic, P. S. (1995). Cellular basis of working memory. *Neuron* 14, 477–485. doi: 10.1016/0896-6273(95)90304-6

Heuer, E., and Bachevalier, J. (2012). Working memory for temporal order is impaired after selective neonatal hippocampal lesions in adult rhesus macaques. *Behav. Brain Res.* 239, 55–62. doi: 10.1016/j.bbr.2012.10.043

Jay, T. M., and Witter, M. P. (1991). Distribution of hippocampal CA1 and subicular efferents in the prefrontal cortex of the rat studied by means of anterograde transport of Phaseolus vulgaris-leucoagglutinin. *J. Comp. Neurol.* 313, 574–586. doi: 10.1002/cne.903130404

Klingberg, T. (2010). Training and plasticity of working memory. *Trends. Cogn. Sci.* 14, 317–324. doi: 10.1016/j.tics.2010.05.002

Kretschmer, B. D., and Fink, S. (1999). Spatial learning deficit after NMDA receptor blockade and state-dependency. *Behav. Pharmacol.* 10, 423–428. doi: 10.1097/00008877-199907000-00009

Lee, I., and Kesner, R. P. (2002). Differential contribution of NMDA receptors in hippocampal subregions to spatial working memory. *Nat. Neurosci.*5, 162–168. doi: 10.1038/nn790

Lee, Y., Lu, M., and Ko, H. (2007). Effects of skill training on working memory capacity. *Learn. Instr.* 17, 336–344. doi: 10.1016/j.learninstruc.2007.02.010

Light, K. R., Kolata, S., Wass, C., Denman-Brice, A., Zagalsky, R., and Matzel, L. D. (2010). Working memory training promotes general cognitive abilities in genetically heterogeneous mice. *Curr. Biol.* 20, 777–782. doi: 10.1016/j.cub.2010.02.034

Lynch, M. A. (2004). Long-term potentiation and memory. *Physiol. Rev.* 84, 87–136. doi: 10.1152/physrev.00014.2003

Manahan-Vaughan, D., von Haebler, D., Winter, C., Juckel, G., and Heinemann, U. (2008). A single application of MK801 causes symptoms of acute psychosis, deficits in spatial memory, and impairment of synaptic plasticity in rats. *Hippocampus* 18, 125–134. doi: 10.1002/hipo.20367

Mondadori, C., Weiskrantz, L., Buerki, H., Petschke, F., and Fagg, G. E. (1989). NMDA receptor antagonists can enhance or impair learning performance in animals. *Exp. Brain Res.* 75, 449–456. doi: 10.1007/BF00249896

Morè, L., Gravius, A., Nagel, J., Valastro, B., Greco, S., and Danysz, W. (2008). Therapeutically relevant plasma concentrations of memantine produce significant L-N-methyl-D-aspartate receptor occupation and do not impair learning in rats. *Behav. Pharmacol.* 19, 724–734. doi: 10.1097/FBP.0b013e3283123cad

Nakazawa, K., Sun, L. D., Quirk, M. C., Rondi-Reig, L., Wilson, M. A., and Tonegawa, S. (2003). Hippocampal CA3 NMDA receptors are crucial for memory acquisition of one-time experience. *Neuron* 38, 305–315. doi: 10.1016/S0896-6273(03)00165-X

Niewoehner, B., Single, F. N., Hvalby, Ø., Jensen, V., Meyer zum Alten Borgloh, S., Seeburg, P. H., et al. (2007). Impaired spatial working memory but spared spatial reference memory following functional loss of NMDA receptors in the dentate gyrus. *Eur. J. Neurosci.* 25, 837–846. doi: 10.1111/j.1460-9568.2007.05312.x

Olesen, P. J., Westerberg, H., and Klingberg, T. (2004). Increased prefrontal and parietal activity after training of working memory. *Nat. Neurosci.* 7, 75–79. doi: 10.1038/nn1165

Paoletti, P., Bellone, C., and Zhou, Q. (2013). NMDA receptor subunit diversity: impact on receptor properties, synaptic plasticity and disease. *Nat. Rev. Neurosci.* 14, 383–400. doi: 10.1038/nrn3504

Parsons, C. G., Quack, G., Bresink, I., Baran, L., Przegalinski, E., Kostowski, W., et al. (1995). Comparison of the potency, kinetics and voltage-dependency of a series of uncompetitive NMDA receptor antagonists *in vitro* with anticonvulsive and motor impairment activity *in vivo*. *Neuropharmacology* 34, 1239–1258. doi: 10.1016/0028-3908(95)00092-K

Parsons, C. G., Stöffler, A., and Danysz, W. (2007). Memantine: a NMDA receptor antagonist that improves memory by restoration of homeostasis in the glutamatergic system–too little activation is bad, too much is even worse. *Neuropharmacology* 53, 699–723. doi: 10.1016/j.neuropharm.2007.07.013

Pastalkova, E., Serrano, P., Pinkhasova, D., Wallace, E., Fenton, A. A., and Sacktor, T. C. (2006). Storage of spatial information by the maintenance mechanism of LTP. *Science* 313, 1141–1144. doi: 10.1126/science.1128657

Phillips, W. A., and Silverstein, S. M. (2003). Convergence of biological and psychological perspectives on cognitive coordination in schizophrenia. Behav. Brain Sci. 26, 65–82. discussion: 82–137. doi: 10.1017/S0140525X03000025

Poldrack, R. A., Prabhakaran, V., Seger, C. A., and Gabrieli, J. D. (1999). Striatal activation during acquisition of a cognitive skill. *Neuropsychology* 13, 564–574. doi: 10.1037/0894-4105.13.4.564

Repovs, G., and Baddeley, A. (2006). The multi-component model of working memory: explorations in experimental cognitive psychology. *Neuroscience* 139, 5–21. doi: 10.1016/j.neuroscience.2005.12.061

Schwarz, A. J., Gass, N., Sartorius, A., Zheng, L., Spedding, M., Schenker, E., et al. (2013). The low-frequency blood oxygenation level-dependent functional connectivity signature of the hippocampal-prefrontal network in the rat brain. *Neuroscience* 228, 243–258. doi: 10.1016/j.neuroscience.2012.10.032

Seidler, R. D., Bo, J., and Anguera, J. A. (2012). Neurocognitive contributions to motor skill learning: the role of working memory. *J. Mot. Behav.* 44, 445–453. doi: 10.1080/00222895.2012.672348

Shapiro, M. L., and O'Connor, C. (1992). N-methyl-D-aspartate receptor antagonist MK-801 and spatial memory representation: working memory is impaired in an unfamiliar environment but not in a familiar environment. *Behav. Neurosci.*106, 604–612. doi: 10.1037/0735-7044.106.4-604

Smith, J. W., Gastambide, F., Gilmour, G., Dix, S., Foss, J., Lloyd, K., et al. (2011). A comparison of the effects of ketamine and phencyclidine with other antagonists of the NMDA receptor in rodent assays of attention and working memory, *Psychopharmacology (Berl)* 217, 255–269. doi: 10.1007/s00213-011-2277-5

Stagg, C. J., Best, J. G., Stephenson, M. C., O'Shea, J., Wylezinska, M., Kincses, Z. T., et al. (2009). Polarity-sensitive modulation of cortical neurotransmitters by transcranial stimulation. *J. Neurosci.* 29, 5202–5206. doi: 10.1523/JNEUROSCI.4432-08.2009

Stuchlík, A., and Vales, K. (2005). Systemic administration of MK-801, a non-competitive NMDA-receptor antagonist, elicits a behavioural deficit of rats in the Active Allothetic Place Avoidance (AAPA) task irrespectively of their intact spatial pretraining. *Behav. Brain Res.* 159, 163–171. doi: 10.1016/j.bbr.2004.10.013

Timofeeva, O. A., and Levin, E. D. (2011). Glutamate and nicotinic receptor interactions in working memory: importance for the cognitive impairment of schizophrenia. *Neuroscience* 195, 21–36. doi: 10.1016/j.neuroscience.2011.08.038

Vales, K., Svoboda, J., Benkovicova, K., Bubenikova-Valesova, V., and Stuchlik, A. (2010). The difference in effect of mGlu2/3 and mGlu5 receptor agonists on cognitive impairment induced by MK-801. *Eur. J. Pharmacol.* 639, 91–98. doi: 10.1016/j.ejphar.2009.11.067

Wang, M., Yang, Y., Wang, C. J., Gamo, N. J., Jin, L. E., Mazer, J. A., et al. (2013). NMDA receptors subserve persistent neuronal firing during working memory in dorsolateral prefrontal cortex. *Neuron* 77, 736–749. doi: 10.1016/j.neuron.2012.12.032

Wegener, N., Nagel, J., Gross, R., Chambon, C., Greco, S., Pietraszek, M., et al. (2011). Evaluation of brain pharmacokinetics of (+) MK-801 in relation to behaviour. *Neurosci Lett.* 503, 68–72. doi: 10.1016/j.neulet.2011.08.012

Wesierska, M., Adamska, I., and Malinowska, M. (2009). Retrosplenial cortex lesion affects segregation of spatial information in the place avoidance task in the rat. *Neurobiol. Learn. Mem.* 91, 41–49. doi: 10.1016/j.nlm.2008.09.005

Wesierska, M., Dockery, C., Fenton, A. A. (2005). Beyond memory, navigation, and inhibition: behavioral evidence for hippocampus-dependent cognitive coordination in the rat. *J. Neurosci.* 25, 2413–2419. doi: 10.1523/JNEUROSCI.3962-04.2005

Westerberg, H., and Klingberg, T. (2007). Changes in cortical activity after training of working memory–a single-subject analysis. *Physiol. Behav.* 92, 186–192. doi: 10.1016/j.physbeh.2007.05.041

Whishaw, I. Q., and Auer, R. N. (1989). Immediate and long-lasting effects of MK-801 on motor activity, spatial navigation in a swimming pool and EEG in the rat. *Psychopharmacology (Berl).* 98, 500–507. doi: 10.1007/BF00441949

White, A. M., and Best, P. J. (1998). The effects of MK-801 on spatial working memory and within-session spatial learning. *Pharmacol. Biochem. Behav.* 59, 613–617. doi: 10.1016/S0091-3057(97)00483-8

Wong, E. H., Kemp, J. A., Priestley, T., Knight, A. R., Woodruff, G. N., and Iversen, L. L. (1986). The anticonvulsant MK-801 is a potent N-methyl-D-aspartate antagonist. *Proc. Natl. Acad. Sci. U.S.A.* 83, 7104–7108. doi: 10.1073/pnas.83.18.7104

Wozniak, D. F., Olney, J. W., Kettinger, L. 3rd., Price, M., and Miller, J. P. (1990). Behavioral effects of MK-801 in the rat. *Psychopharmacology (Berl).*101, 47–56. doi: 10.1007/BF02253717

Yoshihara, T., and Ichitani, Y. (2004). Hippocampal N-methyl-D-aspartate receptor-mediated encoding and retrieval processes in spatial working memory: delay-interposed radial maze performance in rats. *Neuroscience* 129, 1–10. doi: 10.1016/j.neuroscience.2004.07.030

Zajaczkowski, W., Hetman, M., Nikolaev, E., Quack, G., Danysz, W., and Kaczmarek, L. (2000). Behavioural evaluation of long-term neurotoxic effects of NMDA receptor antagonists. *Neurotox. Res.* 1, 299–310. doi: 10.1007/BF03033259

Zajaczkowski, W., Quack, G., and Danysz, W. (1996). Infusion of (+) -MK-801 and memantine – contrasting effects on radial maze learning in rats with entorhinal cortex lesion. *Eur. J. Pharmacol.* 296, 239–246. doi: 10.1016/0014-2999(95)00716-4

Zemanova, A., Stankova, A., Lobellova, V., Svoboda, J., Vales, K., Vlcek, K., et al. (2013). Visuospatial working memory is impaired in an animal model of schizophrenia induced by acute MK-801: an effect of pretraining. *Pharmacol. Biochem. Behav.* 106, 117–123. doi: 10.1016/j.pbb.2013.03.014

Zoladz, P. R., Campbell, A. M., Park, C. R., Schaefer, D., Danysz, W., and Diamond, D. M. (2006). Enhancement of long-term spatial memory in adult rats by the noncompetitive NMDA receptor antagonists, memantine and neramexane. *Pharmacol. Biochem. Behav.* 85, 298–306. doi: 10.1016/j.pbb.2006.08.011

13

Neurosonological examination: a non-invasive approach for the detection of cerebrovascular impairment in AD

Barbora Urbanova[1]*, Ales Tomek[1], Robert Mikulik[2], Hana Magerova[1], Daniel Horinek[3,4] and Jakub Hort[1,4]

[1] *Department of Neurology, 2nd Faculty of Medicine, Motol University Hospital, Charles University, Prague, Czech Republic*
[2] *Department of Neurology, International Clinical Research Center, St. Anne's University Hospital, Brno, Czech Republic*
[3] *Department of Neurosurgery, 1st Faculty of Medicine, Central Military Hospital, Charles University, Prague, Czech Republic*
[4] *International Clinical Research Center, St. Anne's University Hospital, Brno, Czech Republic*

Edited by:
Ales Stuchlik, Academy of Sciences of the Czech Republic, Czech Republic

***Correspondence:**
Barbora Urbanova, Department of Neurology, 2nd Faculty of Medicine, Motol University Hospital, Charles University, V Uvalu 84, 15000 Prague 5, Czech Republic
e-mail: barbora.urbanova@gmail.com

There has been a growing interest in vascular impairment associated with Alzheimer's disease (AD). This interest was stimulated by the findings of higher incidence of vascular risk factors in AD. Signs of vascular impairment were investigated notably in the field of imaging methods. Our aim was to explore ultrasonographic studies of extra- and intracranial vessels in patients with AD and mild cognitive impairment (MCI) and define implications for diagnosis, treatment, and prevention of the disease. The most frequently studied parameters with extracranial ultrasound are intima-media thickness in common carotid artery, carotid atherosclerosis, and total cerebral blood flow. The transcranial ultrasound concentrates mostly on flow velocities, pulsatility indices, cerebrovascular reserve capacity, and cerebral microembolization. Studies suggest that there is morphological and functional impairment of cerebral circulation in AD compared to healthy subjects. Ultrasound as a non-invasive method could be potentially useful in identifying individuals in a higher risk of progression of cognitive decline.

Keywords: Alzheimer's disease, carotid ultrasound, cerebrovascular reserve capacity, neurosonology, transcranial ultrasound

VASCULAR CHANGES AND ALZHEIMER'S DISEASE

In an effort to reveal an etiopathogenic mechanism responsible for Alzheimer's disease (AD) many hypotheses have been postulated. Recent failures of candidate disease-modifying medications have led to many alternative theories of AD pathophysiology. Multiple studies suggest that the risk of AD is apart from other factors associated with midlife hypertension, diabetes mellitus, hypercholesterolemia, and other vascular risk factors (Breteler, 2000; Casserly and Topol, 2004; Gorelick, 2004; Shah et al., 2012). This association has led to a hypothesis that the vascular risk factors could play an important role in the genesis or in the progression of the disease, but even after years of research the role of vascular risk factors in AD remains a subject of discussion. Two principal theories were postulated. First, an impaired cerebral circulation from any cause leads to neurodegeneration (de la Torre, 2010). Second, vascular impairment from any cause (e.g., atherosclerosis) accelerates the rate of progression of neurodegeneration (Kalaria, 2002). The second theory is generally more accepted.

Various imaging methods were used to explore the signs of vascular impairment in AD. White matter lesions in people above 65 years are associated with typical vascular risk factors and cognitive decline (Breteler et al., 1994; DeCarli et al., 2001; Wu et al., 2002). Higher extent of white matter lesions in MCI patients is associated with higher risk of progression of MCI to dementia of any kind (Wolf et al., 2000). In MCI patients, there is a regional hypoperfusion on SPECT examination in hippocampus, amygdala, and prefrontal cortex (Johnson et al., 1998), and in AD patients the perfusion is decreased in whole temporoparietal region and correlates with the disease severity (DeKosky et al., 1990) [AD patient with varying disease severity were divided into four groups according to mini-mental state examination (MMSE): >24; 22–24; 15–21; <15].

The objective of this review was to explore extracranial and transcranial ultrasound projects in AD patients. We tried to describe the pattern of functional or structural cerebrovascular impairment in AD as characterized by ultrasonography, and to summarize ultrasound parameters of cerebral circulation in AD vs. healthy control subjects or in AD patients longitudinally. We have discussed to what extent neurosonological examination could contribute to diagnosis, prevention, or treatment of AD. We have also discussed whether there is a special pattern of circulation impairment, namely: Is AD associated with large vessel or, rather, small vessel disease? Are there predominant changes in a specific region of the brain? Is the incidence of microembolization higher in AD, or is there a correlation of any parameter with disease progression?

EXTRACRANIAL ULTRASOUND IN AD

Main parameters that can be assessed by extracranial ultrasound are parameters of arterial wall [carotid intima-media thickness (IMT) and atherosclerotic plaques] and cerebral perfusion [total cerebral blood flow (CBF)].

IMT AND CAROTID ATHEROSCLEROSIS

Carotid IMT is defined as a distance between media–adventitia interface and intima–lumen interface measured on the common carotid artery, 1–2 cm proximally from bifurcation or, less frequently, on the internal carotid artery using automated analyzers implemented in most of the recent ultrasound devices. IMT is generally regarded as a marker of atherosclerosis and is a good predictor of future vascular events (Lorenz et al., 2007). To ensure the accuracy of IMT measurements, it is necessary to meet the technical, methodological, and operator related criteria (Gonzalez et al., 2008; Stein et al., 2009; Dogan et al., 2010; Society of Atherosclerosis Imaging and Prevention Developed in collaboration with the International Atherosclerosis Society, 2011; Touboul et al., 2012). Thanks to these criteria, the validity and reproducibility of IMT measurement are sufficient and IMT measurement is widely used in clinical practice as well as in the research, and is implemented in several guidelines for cardiovascular risk assessment (National Cholesterol Education Program (NCEP) Expert Panel on Detection, Evaluation, and Treatment of High Blood Cholesterol in Adults (Adult Treatment Panel III), 2002; de la Sierra et al., 2009; Stein et al., 2009; Greenland et al., 2010; Society of Atherosclerosis Imaging and Prevention Developed in collaboration with the International Atherosclerosis Society, 2011).

Atherosclerotic plaque is defined as a focal structure at a vessel wall protruding into the arterial lumen showing a thickness of more than 1.5 mm from the adventitia–media interface (Touboul et al., 2012). Number, proportions, and location of plaques as well as the presence of carotid stenosis caused by plaques need to be considered in the assessment of carotid atherosclerosis severity. The severity of carotid stenosis is quantified according to the flow velocities in the stenosis, residual lumen, and internal carotid artery/common carotid artery flow velocities ratio (Grant et al., 2003). There was a great emphasis on the standardization of the stenosis assessment for the reason of legitimate indication of carotid endarterectomy. The validity and reproducibility of the examination are sufficient for clinical as well as research purposes as long as the technical and personnel conditions are fulfilled (Mohler et al., 2012).

Epidemiological studies have evidenced that AD and VD share common risk factors, which include vascular risk factors such as hypertension, smoking, diabetes mellitus, and hypercholesterolemia (Casserly and Topol, 2004; Gorelick, 2004). These risk factors are also the principal risk factors of atherosclerosis (Greco et al., 2013); considering this, we would expect higher prevalence of large vessel disease in AD than in general population. The results of two large substudies of the prospective cohort of population-based Rotterdam study are in accordance with this hypothesis (Hofman et al., 1997; van Oijen et al., 2007). Both of these substudies were focused on IMT and the degree of carotid (and generally peripheral) atherosclerosis in demented, both AD and vascular dementia (VD), and non-demented subjects. The cross-sectional analysis indicated that the more prominent carotid atherosclerosis the higher probability of dementia. This finding applies for VD, where the association is strong because the atherosclerosis is the principle of the dementia itself, as well as for AD. The longitudinal analysis included measurements at baseline and after 7–9 years and showed that the increased IMT is in the short-term period associated with an increased risk of developing AD. Due to the increased mortality in population with increased IMT, the effect was attenuated in the long-term follow-up (van Oijen et al., 2007). No difference in carotid atherosclerosis is found between AD and high vascular risk patients with VD. This implies that a certain level of impairment is present in both. Concerning the IMT, considered the incipient form of atherosclerosis, also no difference between AD and VD patients was found (Morovic et al., 2009).

In this context, the studies of cognitive decline in asymptomatic carotid stenosis are very interesting. High-degree carotid stenosis (70–99%) or carotid occlusion can be associated with cognitive decline in patients without otherwise clinically evident cerebrovascular disease, making the term "asymptomatic" stenosis somewhat arguable (Johnston et al., 2004; Balucani et al., 2012; Chang et al., 2013). The severity of impairment depends on the quality of collateral blood supply; the character of cognitive decline is influenced by the side of stenosis given by the distinctive functions of cerebral hemispheres. In left-sided stenosis, the verbal memory impairment is more frequent, and in right-sided stenosis there is more prominent visuospatial deficit (Balucani et al., 2012; Zavoreo et al., 2013). Two possible processes are considered in the pathophysiology – silent microembolism or hypoperfusion (Sztriha et al., 2009; Demarin et al., 2012). The carotid endarterectomy or carotid stenting and following reperfusion can improve the mental functions; on the other hand, during both procedures, the microembolism and hypoperfusion can occur as well and cause worsening of the cognitive decline.

Although the IMT in AD is generally increased as compared to healthy population, it does not correlate with cognitive performance in cross-sectional trials (Modrego et al., 2008). In longitudinal studies, IMT and atherosclerosis severity in AD patients correlate with the progression of cognitive impairment (Silvestrini et al., 2009). The progression is faster in AD patients with higher degree of carotid stenosis than in AD patients without stenosis (Silvestrini et al., 2011). Abnormal values of IMT also significantly increase the risk of conversion from amnestic MCI to AD (Viticchi et al., 2012). In a longitudinal study involving a 6-month galantamine treatment of AD, the patients with lower values of IMT at baseline had better response to treatment (Modrego et al., 2009), which suggests that AD patients with lower cerebrovascular burden have slower progression of disease. Details of ultrasound projects focused on IMT and carotid atherosclerosis in AD are listed in **Table 1**.

TOTAL CBF

Total CBF can be assessed by ultrasonography when measuring flow velocities in carotid and vertebral arteries and multiplying the result by the cross-sectional area of the vessels (average of systolic and diastolic areas). The results gained by this method are comparable to nitrous oxide and SPECT measurements giving the average CBF in a healthy subject of approximately 54 ml/100 g/min (Schoning et al., 1994). Insignificant errors in the measurement of flow velocities and vessel diameter can give significant errors in the final blood flow, up to 10%, but the accuracy and reproducibility of measurement are acceptable when repeated measurements are done and the average is calculated (Gill, 1985; Schoning and Scheel, 1996).

Total CBF reduces with age (Dorfler et al., 2000) and brain parenchymal volume (van Es et al., 2010). According to ultrasound

Table 1 | IMT and carotid atherosclerosis.

Reference	Aim of study	Type of study	n MCI	n AD	n VD	n Controls	Parameters	Outcome
Hofman et al. (1997)	Frequency of dementia and its subtypes in relation to atherosclerosis and apo-E	Cross-sectional		207	50	1698	IMT and atherosclerotic plaques in CCA and ICA, ankle and brachial systolic pressure	The risk of dementia of any type increases with the severity of atherosclerosis
Modrego et al. (2008)	Correlation of cognitive decline, WML and IMT in AD	Cross-sectional		51			Neuropsychological tests, WML on MRI, IMT in CCA	No correlation of clinical scales with WML or IMT
Modrego et al. (2009)	Association of IMT and response to ACHEI treatment in AD	Longitudinal		50			IMT in CCA and neuropsychological tests at time 0 and after 6 months while on galantamine treatment	Better response to galantamine treatment in lower IMT
Morovic et al. (2009)	Difference in IMT, beta stiffness index and CCA diameter between AD and VD	Cross-sectional		16	22		IMT, beta stiffness index and lumen diameter in CCA	No significant difference in any parameter between AD and VD
Purandare et al. (2005)	Frequency of cerebral emboli, v-a circulation shunts and carotid artery disease in dementia and controls	Cross-sectional		24	17	16	Spontaneus cerebral emboli in MCAs, bubbles in MCAs, PSV in ICA	More cerebral microemboli in VD than controls, in AD not significant, no difference in v-a shunt or carotid stenosis between dementia and controls
Silvestrini et al. (2009)	Correlation of carotid atherosclerosis progression and cognitive impairment in AD	Longitudinal		66			Carotid plaques, flow velocities, PI and IMT in CCA in time 0 and 12 month, while treated with galantamine	Significant correlation of cognitive decline with baseline IMT, IMT change, PI change, antihypertensive drugs
Silvestrini et al. (2011)	Association of ICA stenosis with cognitive decline progression in AD	Longitudinal		411			ICA plaques and flow velocities at baseline and in 12 months	Faster progression of cognitive decline in severe stenosis
van Oijen et al. (2007)	Association of atherosclerosis with dementia subtypes	Longitudinal		476	78		IMT and plaques in CCA and ICA	Higher IMT associated with greater risk of AD
Viticchi et al. (2012)	Association of carotid atherosclerosis and cerebrovascular reactivity with the risk of conversion from MCI to AD	Longitudinal	117	21			IMT and plaques in CCA, BHI in MCAs	Association of higher IMT and lower BHI with faster progression from MCI to dementia

ACHEI, acetylcholine esterase inhibitor; AD, Alzheimer's disease; BHI, breath holding index; CCA, common carotid artery; ICA, internal carotid artery; IMT, intima-media thickness; MCA, middle cerebral artery; MCI, mild cognitive impairment; MRI, magnetic resonance imaging; PI, pulsatility index; PSV, peak systolic velocity; v-a, venous-to-arterial; VD, vascular dementia; WML, white matter lesions.

studies, the total CBF is significantly lower in both AD and VD than in healthy controls of the same age (Maalikjy Akkawi et al., 2003; Schreiber et al., 2005; Doepp et al., 2006). This corresponds with changes described for an ICA flow curve in AD, where both systolic and diastolic velocities are lower compared to healthy individuals (Gusti et al., 2004). The association of total CBF with percentage of brain atrophy is weak (van Es et al., 2010). In an ultrasound study of three groups of patients with documented cerebral atrophy (AD, VD, and cognitively normal subjects), the total CBF was significantly lower in patients with dementia than in those without a cognitive impairment. There was no significant difference between two types of dementia (Albayrak et al., 2006). Details of ultrasound projects focused on total CBF in AD are listed in **Table 2.**

TRANSCRANIAL ULTRASOUND IN AD

FLOW VELOCITIES, CEREBROVASCULAR RESISTANCE, AND CEREBROVASCULAR RESERVE CAPACITY

The CBF curve in a transcranial ultrasound examination is characterized by two main flow velocities – peak systolic velocity and end diastolic velocity. These velocities can be measured in all major intracranial vessels – anterior, middle, and posterior cerebral arteries, vertebral arteries; and basilar artery. The mean flow velocity and indices describing the resistance of intracranial vessels can be derived from the flow curve. The reproducibility of flow velocities measurement is good when done by an experienced examiner (McMahon et al., 2007).

Many studies have found significantly lower flow velocities in AD compared to controls (Caamano et al., 1993; Roher et al., 2006, 2011; Sun et al., 2007; Vicenzini et al., 2007; Claassen et al., 2009; Stefani et al., 2009; Gucuyener et al., 2010). The most often studied vessel was the middle cerebral artery (MCA) while other major intracranial arteries were studied less frequently. The most often decreased velocity in MCA in AD patients compared to healthy controls was the mean flow velocity (Roher et al., 2006, 2011; Vicenzini et al., 2007; Claassen et al., 2009; Stefani et al., 2009), although not all results support these findings (Ries et al., 1993). Decreases in peak systolic and end diastolic velocities varied in different arteries (Caamano et al., 1993; Sun et al., 2007; Gucuyener et al., 2010). According to a large longitudinal study (Ruitenberg et al., 2005), subjects with higher velocities in MCA

Table 2 | Total cerebral blood flow.

Reference	Aim of study	Type of study	n MCI	n AD	n VD	n Controls	Parameters	Outcome
Albayrak et al. (2006)	Comparison of cerebral blood flow in demented (AD, VD) and cognitively normal subjects, both with brain atrophy	Cross-sectional		9	9	10	Flow velocities and cross-sectional area of the vessel in ICAs and VAs	Total, anterior and right CBF lower in dementia, no difference between two types of dementia
Doepp et al. (2006)	Possible differentiation of AD and VD by various extra- and intracranial ultrasound parameters	Cross-sectional		20	20	12	Flow velocities and PI in MCAs, flow velocities and cross-sectional area in ICAs and VAs, cerebral circulation time, global cerebral blood volume	No significant difference in trans- and extracranial ultrasound between AD and VD
Gusti et al. (2004)	Comparison of carotid flow velocities and flow curve in AD and controls	Cross-sectional		18		40	Flow velocities in carotid arteries	Lower cerebral vascular filling in AD
Maalikjy Akkawi et al. (2003)	Possibility of CBF volume assessment by TCD, difference between AD and controls, correlation with cognitive decline	Cross-sectional		50		50	Flow velocities and vessel diameter in ICA and VA, calculation of cerebral blood flow	Decrease in CBF volume in AD compared to controls, positive correlation between dementia severity and CBF
Schreiber et al. (2005)	CBF, cerebral circulation time and cerebral blood volume in AD, VD and controls	Cross-sectional		20	20	12	Flow velocity and cross-sectional area of ICA and VA, time of contrast agent transfer from ICA to IJV	Difference in CBF and transit time between dementia and controls, no difference in CBF volume or between AD and VD

AD, Alzheimer's disease; CBF, cerebral blood flow; ICA, internal carotid artery; IJV, internal jugular vein; MCA, middle cerebral artery; MCI, mild cognitive impairment; PI, pulsatility index; TCD, transcranial Doppler; VA, vertebral artery; VD, vascular dementia.

were less likely to develop AD. The question is – why the decrease should be most prominent in the MCA. We speculate this could be a consequence of pathological changes in AD, where temporal and parietal lobes supplied by MCA are most affected. In this context, a comparison of healthy subjects and patients with MCI would be interesting, but the results are ambiguous (Roher et al., 2011). No significant difference in flow velocities was found between AD and VD, neither there is a significant side asymmetry.

Unlike SPECT, the transcranial Doppler measures only flow velocities and not absolute blood flow, and the assessment of flow velocities is not helpful in an individual patient due to the wide range of normal values of flow velocities. The methods for assessment of regional cerebral perfusion or metabolism (SPECT, PET) have high sensitivity and specificity in distinguishing AD vs. normal controls (depending on the stage of the disease and method employed) based on characteristic perfusion or metabolism reduction in temporoparietal association cortex: SPECT can reach sensitivity of 65–96% and specificity of 80–87%, PET can reach even sensitivity of 93–94% and specificity of 63–73% (Wollman and Prohovnik, 2003; Matsuda, 2007). These two methods can be used to make the clinical diagnosis of AD more accurate in some unclear cases.

A parameter describing autoregulation of cerebral perfusion is cerebrovascular reserve capacity, which reflects the capability of brain microvasculature to regulate cerebral perfusion in a reaction to various stimuli, thanks to constriction or dilatation. The most often used stimulus is a change of the arterial CO_2 level that can be induced using breath holding, CO_2 inhalation, or intravenous acetazolamide injection. Other less often used stimuli include hand movement, cognitive exercise, or blood pressure challenge (i.e., physical exercise). The cerebrovascular reserve capacity is expressed as the ratio of mean flow velocity in basal conditions and mean flow velocity in the conditions of a higher CO_2 level. In normal brain, there is an increase in flow velocities. When breath holding is the stimulus, the ratio can be multiplied by the duration of breath holding and expressed as breath holding index (BHI). Cerebrovascular reserve capacity decreases with age (Peisker et al., 2010).

The cerebrovascular reserve capacity is in clinical practice routinely tested before revascularization procedures in carotid stenosis or occlusion. The established methods for cerebrovascular reserve capacity assessment are scintigraphic techniques such as SPECT and PET with the use of various radioactive tracer compounds, all of them evaluating the cerebral perfusion in basal conditions and after vasodilatory stimulus (acetazolamide injection or CO_2 inhalation). In comparison with these direct techniques, the transcranial Doppler examination is an indirect assessment based on the relative increase in flow velocities after vasodilatory stimulus (usually acetazolamide injection, CO_2 inhalation or breath holding). All three transcranial Doppler methods correlate very well to 133Xe SPECT (Bishop et al., 1986; Dahl et al., 1992; Muller et al., 1995) with the breath-holding method being the less accurate but sufficient for first screening examination (Markus and Harrison, 1992; Muller et al., 1995). Compared to scintigraphic techniques the ultrasound examination is non-invasive and inexpensive.

Concerning the cerebrovascular reserve capacity measured by transcranial Doppler in the MCA in AD patients, the results are more consistent than those for solely flow velocities. In AD patients, the reactivity to different stimuli in the MCA is significantly lower than in healthy controls (Provinciali et al., 1990; Bar et al., 2007; Lee et al., 2007; Vicenzini et al., 2007; Stefani et al., 2009). Only some studies with fewer subjects do not fully support these findings (Matteis et al., 1998; Claassen et al., 2009). In one of these studies, the result could be influenced by the selection of very mild AD cases (MMSE 25) (Claassen et al., 2009). In another study, it is not sufficiently described how the cognitive impairment was ruled out in control subjects (Matteis et al., 1998). One study proved a better cerebrovascular reserve capacity in AD than VD, but the result was not statistically significant (Likitjaroen et al., 2009). Healthy subjects with higher cerebrovascular reserve capacity are less likely to develop a cognitive decline (AD or VD) (Ruitenberg et al., 2005). Although the impairment of cerebrovascular reserve capacity is more serious in VD, it seems that the microvasculature is altered in both main types of dementia (Bar et al., 2007; Vicenzini et al., 2007).

On the other hand, the hypercapnia challenge in SPECT and PET studies give ambiguous results without convincing evidence of decreased cerebrovascular reserve capacity in AD (Yamaguchi et al., 1980; Bonte et al., 1989; Kuwabara et al., 1992; Stoppe et al., 1995; Knapp et al., 1996; Jagust et al., 1997; Oishi et al., 1999; Pavics et al., 1999). However, it must be taken into account that in earlier publications, the diagnostic criteria for AD may differ from nowadays criteria and older devices may not give very accurate results (Glodzik et al., 2013).

Again the comparison with asymptomatic carotid stenosis or occlusion is interesting. In cases of high degree stenosis or occlusion with insufficient collateral blood supply, the chronic hypoperfusion exhausts the cerebrovascular reserve. This can be observed in different examination methods (Oka et al., 2013) including transcranial Doppler ultrasound examination using BHI (Balestrini et al., 2013; Zavoreo et al., 2013). The decrease of cerebrovascular reserve capacity correlates with the cognitive decline (Zavoreo et al., 2013).

The cerebrovascular reserve capacity of posterior cerebral artery in reaction to a visual stimulus was often tested. The function of occipital lobe should be preserved until late stages of AD. The results of such projects were ambiguous (Asil and Uzuner, 2005; Rosengarten et al., 2006, 2007; Gucuyener et al., 2010) and, thus, not differentiating AD from VD.

The reason for the decreased cerebrovascular reserve capacity is not entirely clear. In VD, the cause is probably a small vessel disease. In AD, amyloid deposits represent the likely culprit – in cerebral amyloid angiopathy, the cerebrovascular reserve capacity is also compromised (Menendez-Gonzalez et al., 2011). Another hypothesis suggests the role of insufficient acetylcholine production necessary for vasodilatation. Therapeutic tests with acetylcholine inhibitors (galantamine or donepezil) demonstrated an increase in flow velocities and improvement of vessel reactivity in both VD and AD (Rosengarten et al., 2006; Bar et al., 2007; Ghorbani et al., 2010). In longitudinal follow-up studies, the BHI significantly correlated with neuropsychological tests – MMSE and Alzheimer's Disease Assessment Scale-cognitive subscale (ADAS-Cog) in AD

Table 3 | Flow velocities, cerebrovascular resistance, and cerebrovascular reserve capacity.

Reference	Aim of study	Type of study	n MCI	n AD	n VD	N Controls	Parameters	Outcome
Asil and Uzuner (2005)	Assessment of CVRC in the occipital lobe in AD	Cross-sectional		15	12	9	Flow velocities in PCAs during eyes opened and eyes closed	No significant difference neither in flow velocities at rest nor at stimuli in three groups; decreased reactivity in VD at stimulus
Bar et al. (2007)	CVRC in AD compared to VD and healthy controls, reactivity after ACHEI treatment	Cross-sectional Longitudinal		17	17	20	Flow velocities in MCA at rest and after CO_2 inhalation in AD and VD repeated after 5 weeks of galantamine treatment	CVRC in MCA decreased in AD and VD in comparison to healthy controls, better CVRC after galantamine treatment on both AD and VD
Caamano et al. (1993)	Comparison of flow velocities in MCA and BA in AD, VD and controls	Cross-sectional		12	12	12	Flow velocities in right and left MCA and BA	Decreased values in demented patients
Claassen et al. (2009)	Assessment of cerebral hemodynamics impairment in early stage AD	Cross-sectional		9		8	Flow velocities in MCA, blood pressure, cerebrovascular resistance index	Significantly reduced flow velocities and increased resistance in AD
Ghorbani et al. (2010)	Assessment of the effect of Donepezil on cerebral blood flow velocity in AD patients	Longitudinal		11			Flow velocities in PCA and MCA at baseline, after 4 weeks of donepezil 5 mg and after another 4 weeks of donepezil 10 mg	Increase in PSV and MFV in MCA, and MFV and EDV in PCA after 10 mg treatment
Gucuyener et al. (2010)	CVRC in PCAs in AD compared to depressive pseudo-dementia	Cross-sectional		11	13	10	Flow velocities in both PCAs simultaneously; in steady state and after a visual stimulus	Lower flow velocities at rest and after stimulus in both AD and depressive pseudodementia then controls. CVRC impaired in AD, not in depressive pseudodementia
Lee et al. (2007)	Assessment of CVRC in AD	Cross-sectional		17		17	Flow velocities and PI in MCA bilaterally in normal conditions and after 5 min of rebreathing	No difference in baseline MFV and PI between subjects and controls, CVRC significantly decreased on both sides in AD
Likitjaroen et al. (2009)	Comparison of CVRC in AD and VD	Cross-sectional		9	9		Flow velocities in MCA in normal conditions and after 1000 mg acetazolamide i.v.	Non-significantly better CVRC in AD than VD

(Continued)

Table 3 | Continued

Reference	Aim of study	Type of study	n MCI	n AD	n VD	N Controls	Parameters	Outcome
Matteis et al. (1998)	Comparison of CVRC in AD and VD	Cross-sectional		10	10	20	Flow velocities in MCA during apnea, hand movement and verbal and design discrimination	CVRC to apnea lower in VD; hand movement – contralateral increase in flow in AD and controls, bilateral in VD; bilateral response on cognitive stimuli in AD and VD, corresponding side response in controls
Provinciali et al. (1990)	Comparison of CVRC in AD, VD and controls	Cross-sectional		20	20	25	Flow velocities in MCA at rest, after hyperventilation, apnea and 5 min air rebreathing	Higher PI, lower velocity decrease in hyperventilation in both dementias; rest flow velocities and response to hypercapnia lower in VD than AD or controls
Ries et al. (1993)	Utility of TCD in differentiation of AD and multi-infarct dementia	Cross-sectional		24	17	64	PSV and EDV in all large intracranial vessels bilaterally, pulse curve in MCA	No difference in PSV in all three groups, difference in MFV, EDV and effective pulsatility range in VD compared to AD or controls
Roher et al. (2006)	Comparison of mean flow velocities and PI in intracranial arteries in AD and controls	Cross-sectional		25		30	Flow velocities in 16 different segments of circle of Willis	Higher PIs in AD, non-significantly lower mean flow velocities in AD
Roher et al. (2011)	Utility of TCD in diagnosing and preventing AD	Cross-sectional	11	42		50	Flow velocities in 16 different segments of circle of Willis	Significant difference in MFV and PI in left siphon, left ICA and right distal MCA between AD and controls
Rosengarten et al. (2006)	Influence of ACHEI treatment on vasoregulation in AD	Longitudinal		8		16	Flow velocities in PCA and MCA in rest and at stimulation (text reading) at baseline, after 4 weeks of donepezil 5 mg and after another 4 weeks of donepezil 10 mg	Decrease in attenuation parameter after 10 mg in AD = dose dependent resolution of functional vascular deficit
Rosengarten et al. (2007)	Comparison of activation-flow coupling in AD, VD and controls	Cross-sectional		15	10	15	Flow velocities in PCA and MCA in rest and at stimulation (text reading)	Lower increase in PSV in VD
Ruitenberg et al. (2005)	Correlation of flow velocities with cognitive decline and hippocampal atrophy	Cross-sectional		13	1	1718	Flow velocities in MCAs at rest and after 5 min of 5% CO_2	Greater PSV, MFV, EDV – less likely dementia and bigger hippocampus and amygdala No association of CVRC and presence of dementia

(Continued)

Table 3 | Continued

Reference	Aim of study	Type of study	n MCI	n AD	n VD	N Controls	Parameters	Outcome
Silvestrini et al. (2006)	Influence of cerebral hemodynamics alterations on the evolution of cognitive impairment	Longitudinal		53			Flow velocities in MCAs at rest and after breath-holding, time 0 and 12 month, during this time donepezil 5 mg daily for 3 month, then 10 mg daily	Positive correlation of neuropsychological tests changes with BHI, age and DM
Silvestrini et al. (2009), Stefani et al. (2009)	Comparison of cerebral hemodynamics in AD and controls	Cross-sectional		40		40	Flow velocities, PI and BHI in MCA	Lower MFV, higher PI and lower BHI in MCA in AD than in controls
Sun et al. (2007)	Changes in cerebral flow velocities in MCI and controls	Cross-sectional	30			30	Flow velocities in MCA, ACA, BA	Decreased PSV, MFV and EDV in MCA and ACA in MCI compared to controls
Vicenzini et al. (2007)	Comparison of flow velocities, PI and CVRC in AD, VD, and controls	Cross-sectional		60	58	62	Flow velocities in MCA in normal conditions, after hyperventilation and CO_2 inhalation	Lower MFV, higher PI and lower CVRC in AD and VD compared to controls
Viticchi et al. (2012)	Association of carotid atherosclerosis and cerebrovascular reserve capacity with the risk of conversion from MCI to AD	Longitudinal	117	21			IMT and plaques in CCA, BHI in MCAs	Association of higher IMT and lower BHI with faster progression from MCI to dementia

ACA, anterior cerebral artery; ACHEI, acetylcholine esterase inhibitor; AD, Alzheimer's disease; BA, basilar artery; CAA, cerebral amyloid angiopathy; CVRC, cerebrovascular reserve capacity; DM, diabetes mellitus; EDV, end diastolic velocity; ICA, internal carotid artery; MCA, middle cerebral artery; MCI, mild cognitive impairment; MFV, mean flow velocity; PCA, posterior cerebral artery; PI, pulsatility index; PSV, peak systolic velocity; VD, vascular dementia.

(Silvestrini et al., 2006). MCI patients with pathological values of BHI have greater risk of converting to dementia than patients with normal values (Viticchi et al., 2012). Details of ultrasound projects focused on flow velocities and cerebrovascular reserve capacity in AD are listed in **Table 3.**

SPONTANEOUS CEREBRAL MICROEMBOLIZATION AND PARADOXICAL EMBOLIZATION VIA RIGHT–LEFT SHUNTS

Recent evidence suggests that cerebral microemboli can lead to a cognitive decline (Pugsley et al., 1994; Gaudet et al., 2009). Cerebral microemboli can originate from arterial sources or venous sources in setting of right–left shunts (intracardiac – foramen ovale patens, atrial septal defects). The spontaneous cerebral embolization can be monitored using a headframe with attached ultrasound probes for time periods of usually 1–24 h. Right–left shunts are examined by intravenous injection of a microbubble agent (agitated saline or hydroxyethyl starch) and observing the presence of microbubbles in brain vessels using transcranial ultrasound at rest and during the Valsalva maneuver. The accuracy of right–left shunt assessment by transcranial Doppler ultrasound compared to the transesophageal echocardiography as a gold standard ranges from 68 to 100% according to the reports in literature, some of them claiming the transcranial Doppler method even more accurate (Nemec et al., 1991; Teague and Sharma, 1991; Di Tullio et al., 1993; Jauss et al., 1994; Job et al., 1994; Sastry et al., 2009). The sensitivity and reproducibility of the examination is highest when performed repeatedly (twice) with the use of Valsalva maneuver (Droste et al., 1999).

There were not many studies focused on spontaneous cerebral embolization in AD. One work suggested that it is more frequent in patients with AD or VD than in healthy controls (Purandare et al., 2005). This suggestion was later confirmed by a larger case–control study (Purandare et al., 2006). In this particular project, there was no significant difference in the

Table 4 | Spontaneous cerebral microembolization and paradoxical embolization via right–left shunts.

Reference	Aim of study	Type of study	n MCI	n AD	n VD	n Controls	Parameters	Outcome
Purandare et al. (2005)	Spontaneous cerebral microemboli, v-a circulation shunts and carotid artery disease in dementia and controls	Cross-sectional		24	17	16	Spontaneus cerebral emboli in MCAs, bubbles in MCAs, PSV in ICA	More cerebral microemboli in VD than controls, in AD not significant, no difference in shunt or carotid stenosis between dementia and controls
Purandare et al. (2006)	Spontaneous cerebral microemboli, v-a circulation shunts and carotid artery disease in dementia and controls	Cross-sectional		85	85	150	Spontaneus cerebral emboli in MCAs, bubbles in MCAs, PSV in ICA	More cerebral microemboli in VD and AD than controls, no difference in shunt or carotid stenosis between dementia and controls
Purandare and Burns (2009)	Association of spontaneous cerebral microembolization with dementia etiology, dementia progression and depression in dementia or controls	Cross-sectional Longitudinal		85	85	150	Spontaneus cerebral emboli in MCAs, bubbles in MCAs, PSV in ICA. Neuropsychological tests in time 0 and 6 months	More cerebral microemboli in AD and VD than controls, more in depression (both dementia and controls). Association with more rapid cognitive decline in dementia

AD, Alzheimer's disease; ICA, internal carotid artery; MCA, middle cerebral artery; MCI, mild cognitive impairment; PSV, peak systolic velocity; v-a, venous-to-arterial; VD, vascular dementia.

Table 5 | Neurosonological parameters in AD – summary.

Ultrasound parameter	Findings in AD	Conclusion
IMT	Increased IMT associated with increased short-term risk of developing AD, converting from MCI to AD, and lower response to galantamine treatment of AD Correlates with the progression of AD	In combination with other neurosonological methods and vascular risks assessment can help to identify patients in higher risk of faster progression of AD
Carotid atherosclerosis	Higher degree of carotid atherosclerosis associated with increased short-term risk of developing AD and converting from MCI to AD Correlates with the progression of AD	In combination with other neurosonological methods and vascular risks assessment can help to identify patients in higher risk of faster progression of AD
Total cerebral blood flow	Decreased in AD Not dependent on brain atrophy Longitudinal data not available	Inconclusive
Flow velocities	Variably decreased MFV in MCA in AD Decreased flow velocities associated with increased risk of developing AD	Inconclusive
Cerebrovascular reserve capacity	Decreased in AD Decreased CVRC associated with increased risk of developing AD	Best correlation with AD incidence and progression among all neurosonological parameters

AD, Alzheimer's disease; IMT, intima-media thickness; MCA, middle cerebral artery; MCI, mild cognitive impairment; MFV, mean flow velocity.

incidence of carotid artery atherosclerosis – i.e., possible source of microembolization. Prevalence of patent foramen ovale in AD and VD cohort was 33% in this study, which is higher than usually reported 20–25% in general population (Hara et al., 2005), but no larger epidemiological studies of prevalence in AD were done. The same author found the association of spontaneous cerebral microembolization with more rapid cognitive decline in dementia (Purandare and Burns, 2009). Details of ultrasound projects focused on spontaneous and paradoxical embolization in AD are listed in **Table 4**.

CONCLUSION

The current evidence suggests that the brain perfusion in AD patients, in general, is impaired compared to healthy non-demented population. The most prominent ultrasonographical findings in extracranial circulation in AD patients show an increased IMT and higher burden of carotid artery atherosclerosis. The most often identified changes in intracranial circulation are lower flow velocities, lower total CBF (not explained by brain atrophy only), and most notably impaired cerebrovascular reserve capacity (**Table 5**). These findings seem to be valid for both AD and VD.

Ultrasonography of extra- and intracranial brain vessels can be helpful in AD patients to identify individuals who are in a higher risk of disease progression. Ultrasonography can be also useful for stratification of MCI patients and can contribute to predict the risk of conversion to AD. The vascular risk factors surveillance and treatment in preclinical stages of AD is of great clinical importance and it could help to delay the development of cognitive decline in susceptible individuals. Ultrasonography is not especially beneficial in differentiating AD and VD, because the microvasculature is altered in both types of dementia.

AUTHOR CONTRIBUTIONS

Barbora Urbanova, Ales Tomek, Robert Mikulik, and Jakub Hort took part in designing the aim and scope of the review. Barbora Urbanova, Ales Tomek, and Hana Magerova did the literature search. All the authors took part in detailed study and interpretation of the reviewed articles. All the authors took part in writing various sections of this article. Barbora Urbanova, Jakub Hort, Robert Mikulik, and Ales Tomek reviewed whole article.

ACKNOWLEDGMENTS

Supported by IGA MZ CR grant (No. NT/13319). Supported by GAUK grant (No 347711). Supported by the project FNUSA-ICRC (no. CZ.1.05/1.1.00/02.0123) from the European Regional Development Fund.

REFERENCES

Albayrak, R., Yaman, M., Uslan, I., Degirmenci, B., Acar, M., and Haktanir, A. (2006). Evaluation of total cerebral blood flow volume in cerebral atrophy. *Neurosci. Lett.* 399, 124–128. doi:10.1016/j.neulet.2006.01.039

Asil, T., and Uzuner, N. (2005). Differentiation of vascular dementia and Alzheimer disease: a functional transcranial Doppler ultrasonographic study. *J. Ultrasound Med.* 24, 1065–1070.

Balestrini, S., Perozzi, C., Altamura, C., Vernieri, F., Luzzi, S., Bartolini, M., et al. (2013). Severe carotid stenosis and impaired cerebral hemodynamics can influence cognitive deterioration. *Neurology* 80, 2145–2150. doi:10.1212/WNL.0b013e318295d71a

Balucani, C., Viticchi, G., Falsetti, L., and Silvestrini, M. (2012). Cerebral hemodynamics and cognitive performance in bilateral asymptomatic carotid stenosis. *Neurology* 79, 1788–1795. doi:10.1212/WNL.0b013e318270402e

Bar, K. J., Boettger, M. K., Seidler, N., Mentzel, H. J., Terborg, C., and Sauer, H. (2007). Influence of galantamine on vasomotor reactivity in Alzheimer's disease and vascular dementia due to cerebral microangiopathy. *Stroke* 38, 3186–3192. doi:10.1161/STROKEAHA.107.492033

Bishop, C. C., Powell, S., Rutt, D., and Browse, N. L. (1986). Transcranial Doppler measurement of middle cerebral artery blood flow velocity: a validation study. *Stroke* 17, 913–915. doi:10.1161/01.STR.17.5.913

Bonte, F. J., Devous, M. D. Sr., Reisch, J. S., Ajmani, A. K., Weiner, M. F., Hom, J., et al. (1989). The effect of acetazolamide on regional cerebral blood flow in patients with Alzheimer's disease or stroke as measured by single-photon emission computed tomography. *Invest. Radiol.* 24, 99–103. doi:10.1097/00004424-198902000-00002

Breteler, M. M. (2000). Vascular risk factors for Alzheimer's disease: an epidemiologic perspective. *Neurobiol. Aging* 21, 153–160. doi:10.1016/S0197-4580(99)00110-4

Breteler, M. M., van Swieten, J. C., Bots, M. L., Grobbee, D. E., Claus, J. J., van den Hout, J. H., et al. (1994). Cerebral white matter lesions, vascular risk factors, and cognitive function in a population-based study: the Rotterdam Study. *Neurology* 44, 1246–1252. doi:10.1212/WNL.44.7.1246

Caamano, J., Gomez, M. J., and Cacabelos, R. (1993). Transcranial Doppler ultrasonography in senile dementia: neuropsychological correlations. *Methods Find. Exp. Clin. Pharmacol.* 15, 193–199.

Casserly, I., and Topol, E. (2004). Convergence of atherosclerosis and Alzheimer's disease: inflammation, cholesterol, and misfolded proteins. *Lancet* 363, 1139–1146. doi:10.1016/S0140-6736(04)15900-X

Chang, X. L., Zhou, H. Q., Lei, C. Y., Wu, B., Chen, Y. C., Hao, Z. L., et al. (2013). Association between asymptomatic carotid stenosis and cognitive function: a systematic review. *Neurosci. Biobehav. Rev.* 37, 1493–1499. doi:10.1016/j.neubiorev.2013.05.011

Claassen, J. A., Diaz-Arrastia, R., Martin-Cook, K., Levine, B. D., and Zhang, R. (2009). Altered cerebral hemodynamics in early Alzheimer disease: a pilot study using transcranial Doppler. *J. Alzheimers Dis.* 17, 621–629. doi:10.3233/JAD-2009-1079

Dahl, A., Lindegaard, K. F., Russell, D., Nyberg-Hansen, R., Rootwelt, K., Sorteberg, W., et al. (1992). A comparison of transcranial Doppler and cerebral blood flow studies to assess cerebral vasoreactivity. *Stroke* 23, 15–19. doi:10.1161/01.STR.23.1.15

de la Sierra, A., Zamorano, J. L., and Ruilope, L. M. (2009). Application of hypertension guidelines in clinical practice: implementation of the 2007 ESH/ESC European practice Guidelines in Spain. *J. Hypertens. Suppl.* 27, S27–S32. doi:10.1097/01.hjh.0000356769.32130.95

de la Torre, J. C. (2010). The vascular hypothesis of Alzheimer's disease: bench to bedside and beyond. *Neurodegener. Dis.* 7, 116–121. doi:10.1159/000285520

DeCarli, C., Miller, B. L., Swan, G. E., Reed, T., Wolf, P. A., and Carmelli, D. (2001). Cerebrovascular and brain morphologic correlates of mild cognitive impairment in the National Heart, Lung, and Blood Institute Twin Study. *Arch. Neurol.* 58, 643–647. doi:10.1001/archneur.58.4.643

DeKosky, S. T., Shih, W. J., Schmitt, F. A., Coupal, J., and Kirkpatrick, C. (1990). Assessing utility of single photon emission computed tomography (SPECT) scan in Alzheimer disease: correlation with cognitive severity. *Alzheimer Dis. Assoc. Disord.* 4, 14–23. doi:10.1097/00002093-199040100-00002

Demarin, V., Zavoreo, I., and Kes, V. B. (2012). Carotid artery disease and cognitive impairment. *J. Neurol. Sci.* 322, 107–111. doi:10.1016/j.jns.2012.07.008

Di Tullio, M., Sacco, R. L., Venketasubramanian, N., Sherman, D., Mohr, J. P., and Homma, S. (1993). Comparison of diagnostic techniques for the detection of a patent foramen ovale in stroke patients. *Stroke* 24, 1020–1024. doi:10.1161/01.STR.24.7.1020

Doepp, F., Valdueza, J. M., and Schreiber, S. J. (2006). Transcranial and extracranial ultrasound assessment of cerebral hemodynamics in vascular and Alzheimer's dementia. *Neurol. Res.* 28, 645–649. doi:10.1179/016164106X130380

Dogan, S., Duivenvoorden, R., Grobbee, D. E., Kastelein, J. J., Shear, C. L., Evans, G. W., et al. (2010). Ultrasound protocols to measure carotid intima-media thickness in trials; comparison of reproducibility, rate of progression, and effect of intervention in subjects with familial hypercholesterolemia and subjects with mixed dyslipidemia. *Ann. Med.* 42, 447–464. doi:10.3109/07853890.2010.499132

Dorfler, P., Puls, I., Schliesser, M., Maurer, M., and Becker, G. (2000). Measurement of cerebral blood flow volume by extracranial sonography. *J. Cereb. Blood Flow Metab.* 20, 269–271. doi:10.1097/00004647-200002000-00007

Droste, D. W., Reisener, M., Kemeny, V., Dittrich, R., Schulte-Altedorneburg, G., Stypmann, J., et al. (1999). Contrast transcranial Doppler ultrasound in the detection of right-to-left shunts. *Stroke* 30, 1014–1018. doi:10.1161/01.STR.30.5.1014

Gaudet, J. G., Meyers, P. M., McKinsey, J. F., Lavine, S. D., Gray, W., Mitchell, E., et al. (2009). Incidence of moderate to severe cognitive dysfunction in patients treated with carotid artery stenting. *Neurosurgery* 65, 325–329. doi:10.1227/01.NEU.0000349920.69637.78 discussion 9–30,

Ghorbani, A., Chitsaz, A., Shishegar, M., and Akbari, M. (2010). Evaluation of the effect of donepezil on cerebral blood flow velocity in Alzheimer's disease. *Neurosciences (Riyadh)* 15, 172–176.

Gill, R. W. (1985). Measurement of blood flow by ultrasound: accuracy and sources of error. *Ultrasound Med. Biol.* 11, 625–641. doi:10.1016/0301-5629(85)90035-3

Glodzik, L., Randall, C., Rusinek, H., and de Leon, M. J. (2013). Cerebrovascular reactivity to carbon dioxide in Alzheimer's disease. *J. Alzheimers Dis.* 35, 427–440. doi:10.3233/JAD-122011

Gonzalez, J., Wood, J. C., Dorey, F. J., Wren, T. A., and Gilsanz, V. (2008). Reproducibility of carotid intima-media thickness measurements in young adults. *Radiology* 247, 465–471. doi:10.1148/radiol.2472070691

Gorelick, P. B. (2004). Risk factors for vascular dementia and Alzheimer disease. *Stroke* 35, 2620–2622. doi:10.1161/01.STR.0000143318.70292.47

Grant, E. G., Benson, C. B., Moneta, G. L., Alexandrov, A. V., Baker, J. D., Bluth, E. I., et al. (2003). Carotid artery stenosis: gray-scale and Doppler US diagnosis – Society of Radiologists in Ultrasound Consensus Conference. *Radiology* 229, 340–346. doi:10.1148/radiol.2292030516

Greco, G., Egorova, N. N., Moskowitz, A. J., Gelijns, A. C., Kent, K. C., Manganaro, A. J., et al. (2013). Model for predicting the risk of carotid artery disease. *Ann. Surg.* 257, 1168–1173. doi:10.1097/SLA.0b013e31827b9761

Greenland, P., Alpert, J. S., Beller, G. A., Benjamin, E. J., Budoff, M. J., Fayad, Z. A., et al. (2010). 2010 ACCF/AHA guideline for assessment of cardiovascular risk in asymptomatic adults: a report of the American College of Cardiology Foundation/American Heart Association Task Force on Practice Guidelines. *J. Am. Coll. Cardiol.* 56, e50–e103. doi:10.1016/j.jacc.2010.09.001

Gucuyener, D. O., Yenilmez, C., Ayranci, U., Ozdemir, F., Uzuner, N., Ozkan, S., et al. (2010). An analysis of changes in cerebral blood flood velocities in depressive pseudo-dementia and Alzheimer disease patients. *Neurologist* 16, 358–363. doi:10.1097/NRL.0b013e3181a2eace

Gusti, S. I., Coteanu, M. I., and Gusti, A. S. (2004). Study of the cerebral vascular Doppler velocimetry and EEG in a group of 18 cases of Alzheimer's disease. *Rom. J. Physiol.* 41, 91–97.

Hara, H., Virmani, R., Ladich, E., Mackey-Bojack, S., Titus, J., Reisman, M., et al. (2005). Patent foramen ovale: current pathology, pathophysiology, and clinical status. *J. Am. Coll. Cardiol.* 46, 1768–1776. doi:10.1016/j.jacc.2005.08.038

Hofman, A., Ott, A., Breteler, M. M., Bots, M. L., Slooter, A. J., van Harskamp, F., et al. (1997). Atherosclerosis, apolipoprotein E, and prevalence of dementia and Alzheimer's disease in the Rotterdam Study. *Lancet* 349, 151–154. doi:10.1016/S0140-6736(96)09328-2

Jagust, W. J., Eberling, J. L., Reed, B. R., Mathis, C. A., and Budinger, T. F. (1997). Clinical studies of cerebral blood flow in Alzheimer's disease. *Ann. N. Y. Acad. Sci.* 826, 254–262. doi:10.1111/j.1749-6632.1997.tb48477.x

Jauss, M., Kaps, M., Keberle, M., Haberbosch, W., and Dorndorf, W. (1994). A comparison of transesophageal echocardiography and transcranial Doppler sonography with contrast medium for detection of patent foramen ovale. *Stroke* 25, 1265–1267. doi:10.1161/01.STR.25.6.1265

Job, F. P., Ringelstein, E. B., Grafen, Y., Flachskampf, F. A., Doherty, C., Stockmanns, A., et al. (1994). Comparison of transcranial contrast Doppler sonography and transesophageal contrast echocardiography for the detection of patent foramen ovale in young stroke patients. *Am. J. Cardiol.* 74, 381–384. doi:10.1016/0002-9149(94)90407-3

Johnson, K. A., Jones, K., Holman, B. L., Becker, J. A., Spiers, P. A., Satlin, A., et al. (1998). Preclinical prediction of Alzheimer's disease using SPECT. *Neurology* 50, 1563–1571. doi:10.1212/WNL.50.6.1563

Johnston, S. C., O'Meara, E. S., Manolio, T. A., Lefkowitz, D., O'Leary, D. H., Goldstein, S., et al. (2004). Cognitive impairment and decline are associated with carotid artery disease in patients without clinically evident cerebrovascular disease. *Ann. Intern. Med.* 140, 237–247. doi:10.7326/0003-4819-140-4-200402170-00005

Kalaria, R. (2002). Similarities between Alzheimer's disease and vascular dementia. *J. Neurol. Sci.* 203-204, 29–34. doi:10.1016/S0022-510X(02)00256-3

Knapp, W. H., Dannenberg, C., Marschall, B., Zedlick, D., Loschmann, K., Bettin, S., et al. (1996). Changes in local cerebral blood flow by neuroactivation and vasoactivation in patients with impaired cognitive function. *Eur. J. Nucl. Med.* 23, 878–888. doi:10.1007/BF01084360

Kuwabara, Y., Ichiya, Y., Otsuka, M., Masuda, K., Ichimiya, A., and Fujishima, M. (1992). Cerebrovascular responsiveness to hypercapnia in Alzheimer's dementia and vascular dementia of the Binswanger type. *Stroke* 23, 594–598. doi:10.1161/01.STR.23.4.594

Lee, S. T., Jung, K. H., and Lee, Y. S. (2007). Decreased vasomotor reactivity in Alzheimer's disease. *J. Clin. Neurol.* 3, 18–23. doi:10.3988/jcn.2007.3.1.18

Likitjaroen, Y., Suwanwela, N. C., and Phanthumchinda, K. (2009). Vasoreactivity induced by acetazolamide in patients with vascular dementia versus Alzheimer's disease. *J. Neurol. Sci.* 283, 32–35. doi:10.1016/j.jns.2009.02.363

Lorenz, M. W., Markus, H. S., Bots, M. L., Rosvall, M., and Sitzer, M. (2007). Prediction of clinical cardiovascular events with carotid intima-media thickness: a systematic review and meta-analysis. *Circulation* 115, 459–467. doi:10.1161/CIRCULATIONAHA.106.628875

Maalikjy Akkawi, N., Borroni, B., Agosti, C., Pezzini, A., Magoni, M., Rozzini, L., et al. (2003). Volume reduction in cerebral blood flow in patients with Alzheimer's disease: a sonographic study. *Dement. Geriatr. Cogn. Disord.* 16, 163–169. doi:10.1159/000071005

Markus, H. S., and Harrison, M. J. (1992). Estimation of cerebrovascular reactivity using transcranial Doppler, including the use of breath-holding as the vasodilatory stimulus. *Stroke* 23, 668–673. doi:10.1161/01.STR.23.5.668

Matsuda, H. (2007). Role of neuroimaging in Alzheimer's disease, with emphasis on brain perfusion SPECT. *J. Nucl. Med.* 48, 1289–1300. doi:10.2967/jnumed.106.037218

Matteis, M., Silvestrini, M., Troisi, E., Bragoni, M., Vernieri, F., and Caltagirone, C. (1998). Cerebral hemodynamic patterns during stimuli tasks in multi-infarct and Alzheimer types of dementia. *Acta Neurol. Scand.* 97, 374–380. doi:10.1111/j.1600-0404.1998.tb05969.x

McMahon, C. J., McDermott, P., Horsfall, D., Selvarajah, J. R., King, A. T., and Vail, A. (2007). The reproducibility of transcranial Doppler middle cerebral artery velocity measurements: implications for clinical practice. *Br. J. Neurosurg.* 21, 21–27. doi:10.1080/02688690701210539

Menendez-Gonzalez, M., Garcia-Garcia, J., Calleja, S., Rojo, J., and Ribacoba, R. (2011). Vasomotor reactivity is similarly impaired in patients with Alzheimer's disease and patients with amyloid hemorrhage. *J. Neuroimaging* 21, e83–e85. doi:10.1111/j.1552-6569.2009.00438.x

Modrego, P. J., Rios, C., Perez Trullen, J. M., Errea, J. M., Garcia-Gomara, M. J., and Sanchez, S. (2008). The cerebrovascular pathology in Alzheimer's disease and its influence on clinical variables. *Am. J. Alzheimers Dis. Other Demen.* 23, 91–96. doi:10.1177/1533317507309274

Modrego, P. J., Rios, C., Perez Trullen, J. M., Garcia-Gomara, M. J., and Errea, J. M. (2009). Carotid intima-media thickness as a predictor of response to cholinesterase inhibitors in Alzheimer's disease: an open-label trial. *CNS Drugs* 23, 253–260. doi:10.2165/00023210-200923030-00006

Mohler, E. R. III, Gornik, H. L., Gerhard-Herman, M., Misra, S., Olin, J. W., and Zierler, E. (2012). ACCF/ACR/AIUM/ASE/ASN/ICAVL/SCAI/SCCT/SIR/SVM/SVS 2012 appropriate use criteria for peripheral vascular ultrasound and physiological testing part I: arterial ultrasound and physiological testing: a report of the American College of Cardiology Foundation Appropriate Use Criteria Task Force, American College of Radiology, American Institute of Ultrasound in Medicine, American Society of Echocardiography, American Society of Nephrology, Intersocietal Commission for the Accreditation of Vascular Laboratories, Society for Cardiovascular Angiography and Interventions, Society of Cardiovascular Computed Tomography, Society for Interventional Radiology, Society for Vascular Medicine, and Society for Vascular Surgery. *J. Vasc. Surg.* 56, e17–e51. doi:10.1016/j.jvs.2012.05.054

Morovic, S., Jurasic, M. J., Martinic Popovic, I., Seric, V., Lisak, M., and Demarin, V. (2009). Vascular characteristics of patients with dementia. *J. Neurol. Sci.* 283, 41–43. doi:10.1016/j.jns.2009.02.330

Muller, M., Voges, M., Piepgras, U., and Schimrigk, K. (1995). Assessment of cerebral vasomotor reactivity by transcranial Doppler ultrasound and breath-holding. *Stroke* 26, 96–100.

National Cholesterol Education Program (NCEP) Expert Panel on Detection, Evaluation, and Treatment of High Blood Cholesterol in Adults (Adult Treatment Panel III). (2002). Third Report of the National Cholesterol Education Program (NCEP) Expert Panel on Detection, Evaluation, and Treatment of High Blood Cholesterol in Adults (Adult Treatment Panel III) final report. *Circulation* 106, 3143–3421.

Nemec, J. J., Marwick, T. H., Lorig, R. J., Davison, M. B., Chimowitz, M. I., Litowitz, H., et al. (1991). Comparison of transcranial Doppler ultrasound and transesophageal contrast echocardiography in the detection of interatrial right-to-left shunts. *Am. J. Cardiol.* 68, 1498–1502. doi:10.1016/0002-9149(91)90285-S

Oishi, M., Mochizuki, Y., and Takasu, T. (1999). Regional differences in cerebrovascular reactivity to acetazolamide in Alzheimer's disease. *J. Clin. Neurosci.* 6, 380–381. doi:10.1054/jocn.1997.0085

Oka, F., Ishihara, H., Kato, S., Oku, T., Yamane, A., Kunitugu, I., et al. (2013). Cerebral hemodynamic benefits after carotid artery stenting in patients with near occlusion. *J. Vasc. Surg.* 58, 1512–1517. doi:10.1016/j.jvs.2013.05.103

Pavics, L., Grunwald, F., Reichmann, K., Horn, R., Kitschenberg, A., Hartmann, A., et al. (1999). Regional cerebral blood flow single-photon emission tomography with 99mTc-HMPAO and the acetazolamide test in the evaluation of vascular and Alzheimer's dementia. *Eur. J. Nucl. Med.* 26, 239–245. doi:10.1007/s002590050383

Peisker, T., Bartos, A., Skoda, O., Ibrahim, I., and Kalvach, P. (2010). Impact of aging on cerebral vasoregulation and parenchymal integrity. *J. Neurol. Sci.* 299, 112–115. doi:10.1016/j.jns.2010.08.064

Provinciali, L., Minciotti, P., Ceravolo, G., Angeleri, F., and Sanguinetti, C. M. (1990). Transcranial Doppler sonography as a diagnostic tool in vascular dementia. *Eur. Neurol.* 30, 98–103. doi:10.1159/000117320

Pugsley, W., Klinger, L., Paschalis, C., Treasure, T., Harrison, M., and Newman, S. (1994). The impact of microemboli during cardiopulmonary bypass on neuropsychological functioning. *Stroke* 25, 1393–1399. doi:10.1161/01.STR.25.7.1393

Purandare, N., and Burns, A. (2009). Cerebral emboli in the genesis of dementia. *J. Neurol. Sci.* 283, 17–20. doi:10.1016/j.jns.2009.02.306

Purandare, N., Burns, A., Daly, K. J., Hardicre, J., Morris, J., Macfarlane, G., et al. (2006). Cerebral emboli as a potential cause of Alzheimer's disease and vascular dementia: case-control study. *BMJ* 332, 1119–1124. doi:10.1136/bmj.38814.696493.AE

Purandare, N., Welsh, S., Hutchinson, S., Riding, G., Burns, A., and McCollum, C. (2005). Cerebral emboli and paradoxical embolisation in dementia: a pilot study. *Int. J. Geriatr. Psychiatry* 20, 12–16. doi:10.1002/gps.1202

Ries, F., Horn, R., Hillekamp, J., Honisch, C., Konig, M., and Solymosi, L. (1993). Differentiation of multi-infarct and Alzheimer dementia by intracranial hemodynamic parameters. *Stroke* 24, 228–235. doi:10.1161/01.STR.24.2.228

Roher, A. E., Garami, Z., Alexandrov, A. V., Kokjohn, T. A., Esh, C. L., Kalback, W. M., et al. (2006). Interaction of cardiovascular disease and neurodegeneration: transcranial Doppler ultrasonography and Alzheimer's disease. *Neurol. Res.* 28, 672–678. doi:10.1179/016164106X130470

Roher, A. E., Garami, Z., Tyas, S. L., Maarouf, C. L., Kokjohn, T. A., Belohlavek, M., et al. (2011). Transcranial Doppler ultrasound blood flow velocity and pulsatility index as systemic indicators for Alzheimer's disease. *Alzheimers Dement.* 7, 445–455. doi:10.1016/j.jalz.2010.09.002

Rosengarten, B., Paulsen, S., Molnar, S., Kaschel, R., Gallhofer, B., and Kaps, M. (2006). Acetylcholine esterase inhibitor donepezil improves dynamic cerebrovascular regulation in Alzheimer patients. *J. Neurol.* 253, 58–64. doi:10.1007/s00415-005-0926-5

Rosengarten, B., Paulsen, S., Molnar, S., Kaschel, R., Gallhofer, B., and Kaps, M. (2007). Activation-flow coupling differentiates between vascular and Alzheimer type of dementia. *J. Neurol. Sci.* 257, 149–154. doi:10.1016/j.jns.2007.01.032

Ruitenberg, A., den Heijer, T., Bakker, S. L., van Swieten, J. C., Koudstaal, P. J., Hofman, A., et al. (2005). Cerebral hypoperfusion and clinical onset of dementia: the Rotterdam Study. *Ann. Neurol.* 57, 789–794. doi:10.1002/ana.20493

Sastry, S., MacNab, A., Daly, K., Ray, S., and McCollum, C. (2009). Transcranial Doppler detection of venous-to-arterial circulation shunts: criteria for patent foramen ovale. *J. Clin. Ultrasound* 37, 276–280. doi:10.1002/jcu.20564

Schoning, M., and Scheel, P. (1996). Color duplex measurement of cerebral blood flow volume: intra- and interobserver reproducibility and habituation to serial measurements in normal subjects. *J. Cereb. Blood Flow Metab.* 16, 523–531. doi:10.1097/00004647-199605000-00020

Schoning, M., Walter, J., and Scheel, P. (1994). Estimation of cerebral blood flow through color duplex sonography of the carotid and vertebral arteries in healthy adults. *Stroke* 25, 17–22. doi:10.1161/01.STR.25.1.17

Schreiber, S. J., Doepp, F., Spruth, E., Kopp, U. A., and Valdueza, J. M. (2005). Ultrasonographic measurement of cerebral blood flow, cerebral circulation time and cerebral blood volume in vascular and Alzheimer's dementia. *J. Neurol.* 252, 1171–1177. doi:10.1007/s00415-005-0826-8

Shah, N. S., Vidal, J. S., Masaki, K., Petrovitch, H., Ross, G. W., Tilley, C., et al. (2012). Midlife blood pressure, plasma beta-amyloid, and the risk for Alzheimer disease: the Honolulu Asia Aging Study. *Hypertension* 59, 780–786. doi:10.1161/HYPERTENSIONAHA.111.178962

Silvestrini, M., Gobbi, B., Pasqualetti, P., Bartolini, M., Baruffaldi, R., Lanciotti, C., et al. (2009). Carotid atherosclerosis and cognitive decline in patients with Alzheimer's disease. *Neurobiol. Aging* 30, 1177–1183. doi:10.1016/j.neurobiolaging.2007.11.008

Silvestrini, M., Pasqualetti, P., Baruffaldi, R., Bartolini, M., Handouk, Y., Matteis, M., et al. (2006). Cerebrovascular reactivity and cognitive decline in patients with Alzheimer disease. *Stroke* 37, 1010–1015. doi:10.1161/01.STR.0000206439.62025.97

Silvestrini, M., Viticchi, G., Falsetti, L., Balucani, C., Vernieri, F., Cerqua, R., et al. (2011). The role of carotid atherosclerosis in Alzheimer's disease progression. *J. Alzheimers Dis.* 25, 719–726. doi:10.3233/JAD-2011-101968

Society of Atherosclerosis Imaging and Prevention Developed in collaboration with the International Atherosclerosis Society. (2011). Appropriate use criteria for carotid intima media thickness testing. *Atherosclerosis* 214, 43–46. doi:10.1016/j.atherosclerosis.2010.10.045

Stefani, A., Sancesario, G., Pierantozzi, M., Leone, G., Galati, S., Hainsworth, A. H., et al. (2009). CSF biomarkers, impairment of cerebral hemodynamics and degree of cognitive decline in Alzheimer's and mixed dementia. *J. Neurol. Sci.* 283, 109–115. doi:10.1016/j.jns.2009.02.343

Stein, J. H., Korcarz, C. E., and Post, W. S. (2009). Use of carotid ultrasound to identify subclinical vascular disease and evaluate cardiovascular disease risk: summary and discussion of the American Society of Echocardiography consensus statement. *Prev. Cardiol.* 12, 34–38. doi:10.1111/j.1751-7141.2008.00021.x

Stoppe, G., Schutze, R., Kogler, A., Staedt, J., Munz, D. L., Emrich, D., et al. (1995). Cerebrovascular reactivity to acetazolamide in (senile) dementia of Alzheimer's type: relationship to disease severity. *Dementia* 6, 73–82.

Sun, Z. W., Zhu, Y. X., Liu, H. Y., Liu, J., Zhu, X. Q., Zhou, J. N., et al. (2007). Decreased cerebral blood flow velocity in apolipoprotein E epsilon4 allele carriers with mild cognitive impairment. *Eur. J. Neurol.* 14, 150–155. doi:10.1111/j.1468-1331.2006.01579.x

Sztriha, L. K., Nemeth, D., Sefcsik, T., and Vecsei, L. (2009). Carotid stenosis and the cognitive function. *J. Neurol. Sci.* 283, 36–40. doi:10.1016/j.jns.2009.02.307

Teague, S. M., and Sharma, M. K. (1991). Detection of paradoxical cerebral echo contrast embolization by transcranial Doppler ultrasound. *Stroke* 22, 740–745. doi:10.1161/01.STR.22.6.740

Touboul, P. J., Hennerici, M. G., Meairs, S., Adams, H., Amarenco, P., Bornstein, N., et al. (2012). Mannheim carotid intima-media thickness and plaque consensus (2004-2006-2011). An update on behalf of the advisory board of the 3rd, 4th and 5th watching the risk symposia, at the 13th, 15th and 20th European Stroke Conferences, Mannheim, Germany, 2004, Brussels, Belgium, 2006, and Hamburg, Germany, 2011. *Cerebrovasc. Dis.* 34, 290–296. doi:10.1159/000343145

van Es, A. C., van der Grond, J., ten Dam, V. H., de Craen, A. J., Blauw, G. J., Westendorp, R. G., et al. (2010). Associations between total cerebral blood flow and age related changes of the brain. *PLoS ONE* 5:e9825. doi:10.1371/journal.pone.0009825

van Oijen, M., de Jong, F. J., Witteman, J. C., Hofman, A., Koudstaal, P. J., and Breteler, M. M. (2007). Atherosclerosis and risk for dementia. *Ann. Neurol.* 61, 403–410. doi:10.1002/ana.21073

Vicenzini, E., Ricciardi, M. C., Altieri, M., Puccinelli, F., Bonaffini, N., Di Piero, V., et al. (2007). Cerebrovascular reactivity in degenerative and vascular dementia: a transcranial Doppler study. *Eur. Neurol.* 58, 84–89. doi:10.1159/000103642

Viticchi, G., Falsetti, L., Vernieri, F., Altamura, C., Bartolini, M., Luzzi, S., et al. (2012). Vascular predictors of cognitive decline in patients with mild cognitive impairment. *Neurobiol. Aging* 33, e1–e9. doi:10.1016/j.neurobiolaging.2011.11.027

Wolf, H., Ecke, G. M., Bettin, S., Dietrich, J., and Gertz, H. J. (2000). Do white matter changes contribute to the subsequent development of dementia in patients with mild cognitive impairment? A longitudinal study. *Int. J. Geriatr. Psychiatry* 15, 803–812. doi:10.1002/1099-1166(200009)15:9<803::AID-GPS190>3.3.CO;2-N

Wollman, D. E., and Prohovnik, I. (2003). Sensitivity and specificity of neuroimaging for the diagnosis of Alzheimer's disease. *Dialogues Clin. Neurosci.* 5, 89–99.

Wu, C. C., Mungas, D., Petkov, C. I., Eberling, J. L., Zrelak, P. A., Buonocore, M. H., et al. (2002). Brain structure and cognition in a community sample of elderly Latinos. *Neurology* 59, 383–391. doi:10.1212/WNL.59.3.383

Yamaguchi, F., Meyer, J. S., Yamamoto, M., Sakai, F., and Shaw, T. (1980). Noninvasive regional cerebral blood flow measurements in dementia. *Arch. Neurol.* 37, 410–418. doi:10.1001/archneur.1980.00500560040003

14

Neural correlates of spatial navigation changes in mild cognitive impairment and Alzheimer's disease

Kamil Vlček [1,2] * and Jan Laczó [2,3]

[1] Department of Neurophysiology of Memory, Institute of Physiology, Academy of Sciences of the Czech Republic, Prague, Czech Republic
[2] International Clinical Research Center, St. Anne's University Hospital Brno, Brno, Czech Republic
[3] Department of Neurology, 2nd Faculty of Medicine, Charles University in Prague and Motol University Hospital, Prague, Czech Republic

Edited by:
Tomiki Sumiyoshi, National Center of Neurology and Psychiatry, Japan

***Correspondence:**
Kamil Vlček, Institute of Physiology, Academy of Sciences of the Czech Republic, Vídenská 1083, Praha 4, 142 20 Prague, Czech Republic
e-mail: kamil@biomed.cas.cz

Although the memory impairment is a hallmark of Alzheimer's disease (AD), AD has also been characterized by spatial disorientation, which is present from its early stages. Spatial disorientation in AD manifests itself in getting lost in familiar and unfamiliar places and have been characterized more specifically using spatial navigation tests in both real space and virtual environments as an impairment in multiple spatial abilities, including allocentric and egocentric navigation strategies, visuo-spatial perception, or selection of relevant information for successful navigation. Patients suffering mild cognitive impairment (MCI), who are at a high risk of development of dementia, show impairment in a subset of these abilities, mainly connected with allocentric and egocentric processing. While spatial disorientation in typical AD patients probably reflects neurodegenerative changes in medial and posterior temporal, parietal, and frontal lobes, and retrosplenial cortex, the impairment of spatial navigation in MCI seem to be connected mainly with the medial temporal and also parietal brain changes. In this review, we will summarize the signs of brain disease in most MCI and AD patients showing in various tasks of spatial memory and navigation.

Keywords: Alzheimer's disease, mild cognitive impairment, spatial navigation, spatial disorientation, brain changes

INTRODUCTION

Spatial disorientation is one of the early manifestations of Alzheimer's disease (AD), besides the clinically mostly used memory impairment. The research in spatial deficits in this neurodegenerative disease has grown rapidly in last years and decline in spatial navigation abilities may become another diagnostic mark for AD in the near future. Spatial navigation is however not a unitary function. This ability to determine and maintain a route from one place to another (Gallistel, 1990) utilizes multiple spatial strategies recruiting distinct brain regions.

This review aims to describe spatial disorientation in AD and mild cognitive impairment (MCI) as a multi-factorial deficit connected with changes in several brain regions. Various described manifestations of these changes in spatial cognitive tasks are the focus of this article. Selected for the review were only studies describing impairment in AD or MCI patients in real or virtual space, in spatial navigation, or associated abilities like perspective taking or object location memory.

CURRENT VIEW ON SPATIAL DEFICITS IN AD AND MCI

A number of studies focusing on visuo-spatial deficits in AD and MCI appeared during last two decades. The main published view on these deficits is broadly dual: one series of studies documented visuo-perceptual nature of the disorientation, its association with optic flow perception, and visuo-spatial attention (e.g., Tetewsky and Duffy, 1999; Cherrier et al., 2001; Mapstone et al., 2003; Kavcic et al., 2006). Another series of investigations stressed, however, the cognitive mapping deficits in these patients, specifically in using the allocentric navigation (Kalova et al., 2005; Hort et al., 2007; Weniger et al., 2011; Nedelska et al., 2012). According to some other reports, the spatial disorientation in AD and MCI patients seem to be associated with both medial temporal and parietal lobe function (Henderson et al., 1989; deIpolyi et al., 2007). Several reviews on this theme published recently support either the latter allocentric view (Iachini et al., 2009) or combination of both cognitive mapping and visuo-perceptual factors (Vlcek, 2011; Gazova et al., 2012) or suggest a multifocal theory of disease developing from temporal to parietal and lateral to frontal brain and midbrain and associated cognitive deficits (Lithfous et al., 2013). One other review proposes the translation between egocentric and allocentric frames, supported by retrosplenial cortex (RSC), being the basis of spatial disorientation deficits in MCI and AD (Serino and Riva, 2013).

BRAIN CHANGES IN MCI AND AD

The anterior medial temporal lobe structures are the first affected by AD pathology. Histopathological changes initially occur in the entorhinal cortex and the hippocampus, further spread throughout parahippocampal gyrus to the temporal pole and inferior and middle temporal gyri in MCI and preclinical AD, and subsequently spread throughout the temporal, parietal, and frontal neocortex by the time of dementia due to AD (Braak and Braak, 1995; Petersen et al., 2006). In agreement with this neuropathological staging, the highest rate of atrophy in the MCI and initial stages of AD has been found in the entorhinal and perirhinal cortices and the hippocampus (Pennanen et al., 2004; Schmidt-Wilcke et al., 2009; Risacher et al., 2010), which also showed accelerated volume loss over the time (Schuff et al., 2012) and hypometabolism (Karow et al., 2010).

The anteromedial temporal atrophy was described even in cognitively normal individuals later converting to MCI (Smith et al., 2007). The posterior part of the gyrus, the parahippocampal cortex, is affected later in the course of AD (Karow et al., 2010; Spulber et al., 2012), followed by atrophy of the fusiform gyrus (McDonald et al., 2009).

A number of neuroimaging studies have also shown structural and metabolic changes in the parietal lobe, early in the course of AD. Cortical atrophy (Fennema-Notestine et al., 2009) in the precuneus and the inferior parietal lobule were reduced in the early MCI stages (McDonald et al., 2009) and volume reduction of these areas is the most consistent finding among the MCI to AD converters (Karas et al., 2008; Whitwell et al., 2008) and was described even in normal individuals later converting to MCI and AD (Smith et al., 2007; Jacobs et al., 2011). Hypometabolism was also found in superior parietal lobules (Li et al., 2008; Nobili et al., 2008) and even more in the inferior parietal lobule (Nobili et al., 2009) in MCI patients, especially those converting later to AD (Drzezga et al., 2003; Hirao et al., 2005).

Within the cingulate gyrus, the posterior cingulate and RSC are affected early in the course of AD. Atrophy of these areas was demonstrated in mild AD patients (Scahill et al., 2002) and patients with early stages of MCI (Chetelat et al., 2002; Fennema-Notestine et al., 2009), especially in those later progressing to AD (Hamalainen et al., 2007; Whitwell et al., 2008; Julkunen et al., 2009; Pengas et al., 2010a). Severe posterior cingulate cortex hypometabolism is a feature of incipient AD (Nestor et al., 2003a,b) and is present already in the MCI patients (Huang et al., 2002; Ishiwata et al., 2006; Johnson et al., 2007; Pappata et al., 2010).

Neuropathological changes occur in the frontal cortex later in the course of AD (Braak and Braak, 1995; Petersen et al., 2006). Frontal lobe atrophy and hypometabolism is not present earlier than at the later stages of MCI and mainly in the prefrontal cortex (Fennema-Notestine et al., 2009; Langbaum et al., 2009; McDonald et al., 2009) but is more pronounced in those MCI patients who later converted to AD (Drzezga et al., 2003; Whitwell et al., 2008).

Although the described the brain changes prevails in AD and MCI patients, in a significant portion of AD patients the underlying neuropathological process follows alternative distribution, representing at least two other clinicopathological subtypes of AD and contrasting with the typical AD (Murray et al., 2011). In the hippocampal sparing AD subtype, found in 11% of patients, the neuronal degeneration results in lower gray matter volumes of lateral parietal, lateral temporal, and lateral frontal cortex, compared to typical AD (Whitwell et al., 2012). In the limbic-predominant AD subtype, found in 14–19% patients, the areas affected more than in the typical AD are the hippocampus and amygdala, with lower gray matter volumes. These differences are associated with distinct cognitive profiles in memory and other cognitive domains and necessarily also in spatial navigation, as well as with the different course of cognitive changes over time. However, the AD subtypes have not been considered in the studies reviewed below and the described deficits in spatial memory applies probably only to the predominating typical AD.

SPATIAL NAVIGATION DEFICITS IN MCI AND AD

ALLOCENTRIC NAVIGATION, OBJECT LOCATION MEMORY, AND SCENE PROCESSING

Allocentric memory enables us to locate a goal in relation to surrounding objects and global landmarks, a function localized to medial temporal lobe, and hippocampus specifically (O'Keefe and Nadel, 1978; Maguire et al., 1998; Astur et al., 2002; Feigenbaum and Morris, 2004; Parslow et al., 2004). Hippocampal role in spatial deficits in AD and MCI have been documented by a series of allocentric navigation studies: AD patients were impaired in a real space analog of Morris water maze, termed blue velvet arena (BVA): only in allocentric trials when the cues on the wall could be used for orientation, but not in trials without cues, when only the start position could be used (Kalova et al., 2005). In the same apparatus, a more strictly defined AD group had problems navigating using both start position and cues on the walls, but an amnestic MCI single-domain group was impaired only in the allocentric trials (Hort et al., 2007), suggesting specific hippocampal impairment. This was supported later in a follow-up study where hippocampal amnestic MCI patients showed no learning in the allocentric trials (Laczo et al., 2009). Virtual analogy was also used in a recent study (Hort et al., 2014), where BVA was termed Urania. Amnestic MCI were also impaired in another allocentric navigation test to find shortest way to hidden targets in a virtual park (Weniger et al., 2011). A connection of allocentric navigation to hippocampal function was supported also in a study correlating real space Morris water maze analogy navigation successfulness with right hippocampal volume (Nedelska et al., 2012).

Successfulness in other spatial tasks is probably also connected to hippocampal function. Memory for temporal sequence of three body turns in a Starmaze was documented to activate left hippocampus (Igloi et al., 2010) and later shown to distinguish well between mild AD patients and controls (Bellassen et al., 2012). Memory for location of objects in space was several time consistently shown to be dependent on hippocampal function (Milner et al., 1997; Kessels et al., 2004; Stepankova et al., 2004) and reported to be deficient in patients suffering AD (Bucks and Willison, 1997; Brandt et al., 2005) and also in MCI patients, although to a lesser degree than in AD (Kessels et al., 2010). In contrast, memory for several positions without objects seem to be preserved even in mild AD (Adelstein et al., 1992; Kalova et al., 2005).

Processing of viewpoint independent spatial representation of a scene during scene matching seem also to be associated with hippocampal function after very short delays and with parahippocampal cortex function even in the presence of the sample scene (Hartley et al., 2007). In the same test, groups of six AD patients and seven amnestic MCI patients were impaired after short delays but not in direct scene matching (Bird et al., 2010), while a larger group of AD patients was impaired even in matching of simultaneously visible scenes (Pengas et al., 2010b). In a similar test, scene discrimination across different views was worsened in a selective hippocampal damage group (Lee et al., 2005) and also in a group of mild AD patients (Lee et al., 2006).

REFERENCE FRAME TRANSLATION

Retrosplenial cortex, a part of the posterior cingulate cortex, is strongly involved in spatial processing, specifically in translation between egocentric and allocentric representations (Byrne et al., 2007). Its damage shows as heading disorientation, an inability to derive directional information from scenes or to estimate spatial relationship between two locations (Aguirre and D'Esposito, 1999). Impairment of head orientation was also documented in AD but not MCI patients, reaching lower score in head orientation test, requiring to indicate directions after a test of navigation within a virtual city (Pengas et al., 2010b). Navigation score in this test correlated with gray matter density and glucose metabolism in RSC, but also hippocampus (Pengas et al., 2012). In another study on virtual as well as real navigation in a hospital lobby, AD patients, but again not MCI patients, were impaired in a test of self-orientation, requiring to indicate directions to scenes from the route (Cushman et al., 2008). The AD patients were also impaired in navigation in a virtual-reality maze using its map, which required translation of allocentric representation in the map to the egocentric direction in the maze (Morganti et al., 2013). Location of scenes on a map could possibly be also regarded as a behavioral measure of RSC function, requiring egocentric to allocentric translation. This ability was impaired in MCI patients in two studies focused on route learning and follow-up set of spatial tests (delpolyi et al., 2007; Cushman et al., 2008).

EGOCENTRIC NAVIGATION

Egocentric memory enables us to remember positions in space in relation to one's own position and heading in space. The brain localization of the navigational strategy using egocentric reference frame seems to be diverse and possibly reflects multiplicity of strategies concealed under the usage of a single egocentric reference frame. The superior and inferior parietal lobe structures have been activated during various egocentric tasks in Morris water maze analogy (Parslow et al., 2004), virtual city (Maguire et al., 1998; Wolbers et al., 2004) as well as in landmark-free environment (Wolbers et al., 2008). The activity in caudated nucleus was associated with a response strategy in a virtual analogy of a radial maze (Iaria et al., 2003) and following a well-learned route in a virtual city (Hartley et al., 2003).

Egocentric navigation was documented to be impaired in AD and also MCI patients in two types of experiments. In a both real space and computer analogy of Morris water maze, amnestic MCI patients with associated non-memory impairment scored similarly to AD patients in finding of hidden goal position using only their starting position (Hort et al., 2007). In landmark-free virtual-reality maze, requiring the subjects to use only the sequence of egocentric turns during navigation, the amnestic MCI subjects were unable to learn a route to a hidden reward (Weniger et al., 2011). In addition, the number of errors in this maze correlated negatively with precuneus volume, supporting the assumption of egocentric strategy use.

VISUAL PERCEPTION

A wealth of reports document the role of visual perception functions in navigational impairment: either perception of optic flow, visuo-spatial attention, or visual perceptual analysis. The optic flow perception is supported by the visual area V5/MT at the junction of occipital, temporal, and parietal lobes (Morrone et al., 2000). Connection of optic flow perception thresholds with navigation impairment in AD patients was described in studies using route learning in a hospital lobby (Tetewsky and Duffy, 1999) or indirectly using left–right orientation in table-top Money Road Map test (MRMT) and sustained driving in On-the-Road Driving test (O'Brien et al., 2001). Similar correlation between MRMT scores and optic flow perception was found also in MCI patients (Mapstone et al., 2003). Even better prediction of the navigation score in a hospital lobby was found in a combined regression model containing contrast sensitivity score and amplitude of the visual ERP N200 responses (Kavcic et al., 2006). This association of navigation score to visual perception could however be confined only to men patients (Cushman and Duffy, 2007), while in women patients the navigation score seem to be better predicted by verbal fluency and figural memory.

The perceptual nature of disorientation could be inferred also from other studies on AD patients. These patients were impaired in recognition of incidental landmarks not mentioned during the walk in a hospital lobby in contrast to correct recognition of the mentioned landmarks (Cherrier et al., 2001). In another study, also using route learning in a hospital lobby, the impairment of AD patients was predicted by MRMT and Line orientation test but not by mostly low memory scores (Monacelli et al., 2003). The impairment of AD patients in all angle categories of turns in MRMT, in combination with their normal left–right discrimination, have also been explained by visual perceptual deficits (Rainville et al., 2002). Similarly, visuoconstructive test scores together with results from a memory test predicted spatial disorientation sub-score from Memory and Behavior Problems Checklist questionnaire (Henderson et al., 1989), supporting the dual roots of AD disorientation.

PLANNING AND PROBLEM SOLVING

Deficits in frontal problem solving functions were documented in a unique experiment (Passini et al., 1995), requiring AD subjects to guide the experimenter to the dental clinic in an unknown hospital and to express verbally everything that went through their mind. To minimize the effect of memory and attentional deficit, the subjects were repeatedly reminded about their task. Their behavior was seemingly more driven by external stimuli than by the goal of the way-finding task, suggesting difficulties to distinguish relevant from irrelevant information and to structure their decision plan.

LANDMARK RECOGNITION

Individual recognition of landmarks, salient features of environment useful for navigation, is an isolated cognitive ability, impaired in landmark agnosia (Aguirre and D'Esposito, 1999) and dependent on the function of the anterior end of the right lingual gyrus (Aguirre et al., 1998; Mendez and Cherrier, 2003). Three real-world navigation studies report different successfulness in AD and MCI patients: in a series of tests after a walk in a hospital lobby, MCI and mild AD patients were similar to controls in landmarks recognition (delpolyi et al., 2007), but were impaired in a more recent study (Benke et al., 2013). The relationship of this impairment to visuospatial attention are suggesting the results of an earlier study, where recognition of landmarks mentioned by experimenter during the walk was least impaired in AD patients, in contrast to their large impairment in recognition of landmarks not mentioned during the walk (Cherrier et al., 2001).

In contrast, in a free recall of landmarks along a route, the AD patients were found to be impaired (Monacelli et al., 2003) and this measure even distinguished reliably between MCI and healthy old subjects (Cushman et al., 2008).

CONCLUSION

Findings of this survey are mainly consistent with the described brain changes during spreading of the disease and suggest its propagation from the anterior medial temporal lobe to posterior temporal and parietal areas in MCI and to frontal and parieto-occipital areas later in AD patients. MCI patients seem to be impaired first in the allocentric navigation and later in the multi-domain stage also in egocentric navigation. Consistently with this double impairment, suggesting their medial temporal as well as posterior parietal damage, they have been found to be impaired also in route learning in both real and virtual environments. Short-term scene memory, visuo-spatial attention, and optic flow perception may also affect their navigational successfulness.

The broad cognitive impairment of even mild AD patients interferes also with other abilities essential for successful navigation, as optic flow perception, reference frame translation, scene matching, spatial planning, visual perceptual analyses, and possibly landmark recognition. Their navigation difficulties seem therefore to be connected with their more wide spread brain damage in other areas of parietal lobes and temporal cortex, RSC, as well as frontal lobes.

AUTHOR CONTRIBUTIONS

Both Kamil Vlček and Jan Laczó wrote and discussed the manuscript, contributed to the final version of the paper and have approved it.

ACKNOWLEDGMENTS

We would like to thank to Jakub Hort for his thorough revisions and comments. The study was supported by MH CR – IGA grant NT13386; ERDF – Project FNUSA-ICRC (No. CZ.1.05/1.1.00/02.0123); ESF and the State Budget of the CR; Young Talent Incubator II (Reg. no. CZ.1.07/2.3.00/20.0117); MH CR – DRO (University Hospital Motol, Prague, Czech Republic, 00064203); Institutional Support of Laboratory Research Grant No. 2/2012 (699002); research projects AV0Z 50110509 and RVO:67985823.

REFERENCES

Adelstein, T. B., Kesner, R. P., and Strassberg, D. S. (1992). Spatial recognition and spatial order memory in patients with dementia of the Alzheimer's type. *Neuropsychologia* 30, 59–67. doi:10.1016/0028-3932(92)90014-D

Aguirre, G. K., and D'Esposito, M. (1999). Topographical disorientation: a synthesis and taxonomy. *Brain* 122, 1613–1628. doi:10.1093/brain/122.9.1613

Aguirre, G. K., Zarahn, E., and D'Esposito, M. (1998). An area within human ventral cortex sensitive to "building" stimuli: evidence and implications. *Neuron* 21, 373–383. doi:10.1016/S0896-6273(00)80546-2

Astur, R. S., Taylor, L. B., Mamelak, A. N., Philpott, L., and Sutherland, R. J. (2002). Humans with hippocampus damage display severe spatial memory impairments in a virtual Morris water task. *Behav. Brain Res.* 132, 77–84. doi:10.1016/S0166-4328(01)00399-0

Bellassen, V., Igloi, K., de Souza, L. C., Dubois, B., and Rondi-Reig, L. (2012). Temporal order memory assessed during spatiotemporal navigation as a behavioral cognitive marker for differential Alzheimer's disease diagnosis. *J. Neurosci.* 32, 1942–1952. doi:10.1523/JNEUROSCI.4556-11.2012

Benke, T., Karner, E., Petermichl, S., Prantner, V., and Kemmler, G. (2013). Neuropsychological deficits associated with route learning in Alzheimer disease, MCI, and normal aging. *Alzheimer Dis. Assoc. Disord.* doi:10.1097/WAD.0000000000000009

Bird, C. M., Chan, D., Hartley, T., Pijnenburg, Y. A., Rossor, M. N., and Burgess, N. (2010). Topographical short-term memory differentiates Alzheimer's disease from frontotemporal lobar degeneration. *Hippocampus* 20, 1154–1169. doi:10.1002/hipo.20715

Braak, H., and Braak, E. (1995). Staging of Alzheimer's disease-related neurofibrillary changes. *Neurobiol. Aging* 16, 271–278. doi:10.1016/0197-4580(95)00021-6

Brandt, J., Shpritz, B., Munro, C. A., Marsh, L., and Rosenblatt, A. (2005). Differential impairment of spatial location memory in Huntington's disease. *J. Neurol. Neurosurg. Psychiatr.* 76, 1516–1519. doi:10.1136/jnnp.2004.059253

Bucks, R. S., and Willison, J. R. (1997). Development and validation of the location learning test (LLT): a test of visuo-spatial learning designed for use with older adults and in dementia. *Clin. Neuropsychol.* 11, 273–286. doi:10.1080/13854049708400456

Byrne, P., Becker, S., and Burgess, N. (2007). Remembering the past and imagining the future: a neural model of spatial memory and imagery. *Psychol. Rev.* 114, 340–375. doi:10.1037/0033-295X.114.2.340

Cherrier, M. M., Mendez, M., and Perryman, K. (2001). Route learning performance in Alzheimer disease patients. *Neuropsychiatry Neuropsychol. Behav. Neurol.* 14, 159–168.

Chetelat, G., Desgranges, B., De La Sayette, V., Viader, F., Eustache, F., and Baron, J. C. (2002). Mapping gray matter loss with voxel-based morphometry in mild cognitive impairment. *Neuroreport* 13, 1939–1943. doi:10.1097/00001756-200210280-00022

Cushman, L. A., and Duffy, C. J. (2007). The sex specificity of navigational strategies in Alzheimer disease. *Alzheimer Dis. Assoc. Disord.* 21, 122–129. doi:10.1097/WAD.0b013e318047df2f

Cushman, L. A., Stein, K., and Duffy, C. J. (2008). Detecting navigational deficits in cognitive aging and Alzheimer disease using virtual reality. *Neurology* 71, 888–895. doi:10.1212/01.wnl.0000326262.67613.fe

delpolyi, A. R., Rankin, K. P., Mucke, L., Miller, B. L., and Gorno-Tempini, M. L. (2007). Spatial cognition and the human navigation network in AD and MCI. *Neurology* 69, 986–997. doi:10.1212/01.wnl.0000271376.19515.c6

Drzezga, A., Lautenschlager, N., Siebner, H., Riemenschneider, M., Willoch, F., Minoshima, S., et al. (2003). Cerebral metabolic changes accompanying conversion of mild cognitive impairment into Alzheimer's disease: a PET follow-up study. *Eur. J. Nucl. Med. Mol. Imaging* 30, 1104–1113. doi:10.1007/s00259-003-1194-1

Feigenbaum, J. D., and Morris, R. G. (2004). Allocentric versus egocentric spatial memory after unilateral temporal lobectomy in humans. *Neuropsychology* 18, 462–472. doi:10.1037/0894-4105.18.3.462

Fennema-Notestine, C., Hagler, D. J. Jr, McEvoy, L. K., Fleisher, A. S., Wu, E. H., Karow, D. S., et al. (2009). Structural MRI biomarkers for preclinical and mild Alzheimer's disease. *Hum. Brain Mapp.* 30, 3238–3253. doi:10.1002/hbm.20744

Gallistel, C. R. (1990). *The Organization of Learning.* Cambridge: The MIT Press.

Gazova, I., Vlcek, K., Laczo, J., Nedelska, Z., Hyncicova, E., Mokrisova, I., et al. (2012). Spatial navigation-a unique window into physiological and pathological aging. *Front. Aging Neurosci.* 4:16. doi:10.3389/fnagi.2012.00016

Hamalainen, A., Tervo, S., Grau-Olivares, M., Niskanen, E., Pennanen, C., Huuskonen, J., et al. (2007). Voxel-based morphometry to detect brain atrophy in progressive mild cognitive impairment. *Neuroimage* 37, 1122–1131. doi:10.1016/j.neuroimage.2007.06.016

Hartley, T., Bird, C. M., Chan, D., Cipolotti, L., Husain, M., Vargha-Khadem, F., et al. (2007). The hippocampus is required for short-term topographical memory in humans. *Hippocampus* 17, 34–48. doi:10.1002/hipo.20240

Hartley, T., Maguire, E. A., Spiers, H. J., and Burgess, N. (2003). The well-worn route and the path less traveled: distinct neural bases of route following and wayfinding in humans. *Neuron* 37, 877–888. doi:10.1016/S0896-6273(03)00095-3

Henderson, V. W., Mack, W., and Williams, B. W. (1989). Spatial disorientation in Alzheimer's disease. *Arch. Neurol.* 46, 391–394. doi:10.1001/archneur.1989.00520400045018

Hirao, K., Ohnishi, T., Hirata, Y., Yamashita, F., Mori, T., Moriguchi, Y., et al. (2005). The prediction of rapid conversion to Alzheimer's disease in mild cognitive impairment using regional cerebral blood flow SPECT. *Neuroimage* 28, 1014–1021. doi:10.1016/j.neuroimage.2005.06.066

Hort, J., Andel, R., Mokrisova, I., Gazova, I., Amlerova, J., Valis, M., et al. (2014). Effect of donepezil in Alzheimer disease can be measured by a computerized human analog of the morris water maze. *Neurodegener. Dis.* 13, 192–196. doi:10.1159/000355517

Hort, J., Laczo, J., Vyhnalek, M., Bojar, M., Bures, J., and Vlcek, K. (2007). Spatial navigation deficit in amnestic mild cognitive impairment. *Proc. Natl. Acad. Sci. U.S.A.* 104, 4042–4047. doi:10.1073/pnas.0611314104

Huang, C., Wahlund, L. O., Svensson, L., Winblad, B., and Julin, P. (2002). Cingulate cortex hypoperfusion predicts Alzheimer's disease in mild cognitive impairment. *BMC Neurol.* 2:9. doi:10.1186/1471-2377-2-9

Iachini, T., Iavarone, A., Senese, V. P., Ruotolo, F., and Ruggiero, G. (2009). Visuospatial memory in healthy elderly, AD and MCI: a review. *Curr. Aging Sci.* 2, 43–59. doi:10.2174/1874612810902010043

Iaria, G., Petrides, M., Dagher, A., Pike, B., and Bohbot, V. D. (2003). Cognitive strategies dependent on the hippocampus and caudate nucleus in human navigation: variability and change with practice. *J. Neurosci.* 23, 5945–5952.

Igloi, K., Doeller, C. F., Berthoz, A., Rondi-Reig, L., and Burgess, N. (2010). Lateralized human hippocampal activity predicts navigation based on sequence or place memory. *Proc. Natl. Acad. Sci. U.S.A.* 107, 14466–14471. doi:10.1073/pnas.1004243107

Ishiwata, A., Sakayori, O., Minoshima, S., Mizumura, S., Kitamura, S., and Katayama, Y. (2006). Preclinical evidence of Alzheimer changes in progressive mild cognitive impairment: a qualitative and quantitative SPECT study. *Acta Neurol. Scand.* 114, 91–96. doi:10.1111/j.1600-0404.2006.00661.x

Jacobs, H. I., Van Boxtel, M. P., Uylings, H. B., Gronenschild, E. H., Verhey, F. R., and Jolles, J. (2011). Atrophy of the parietal lobe in preclinical dementia. *Brain Cogn.* 75, 154–163. doi:10.1016/j.bandc.2010.11.003

Johnson, K. A., Moran, E. K., Becker, J. A., Blacker, D., Fischman, A. J., and Albert, M. S. (2007). Single photon emission computed tomography perfusion differences in mild cognitive impairment. *J. Neurol. Neurosurg. Psychiatr.* 78, 240–247. doi:10.1136/jnnp.2006.096800

Julkunen, V., Niskanen, E., Muehlboeck, S., Pihlajamaki, M., Kononen, M., Hallikainen, M., et al. (2009). Cortical thickness analysis to detect progressive mild cognitive impairment: a reference to Alzheimer's disease. *Dement. Geriatr. Cogn. Disord.* 28, 404–412. doi:10.1159/000256274

Kalova, E., Vlcek, K., Jarolimova, E., and Bures, J. (2005). Allothetic orientation and sequential ordering of places is impaired in early stages of Alzheimer's disease: corresponding results in real space tests and computer tests. *Behav. Brain Res.* 159, 175–186. doi:10.1016/j.bbr.2004.10.016

Karas, G., Sluimer, J., Goekoop, R., van der Flier, W., Rombouts, S. A., Vrenken, H., et al. (2008). Amnestic mild cognitive impairment: structural MR imaging findings predictive of conversion to Alzheimer disease. *AJNR Am. J. Neuroradiol.* 29, 944–949. doi:10.3174/ajnr.A0949

Karow, D. S., McEvoy, L. K., Fennema-Notestine, C., Hagler, D. J. Jr, Jennings, R. G., Brewer, J. B., et al. (2010). Relative capability of MR imaging and FDG PET to depict changes associated with prodromal and early Alzheimer disease. *Radiology* 256, 932–942. doi:10.1148/radiol.10091402

Kavcic, V., Fernandez, R., Logan, D., and Duffy, C. J. (2006). Neurophysiological and perceptual correlates of navigational impairment in Alzheimer's disease. *Brain* 129, 736–746. doi:10.1093/brain/awh727

Kessels, R. P., Hendriks, M., Schouten, J., Van Asselen, M., and Postma, A. (2004). Spatial memory deficits in patients after unilateral selective amygdalohippocampectomy. *J. Int. Neuropsychol. Soc.* 10, 907–912. doi:10.1017/S1355617704106140

Kessels, R. P., Rijken, S., Joosten-Weyn Banningh, L. W., Van Schuylenborgh-VAN Es, N., and Olde Rikkert, M. G. (2010). Categorical spatial memory in patients with mild cognitive impairment and Alzheimer dementia: positional versus object-location recall. *J. Int. Neuropsychol. Soc.* 16, 200–204. doi:10.1017/S1355617709990944

Laczo, J., Vlcek, K., Vyhnalek, M., Vajnerova, O., Ort, M., Holmerova, I., et al. (2009). Spatial navigation testing discriminates two types of amnestic mild cognitive impairment. *Behav. Brain Res.* 202, 252–259. doi:10.1016/j.bbr.2009.03.041

Langbaum, J. B., Chen, K., Lee, W., Reschke, C., Bandy, D., Fleisher, A. S., et al. (2009). Categorical and correlational analyses of baseline fluorodeoxyglucose positron emission tomography images from the Alzheimer's Disease Neuroimaging Initiative (ADNI). *Neuroimage* 45, 1107–1116. doi:10.1016/j.neuroimage.2008.12.072

Lee, A. C., Buckley, M. J., Gaffan, D., Emery, T., Hodges, J. R., and Graham, K. S. (2006). Differentiating the roles of the hippocampus and perirhinal cortex in processes beyond long-term declarative memory: a double dissociation in dementia. *J. Neurosci.* 26, 5198–5203. doi:10.1523/JNEUROSCI.3157-05.2006

Lee, A. C., Buckley, M. J., Pegman, S. J., Spiers, H., Scahill, V. L., Gaffan, D., et al. (2005). Specialization in the medial temporal lobe for processing of objects and scenes. *Hippocampus* 15, 782–797. doi:10.1002/hipo.20101

Li, Y., Rinne, J. O., Mosconi, L., Pirraglia, E., Rusinek, H., DeSanti, S., et al. (2008). Regional analysis of FDG and PIB-PET images in normal aging, mild cognitive impairment, and Alzheimer's disease. *Eur. J. Nucl. Med. Mol. Imaging* 35, 2169–2181. doi:10.1007/s00259-008-0833-y

Lithfous, S., Dufour, A., and Despres, O. (2013). Spatial navigation in normal aging and the prodromal stage of Alzheimer's disease: insights from imaging and behavioral studies. *Ageing Res. Rev.* 12, 201–213. doi:10.1016/j.arr.2012.04.007

Maguire, E. A., Burgess, N., Donnett, J. G., Frackowiak, R. S., Frith, C. D., and O'Keefe, J. (1998). Knowing where and getting there: a human navigation network. *Science* 280, 921–924. doi:10.1126/science.280.5365.921

Mapstone, M., Steffenella, T. M., and Duffy, C. J. (2003). A visuospatial variant of mild cognitive impairment: getting lost between aging and AD. *Neurology* 60, 802–808. doi:10.1212/01.WNL.0000049471.76799.DE

McDonald, C. R., McEvoy, L. K., Gharapetian, L., Fennema-Notestine, C., Hagler, D. J. Jr, Holland, D., et al. (2009). Regional rates of neocortical atrophy from normal aging to early Alzheimer disease. *Neurology* 73, 457–465. doi:10.1212/WNL.0b013e3181b16431

Mendez, M. F., and Cherrier, M. M. (2003). Agnosia for scenes in topographagnosia. *Neuropsychologia* 41, 1387–1395. doi:10.1016/S0028-3932(03)00041-1

Milner, B., Johnsrude, I., and Crane, J. (1997). Right medial temporal-lobe contribution to object-location memory. *Philos. Trans. R. Soc. Lond. B Biol. Sci.* 352, 1469–1474. doi:10.1098/rstb.1997.0133

Monacelli, A. M., Cushman, L. A., Kavcic, V., and Duffy, C. J. (2003). Spatial disorientation in Alzheimer's disease: the remembrance of things passed. *Neurology* 61, 1491–1497. doi:10.1212/WNL.61.11.1491

Morganti, F., Stefanini, S., and Riva, G. (2013). From allo- to egocentric spatial ability in early Alzheimer's disease: a study with virtual reality spatial tasks. *Cogn. Neurosci.* 4, 171–180. doi:10.1080/17588928.2013.854762

Morrone, M. C., Tosetti, M., Montanaro, D., Fiorentini, A., Cioni, G., and Burr, D. C. (2000). A cortical area that responds specifically to optic flow, revealed by fMRI. *Nat. Neurosci.* 3, 1322–1328. doi:10.1038/81860

Murray, M. E., Graff-Radford, N. R., Ross, O. A., Petersen, R. C., Duara, R., and Dickson, D. W. (2011). Neuropathologically defined subtypes of Alzheimer's disease with distinct clinical characteristics: a retrospective study. *Lancet Neurol.* 10, 785–796. doi:10.1016/S1474-4422(11)70156-9

Nedelska, Z., Andel, R., Laczo, J., Vlcek, K., Horinek, D., Lisy, J., et al. (2012). Spatial navigation impairment is proportional to right hippocampal volume. *Proc. Natl. Acad. Sci. U.S.A.* 109, 2590–2594. doi:10.1073/pnas.1121588109

Nestor, P. J., Fryer, T. D., Ikeda, M., and Hodges, J. R. (2003a). Retrosplenial cortex (BA 29/30) hypometabolism in mild cognitive impairment (prodromal Alzheimer's disease). *Eur. J. Neurosci.* 18, 2663–2667. doi:10.1046/j.1460-9568.2003.02999.x

Nestor, P. J., Fryer, T. D., Smielewski, P., and Hodges, J. R. (2003b). Limbic hypometabolism in Alzheimer's disease and mild cognitive impairment. *Ann. Neurol.* 54, 343–351. doi:10.1002/ana.10669

Nobili, F., De Carli, F., Frisoni, G. B., Portet, F., Verhey, F., Rodriguez, G., et al. (2009). SPECT predictors of cognitive decline and Alzheimer's disease in mild cognitive impairment. *J. Alzheimers Dis.* 17, 761–772. doi:10.3233/JAD-2009-1091

Nobili, F., Frisoni, G. B., Portet, F., Verhey, F., Rodriguez, G., Caroli, A., et al. (2008). Brain SPECT in subtypes of mild cognitive impairment. Findings from the DESCRIPA multicenter study. *J. Neurol.* 255, 1344–1353. doi:10.1007/s00415-008-0897-4

O'Brien, H. L., Tetewsky, S. J., Avery, L. M., Cushman, L. A., Makous, W., and Duffy, C. J. (2001). Visual mechanisms of spatial disorientation in Alzheimer's disease. *Cereb. Cortex* 11, 1083–1092. doi:10.1093/cercor/11.11.1083

O'Keefe, J., and Nadel, L. (1978). *The Hippocampus as a Cognitive Map.* Oxford: Clarendon Press.

Pappata, S., Varrone, A., Vicidomini, C., Milan, G., De Falco, C., Sansone, V., et al. (2010). SPECT imaging of GABA(A)/benzodiazepine receptors and cerebral perfusion in mild cognitive impairment. *Eur. J. Nucl. Med. Mol. Imaging* 37, 1156–1163. doi:10.1007/s00259-010-1409-1

Parslow, D. M., Rose, D., Brooks, B., Fleminger, S., Gray, J. A., Giampietro, V., et al. (2004). Allocentric spatial memory activation of the hippocampal formation measured with fMRI. *Neuropsychology* 18, 450–461. doi:10.1037/0894-4105.18.3.450

Passini, R., Rainville, C., Marchand, N., and Joanette, Y. (1995). Wayfinding in dementia of the Alzheimer type: planning abilities. *J. Clin. Exp. Neuropsychol.* 17, 820–832. doi:10.1080/01688639508402431

Pengas, G., Hodges, J. R., Watson, P., and Nestor, P. J. (2010a). Focal posterior cingulate atrophy in incipient Alzheimer's disease. *Neurobiol. Aging* 31, 25–33. doi:10.1016/j.neurobiolaging.2008.03.014

Pengas, G., Patterson, K., Arnold, R. J., Bird, C. M., Burgess, N., and Nestor, P. J. (2010b). Lost and found: bespoke memory testing for Alzheimer's disease and semantic dementia. *J. Alzheimers Dis.* 21, 1347–1365. doi:10.3233/JAD-2010-100654

Pengas, G., Williams, G. B., Acosta-Cabronero, J., Ash, T. W., Hong, Y. T., Izquierdo-Garcia, D., et al. (2012). The relationship of topographical memory performance to regional neurodegeneration in Alzheimer's disease. *Front. Aging Neurosci.* 4:17. doi:10.3389/fnagi.2012.00017

Pennanen, C., Kivipelto, M., Tuomainen, S., Hartikainen, P., Hanninen, T., Laakso, M. P., et al. (2004). Hippocampus and entorhinal cortex in mild cognitive impairment and early AD. *Neurobiol. Aging* 25, 303–310. doi:10.1016/S0197-4580(03)00084-8

Petersen, R. C., Parisi, J. E., Dickson, D. W., Johnson, K. A., Knopman, D. S., Boeve, B. F., et al. (2006). Neuropathologic features of amnestic mild cognitive impairment. *Arch. Neurol.* 63, 665–672. doi:10.1001/archneur.63.5.665

Rainville, C., Marchand, N., and Passini, R. (2002). Performances of patients with a dementia of the Alzheimer type in the Standardized Road-Map test of Direction Sense. *Neuropsychologia* 40, 567–573. doi:10.1016/S0028-3932(01)00133-6

Risacher, S. L., Shen, L., West, J. D., Kim, S., McDonald, B. C., Beckett, L. A., et al. (2010). Longitudinal MRI atrophy biomarkers: relationship to conversion in the ADNI cohort. *Neurobiol. Aging* 31, 1401–1418. doi:10.1016/j.neurobiolaging.2010.04.029

Scahill, R. I., Schott, J. M., Stevens, J. M., Rossor, M. N., and Fox, N. C. (2002). Mapping the evolution of regional atrophy in Alzheimer's disease: unbiased analysis of fluid-registered serial MRI. *Proc. Natl. Acad. Sci. U.S.A.* 99, 4703–4707. doi:10.1073/pnas.052587399

Schmidt-Wilcke, T., Poljansky, S., Hierlmeier, S., Hausner, J., and Ibach, B. (2009). Memory performance correlates with gray matter density in the ento-/perirhinal cortex and posterior hippocampus in patients with mild cognitive impairment and healthy controls – a voxel based morphometry study. *Neuroimage* 47, 1914–1920. doi:10.1016/j.neuroimage.2009.04.092

Schuff, N., Tosun, D., Insel, P. S., Chiang, G. C., Truran, D., Aisen, P. S., et al. (2012). Nonlinear time course of brain volume loss in cognitively normal and impaired elders. *Neurobiol. Aging* 33, 845–855. doi:10.1016/j.neurobiolaging.2010.07.012

Serino, S., and Riva, G. (2013). Getting lost in Alzheimer's disease: a break in the mental frame syncing. *Med. Hypotheses* 80, 416–421. doi:10.1016/j.mehy.2012.12.031

Smith, C. D., Chebrolu, H., Wekstein, D. R., Schmitt, F. A., Jicha, G. A., Cooper, G., et al. (2007). Brain structural alterations before mild cognitive impairment. *Neurology* 68, 1268–1273. doi:10.1212/01.wnl.0000259542.54830.34

Spulber, G., Niskanen, E., Macdonald, S., Kivipelto, M., Padilla, D. F., Julkunen, V., et al. (2012). Evolution of global and local grey matter atrophy on serial MRI scans during the progression from MCI to AD. *Curr. Alzheimer Res.* 9, 516–524. doi:10.2174/156720512800492486

Stepankova, K., Fenton, A. A., Pastalkova, E., Kalina, M., and Bohbot, V. D. (2004). Object-location memory impairment in patients with thermal lesions to the right or left hippocampus. *Neuropsychologia* 42, 1014–1028. doi:10.1016/j.neuropsychologia.2004.01.002

Tetewsky, S. J., and Duffy, C. J. (1999). Visual loss and getting lost in Alzheimer's disease. *Neurology* 52, 958–965. doi:10.1212/WNL.52.5.958

Vlcek, K. (2011). "Spatial navigation impairment in healthy aging and Alzheimer's disease," in *The Clinical Spectrum of Alzheimer's Disease – The Charge Toward Comprehensive Diagnostic and Therapeutic Strategies*, ed. S. De La Monte (Rijeka, Croatia: InTech), 75–100.

Weniger, G., Ruhleder, M., Lange, C., Wolf, S., and Irle, E. (2011). Egocentric and allocentric memory as assessed by virtual reality in individuals with amnestic mild cognitive impairment. *Neuropsychologia* 49, 518–527. doi:10.1016/j.neuropsychologia.2010.12.031

Whitwell, J. L., Dickson, D. W., Murray, M. E., Weigand, S. D., Tosakulwong, N., Senjem, M. L., et al. (2012). Neuroimaging correlates of pathologically defined subtypes of Alzheimer's disease: a case-control study. *Lancet Neurol.* 11, 868–877. doi:10.1016/S1474-4422(12)70200-4

Whitwell, J. L., Shiung, M. M., Przybelski, S. A., Weigand, S. D., Knopman, D. S., Boeve, B. F., et al. (2008). MRI patterns of atrophy associated with progression to AD in amnestic mild cognitive impairment. *Neurology* 70, 512–520. doi:10.1212/01.wnl.0000280575.77437.a2

Wolbers, T., Hegarty, M., Buchel, C., and Loomis, J. M. (2008). Spatial updating: how the brain keeps track of changing object locations during observer motion. *Nat. Neurosci.* 11, 1223–1230. doi:10.1038/nn.2189

Wolbers, T., Weiller, C., and Buchel, C. (2004). Neural foundations of emerging route knowledge in complex spatial environments. *Brain Res. Cogn. Brain Res.* 21, 401–411. doi:10.1016/j.cogbrainres.2004.06.013

15

Effect of meditation on cognitive functions in context of aging and neurodegenerative diseases

Rafał Marciniak[1]*, Katerina Sheardova[1], Pavla Čermáková[1,2], Daniel Hudeček[1], Rastislav Šumec[1] and Jakub Hort[1,3]

[1] *International Clinical Research Center, St. Anne's University Hospital Brno, Brno, Czech Republic*
[2] *Alzheimer's Disease Research Center, Department of Neurobiology, Care Sciences and Society, Karolinska Institutet, Stockholm, Sweden*
[3] *Memory Disorders Clinic, Department of Neurology, 2nd Faculty of Medicine, Charles University in Prague and University Hospital Motol, Prague, Czech Republic*

Edited by:
Ales Stuchlik, Institute of Physiology Academy of Sciences of the Czech Republic, Czech Republic

***Correspondence:**
Rafał Marciniak, International Clinical Research Center, St. Anne's University Hospital, Pekařská 53, Brno 656 91, Czech Republic
e-mail: rafal.marciniaq@gmail.com

Effect of different meditation practices on various aspects of mental and physical health is receiving growing attention. The present paper reviews evidence on the effects of several mediation practices on cognitive functions in the context of aging and neurodegenerative diseases. The effect of meditation in this area is still poorly explored. Seven studies were detected through the databases search, which explores the effect of meditation on attention, memory, executive functions, and other miscellaneous measures of cognition in a sample of older people and people suffering from neurodegenerative diseases. Overall, reviewed studies suggested a positive effect of meditation techniques, particularly in the area of attention, as well as memory, verbal fluency, and cognitive flexibility. These findings are discussed in the context of MRI studies suggesting structural correlates of the effects. Meditation can be a potentially suitable non-pharmacological intervention aimed at the prevention of cognitive decline in the elderly. However, the conclusions of these studies are limited by their methodological flaws and differences of various types of meditation techniques. Further research in this direction could help to verify the validity of the findings and clarify the problematic aspects.

Keywords: meditation, cognition, dementia, aging, neurodegenerative diseases, Alzheimer's disease, mild cognitive impairment, elderly

INTRODUCTION

Increasing age of the world's population leads to a high number of people suffering from dementia. Alzheimer's Disease International association estimated that there are nearly 36 million people suffering from dementia. The number is expected to double every 20 years, therefore 66 million people could be affected by dementia in 2030 (Prince et al., 2013). This highlights the need for an appropriate therapy for patients with dementia, which is based both on pharmacotherapy and non-pharmacological interventions.

One kind of non-pharmacological approach is represented by cognitive training or stimulation aimed at impacting cognitive functions, most commonly memory, attention, orientation, or language. However, the effects of such interventions are not consistent. They seem to be more efficient in motivated patients in early or intermediate stages of dementia (Hulme et al., 2010; Olazaran et al., 2010). Other non-pharmacological ways include behavioral interventions aimed at improving skills in activities of daily living (ADL) or management of stimuli exposed to patients. Patients are encouraged to engage in appropriate physical activity and their emotional health is supported individually or in the form of group sessions. Attention is paid to the reduction of anxiety or sleep disorders. Other options of intervention with a positive impact on multiple domains (cognition, emotivity, ADL) are represented by ergotherapy, reminiscensce therapy, art therapy, relaxation, movement therapy, or musicotherapy (Gauthier et al., 2010; Olazaran et al., 2010). An important aspect of non-pharmacological approaches is the attempt to postpone the institutionalization of patients and the support of caregivers (education, self-supporting groups) in order to reduce a great burden to which they are exposed in later stages of the disease (Chien et al., 2011).

Other possibilities of non-pharmacological interventions are based on various meditation techniques. The impact of meditation on human health has been recently a subject of great scientific interest. The effect of these techniques has been studied from different perspectives (depression, anxiety disorders, eating disorders, addictions, and disorders caused by the use of psychoactive drugs) (Ospina et al., 2007; Balaji et al., 2012; Khanna and Greeson, 2013; Lakhan and Schofield, 2013). The impact of meditation on stress reduction, the prevention of psychosomatic disorders, blood pressure, and other cardiovascular diseases is a subject of several studies as well (Barnes et al., 2001; Grossman et al., 2004). Meditation can help with chronic pain and musculoskeletal disorders, respiratory diseases, and dermatological problems. It may be beneficial as a support of the immune system or as a symptomatic treatment of cancer (Ospina et al., 2007). Recently, there have been studies on the effect of meditation techniques on cognitive skills, which are reviewed in this paper in a specific context of aging and neurodegenerative diseases. Meditation techniques are considered to be specific cognitively stimulating activities. The effect of meditation on cognition is studied directly as well as from the perspective of the reduction of depressive symptoms and anxiety. There is a growing interest in meditation as one of the potential strategies for the prevention of Alzheimer's disease (Horrigan, 2007).

MEDITATION

Even though scientists have been investigating meditation for a long time, there has not been consensus on its definition. Diversity in the range of possible definitions reflects the vast number of different methods of meditation. Western definitions emphasize that meditation is a self-regulatory technique focused on maintaining one's attention. However, in the spiritual tradition, meditation is perceived as a tool for spiritual development, the growth of inner peace, concentration, positive emotions, such as love and happiness, and on reduction of negative emotions, such as fear and anger. Walsh and Shapiro (2006) integrate those two views and propose a new definition. It characterizes meditation as a group of self-regulatory techniques focused on maintaining attention and awareness. The main goal is to achieve a greater rate of well-being, serenity, and concentration through the enhancement of control over spiritual processes. This definition distinguishes meditation from other methods, for example hypnosis, imagination, or psychotherapy. These techniques are not based on development of awareness or attention, but they rather focus on changing mental content of thoughts, images, and emotions.

Walsh and Shapiro (2006) suggest a classification of meditation according (1) to its area of interest: there are techniques, which primarily focus on a single object, such as breath or sounds. They are known as concentration meditations. Another type is represented by meditation, which aspires to gain open attention, containing more objects at once or selected in a consecutive order. This type is called awareness or open meditation. In addition, we can divide meditation techniques according to its relation to cognitive processes (thoughts, images) (2). This classification is consistent with the categories proposed by Lutz et al. (2008), who speaks about openly monitoring meditation (open monitoring, OM) and meditation with focused attention (focused attention, FA). The third type of classification relies on the targets (3). While some practices focus on supporting a general mental development and the state of well-being, others concentrate primarily on the growth of specific mental qualities, such as concentration, love, or wisdom. The most scientifically exploited techniques are described thoroughly below.

MINDFULNESS

One of the most researched meditation techniques is based on the concept of mindfulness (in Pāli language *Satí*). Traditionally this method has its origin in Buddhist meditation of mindfulness and insight (in Pāli language "*satipatthana-vipassana*"). Mindfulness practice includes a number of meditational techniques, such as activities focused on breath and physical awareness or using metaphors enlightening the essence of mindfulness. All these techniques have a common goal, which is expanding a subject's mindfulness – i.e., the ability to focus on the present moment and to perceive without any judgment or choice current internal or external impulses, which are emerging at a given moment of consciousness. Mindfulness thus allows one to stay "above" the particular content of thoughts, emotions, or imaginations and enables one to become aware of the process of consciousness itself (Kabat-Zinn, 2005). Mindfulness allows one's active approach, which can alter current categories and distinctions through focusing on new impulses, which would otherwise remain unconsciously unnoticed. This conscious processing of impulses impacts a person's behavior and supports a change of habitual behavioral patterns (Langer, 1989).

Personal experience of many western psychologists leads them to establish meditational techniques as a part of their psychotherapeutic praxis, in which they use the techniques based on mindfulness very frequently. There are many psychotherapeutic schools and approaches, which use the techniques based on the concept of mindfulness, for example, Gestalt therapy or Morit's therapy. There are several new areas combining a mindfulness approach with cognitively behavioral therapy, such as mindfulness-based cognitive therapy, dialectical behavior therapy, and acceptance and commitment therapy (Germer et al., 2005).

Zen meditation

Zen meditation is often classified as a meditational technique based on fundamentals of mindfulness. It comes from Zen Buddhism, Mahayan Buddhism's offshoot, which originated in the fifth century in China. It is performed sitting with legs crossed (lotus position) and the meditating person tries to maintain straight position of the body and a regular speed of breathing. On the mental level, they focus on their breath while their mind is open to emerging spiritual processes and contents, which they neither judge, conceptualize nor evolve. There upon moments of completely content-free consciousness occur (Pagnoni and Cekic, 2007).

TRANSCENDENTAL MEDITATION

Transcendental meditation represents another frequently used scientific method. It was developed by Maharishi Mahesh Yogi in the second half of the twentieth century, but it is based on ancient Indian Vedic tradition. This practice is based on the repetition of mantra for 15–20 min twice a day with closed eyes. Mantras in other words are sounds or simple sentences usually in Sanskrit facilitating the process of "inlaying" of attention. Attention is paid on inner psychological processes with the aim of overcoming even the mildest forms of thinking and to discover the source of thoughts, which is felt as a moment of pure consciousness, absolutely free of any content (Forem, 2012).

VIHANGAM YOGA

Another method, which has been investigated by researchers is Vihangam yoga. Its roots arise from the teaching of Sadguru Sadafaldeo Ji Maharaj. In theory and practice, it relates to the Indian Vedic tradition. The practice of this meditation is divided into five levels, but in scientific studies the most examined is the first one. In the first level, the meditating person tries through the training of concentration (for example, by repetition of mantra) to develop conscious reflexion, the ability to observe his mind's own tendencies. This helps to get better orientation in one's own inner world and to take better control of it. This state of mind allows subjective feelings of harmony and satisfaction.

KIRTAN KIRYA

Experiments with the method of Kirtan Kirya are often performed in the context of neurodegenerative diseases. This technique originates in the tradition of Kundalini yoga school. The technique itself is based on repetition of sounds "sa ta na ma," loudly, in a whisper and silently in 2 min periods. Meanwhile the meditator touches the rest of the fingers with their thumb. According to Kundalini yoga, 84 acupuncture points are being stimulated while performing this technique. This leads to a positive bio-chemical transformation in the brain. From a neuropsychological point of view the effect of this method is explained as the activation of the brain areas associated with attention and exclusive functions (frontal area, cingulate cortex), which takes places during the meditation (Newberg et al., 2010a).

RELAXATION

The effect of meditation is often compared with the effect of relaxation. Relaxation can be understood as a reduction of neurophysiological agitation (Benson et al., 1975). Meditation as a certain type of mental exercise can be included in such a broadly defined framework. But in the context of studies mentioned below, relaxation is a physical exercise focused on releasing muscles, which reduces somatic stress (Schwartz et al., 1978), or a mental relaxation, which does not cooperate with conscious focus of attention, but only instructs the subject to sit calmly with closed eyes (Alexander et al., 1989). However meditation has some additional features and can be defined as a group of self-regulatory techniques focused on maintaining attention and awareness, where the main goal is developing voluntary control over mental processes to achieve a higher overall level of well-being and also to achieve peace and concentration (Walsh and Shapiro, 2006).

RESEARCH

There is an increasing amount of literature suggesting that there are many areas, which can be influenced by meditation. The most commonly studied topics include physiological, psychiatrical, and psychological conditions (e.g., anxiety, depression, quality of life, or impact on ADL) or a general medical condition (Ospina et al., 2007). Another subject of research is the effect of meditation techniques on cognition and neuropsychological functions. Various types of mindfulness meditation seem to positively influence cognitive functions. A review by Chiesa et al. (2011) suggests a significant improvement of selective and executive attention in early stages of meditation, which aims at cultivating focused attention. Non-focused, long-term attention can be improved during following stages of meditation, which are characterized by non-judgmental observation of external and internal stimuli. Besides, this technique can increase the capacity of working memory and several executive functions. However, many studies are biased due to methodological mistakes and connections of researchers with institutions which propagate a specific type of meditation.

The studies in this review were selected through a search in scientific databases (PubMed, SpringerLink, JSTOR, EBSCO, ISI, ScienceDirect, SCOPUS, Wiley, ProQuest) by using relevant keywords (meditation, neurodegenerative disorders, dementia, Alzheimer's disease, aging, etc.). Studies investigating the effect of meditation on cognition in which aging people and people with neurodegenerative diseases were included.

MEDITATION AS A PREVENTIVE STRATEGY AGAINST ALZHEIMER'S DISEASE

Alzheimer's disease is the most common cause of dementia and is strongly related to age (Wallin et al., 2013). Other risk factors include family history, hypertension and hypotension, high levels of cholesterol, low physical activity, obesity, low level of education, and the presence of ApoE4 (Kivipelto et al., 2001, 2005; Huang et al., 2004). At least five studies have been published during the past 2 years suggesting that the incidence of dementia may have decreased over the last two decades (Rocca et al., 2011; Schrijvers et al., 2012; Christensen et al., 2013; Matthews et al., 2013; Qiu et al., 2013). The mortality improvements are generally attributed to better awareness and successful management of its risk factors. It was estimated that delaying the onset of AD by a mere year would yield nine million fewer cases by 2050 (Brookmeyer et al., 2007). The prevention of dementia may to be more effective than current pharmacological treatment (Forette et al., 1998; Khachaturian et al., 2006). A general agreement concerning cognitive decline at advanced age motivates many scientists to search for new preventive strategies to maintain cognitive functions until the end of life (Salthouse, 2011). There is a growing evidence that meditation can serve as a potential tool for the prevention of Alzheimer's disease (Horrigan, 2007).

It has been revealed that meditation can influence risk factors of Alzheimer's disease such as hypertension (Anderson et al., 2008) and high levels of cholesterol (Walton et al., 2004; Khatri et al., 2007). Besides, the impact of meditation on the cerebral blood flow (Newberg et al., 2001, 2010b; Khalsa et al., 2009) could play a role in Alzheimer's disease as well (Roher et al., 2012) (**Figure 1**).

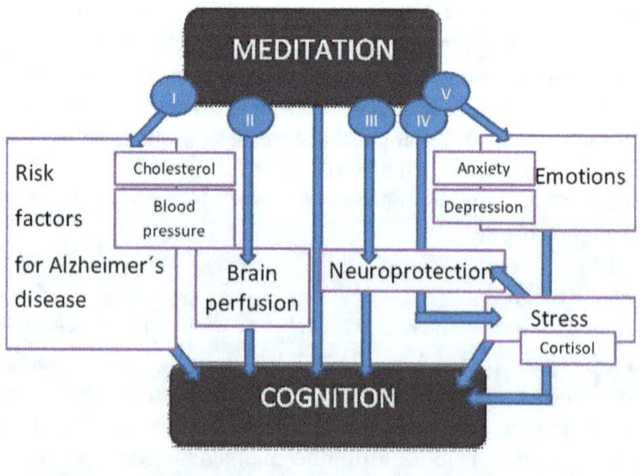

FIGURE 1 | Suggested influence of meditation on cognitive functions. The figure shows proposed ways how meditation impacts cognitive functions. The effect of meditation on cognition is both direct and indirect (I–V): meditation positively influences hypercholesterolemia and hypertension which represent risk factors for Alzheimer's disease (I). Further it increases cerebral blood flow (II) and has a protective effect on the cortical thickness (III). Meditation further reduces stress (IV), anxiety, and depression (V). All these mechanisms lead to better cognitive functions.

MEDITATION AND COGNITION IN AGING POPULATION

Research on preventive strategies against abnormal aging usually focuses on life style, in particular on physical activity and healthy diet. Only a few studies emphasize the potentially protective effect of meditation on cognition.

One of the first studies on the effect of meditation in elderly was performed by Alexander et al. (1989). The population was represented by 73 seniors (mean age 81 years) who were randomly divided into three groups based on the meditation technique they underwent. A control group without any intervention was also included. Seniors were trained in the following meditation techniques: transcendental meditation, mindfulness (*mindfulness training in active distinction making*) and a relaxation program which they performed twice a day for 20 min a period of 12 weeks. This study examined the effect of the intervention on cognitive flexibility (*Stroop's test*), memory (*Associate Learning subtest*), and verbal fluency of the elderly (*Word Fluency Scale, Overlearned Verbal Task*). These were measured before and immediately after the meditation, after 18 months and finally after 36 months. The results suggest a strong improvement in measured variables in the group of subjects using transcendental meditation, followed by mindfulness. Worse results were shown in the control group and in the group with the relaxation program. In addition, testing after 3 years revealed 100% maintained effect in persons using transcendental meditation and 87.5% in those within the mindfulness program. Other groups had lower scores (65 and 75%). Even though the described study suggested a potentially positive impact of meditation on cognitive decline in the elderly, no other studies had been performed until recently.

A study by Pagnoni and Cekic (2007) examined in a case–control study ($n = 26$) the effect of regular Zen meditation on the decrease in gray matter thickness and ability to solve tasks demanding focused attention. While the study showed age-related decrease in gray matter thickness in the case of 13 subjects in the control group (without any intervention), there was no correlation between any studied variable and age in the case of the 13 subjects who regularly meditated. The effect of meditation on gray matter was the most significant in putamen, which is a structure involved in attention processing.

Another case–control study (van Leeuwen et al., 2009) compared long-term meditating seniors using mindfulness with two groups of control participants, who had never engaged in any meditation practice. In the first one, there were people of the same age. Younger people belonged to the second control group. The groups were compared on the basis of their performance in *attentional blink*. The results of meditating group were significantly better compared to the age-matched control group. Furthermore, they performed better also in comparison with the control group consisting of young people, even though several studies have proved that attention ability decreases with age (Maciokas and Crognale, 2003; Georgiou-Karistianis et al., 2007).

A recent cross-sectional study (Prakash et al., 2012) compared cognitive skills between long-term meditating and non-meditating seniors. Twenty seniors with more than 10 years of experience with Vihanam yoga meditation underwent a battery of tests on short-term memory, psychomotoric tempo, attention, and executive functions (*Digit Span test, Stroop's test, Trail Making test, Letter Cancelation Task, Digit symbol substitution test*, and *Rule Shift Card Test*). The results were compared with the performance of non-meditating seniors. Meditating seniors showed significantly better results in all attentional tests. The study revealed that long-term meditation of Vihanagam yoga impacted positively on the extent of attention, the speed of processing, the ability of attentional shift, and performance in tests using distracting factors.

IMAGING STUDIES

MRI studies provide an interesting insight into morphological changes of the brain resulting from meditation. Even though they do not investigate elderly population, they reveal structural changes in several regions, such as increased cortical thickness. Most frequently reported are structural alterations in anterior cingulate cortex, superior and inferior frontal cortex, and prefrontal cortex. These regions are involved in attention, perceiving internal experience, sensory processing, and executive functions. Some studies report increased volume of hippocampi, which are important for memory. For an overview of MRI studies on meditation and their findings, see **Table 1**. Similar regions of activation are reported from functional imaging studies. SPECT performed during meditation showed increased regional cerebral blood flow in the prefrontal cortex, superior frontal, and cingulate cortex, and the right temporal lobe (Wang et al., 2011).

Moreover, in the study by Lazar et al. (2005), the biggest effect of mindfulness meditation on the thickness of the prefrontal cortex was surprisingly found in older participants. This suggests that meditation can have a compensatory effect on the decrease of cortical thickness related to aging. The increased cortical thickness found in meditators can be explained by several mechanisms: neuronal arborization, multiplication of glial cells, or formation of vessels (Lazar et al., 2005). This also implies that meditation could potentially lead to neuroregeneration.

Study by Luders et al. (2011) explores the fractional anisotropy for 20 different fiber tracts on sample of long-term meditators (Shamatha, Vipassana, and Zazen) and controls ($n = 54$). Results showed stronger structural connections in meditators compared to controls throughout the brain in large projection pathways, commissural pathways, and association pathways. Although fractional anisotropy and age were negatively correlated in both groups, regression lines of age-related decline in meditators were much less marked than in controls.

INTERVENTIONS STUDIES AND NEURODEGENERATIVE DISEASES

Research of meditation from the perspective of neurodegenerative disorders is still in its infancy. It includes studies on the effect of meditation on well-being of caregivers (Waelde et al., 2004; Lavretsky et al., 2013) as well as on patients suffering from dementia. As Newberg et al. (2013) summarized, current knowledge about meditation, memory, and attention supports the application of meditation techniques in patients with neurodegenerative diseases. Below are presented concrete studies investigating the effect of meditation on cognition on a sample of patients with neurodegenerative diseases.

An article by Newberg et al. (2010b) examined the effect of an 8-week meditation program using a simple method of Kirtan Kirya. The control group was listening to music instead of performing

Table 1 | List of brain imaging studies using MRI.

Study	Intervention	n	Mean age ± SD	Experience with meditation	Loci with increased cortical thickness	Interpretation
Lazar et al. (2005)	Various	20	38.2	9.1 ± 7.1 years, 6.2 ± 4 h per week	Anterior insula, parts of frontal lobe, auditory cortex in temporal lobe	Somato-sensory, auditory, and interceptive processes
Pagnoni and Cekic (2007)	Zen	13	37.2 ± 6.9	>3 years per day	Putamen	Attention
Holzel et al. (2008)	Vipassana	20	34.1 ± 4.7	8.6 years, 2 h daily	Anterior insula, right hippocampus, left inferior temporal gyrus	Anterior insula – awareness of internal experience
Vestergaard-Poulsen et al. (2009)	Tibetan buddhism	10	55 ± 6.2	16.5 ± 5.1 years	Medulla oblongata, anterior cerebellum, superior, and inferior frontal gyrus	Breath control, resistance to stress, attention, calmness
Luders et al. (2009)	Various	22	53 ± 11.5	24 ± 12 years	Orbito-frontal cortex, right talamus, left inferior temporal gyrus	Regulation of emotions and sensory functions
Grant et al. (2010)	Zen	17	37.6 ± 10.9	>1000 h	Anterior cingulate cortex, secondary somato-sensory cortex	Anterior cingulate cortex – adaptive control of behavior
Holzel et al. (2011)	MBSR	16	39 ± 4	0	Left hippocampus, posterior cingulate cortex, temporo-parietal junction, cerebellum	Learning, memory, regulation of emotions, empathy
Luders et al. (2013b)	Various	50	51.4 ± 12.8	20 years	Hippocampus, especially subiculum	Subiculum – regulation of stress
Grant et al. (2013)	Zen	18	37.1 ± 10.9	>1000 h	Cingulo-fronto-parietal network	Attention

n, number of subjects, SD, standard deviation, MBSR, mindfulness-based stress reduction, IBMT, integrative body mind training.

meditation. Fifteen seniors with age-related cognitive impairment ($n=7$), mild cognitive impairment ($n=5$), and Alzheimer's disease ($n=3$) were included in the study. Cerebral blood flow and performance in cognitive tests were examined. The effect of the 8-week long meditation program showed a significant increase in cerebral perfusion in prefrontal, parietal, and auditory cortex. The results of neuropsychological tests showed an improvement in verbal fluency, part B in *Trail making test* (test on working memory and attention) and logical memory in the meditating group. Most of the participants also expressed a significant subjective improvement in cognitive functions.

Similar research by Moss et al. (2012) studied the effect of an 8-week meditation program in Kirtan Kirya technique. They measured the effect of this program on depression and anxiety. Cerebral perfusion, level of spirituality, cognitive functions in categorical fluency, *Trail making test* (part B), and logical memory was also examined. The participants consisted of seniors with impaired memory ($n=7$), mild cognitive impairment ($n=5$), and Alzheimer's disease ($n=3$). The control group listened to music in this study as well. The results in the meditating group revealed a significant improvement in depression, anxiety, internal tension, and fatigue. Increased cerebral perfusion in the frontal lobe and right parietal lobe has also been found. However, in this research, there was no significant effect of meditation on cognitive functions. Interestingly, there were no significant changes in spirituality scores [index of core spiritual experiences (INSPIRIT), the purpose in life scale, the mysticism scale, the quest scale, and mindful attention awareness scale] over the 8-week period.

A recent study by Innes et al. (2012) examined the effect of Kirtan Kirya on stress, quality of sleep, mood, sympathetic activation, and memory functions in adults suffering from cognitive decline. The effect was also studied on their caregivers. Six patients in early stages of Alzheimer's disease and their caregivers were tested before and after undergoing an 8-week meditation program. The participants showed a significant improvement in retrospective memory (tested by *Memory Functioning Questionnaire*) and also in other measured variables, such as stress, mood disorders, quality of sleep, and blood pressure.

DISCUSSION

Insufficient amount of research on the effect of meditation on age-related cognitive decline and neurodegenerative diseases makes any generalization of the results very difficult. However, the reviewed studies suggest a positive effect of various meditation techniques on particular cognitive functions. There is evidence that meditation enhances attention (Pagnoni and Cekic, 2007; van Leeuwen et al., 2009; Prakash et al., 2012), improves verbal fluency (Alexander et al., 1989; Newberg et al., 2010a), memory (Alexander et al., 1989; Newberg et al., 2010a; Innes et al., 2012), and cognitive flexibility (Alexander et al., 1989; Newberg et al., 2010a).

Results mentioned above suggest a possible explanation of the impact of meditation on processes in the human brain (see **Figure 1**). The mechanisms include increased cerebral perfusion in prefrontal, parietal and auditory cortex (Newberg et al., 2010a), a protective effect on gray matter thickness (Pagnoni and Cekic, 2007), and enhancing of the function of areas involved in attention (Lazar et al., 2005). In addition, meditation can potentially enhance the power of cognitive circuits and increase cognitive capacity (Xiong and Doraiswamy, 2009). Moreover, it can improve myelination or restructuralization of white-matter tracts in the involved areas such as anterior corona radiate associated with the anterior cingulate cortex (Tang et al., 2010).

Another explanation of the neuroprotective effect of meditation can be the decrease in cortisol level (Jacobs et al., 2013; Turakitwanakan et al., 2013) caused by stress, which may be related to a higher hippocampal volume in meditators (Luders et al., 2013a). Epel et al. (2009) emphasize the correlation between the maintenance of the length of telomeres and decreased cognitive stress and tension due to meditation (Jacobs et al., 2011; Hoge et al., 2013) Meditation can positively impact dyslipidemia and oxidative stress, which further decreases the risk of vascular diseases of the brain as well as Alzheimer's disease (Reitz, 2013).

From a psychological point of view, the effects on cognitive functions can be explained by enhancing the ability of mindfulness (in the case of mindfulness meditation). Mindfulness enables a non-judgmental reflexion of processes happening in consciousness "beyond" concrete contents of thoughts and feelings. This leads to experiencing a relativity and transient nature of these contents, which can (from the long-term point of view) lead to weakening of affective power of these perceptions in consciousness (e.g., as in anxiety) and enlarging the capacity for focused processing. This ability can lead to improvement in attentional and working memory tasks. Similarly, we can look at the effect of meditation based on mantra repetition (transcendental meditation, Kirtan Kirya, etc.). This method aims at releasing consciousness from constantly appearing language based thoughts. Short-lasting experience of the relief of consciousness from its contents (thoughts and feelings) can lead to understanding of their relativity and transience (Alexander et al., 1989). It is necessary to emphasize the potential of various meditation techniques in the enhancement of flexibility, contrasts with its decrease during aging. This is related to higher perception of new stimuli, which are not in line with old cognitive schemes and habitual behavioral patterns. This supports adaptive behavior based on one's own decisions (Alexander et al., 1989; Langer, 1989). An important aspect, which is enhanced by all the mentioned types of meditation, is self-reflexion and cultivation of the ability to deal with one's own mental processes. Such skills can contribute to decreased depressivity and anxiety, which have negative effect on cognitive functions (Beaudreau and O'Hara, 2008).

The positive potential of meditation, which is suggested from research reported here, has to be related to the limitation of these studies, which are often preliminary capture. Many papers included too few subjects, control groups were missing or the research has been performed by institutions supporting a special type of meditation. In many studies, the effect of meditation on cognition was often measured by many cognitive tests, authors of the studies pointed out significant positive changes, but there should be also emphasized fact, that in some tests, the effect on specific cognitive functions has not been proved, as you can see in **Table 2**. For example, in study of Moss et al. has not been proved significant effect of meditation on cognitive functions, only on the other measured variables.

An attempt to generalize such results is in contrast with the fact that meditation comprises a heterogeneous group of practices. It is becoming evident that in the context of neurodegenerative disorders there is a lack of studies using methods other than Kirtan Kriya. The key tasks for future studies will be identification of a potential common element of different meditation techniques, establishment of a valid tool to measure meditation techniques, better control of life style factors, genetics, and eating habits, applying findings on larger randomized population samples and finding out whether the results observed in highly experienced meditation practitioners can be found in a wider population.

Various types of meditation were traditionally established among religious systems, which related a close connection between meditation and the spiritual part of human beings. It is becoming evident that, despite the loss of intellectual and memory skills, patients with Alzheimer's disease often maintain spiritual consciousness and intuition (Dopson, 2005). Such patients still manage, despite a significant memory loss, to learn to use simple meditation techniques. Involving patients with Alzheimer's disease in activities, such as prayers or meditation, can positively impact on the quality of their life, spiritual well-being, feelings of self-value and belonging (Lindberg, 2005).They can also decrease

Table 2 | List of studies investigating the effect of meditation on cognition on a sample of elderly people and people with neurodegenerative diseases.

Study	Participants	Significant effect on cognitive functions	Memory	Attention	Executive functions[a]
Alexander et al. (1989)	Elderly		Yes	Yes	Yes
Pagnoni and Cekic (2007)	Elderly		–	Yes	–
van Leeuwen et al. (2009)	Elderly		–	Yes	–
Newberg et al. (2010a)	Elderly, MCI, Alzheimer's disease		Yes	Yes	Yes
Newberg et al. (2013)	Elderly, MCI, Alzheimer's disease		No	No	No
Grant et al. (2010)	MCI, Alzheimer's disease, caregivers		Yes	–	–

[a] *Into executive functions are assigned cognitive flexibility and verbal fluency.*

anxiety related to this disease and serve as a potentially useful intervention for improving negative symptoms and behavior. Studies by Kaufman et al. (2007) emphasize slower cognitive decline and progression of Alzheimer's disease in patients with higher level of spirituality or personal religious practice, however, another study (Levin et al., 1994) did not show that regular visits to church slow down the progression of Alzheimer's disease. These findings imply an alternative explanation of the impact of meditation, which is by enhancing a spiritual dimension of the elderly. Even though researchers suggest a different effect of secularly and spiritually aimed meditation on the health and well-being of meditators (Wachholtz and Pargament, 2005), spirituality has been among measured variables in only one of the reported studies (Moss et al., 2012). However, there was no significant association with the effect of meditation, therefore the question of the relationship between meditation and spirituality remains open to further research.

CONCLUSION

There is an increasing amount of literature suggesting a positive impact of meditation on physical and psychological health. Recently, there have been studies on the influence of meditation on cognitive functions in the context of aging and neurodegenerative diseases. The results imply a positive effect especially on attention, memory, verbal fluency, and cognitive flexibility. Meditation can represent an appropriate non-pharmacological intervention aiming at the prevention of cognitive decline in the elderly. Conclusions of such studies are limited due to their methodological problems and differences among various meditation techniques. Further research in this area could help to confirm the validity of recent results and clarify problematical aspects.

REFERENCES

Alexander, C. N., Langer, E. J., Newman, R. I., Chandler, H. M., and Davies, J. L. (1989). Transcendental meditation, mindfulness, and longevity: an experimental study with the elderly. *J. Pers. Soc. Psychol.* 57, 950–964. doi:10.1037/0022-3514.57.6.950

Anderson, J. W., Liu, C., and Kryscio, R. J. (2008). Blood pressure response to transcendental meditation: a meta-analysis. *Am. J. Hypertens.* 21, 310–316. doi:10.1038/ajh.2007.65

Balaji, P. A., Varne, S. R., and Ali, S. S. (2012). Physiological effects of yogic practices and transcendental meditation in health and disease. *N. Am. J. Med. Sci.* 4, 442–448. doi:10.4103/1947-2714.101980

Barnes, V. A., Treiber, F. A., and Davis, H. (2001). Impact of transcendental meditation on cardiovascular function at rest and during acute stress in adolescents with high normal blood pressure. *J. Psychosom. Res.* 51, 597–605. doi:10.1016/S0022-3999(01)00261-6

Beaudreau, S. A., and O'Hara, R. (2008). Late-life anxiety and cognitive impairment: a review. *Am. J. Geriatr. Psychiatry* 16, 790–803. doi:10.1097/JGP.0b013e31817945c3

Benson, H., Greenwood, M. M., and Klemchuk, H. (1975). The relaxation response: psychophysiologic aspects and clinical applications. *Int. J. Psychiatry Med.* 6, 87–98. doi:10.2190/376W-E4MT-QM6Q-H0UM

Brookmeyer, R., Johnson, E., Ziegler-Graham, K., and Arrighi, H. M. (2007). Forecasting the global burden of Alzheimer's disease. *Alzheimers Dement.* 3, 186–191. doi:10.1016/j.jalz.2007.04.381

Chien, L. Y., Chu, H., Guo, J. L., Liao, Y. M., Chang, L. I., Chen, C. H., et al. (2011). Caregiver support groups in patients with dementia: a meta-analysis. *Int. J. Geriatr. Psychiatry* 26, 1089–1098. doi:10.1002/gps.2660

Chiesa, A., Calati, R., and Serretti, A. (2011). Does mindfulness training improve cognitive abilities? A systematic review of neuropsychological findings. *Clin. Psychol. Rev.* 31, 449–464. doi:10.1016/j.cpr.2010.11.003

Christensen, K., Thinggaard, M., Oksuzyan, A., Steenstrup, T., Andersen-Ranberg, K., Jeune, B., et al. (2013). Physical and cognitive functioning of people older than 90 years: a comparison of two Danish cohorts born 10 years apart. *Lancet* 382, 1507–1513. doi:10.1016/S0140-6736(13)60777-1

Dopson, L. (2005). Spirituality and Alzheimer's. *Nurs. Older People* 17, 39. doi:10.7748/nop2005.05.17.3.39.c2374

Epel, E., Daubenmier, J., Moskowitz, J. T., Folkman, S., and Blackburn, E. (2009). Can meditation slow rate of cellular aging? Cognitive stress, mindfulness, and telomeres. *Ann. N. Y. Acad. Sci.* 1172, 34–53. doi:10.1111/j.1749-6632.2009.04414.x

Forem, J. (2012). *Transcendental Meditation.* London: Hay House Inc.

Forette, F., Seux, M. L., Staessen, J. A., Thijs, L., Birkenhager, W. H., Babarskiene, M. R., et al. (1998). Prevention of dementia in randomised double-blind placebo-controlled systolic hypertension in Europe (Syst-Eur) trial. *Lancet* 352, 1347–1351. doi:10.1016/S0140-6736(98)03086-4

Gauthier, S., Cummings, J., Ballard, C., Brodaty, H., Grossberg, G., Robert, P., et al. (2010). Management of behavioral problems in Alzheimer's disease. *Int. Psychogeriatr.* 22, 346–372. doi:10.1017/S1041610209991505

Georgiou-Karistianis, N., Tang, J., Vardy, Y., Sheppard, D., Evans, N., Wilson, M., et al. (2007). Progressive age-related changes in the attentional blink paradigm. *Neuropsychol. Dev. Cogn. B Aging Neuropsychol. Cogn.* 14, 213–226. doi:10.1080/13825580500320681

Germer, C. K., Siegel, R. D., and Fulton, P. R. (2005). *Mindfulness and Psychotherapy.* New York: Guilford Press.

Grant, J. A., Courtemanche, J., Duerden, E. G., Duncan, G. H., and Rainville, P. (2010). Cortical thickness and pain sensitivity in Zen meditators. *Emotion* 10, 43–53. doi:10.1037/a0018334

Grant, J. A., Duerden, E. G., Courtemanche, J., Cherkasova, M., Duncan, G. H., and Rainville, P. (2013). Cortical thickness, mental absorption and meditative practice: possible implications for disorders of attention. *Biol. Psychol.* 92, 275–281. doi:10.1016/j.biopsycho.2012.09.007

Grossman, P., Niemann, L., Schmidt, S., and Walach, H. (2004). Mindfulness-based stress reduction and health benefits. A meta-analysis. *J. Psychosom. Res.* 57, 35–43. doi:10.1016/S0022-3999(03)00573-7

Hoge, E. A., Chen, M. M., Orr, E., Metcalf, C. A., Fischer, L. E., Pollack, M. H., et al. (2013). Loving-Kindness Meditation practice associated with longer telomeres in women. *Brain Behav. Immun.* 32, 159–163. doi:10.1016/j.bbi.2013.04.005

Holzel, B. K., Carmody, J., Vangel, M., Congleton, C., Yerramsetti, S. M., Gard, T., et al. (2011). Mindfulness practice leads to increases in regional brain gray matter density. *Psychiatry Res.* 191, 36–43. doi:10.1016/j.pscychresns.2010.08.006

Holzel, B. K., Ott, U., Gard, T., Hempel, H., Weygandt, M., Morgen, K., et al. (2008). Investigation of mindfulness meditation practitioners with voxel-based morphometry. *Soc. Cogn. Affect. Neurosci.* 3, 55–61. doi:10.1093/scan/nsm038

Horrigan, B. J. (2007). New studies support the therapeutic value of meditation. *Explore (NY)* 3, 449–450. doi:10.1016/j.explore.2007.07.003

Huang, W., Qiu, C., von Strauss, E., Winblad, B., and Fratiglioni, L. (2004). APOE genotype, family history of dementia, and Alzheimer disease risk: a 6-year follow-up study. *Arch. Neurol.* 61, 1930–1934. doi:10.1001/archneur.61.12.1930

Hulme, C., Wright, J., Crocker, T., Oluboyede, Y., and House, A. (2010). Non-pharmacological approaches for dementia that informal carers might try or access: a systematic review. *Int. J. Geriatr. Psychiatry* 25, 756–763. doi:10.1002/gps.2429

Innes, K. E., Selfe, T. K., Brown, C. J., Rose, K. M., and Thompson-Heisterman, A. (2012). The effects of meditation on perceived stress and related indices of psychological status and sympathetic activation in persons with Alzheimer's disease and their caregivers: a pilot study. *Evid. Based Complement. Altern. Med.* 2012, 927509. doi:10.1155/2012/927509

Jacobs, T. L., Epel, E. S., Lin, J., Blackburn, E. H., Wolkowitz, O. M., Bridwell, D. A., et al. (2011). Intensive meditation training, immune cell telomerase activity, and psychological mediators. *Psychoneuroendocrinology* 36, 664–681. doi:10.1016/j.psyneuen.2010.09.010

Jacobs, T. L., Shaver, P. R., Epel, E. S., Zanesco, A. P., Aichele, S. R., Bridwell, D. A., et al. (2013). Self-reported mindfulness and cortisol during a Shamatha meditation retreat. *Health Psychol.* 32, 1104–1109. doi:10.1037/a0031362

Kabat-Zinn, J. (2005). Bringing mindfulness to medicine: an interview with Jon Kabat-Zinn, PhD. Interview by Karolyn Gazella. *Adv. Mind Body Med.* 21, 22–27.

Kaufman, Y., Anaki, D., Binns, M., and Freedman, M. (2007). Cognitive decline in Alzheimer disease: impact of spirituality, religiosity, and QOL. *Neurology* 68, 1509–1514. doi:10.1212/01.wnl.0000260697.66617.59

Khachaturian, A. S., Zandi, P. P., Lyketsos, C. G., Hayden, K. M., Skoog, I., Norton, M. C., et al. (2006). Antihypertensive medication use and incident Alzheimer disease: the Cache County Study. *Arch. Neurol.* 63, 686–692. doi:10.1001/archneur.63.5.noc60013

Khalsa, D. S., Amen, D., Hanks, C., Money, N., and Newberg, A. (2009). Cerebral blood flow changes during chanting meditation. *Nucl. Med. Commun.* 30, 956–961. doi:10.1097/MNM.0b013e32832fa26c

Khanna, S., and Greeson, J. M. (2013). A narrative review of yoga and mindfulness as complementary therapies for addiction. *Complement. Ther. Med.* 21, 244–252. doi:10.1016/j.ctim.2013.01.008

Khatri, D., Mathur, K. C., Gahlot, S., Jain, S., and Agrawal, R. P. (2007). Effects of yoga and meditation on clinical and biochemical parameters of metabolic syndrome. *Diabetes Res. Clin. Pract.* 78, e9–e10. doi:10.1016/j.diabres.2007.05.002

Kivipelto, M., Helkala, E. L., Laakso, M. P., Hanninen, T., Hallikainen, M., Alhainen, K., et al. (2001). Midlife vascular risk factors and Alzheimer's disease in later life: longitudinal, population based study. *BMJ* 322, 1447–1451. doi:10.1136/bmj.322.7300.1447

Kivipelto, M., Ngandu, T., Fratiglioni, L., Viitanen, M., Kareholt, I., Winblad, B., et al. (2005). Obesity and vascular risk factors at midlife and the risk of dementia and Alzheimer disease. *Arch. Neurol.* 62, 1556–1560. doi:10.1001/archneur.62.10.1556

Lakhan, S. E., and Schofield, K. L. (2013). Mindfulness-based therapies in the treatment of somatization disorders: a systematic review and meta-analysis. *PLoS ONE* 8:e71834. doi:10.1371/journal.pone.0071834

Langer, E. J. (1989). Minding matters: the consequences of mindlessness-mindfulness. *Adv. Exp. Soc. Psychol.* 22, 137–173.

Lavretsky, H., Epel, E. S., Siddarth, P., Nazarian, N., Cyr, N. S., Khalsa, D. S., et al. (2013). A pilot study of yogic meditation for family dementia caregivers with depressive symptoms: effects on mental health, cognition, and telomerase activity. *Int. J. Geriatr. Psychiatry* 28, 57–65. doi:10.1002/gps.3790

Lazar, S. W., Kerr, C. E., Wasserman, R. H., Gray, J. R., Greve, D. N., Treadway, M. T., et al. (2005). Meditation experience is associated with increased cortical thickness. *Neuroreport* 16, 1893–1897. doi:10.1097/01.wnr.0000186598.66243.19

Levin, J. S., Taylor, R. J., and Chatters, L. M. (1994). Race and gender differences in religiosity among older adults: findings from four national surveys. *J. Gerontol.* 49, S137–S145. doi:10.1093/geronj/49.3.S137

Lindberg, D. A. (2005). Integrative review of research related to meditation, spirituality, and the elderly. *Geriatr. Nurs.* 26, 372–377. doi:10.1016/j.gerinurse.2005.09.013

Luders, E., Clark, K., Narr, K. L., and Toga, A. W. (2011). Enhanced brain connectivity in long-term meditation practitioners. *Neuroimage* 57, 1308–1316. doi:10.1016/j.neuroimage.2011.05.075

Luders, E., Thompson, P. M., Kurth, F., Hong, J. Y., Phillips, O. R., Wang, Y., et al. (2013a). Global and regional alterations of hippocampal anatomy in long-term meditation practitioners. *Hum. Brain Mapp.* 34, 3369–3375. doi:10.1002/hbm.22153

Luders, E., Kurth, F., Toga, A. W., Narr, K. L., and Gaser, C. (2013b). Meditation effects within the hippocampal complex revealed by voxel-based morphometry and cytoarchitectonic probabilistic mapping. *Front. Psychol.* 4:398. doi:10.3389/fpsyg.2013.00398

Luders, E., Toga, A. W., Lepore, N., and Gaser, C. (2009). The underlying anatomical correlates of long-term meditation: larger hippocampal and frontal volumes of gray matter. *Neuroimage* 45, 672–678. doi:10.1016/j.neuroimage.2008.12.061

Lutz, A., Slagter, H. A., Dunne, J. D., and Davidson, R. J. (2008). Attention regulation and monitoring in meditation. *Trends Cogn. Sci.* 12, 163–169. doi:10.1016/j.tics.2008.01.005

Maciokas, J. B., and Crognale, M. A. (2003). Cognitive and attentional changes with age: evidence from attentional blink deficits. *Exp. Aging Res.* 29, 137–153. doi:10.1080/03610730303715

Matthews, F. E., Arthur, A., Barnes, L. E., Bond, J., Jagger, C., Robinson, L., et al. (2013). A two-decade comparison of prevalence of dementia in individuals aged 65 years and older from three geographical areas of England: results of the Cognitive Function and Ageing Study I and II. *Lancet* 382, 1405–1412. doi:10.1016/S0140-6736(13)61570-6

Moss, A. S., Wintering, N., Roggenkamp, H., Khalsa, D. S., Waldman, M. R., Monti, D., et al. (2012). Effects of an 8-week meditation program on mood and anxiety in patients with memory loss. *J. Altern. Complement. Med.* 18, 48–53. doi:10.1089/acm.2011.0051

Newberg, A., Alavi, A., Baime, M., Pourdehnad, M., Santanna, J., and d'Aquili, E. (2001). The measurement of regional cerebral blood flow during the complex cognitive task of meditation: a preliminary SPECT study. *Psychiatry Res.* 106, 113–122. doi:10.1016/S0925-4927(01)00074-9

Newberg, A. B., Serruya, M., Wintering, N., Moss, A. S., Reibel, D., and Monti, D. A. (2013). Meditation and neurodegenerative diseases. *Ann. N. Y. Acad. Sci.* 1307, 112–123. doi:10.1111/nyas.12187

Newberg, A. B., Wintering, N., Khalsa, D. S., Roggenkamp, H., and Waldman, M. R. (2010a). Meditation effects on cognitive function and cerebral blood flow in subjects with memory loss: a preliminary study. *J. Alzheimers Dis.* 20, 517–526. doi:10.3233/JAD-2010-1391

Newberg, A. B., Wintering, N., Waldman, M. R., Amen, D., Khalsa, D. S., and Alavi, A. (2010b). Cerebral blood flow differences between long-term meditators and non-meditators. *Conscious. Cogn.* 19, 899–905. doi:10.1016/j.concog.2010.05.003

Olazaran, J., Reisberg, B., Clare, L., Cruz, I., Pena-Casanova, J., Del Ser, T., et al. (2010). Nonpharmacological therapies in Alzheimer's disease: a systematic review of efficacy. *Dement. Geriatr. Cogn. Disord.* 30, 161–178. doi:10.1159/000316119

Ospina, M. B., Bond, K., Karkhaneh, M., Tjosvold, L., Vandermeer, B., Liang, Y., et al. (2007). Meditation practices for health: state of the research. *Evid. Rep. Technol. Assess.* 155, 1–263.

Pagnoni, G., and Cekic, M. (2007). Age effects on gray matter volume and attentional performance in Zen meditation. *Neurobiol. Aging* 28, 1623–1627. doi:10.1016/j.neurobiolaging.2007.06.008

Prakash, R., Rastogi, P., Dubey, I., Abhishek, P., Chaudhury, S., and Small, B. J. (2012). Long-term concentrative meditation and cognitive performance among older adults. *Neuropsychol Dev Cogn B Aging Neuropsychol Cogn.* 19, 479–494. doi:10.1080/13825585.2011.630932

Prince, M., Bryce, R., Albanese, E., Wimo, A., Ribeiro, W., and Ferri, C. P. (2013). The global prevalence of dementia: a systematic review and metaanalysis. *Alzheimers Dement.* 9, 63e–75e. doi:10.1016/j.jalz.2012.11.007

Qiu, C., von Strauss, E., Backman, L., Winblad, B., and Fratiglioni, L. (2013). Twenty-year changes in dementia occurrence suggest decreasing incidence in central Stockholm, Sweden. *Neurology* 80, 1888–1894. doi:10.1212/WNL.0b013e318292a2f9

Reitz, C. (2013). Dyslipidemia and the risk of Alzheimer's disease. *Curr. Atheroscler. Rep.* 15, 307. doi:10.1007/s11883-012-0307-3

Rocca, W. A., Petersen, R. C., Knopman, D. S., Hebert, L. E., Evans, D. A., Hall, K. S., et al. (2011). Trends in the incidence and prevalence of Alzheimer's disease, dementia, and cognitive impairment in the United States. *Alzheimers Dement.* 7, 80–93. doi:10.1016/j.jalz.2010.11.002

Roher, A. E., Debbins, J. P., Malek-Ahmadi, M., Chen, K., Pipe, J. G., Maze, S., et al. (2012). Cerebral blood flow in Alzheimer's disease. *Vasc. Health Risk Manag.* 8, 599–611. doi:10.2147/VHRM.S34874

Salthouse, T. A. (2011). Neuroanatomical substrates of age-related cognitive decline. *Psychol. Bull.* 137, 753. doi:10.1037/a0023262

Schrijvers, E. M., Verhaaren, B. F., Koudstaal, P. J., Hofman, A., Ikram, M. A., and Breteler, M. M. (2012). Is dementia incidence declining? Trends in dementia incidence since 1990 in the Rotterdam Study. *Neurology* 78, 1456–1463. doi:10.1212/WNL.0b013e3182553be6

Schwartz, G. E., Davidson, R. J., and Goleman, D. J. (1978). Patterning of cognitive and somatic processes in the self-regulation of anxiety: effects of meditation versus exercise. *Psychosom. Med.* 40, 321–328.

Tang, Y. Y., Lu, Q., Geng, X., Stein, E. A., Yang, Y., and Posner, M. I. (2010). Short-term meditation induces white matter changes in the anterior cingulate. *Proc. Natl. Acad. Sci. U.S.A.* 107, 15649–15652. doi:10.1073/pnas.1011043107

Turakitwanakan, W., Mekseepralard, C., and Busarakumtragul, P. (2013). Effects of mindfulness meditation on serum cortisol of medical students. *J. Med. Assoc. Thai.* 96(Suppl. 1), S90–S95.

van Leeuwen, S., Muller, N. G., and Melloni, L. (2009). Age effects on attentional blink performance in meditation. *Conscious. Cogn.* 18, 593–599. doi:10.1016/j.concog.2009.05.001

Vestergaard-Poulsen, P., van Beek, M., Skewes, J., Bjarkam, C. R., Stubberup, M., Bertelsen, J., et al. (2009). Long-term meditation is associated with increased gray matter density in the brain stem. *Neuroreport* 20, 170–174. doi:10.1097/WNR.0b013e328320012a

16

Pregnanolone glutamate, a novel use-dependent NMDA receptor inhibitor, exerts antidepressant-like properties in animal models

Kristina Holubova[1], Tereza Nekovarova[1], Jana Pistovcakova[2], Alexandra Sulcova[3], Ales Stuchlík[1] and Karel Vales[1]*

[1] *Institute of Physiology, Academy of Sciences of the Czech Republic, Prague, Czech Republic*
[2] *Faculty of Medicine, Department of Pharmacology, Masaryk University, Brno, Czech Republic*
[3] *Central European Institute of Technology, Masaryk University, Brno, Czech Republic*

Edited by:
Tomiki Sumiyoshi, National Center of Neurology and Psychiatry, Japan

***Correspondence:**
Karel Vales, Department of Neurophysiology of Memory, Institute of Physiology, v.v.i. Academy of Sciences of the Czech Republic, Videnska 1083, Prague CZ-14220, Czech Republic
e-mail: vales@biomed.cas.cz; vales@fgu.cas.cz

A number of studies demonstrated a rapid onset of an antidepressant effect of non-competitive *N*-methyl-D-aspartic acid receptor (NMDAR) antagonists. Nonetheless, its therapeutic potential is rather limited, due to a high coincidence of negative side-effects. Therefore, the challenge seems to be in the development of NMDAR antagonists displaying antidepressant properties, and at the same time maintaining regular physiological function of the NMDAR. Previous results demonstrated that naturally occurring neurosteroid 3α5β-pregnanolone sulfate shows pronounced inhibitory action by a use-dependent mechanism on the tonically active NMDAR. The aim of the present experiments is to find out whether the treatment with pregnanolone 3αC derivatives affects behavioral response to chronic and acute stress in an animal model of depression. Adult male mice were used throughout the study. Repeated social defeat and forced swimming tests were used as animal models of depression. The effect of the drugs on the locomotor/exploratory activity in the open-field test was also tested together with an effect on anxiety in the elevated plus maze. Results showed that pregnanolone glutamate (PG) did not induce hyperlocomotion, whereas both dizocilpine and ketamine significantly increased spontaneous locomotor activity in the open field. In the elevated plus maze, PG displayed anxiolytic-like properties. In forced swimming, PG prolonged time to the first floating. Acute treatment of PG disinhibited suppressed locomotor activity in the repeatedly defeated group-housed mice. Aggressive behavior of isolated mice was reduced after the chronic 30-day administration of PG. PG showed antidepressant-like and anxiolytic-like properties in the used tests, with minimal side-effects. Since PG combines $GABA_A$ receptor potentiation and use-dependent NMDAR inhibition, synthetic derivatives of neuroactive steroids present a promising strategy for the treatment of mood disorders.

Highlights:

- 3α5β-pregnanolone glutamate (PG) is a use-dependent antagonist of NMDA receptors.
- We demonstrated that PG did not induce significant hyperlocomotion.
- We showed that PG displayed anxiolytic-like and antidepressant-like properties.

Keywords: depression, anxiety, NMDA channel blocker, neuroactive steroid, 3α5β-pregnanolone glutamate

INTRODUCTION

Depressive disorders are among the most common and the most disabling mental diseases. There exist various and widely used antidepressants; however, one of their major limitations is a relatively long onset of antidepressant effect. But several studies demonstrate antidepressant properties of a single administration of ketamine – the non-competitive *N*-methyl-D-aspartic acid receptor (NMDAR) antagonist (Berman et al., 2000; Zarate et al., 2006, 2012; Diazgranados et al., 2010). Both subjective and objective evaluation of the mood after ketamine administration showed a significant improvement of the mood in the interval spanning from 2 h to 7 days (Entsuah et al., 2001; Thase et al., 2005). The minimum treatment of 2–4 weeks (often even more) is required to produce significant improvement in symptomatology with common antidepressants (Lam, 2012), while an infusion of ketamine

Abbreviations: ACTH, adrenocorticotropic hormone; β-CD, hydroxypropyl-β-cyclodextrin; CNS, central nervous system; CRH, corticotropin-releasing hormone; DHEA/S, dehydroepiandrosterone sulfate; GABA, γ-aminobutyric acid; HPA axis, hypothalamic–pituitary–adrenal axis; MK-801, dizocilpine; NMDA, *N*-methyl-D-aspartic acid; NMDAR, *N*-methyl-D-aspartic acid receptor; PG, 3α5β-pregnanolone glutamate; SSRI, selective serotonin reuptake inhibitor.

to pharmaco-resistant patients show a similar effect (Murrough et al., 2013). The current hypothesis for the mechanism of ketamine action focuses on a complex cascade of neurochemical events that are induced by ketamine administration. These consequences persist for days after the ketamine elimination. First of all, ketamine administration blocks NMDAR. In all the cases, the protracted antidepressant effect is mediated by the consequent neuroplastic alterations (see Browne and Lucki, 2013; Hayley and Litteljohn, 2014).

It has been more than 20 years since the first proof of antidepressant action of the NMDAR antagonist emerged (Trullas and Skolnick, 1990). Since then, a growing number of evidence confirms that glutamate neurotransmission plays a crucial role in the neuropathology of the depression. Researchers have found that various types of drugs impairing NMDAR functioning (competitive, non-competitive and uncompetitive antagonists, and allosteric modulators) display antidepressant effects in the preclinical (Layer et al., 1995; Rogóz et al., 2002; Li et al., 2011; Burgdorf et al., 2013; Lapidus et al., 2013; Pilc et al., 2013) as well as in the clinical trials (Zarate et al., 2006, 2012). However, the clinical use of NMDA antagonists in pharmacotherapy of mood disorders is hampered by severe side-effects, particularly by psychotic symptoms in humans (Krystal et al., 1994). For this reason, research of the NMDA antagonists is a prominent topic in current neurobiology of the depressive disorder. It focuses on the elucidation of mechanisms of their antidepressant effect, and on the development of novel antidepressants – drugs with antidepressant properties and minimal side-effects, i.e., with more favorable benefit/risk ratio.

Therefore, the research and development of the novel therapeutics based on the NMDA antagonists is necessary in order to avoid psychotomimetic effects. These negative behavioral effects are most pronounced in the case of non-competitive antagonists. Conversely, the behavioral side-effects of the uncompetitive antagonists (antagonists selective for NMDAR containing a NR2B subunit or NMDAR glycine binding site antagonists) are less severe (Danysz et al., 1998; Popik et al., 1998; Karcz-Kubicha et al., 1999; Parsons, 2001; Kemp and McKernan, 2002; Chen and Lipton, 2006).

Neurosteroids are involved in several CNS physiological and pathological processes, such as the response to stress, depression, anxiety, sleep, or memory deficit (see more Morrow, 2007). Antidepressant effects of neuroactive steroids were described in animal models (Urani et al., 2001) as well as in patients (Wolkowitz et al., 1997, 1999). It has been shown that antidepressant treatment normalized the imbalance of 3α and 3β pregnanolone in patients suffering from depression (Romeo et al., 1998; Schüle et al., 2011). During social isolation, an animal model of depression-like behavior, biosynthesis of pregnanolone is significantly decreased (Pinna et al., 2008). SSRI are able to reverse the decreased brain pregnanolone level, and to correct behavioral deficits (Pinna et al., 2006).

The neurosteroids are known for their potentiation as well as inhibition of NMDA and GABA receptors. Naturally occurring 3α5β-pregnanolone sulfate has a substantial inhibitory activity (Irwin et al., 1994; Weaver et al., 2000; Kussius et al., 2009) on tonically activated NMDAR (Petrovic et al., 2005). Therefore, we introduced the development and testing of a novel synthetic NMDA antagonists derived from the 3αC pregnanolone having improved pharmacokinetic properties (Rambousek et al., 2011).

The newly synthesized neuroactive steroid 3α5β-pregnanolone glutamate (PG) is a representative member of a group of the steroids exerting effects on $GABA_A$, AMPA, kainate, and NMDAR. Concerning the NMDAR, the mechanism of an action is not fully understood in detail, but it can be stated that it displays specific properties. The drug is an allosteric inhibitor of the NMDAR. Its degree of inhibition of the NMDAR currents is independent of the cell membrane potential. On the other hand, the binding to its inhibitory binding site is pre-conditioned by the activation of NMDAR by agonists. Therefore, it is so-called a use-dependent allosteric inhibitor of NMDAR (see Korinek et al., 2011) with more potent inhibition of responses mediated by NR1/NR2C-D receptors, compared to those mediated by the NR1/NR2A-B receptors (Petrovic et al., 2005) and $GABA_A$ agonist (unpublished data). On the contrary to the non-competitive NMDA antagonists, 3α5β-PG is devoid of its adverse side-effects. 3α5β-PG binds only to the extrasynaptic and tonically activated NMDAR, which results in use-dependent selectivity (Rambousek et al., 2011).

In the present study, we examined potential antidepressant activity of PG. The effect of a single dose administration of PG was assessed by the Porsolt forced swim test, and by the repeated stress of social defeat, both used as common animal models of depression. The locomotor activity and the anxiolytic properties of PG were evaluated together with an open field and elevated plus maze tests. The effect of the chronic administration of PG on the aggressive behavior of singly housed male mice was evaluated by paired agonistic interactions with the non-aggressive group-housed partners.

MATERIALS AND METHODS

ANIMALS

Open field, elevated plus maze, and forced swimming studies

Naive adult male ICR mice (VELAZ s.r.o., Prague, Czech Republic), 15 weeks old and weighing 25–35 g, were used for the experiments. The animals were housed in groups of five in the plastic cages in a keeping of Institute of Physiology, Academy of Sciences of the Czech Republic. The mice had *ad libitum* access to the laboratory chow and water, except during behavioral experiments, and they were kept in a regulated environment (22°C, 50% humidity) under a 12-h light/dark cycle (lights on at 06:00 a.m.).

Social defeat and agonistic interaction studies

Naive adult male mice (ICR strain, VELAZ s.r.o., Prague, Czech Republic, 30–37 g) were used in this study. Food and water were available *ad libitum*. Mice were housed in a keeping of Department of Pharmacology, Faculty of Medicine of Masaryk University, Brno, either individually without any handling in self-cleaning cages with a grid floor (8 cm × 6 cm × 13 cm), or in groups of 17–20 in standard plastic cages (38 cm × 22 cm × 14 cm) with the floors covered with wooden shavings. The animals were housed, and behavioral testing was performed in a different room during the light phase of the constant light–dark cycle, with lights on at 06:00 and off at 18:00 h. The temperature was maintained at 21°C, and relative humidity was 50%. The group-housed mice were not handled, except on the experimental days. Singly housed mice were handled after 3 weeks of isolation, just during oral administration of PG.

Experiments were carried out between 09:00 a.m. and 06:00 p.m. All animal procedures were conducted in accordance with the European Community Council Directives of November 24, 1986 (86-609/EEC), and the Decree of October 20, 1987 (87–848). The study protocol was approved by the Animal Care Committee of the Institute of Physiology of Academy of Sciences of the Czech Republic and Masaryk University Brno, Faculty of Medicine, Czech Republic.

DRUG ADMINISTRATION

Drugs and chemicals used in the study were purchased from Sigma-Aldrich (Germany). PG was prepared by the esterification of 3α-hydroxy-5β-pregnan-20-one (Steraloids Inc., USA) with a protected glutamic acid. The synthesis is thoroughly described in Rambousek et al. (2011). PG solutions were prepared by dissolution of PG in hydroxypropyl-β-cyclodextrin (β-CD, 72 mM saline solution, pH adjusted to 7.4 by 1 M NaOH). MK-801 and ketamine were prepared by dissolution in saline. β-CD was administered as a control for PG, and saline as a control for dizocilpine (MK-801) and ketamine. Dizocilpine was used as a representative of non-competitive highly selective NMDA antagonists. In addition, ketamine was used as a non-competitive NMDA antagonist possessing antidepressant activity. In the open-field test, PG was applied i.p. at doses of 0.1, 1, and 10 mg/kg, and dizocilpine at the dose of 0.3 mg/kg, and ketamine at the dose of 10 mg/kg. In the elevated plus maze test, PG was injected i.p. at doses of 1 and 10 mg/kg. In the forced swim test, PG was administered i.p. at doses of 0.1, 1, and 10 mg/kg, and in the social defeat test and agonistic interactions orally at the dose of 1 mg/kg via gastric tube. In these tests, PG was administered 30 min prior to behavioral testing at a volume of 1 ml/kg, except for the social defeat test and agonistic interactions, where PG was administered 60 min prior to testing. In agonistic interactions, PG at the dose of 1 mg/kg/day was administered orally once daily for 30 days at a volume of 1 ml/kg. All animals received the same volume of liquid per 1 kg of body weight.

BEHAVIORAL PROCEDURES

Open-field test

The animals were placed individually into a circular open-field arena (82 cm in diameter), located in a soundproof room. The locomotor activity in the open field was assessed by placing the animal in the arena immediately after i.p. application of PG, MK-801, ketamine, and their vehicles, and monitoring their activity over 50 min using a video tracking system (iTrack, Biosignal Group, USA). We analyzed the locomotor activity, expressed as a total distance traveled (**Figure 1**). The number of animals per group was as follows: five animals in ketamine, MK-801 and PG 10 mg/kg group, seven mice in PG 0.1 mg/kg group, eight mice in saline and PG 1 mg/kg group, and nine mice in β-CD group.

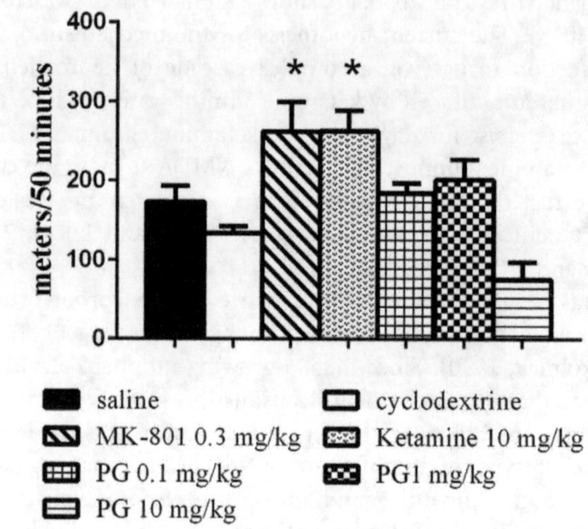

FIGURE 1 | Locomotor activity in the open field was assessed by placing an animal in the arena immediately after i.p. application of PG, MK-801, ketamine, and their vehicles. Locomotor activity was monitored over 50 min. Ketamine and dizocilpine administration resulted in hyperlocomotion. Animals treated with these non-competitive NMDA antagonists significantly increased distance traveled. PG administration did not lead to significant changes in locomotion. All values represent group means ± SEM. $*p < 0.05$ compared to the saline group.

Elevated plus maze

The apparatus consisted of open arms (30 cm × 6.5 cm), crossed at right angles, with two arms of the same length enclosed by walls of 15.5 cm high (closed arms). The whole apparatus was raised 50 cm above the floor. At the beginning of each session, the mouse was placed on the central platform (6.5 cm × 6.5 cm) facing the closed arm. The time spent in the open, close arms, and central platform was recorded over a 10-min test session by a video recorder positioned above the maze, tracked, and analyzed by software (iTrack, Biosignal Group, USA). Each experimental group consisted of 10 mice.

Forced swimming

The forced swimming test was carried out in accordance with the methods described by Porsolt et al. (1978), only with slight modifications. Mice were randomly assigned into the three groups – vehicle treated (10 mice), PG 0.1 mg/kg treated (10 mice), PG 1 mg/kg (8 mice), and PG 10 mg/kg (8 mice) treated mice. Each mouse was placed in a 25-cm plastic transparent cylinder (12 cm in diameter) containing 10 cm of water at 24 ± 1°C. The mice were left in the cylinder for 6 min, and their behavior was recorded. The duration of immobility was scored in the last 4 min of the swimming test. Mice were considered to be immobile if they floated while making only necessary movements to keep the head above water (Porsolt et al., 1978). In addition to immobility duration, we analyzed time to the first floating. Latency was measured immediately after the mice were put into the water. Recorded videos were analyzed by two independent observers, blind to the treatment conditions. Analysis was performed by Observer 3.0 (Noldus Information Technology, The Netherlands) software, and the results were displayed as ethograms in excel tables.

Social defeat

The chronic social defeat stress procedure was carried out using a similar method, described by Sulcova and Krsiak (1987) and Pistovcakova et al. (2005). In the first part of the experiment, mice were given β-CD (14 mice) or PG (18 mice) orally via a gastric tube. Administration was carried out in a randomized order, 60 min prior to the open-field test observations performed in the identical animal cage, but in a different room from that used for the social defeat interactions. Each animal was placed singly into the center of a novel environment (arena 30 cm × 30 cm) of the PC-controlled tracking apparatus Acti-track (Panlab, S.L., Spain) with the infrared beam sensors. Over the 8-min testing period, the overall distance traveled (as a marker of locomotor/exploratory behavior) in the open field was measured. Two days later, each mouse was defeated with a singly housed mouse exhibiting an aggressive behavior in a 4-min paired agonistic interaction. The procedure was repeated four times, 7 days apart. Immediately after the last (fourth) agonistic interaction, each mouse was randomly assigned to the vehicle (12 mice), or the treatment group (6 mice). Sixty minutes following the drug administration, the animal was placed into the open-field arena, and the overall distance traveled was measured, as described above. Mice that received a timid partner instead of an aggressive one were excluded from the experiment, since they were not defeated.

Agonistic interactions

Prior to the experiment, mice were housed individually for 3 weeks. Each individually singly housed mouse was allowed 30 min adaptation in a Plexiglas neutral observation cage (20 cm × 20 cm × 30 cm) with clean wood shavings before it was coupled with a group-housed non-aggressive male partner for 4 min interaction. On the first day of the experiment, each animal received vehicle orally via a gastric tube 60 min prior to the agonistic interaction. Singly housed mice were divided into two groups, according to their behavior during the control interaction (vehicle treatment) with the group-housed partner: (a) an aggressive one (attacking group-housed mouse at least once), and (b) a timid one [exhibiting no attacks, displaying defensive-escape (timid) behavior toward the group-housed mouse]. The number, latency, and duration of attacks, tail rattles, unrests (aggressive activities), defenses, escapes, alert postures (timid activities), social sniffing, climbing, and following the partner (sociable behavior) exhibited by singly housed mice were recorded and evaluated by the hardware/software Observer 3.1, Noldus Technology, Holland. Aggressive singly housed mice were subdivided into the two groups – one receiving vehicle (9 mice) and one receiving PG (11 mice). The agonistic interactions with group-housed mice were video-recorded after 14 and 30 days of vehicle/drug administration. The test protocol was adopted from Sulcova and Krsiak (1987).

STATISTICAL ANALYSIS

Data are presented as the group means ± standard error of mean (SEM). Statistical analyses were performed by the program GraphPad Prism 6.0 (San Diego, CA, USA). The statistical significance for the social defeat test was detected by the two-way ANOVA, followed by Sidak's *post hoc* test. The treatment (two factor level) and the stress (two factor levels) served as independent variables. In the agonistic interaction test, the effect of the treatment (two factor level) and the length of administration (three factor levels) of PG/vehicle were assessed by the two-way repeated measures ANOVA (control interaction first day vs. interactions days 14th and 30th). In the other tests, where the treatment effect was assessed alone, the one-way ANOVA was conducted. Sidak's *post hoc* test was used when appropriate. The significant level was set at $p < 0.05$.

RESULTS

OPEN FIELD

Statistical analysis of the locomotor activity in the open field by the one-way ANOVA showed significant differences in total distance traveled $F(6, 40) = 8.034$, $p < 0.0001$. MK-801 0.3 mg/kg and ketamine 10 mg/kg induced hyperlocomotion (**Figure 1**) during 50 min of an exploration. PG plasma levels were highest 15 min after i.p. administration, and brain neurosteroid level peaks occurred 60 min after i.p. application (Rambousek et al., 2011). Therefore, we chose a time interval of 30 min after i.p. application of PG for the subsequent tests.

ELEVATED PLUS MAZE

One-way ANOVAs revealed that PG administered at the dose of 1 mg/kg significantly increased the time spent in the open arms, $F(2, 24) = 7.654$, $p = 0.0027$ and decreased the time spent in the central platform, $F(2, 24) = 10.01$, $p = 0.0007$. Mice treated with PG 10 mg/kg did not display anxiolytic behavior, and their times spent in the open arms and central platform did not differ from the control group treated with only the vehicle. The treatment had no effect at all on the time spent in the closed arms (**Figure 2A**). Time spent in the central platform may be indicative of risk assessment behavior. Increased time spent in the central platform may be a sign of hesitation before entering either arm. In order to evaluate locomotor activity in the elevated plus maze, an analysis of open to close arms entries was conducted as well. However, no significant difference was revealed (**Figure 2B**), probably due to a big variance within each treatment group.

FORCED SWIMMING

Even though PG treatment led to the slight decrease in immobility time (**Figure 3A**), none of the doses used significantly reduced the immobility in comparison with the controls. As the next parameter, we assessed the time of the first floating (latency, **Figure 3B**). One-way ANOVA detected significant elongation of the latency after PG 1 mg/kg treatment $F(3, 29) = 5.248$, $p = 0.0051$. The discrepancy between results obtained from immobility and the latency analyses remains to be clarified. Sensitivity of the two parameters to antidepressant treatment may differ.

SOCIAL DEFEAT

Group-housed mice repeatedly defeated on aggressive agonistic interactions with singly housed partners exhibited decreased locomotor activity in the open field. Two-way ANOVA revealed significant effect of treatment vs. stress interaction $F(1, 46) = 4.687$, $p = 0.0356$. No significance was found for the effect of factor stress and factor treatment. PG 1 mg/kg administration normalized the stress-induced inhibition of locomotor activity in the open field, expressed as an overall distance traveled (**Figure 4**).

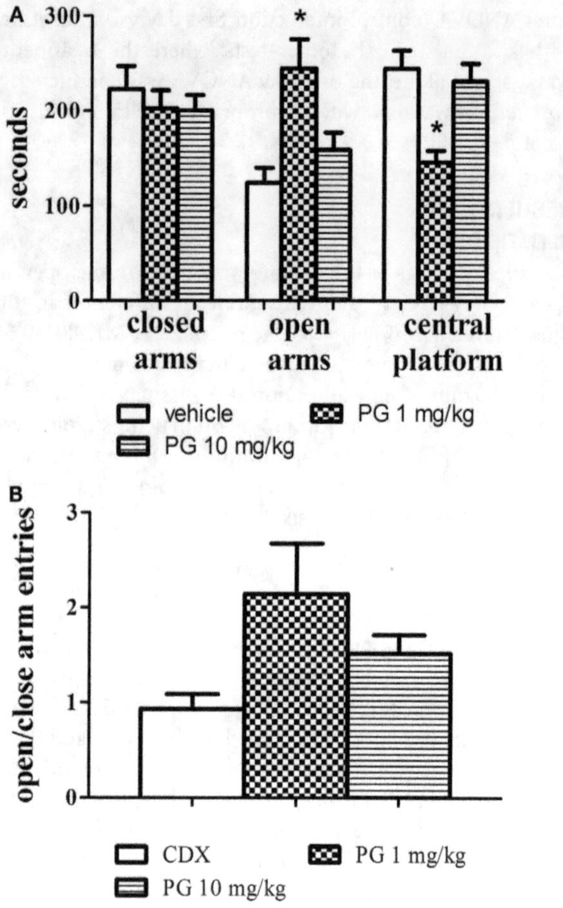

FIGURE 2 | Anxiolytic effect of PG was assessed in an elevated plus maze. **(A)** PG administered at the dose of 1 mg/kg significantly increased the time spent in the open arms, and decreased the time spent in the central platform. Mice treated with PG at the dose of 10 mg/kg did not display anxiolytic behavior. All values represent group means ± SEM. $^{*}p < 0.005$ compared to the vehicle, β-CD group. **(B)** The analysis of open to close arm entries did not reveal differences between treatment groups, probably due to big differences in variance within each group. All values represent group means ± SEM.

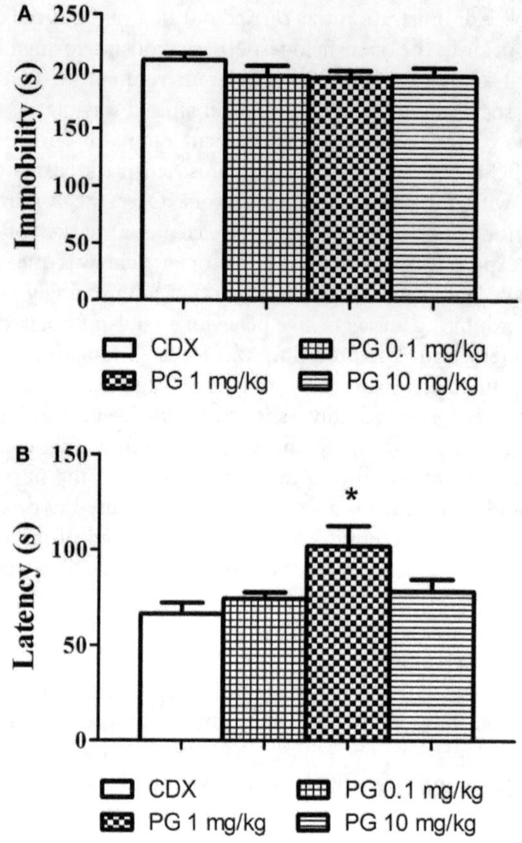

FIGURE 3 | In the forced swim test, we evaluated the possible antidepressant effect of PG. **(A)** Immobility time in the forced swim test was assessed 30 min after i.p. administration of PG and vehicle. None of the doses applied significantly influenced floating. Average group values ± SEM. **(B)** In addition to immobility duration in the forced swimming test, we measured time to the first floating as well. Administration of PG at the dose of 1 mg/kg significantly prolonged the latency to the first floating compared to controls. All values represent group means ± SEM. $^{*}p < 0.005$ compared to the vehicle group.

AGONISTIC INTERACTIONS

Chronic administration of PG at the dose of 1 mg/kg over 30 days reduced aggressive actions in singly housed mice exhibiting aggressive behavior on the first interaction. Two-way repeated measures ANOVA detected significant effect of the treatment vs. the length of administration interaction in the parameter duration $F(2, 116) = 5.407$, $p = 0.0057$. Length of the administration showed significant effect $F(2, 116) = 11.97$, $p < 0.0001$, whereas treatment showed no influence on the duration of aggression. Aggression was significantly reduced after 14 and 30 days of PG 1 mg/kg administration, compared to the scores of vehicle treated controls in the first day (**Figure 5A**). This reduction was more pronounced after 30 days of PG treatment ($p < 0.0001$ *post hoc* analysis), compared to only 2 weeks treatment ($p = 0.0037$). The time spent in aggressive interactions dropped in PG treated animals.

Time to the first aggressive action (the latency) was prolonged in PG treated mice. Two-way repeated measures ANOVA revealed the effect of the factor treatment $F(1,58) = 4.55$, $p = 0.0372$ and the factor of administration length $F(2, 116) = 8.652$, $p = 0.0003$ on the latency. Interaction between the two factors was not significant. It took more time for the PG treated animals to attack the intruder after 14 and 30 days of PG application in comparison to the controls (**Figure 5B**). Again, this effect was greater after longer administration ($p < 0.0001$ after 30 days vs. $p = 0.0275$ after 14 days, revealed by *post hoc* test).

The frequency of aggressive actions decreased over the course of an experiment. Interaction between the two factors, treatment, and length of administration, came out significant [$F(2, 116) = 8.505$, $p = 0.0004$] when analyzed by the two-way repeated measures ANOVA. The length of administration had a significant effect $F(2, 116) = 30.04$, $p < 0.0001$ on the frequency. The kind of treatment we used had no effect. Frequency expressed as a number of aggressive actions decreased after 14 and 30 days of PG treatment. Vehicle

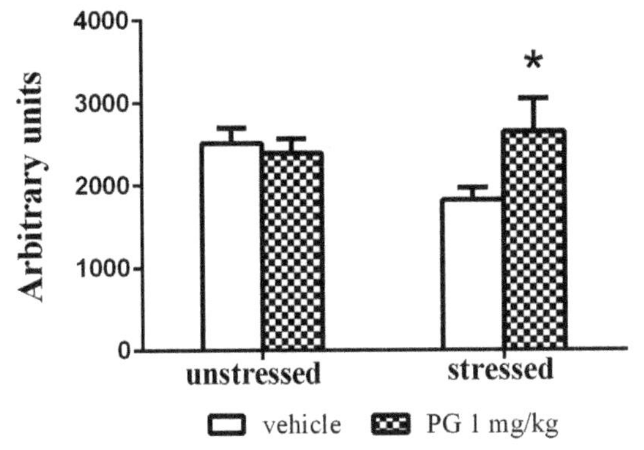

FIGURE 4 | Group-housed mice repeatedly stressed by defeat on four agonistic interactions (7 days apart) with aggressive singly housed partners exhibited depressed locomotor activity in the open field. This effect was disinhibited by treatment with PG at the dose of 1 mg/kg. There was no difference in unstressed animals between two treatment groups in the open-field activity. All values represent group means ± SEM. *$p < 0.05$ compared to the stressed vehicle treated animals.

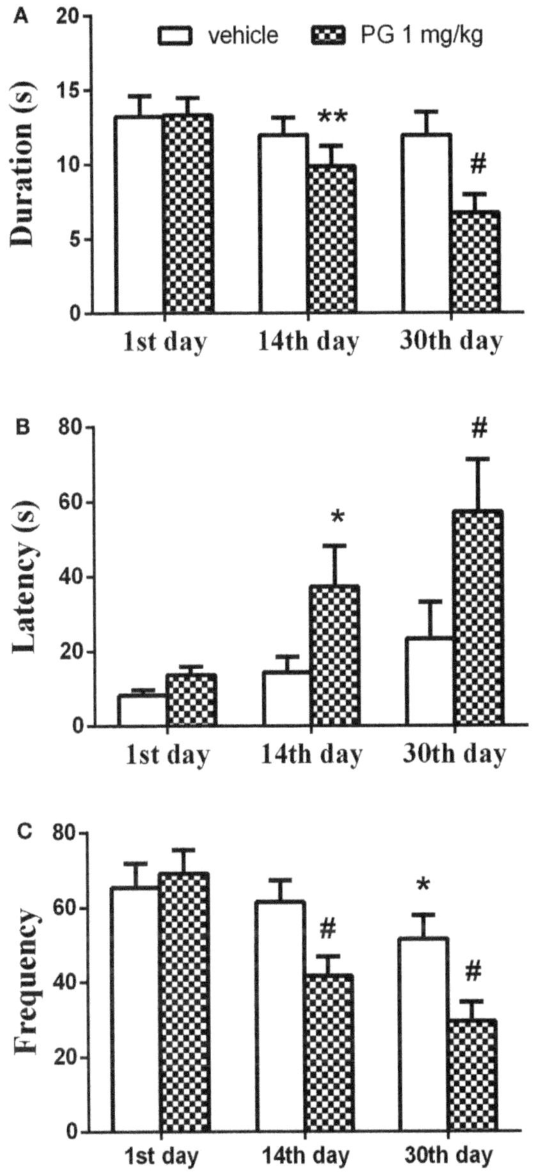

FIGURE 5 | In 4-min paired agonistic interactions, singly housed mice were confronted with non-aggressive group-housed partners. Chronic administration of PG at the dose of 1 mg/kg over 30 days reduced aggressive behavior in singly housed mice exhibiting aggressive behavior during the first agonistic interaction. **(A)** Graph shows the duration of aggressive activities. The duration was significantly reduced after 14 and 30 days of PG 1 mg/kg administration, compared to the scores of vehicle treated controls in the first day. The effect was more prominent after 30 days. **(B)** Graph shows latency to the first aggressive action. Latency prolonged in PG treated mice after 14 and 30 days of PG application in comparison to controls. Again this effect was greater after longer administration. **(C)** Graph displays number of aggressive actions. Frequency decreased over the course of the experiment. Vehicle treated mice also showed significant reduction in the frequency of aggressive actions between the 1st and 30th day. However, this change in frequency was not as prominent as in PG treated animals. All values represent group means ± SEM. *$p < 0.05$, **$p < 0.005$, #$p < 0.0001$ compared to the vehicle treated animals on the first day of agonistic interaction.

treated mice also showed significant reduction in the frequency of aggressive actions between the 1st and 30th day. However, this change in frequency was not as prominent ($p = 0.0163$) as in PG treated animals ($p < 0.0001$ for both time intervals) (**Figure 5C**). Taken altogether, mice treated daily with PG at the dose of 1 mg/kg over the course of 30 days indulged less in aggressive interactions.

DISCUSSION

The present study focused on the evaluation of antidepressant-like and anxiolytic-like effects of newly synthesized neurosteroid PG. Neurosteroids are known for their neuroprotective and antipsychotic effects (Pringle et al., 2003; Veiga et al., 2003; MacKenzie et al., 2007; Rambousek et al., 2011; Vales et al., 2012), and alternation of their brain levels is well-documented in various neurodegenerative diseases and aging (Vallée et al., 1997; Nafziger et al., 1998; Kim et al., 2003; Aldred and Mecocci, 2010; Luchetti et al., 2010; Sorwell and Urbanski, 2010). Similarly, the down-regulation of neurosteroid synthesis possibly contributes to the development of depressive disorders and anxiety (Morrow, 2007; Schüle et al., 2011, 2014). Neurosteroids as potent NMDAR antagonist and GABA receptor agonists might be promising therapeutic agents in depressive disorders (Zorumski et al., 2013).

Our results from the open-field test indicate that hyperlocomotion found in MK-801 and ketamine treated animals is not present after PG application (**Figure 1**). It is in concordance with our previous results (Vales et al., 2012). As opposed to non-competitive NMDA antagonists such as dizocilpine (MK-801), ketamine, and PCP often used for induction of schizophrenia-like behavior (Bubeníková-Valesová et al., 2008), PG does not display psychotomimetic properties, but quite the contrary. Administration of PG at the doses of 0.1 and 1 mg/kg did not significantly influence spontaneous locomotor activity in comparison to the control (**Figure 1**). Furthermore, PG at the highest dose of 10 mg/kg exhibited hypolocomotion after i.p. administration.

It cannot be interpreted as an unexpected effect, because GABA agonists as well as NMDA antagonists are drugs, which produce typically sedative and anesthetic effects.

The lower risk of hyperlocomotion can be explained by the different mechanism of action. PG is a use-dependent NMDA inhibitor, which has a more pronounced inhibitory action on the tonically active NMDAR (Petrovic et al., 2005). The hypothesis underlying the ability of use-dependent inhibitors to differentiate between phasic physiological and tonic pathological activation of NMDAR during pathological states have gained relatively wide acceptance. However, it is still unclear how such compounds could differentiate between normal and abnormal synaptic activation of NMDAR (Borovska et al., 2012). The lowered risk of hyperlocomotion displays memantine as well. Memantine has been shown to result in the preferential blockade of excessive NMDAR activity, while sparing normal excitatory synaptic function (Lipton, 2006, 2007).

Anxiolytic performance of PG was assessed in the elevated plus maze test. Agonists of GABA receptors are recognized for their anxiolytic properties (Brot et al., 1997), and in the elevated plus maze test they increase the time spent in open arms (Rodgers and Johnson, 1998). PG at the dose of 1 mg/kg exhibited anxiolytic-like activity clearly indicated by significant increase in time spent in open arms (**Figure 2A**). Anxiolytic-like properties of PG were also previously confirmed by decreased shock-induced ultrasonic vocalization in rats after PG application (Vales et al., 2012). The analysis of open to close arm entries did not reveal differences between treatment groups (**Figure 2B**), however the decrease in locomotion in the PG of 10 mg/kg treated group was not as prominent as in the open field. It can be explained by the decreased habituation to the maze, since animals spent considerably less time in the elevated plus maze than in the open field, and the activity of the mice is enforced by the nature of the task.

Pregnenolone glutamate at all doses slightly reduced floating when applied 30 min prior to the test, however this decrease was not significant (**Figure 3A**). We analyzed not only the overall time of floating in the session, but also the time to the first floating. In our experiment, PG 1 mg/kg significantly prolonged the latency to the first immobility (**Figure 3B**). Time to the first floating analysis produced more robust results, at least in our experimental set-up. According to literature available and our experience, the forced swim test is sensitive to various independent variables, such as mouse strains (Lucki et al., 2001; Mason et al., 2009), age of mice used (Mason et al., 2009; Sequeira-Cordero et al., 2013), water temperature (Pintér et al., 2011), 2 days vs. 1 day protocol, water depth (Pintér et al., 2011), diameter of cylinders animals swim in, seasonal changes, etc. (Petit-Demouliere et al., 2005). We probably failed to find the optimal protocol where the differences between the groups would be more distinct.

3α-reduced neuroactive steroids have anxiolytic and antidepressant-like effects in the preclinical studies (Eser et al., 2006). Even though PG meets this effect, it failed to improve immobility scores in the forced swim test. Similar results were obtained after progesterone application (Urani et al., 2001). However, the administration of allopregnanolone significantly reduced the time spent by immobilization (Rodríguez-Landa et al., 2009), indicating that allopregnanolone is a more potent GABA activator, compared to progesterone. The mechanism of action of PG on GABA neurons is not fully known. If the failure to decrease immobility in the forced swimming could be ascribed to the lower affinity of PG to GABA receptors, or if it is caused by the methodological drawbacks in the test, remains to be clarified.

Pregnenolone glutamate at the particular dose of 1 mg/kg had the most pronounced effect in the tests mentioned above. Therefore, we decided to use this concentration in the repeated social defeat model. This animal model of depressive disorder is more plausible than the forced swim test, since it mimics a different aspect of depression by prolonged exposure to psychosocial stress (Chaouloff, 2013; Venzala et al., 2013). In the social defeat test, PG at 1 mg/kg normalized the locomotor activity in the open field in mice exposed to aggressive conspecific prior to open-field testing (**Figure 4**). Stressed mice receiving no PG exhibited stress-induced reduction in locomotion measured by distance passed. There was no difference in unstressed animals between the two treatment groups in the open-field activity. The spontaneous locomotor activity was not affected by PG administration; this conclusion is also supported by the results from the open field.

The social defeat stress leads to depression-like abnormalities in defeated animals, lasting for weeks, such as anxiety, social avoidance, anhedonia, and changes in body weight, increased blood pressure, suppressed immune responses, and others (Blanchard et al., 2001; Huhman, 2006; Chaouloff, 2013). Among the most often noted behavioral responses is the decrease in activity and exploration in the open field (Meerlo et al., 1996; Rygula et al., 2005; Razzoli et al., 2009). Chronic, but not acute, treatment with antidepressants, both SSRI and tricyclics, can reverse the consequences of social stress exposure (van Bokhoven et al., 2011; Olivares et al., 2012; Venzala et al., 2012). Similarly, NMDAR antagonist (Jasnow et al., 2004) and GABA receptor agonist (Jasnow and Huhman, 2001) microinjected to the amygdala block conditioned defeat.

Aggressive mice after 30 days of single-housing were receiving PG of 1 mg/kg chronically over 30 days. PG administration led to the significant decrease of aggressive behavior in the agonistic interactions with non-aggressive group-housed partners, when compared to the control interaction in the first day of the experiment. The duration and frequency of the aggressive behavior decreased after 14 days of chronic application of PG. An even more profound effect was reached after 30 days of application (**Figures 5A,C**). The significant decrease in frequency was also detected in vehicle treated animals 30 days after β-CD administration. However, this effect was less prominent, compared to PG treated animals (**Figure 5C**), and it might be caused by habituation to intruder. The latency to the first aggressive action was prolonged 14 days after PG administration, and it was again accompanied by a more profound effect 30 days after (**Figure 5B**). Taken together, the mice treated daily with PG at the dose level of 1 mg/kg over the course of 30 days indulged less in aggressive interactions.

Stress induced by social isolation causes a significant decrease in pregnenolone, progesterone, allotetrahydrodeoxycorticosterone, and allopregnanolone concentrations in the cerebral cortex, compared to the group-housed controls (Serra et al., 2000). The neuroactive steroid changes were not evident after 48 h of chronic stress exposure, but their decrease was present 7 days after the chronic stress, with the most prominent change 30 days after (Serra et al., 2000). Stress and depression are associated with a decrease in GABAergic function in the PFC and hippocampus (Benes et al., 2008; Croarkin et al., 2011). Administration of PG could lead to normalization of the level of GABA potentiating neurosteroids, and therefore contribute to the homeostasis restoration (aggression reduction/normal locomotor activity) by enhancement of the GABA neurotransmission.

Chronic stress reduces the production of allopregnanolone, as well as other GABAergic neurosteroids (Serra et al., 2000). Decreased levels of neurosteroids in the plasma and CSF are found in patients with major depression (Romeo et al., 1998; Uzunova et al., 1998). Prolonged exposure to stress may induce a reduction in pituitary responsiveness to high concentrations of CRH, leading to desensitization, and consequently to decreased ACTH secretion (Hoffman et al., 1985), affecting neurosteroid synthesis. A reduced ACTH response to chronic stress leads to hyper-responsiveness of the hypothalamic–pituitary–adrenal axis (HPA) axis to the new stimuli, and confers vulnerability to mood and anxiety-related disorders, as well as depression (Biggio and Purdy, 2001). Antidepressant treatment normalizes the altered allopregnanolone levels (Uzunov et al., 1996; Uzunova et al., 1998; Schüle et al., 2014) suggesting that GABAergic neurotransmission alteration by the neurosteroids has a therapeutic effect.

The increasing number of evidence shows that the NMDARs play a crucial role in the neurobiology and treatment of depression. PG as the use-dependent inhibitor of NMDARs binds only to the extrasynaptic and tonically activated NMDARs, leaving normal neurotransmission unaffected (Rambousek et al., 2011), and therefore causing less severe side-effects. The effect of neuroactive steroids appears to be subtype selective (Gibbs et al., 2006). Similarly, PG displays more potent inhibition of responses mediated by NR1/NR2C-D receptors, compared to those mediated by NR1/NR2A-B receptors (Petrovic et al., 2005). The current challenge in development of steroidal NMDA antagonists suitable for clinical use is in the low potency of existing drugs. Nonetheless, if both the $GABA_A$ enhancers and NMDA antagonists have antidepressant potential, the ideal agent might be the one that combines all these effects in a single molecule (Zorumski et al., 2013). Therefore, it might be surprising that DHEA and DHEAS as positive NMDA and negative $GABA_A$ modulators exert antidepressant activity (Wolkowitz et al., 1997, 1999; Urani et al., 2001). However, the mechanism of action of DHEA/S suggests an indirect way of normalizing HPA axis activity (via MAP2C protein activity, serotonin turn-over, anti-glucocorticoid effects, MAO inhibitory effect, promotion of neurogenesis, etc.) (Maninger et al., 2009; Pérez-Neri et al., 2009; Felice et al., 2012).

Taken altogether, these results showed that 3α5β-PG activity at NMDARs lacks negative side-effects accompanying treatment with non-competitive NMDA antagonists that impair normal neurotransmission. Since PG combines both effects – $GABA_A$ receptor potentiation and the NMDAR inhibition – it has a potential as an antidepressant in the treatment of depressive symptoms.

In conclusion, we demonstrated in animal models antidepressant-like and anxiolytic-like activities of 3α5β-PG – an analog of naturally occurring 3α5β-pregnanolone sulfate. PG is an example of a promising neurosteroid showing possible potential for development of a novel antidepressant, procognitive, and neuroprotective agents. This branch of research gives rise to a possibility of obtaining drugs with antidepressant/anxiolytic properties and minimal side-effects, i.e., with a more favorable risk/benefit ratio.

ACKNOWLEDGMENTS

This study was supported by GACR grants P304/12/G069, P303/12/1464 IGA MZCR NT 13403-4/2012; TACR-TE01020028, institutional support RVO: 67985823, ACIU LM2011017 and by the project "CEITEC – Central European Institute of Technology" (CZ.1.05/1.1.00/02.0068) from the European Regional Development Fund. We would like to thank Michaela Fialova and Zdenka Oplatkova for their technical assistance. Next, we are appreciative to Dr. Ladislav Vyklicky, Dr. Hana Chodounska, and Dr. Eva Kudova for scientific inspiration and for steroid synthesis. Finally, we want to express thanks to Ms. Thuy Hua for proofreading.

REFERENCES

Aldred, S., and Mecocci, P. (2010). Decreased dehydroepiandrosterone (DHEA) and dehydroepiandrosterone sulfate (DHEAS) concentrations in plasma of Alzheimer's disease (AD) patients. *Arch. Gerontol. Geriatr.* 51, e16–e18. doi:10.1016/j.archger.2009.07.001

Benes, F. M., Lim, B., Matzilevich, D., Subburaju, S., and Walsh, J. P. (2008). Circuitry-based gene expression profiles in GABA cells of the trisynaptic pathway in schizophrenics versus bipolars. *Proc. Natl. Acad. Sci. U.S.A.* 105, 20935–20940. doi:10.1073/pnas.0810153105

Berman, R. M., Cappiello, A., Anand, A., Oren, D. A., Heninger, G. R., Charney, D. S., et al. (2000). Antidepressant effects of ketamine in depressed patients. *Biol. Psychiatry* 47, 351–354. doi:10.1016/S0006-3223(99)00230-9

Biggio, G., and Purdy, R. H. (2001). *Neurosteroids and Brain Function.* San Diego, CA: Academic Press.

Blanchard, R. J., McKittrick, C. R., and Blanchard, D. C. (2001). Animal models of social stress: effects on behavior and brain neurochemical systems. *Physiol. Behav.* 73, 261–271. doi:10.1016/S0031-9384(01)00449-8

Borovska, J., Vyklicky, V., Stastna, E., Kapras, V., Slavikova, B., Horak, M., et al. (2012). Access of inhibitory neurosteroids to the NMDA receptor. *Br. J. Pharmacol.* 166, 1069–1083. doi:10.1111/j.1476-5381.2011.01816.x

Brot, M. D., Akwa, Y., Purdy, R. H., Koob, G. F., and Britton, K. T. (1997). The anxiolytic-like effects of the neurosteroid allopregnanolone: interactions with GABA(A) receptors. *Eur. J. Pharmacol.* 325, 1–7. doi:10.1016/S0014-2999(97)00096-4

Browne, C. A., and Lucki, I. (2013). Antidepressant effects of ketamine: mechanisms underlying fast-acting novel antidepressants. *Front. Pharmacol.* 4:161. doi:10.3389/fphar.2013.00161

Bubeníková-Valesová, V., Horácek, J., Vrajová, M., and Höschl, C. (2008). Models of schizophrenia in humans and animals based on inhibition of NMDA receptors. *Neurosci. Biobehav. Rev.* 32, 1014–1023. doi:10.1016/j.neubiorev.2008.03.012

Burgdorf, J., Zhang, X. L., Nicholson, K. L., Balster, R. L., Leander, J. D., Stanton, P. K., et al. (2013). GLYX-13, a NMDA receptor glycine-site functional partial agonist, induces antidepressant-like effects without ketamine-like side effects. *Neuropsychopharmacology* 38, 729–742. doi:10.1038/npp.2012.246

Chaouloff, F. (2013). Social stress models in depression research: what do they tell us? *Cell Tissue Res.* 354, 179–190. doi:10.1007/s00441-013-1606-x

Chen, H. S., and Lipton, S. A. (2006). The chemical biology of clinically tolerated NMDA receptors antagonist. *J. Neurochem.* 97, 1611–1626. doi:10.1111/j.1471-4159.2006.03991.x

Croarkin, P. E., Levinson, A. J., and Daskalakis, Z. J. (2011). Evidence for GABAergic inhibitory deficits in major depressive disorder. *Neurosci. Biobehav. Rev.* 35, 818–825. doi:10.1016/j.neubiorev.2010.10.002

Danysz, W., Parsons, C. G., Karcz-Kubicha, M., Schwaier, A., Popik, P., Wedzony, K., et al. (1998). GlycineB antagonists as potential therapeutic agents. Previous hopes and present reality. *Amino Acids* 14, 235–239. doi:10.1007/BF01345268

Diazgranados, N., Ibrahim, L. A., Brutsche, N. E., Ameli, R., Henter, I. D., Luckenbaugh, D. A., et al. (2010). Rapid resolution of suicidal ideation after a single infusion of an N-methyl-D-aspartate antagonist in patients with treatment-resistant major depressive disorder. *J. Clin. Psychiatry* 71, 1605–1611. doi:10.4088/JCP.09m05327blu

Entsuah, A. R., Huang, H., and Thase, M. E. (2001). Response and remission rates in different subpopulations with major depressive disorder administered venlafaxine, selective serotonin reuptake inhibitors, or placebo. *J. Clin. Psychiatry* 62, 869–877. doi:10.4088/JCP.v62n1106

Eser, D., Romeo, E., Baghai, T. C., di Michele, F., Schüle, C., Pasini, A., et al. (2006). Neuroactive steroids as modulators of depression and anxiety. *Neuroscience* 138, 1041–1048. doi:10.1016/j.neuroscience.2005.07.007

Felice, D., O'Leary, O. F., Pizzo, R. C., and Cryan, J. F. (2012). Blockade of the GABA(B) receptor increases neurogenesis in the ventral but not dorsal adult hippocampus: relevance to antidepressant action. *Neuropharmacology* 63, 1380–1388. doi:10.1016/j.neuropharm.2012.06.066

Gibbs, T. T., Russek, S. J., and Farb, D. H. (2006). Sulfated steroids as endogenous neuromodulators. *Pharmacol. Biochem. Behav.* 84, 555–567. doi:10.1016/j.pbb.2006.07.031

Hayley, S., and Litteljohn, D. (2014). Neuroplasticity and the next wave of antidepressant strategies. *Front. Cell Neurosci.* 7:218. doi:10.3389/fncel.2013.00218

Hoffman, A. R., Ceda, G., and Reisine, T. D. (1985). Corticotropin-releasing factor desensitization of adrenocorticotropic hormone release is augmented by arginine vasopressin. *J. Neurosci.* 5, 234–242.

Huhman, K. L. (2006). Social conflict models: can they inform us about human psychopathology? *Horm. Behav.* 50, 640–646. doi:10.1016/j.yhbeh.2006.06.022

Irwin, R. P., Lin, S. Z., Rogawski, M. A., Purdy, R. H., and Paul, S. M. (1994). Steroid potentiation and inhibition of N-methyl-D-aspartate receptor-mediated intracellular Ca++ responses: structure-activity studies. *J. Pharmacol. Exp. Ther.* 271, 677–682.

Jasnow, A. M., Cooper, M. A., and Huhman, K. L. (2004). N-methyl-D-aspartate receptors in the amygdala are necessary for the acquisition and expression of conditioned defeat. *Neuroscience* 123, 625–634. doi:10.1016/j.neuroscience.2003.10.015

Jasnow, A. M., and Huhman, K. L. (2001). Activation of GABA(A) receptors in the amygdala blocks the acquisition and expression of conditioned defeat in Syrian hamsters. *Brain Res.* 920, 142–150. doi:10.1016/S0006-8993(01)03054-2

Karcz-Kubicha, M., Wedzony, K., Zajaczkowski, W., and Danysz, W. (1999). NMDA receptor antagonists acting at the glycineB site in rat models for antipsychotic-like activity. *J. Neural. Transm.* 106, 1189–1204. doi:10.1007/s007020050233

Kemp, J. A., and McKernan, R. M. (2002). NMDA receptor pathways as drug targets. *Nat. Neurosci.* 5(Suppl.), 1039–1042. doi:10.1038/nn936

Kim, S. B., Hill, M., Kwak, Y. T., Hampl, R., Jo, D. H., and Morfin, R. (2003). Neurosteroids: cerebrospinal fluid levels for Alzheimer's disease and vascular dementia diagnostics. *J. Clin. Endocrinol. Metab.* 88, 5199–5206. doi:10.1210/jc.2003-030646

Korinek, M., Kapras, V., Vyklicky, V., Adamusova, E., Borovska, J., Vales, K., et al. (2011). Neurosteroid modulation of N-methyl-D-aspartate receptors: molecular mechanism and behavioral effects. *Steroids* 76, 1409–1418. doi:10.1016/j.steroids.2011.09.002

Krystal, J. H., Karper, L. P., Seibyl, J. P., Freeman, G. K., Delaney, R., Bremner, J. D., et al. (1994). Subanesthetic effects of the noncompetitive NMDA antagonist, ketamine, in humans. Psychotomimetic, perceptual, cognitive, and neuroendocrine responses. *Arch. Gen. Psychiatry* 51, 199–214. doi:10.1001/archpsyc.1994.03950030035004

Kussius, C. L., Kaur, N., and Popescu, G. K. (2009). Pregnanolone sulfate promotes desensitization of activated NMDA receptors. *J. Neurosci.* 29, 6819–6827. doi:10.1523/JNEUROSCI.0281-09.2009

Lam, R. W. (2012). Onset, time course and trajectories of improvement with antidepressants. *Eur. Neuropsychopharmacol.* 22(Suppl. 3), S492–S498. doi:10.1016/j.euroneuro.2012.07.005

Lapidus, K. A., Soleimani, L., and Murrough, J. W. (2013). Novel glutamatergic drugs for the treatment of mood disorders. *Neuropsychiatr. Dis. Treat.* 9, 1101–1112. doi:10.2147/NDT.S36689

Layer, R. T., Popik, P., Olds, T., and Skolnick, P. (1995). Antidepressant-like actions of the polyamine site NMDA antagonist, eliprodil (SL-82.0715). *Pharmacol. Biochem. Behav.* 52, 621–627. doi:10.1016/0091-3057(95)00155-P

Li, N., Liu, R. J., Dwyer, J. M., Banasr, M., Lee, B., Son, H., et al. (2011). Glutamate N-methyl-D-aspartate receptor antagonists rapidly reverse behavioral and synaptic deficits caused by chronic stress exposure. *Biol. Psychiatry* 69, 754–761. doi:10.1016/j.biopsych.2010.12.015

Lipton, A. S. (2006). NMDA receptors, glial cells, and clinical medicine. *Neuron* 50, 9–11. doi:10.1016/j.neuron.2006.03.026

Lipton, A. S. (2007). Pathologically activated therapeutics for neuroprotection. *Nat. Rev. Neurosci.* 8, 803–808. doi:10.1038/nrn2260

Luchetti, S., Bossers, K., Frajese, G. V., and Swaab, D. F. (2010). Neurosteroid biosynthetic pathway changes in substantia nigra and caudate nucleus in Parkinson's disease. *Brain Pathol.* 20, 945–951. doi:10.1111/j.1750-3639.2010.00396.x

Lucki, I., Dalvi, A., and Mayorga, A. J. (2001). Sensitivity to the effects of pharmacologically selective antidepressants in different strains of mice. *Psychopharmacology (Berl.)* 155, 315–322. doi:10.1007/s002130100694

MacKenzie, E. M., Odontiadis, J., Le Mellédo, J. M., Prior, T. I., and Baker, G. B. (2007). The relevance of neuroactive steroids in schizophrenia, depression, and anxiety disorders. *Cell. Mol. Neurobiol.* 27, 541–574. doi:10.1007/s10571-006-9086-0

Maninger, N., Wolkowitz, O. M., Reus, V. I., Epel, E. S., and Mellon, S. H. (2009). Neurobiological and neuropsychiatric effects of dehydroepiandrosterone (DHEA) and DHEA sulfate (DHEAS). *Front. Neuroendocrinol.* 30:65–91. doi:10.1016/j.yfrne.2008.11.002

Mason, S. S., Baker, K. B., Davis, K. W., Pogorelov, V. M., Malbari, M. M., Ritter, R., et al. (2009). Differential sensitivity to SSRI and tricyclic antidepressants in juvenile and adult mice of three strains. *Eur. J. Pharmacol.* 602, 306–315. doi:10.1016/j.ejphar.2008.11.010

Meerlo, P., Overkamp, G. J., Benning, M. A., Koolhaas, J. M., and Van den Hoofdakker, R. H. (1996). Long-term changes in open field behaviour following a single social defeat in rats can be reversed by sleep deprivation. *Physiol. Behav.* 60, 115–119. doi:10.1016/0031-9384(95)02271-6

Morrow, A. L. (2007). Recent developments in the significance and therapeutic relevance of neuroactive steroids – introduction to the special issue. *Pharmacol. Ther.* 116, 1–6. doi:10.1016/j.pharmthera.2007.04.003

Murrough, J. W., Perez, A. M., Pillemer, S., Stern, J., Parides, M. K., Aan Het Rot, M., et al. (2013). Rapid and longer-term antidepressant effects of repeated ketamine infusions in treatment-resistant major depression. *Biol. Psychiatry* 74, 250–256. doi:10.1016/j.biopsych.2012.06.022

Nafziger, A. N., Bowlin, S. J., Jenkins, P. L., and Pearson, T. A. (1998). Longitudinal changes in dehydroepiandrosterone concentrations in men and women. *J. Lab. Clin. Med.* 131, 316–323. doi:10.1016/S0022-2143(98)90181-0

Olivares, E. L., Silva-Almeida, C., Pestana, F. M., Sonoda-Côrtes, R., Araujo, I. G., Rodrigues, N. C., et al. (2012). Social stress-induced hypothyroidism is attenuated by antidepressant treatment in rats. *Neuropharmacology* 62, 446–456. doi:10.1016/j.neuropharm.2011.08.035

Parsons, C. G. (2001). NMDA receptors as targets for drug action in neuropathic pain. *Eur. J. Pharmacol.* 429, 71–78. doi:10.1016/S0014-2999(01)01307-3

Pérez-Neri, I., Montes, S., and Ríos, C. (2009). Inhibitory effect of dehydroepiandrosterone on brain monoamine oxidase activity: in vivo and in vitro studies. *Life Sci.* 85, 652–656. doi:10.1016/j.lfs.2009.09.008

Petit-Demouliere, B., Chenu, F., and Bourin, M. (2005). Forced swimming test in mice: a review of antidepressant activity. *Psychopharmacology (Berl.)* 177, 245–255. doi:10.1007/s00213-004-2048-7

Petrovic, M., Sedlacek, M., Horak, M., Chodounska, H., and Vyklický, L. Jr. (2005). 20-oxo-5beta-pregnan-3alpha-yl sulfate is a use-dependent NMDA receptor inhibitor. *J. Neurosci.* 25, 8439–8450. doi:10.1523/JNEUROSCI.1407-05.2005

Pilc, A., Wieronska, J. M., and Skolnick, P. (2013). Glutamate-based antidepressants: preclinical psychopharmacology. *Biol. Psychiatry* 73, 1125–1132. doi:10.1016/j.biopsych.2013.01.021

Pinna, G., Agis-Balboa, R. C., Pibiri, F., Nelson, M., Guidotti, A., and Costa, E. (2008). Neurosteroid biosynthesis regulates sexually dimorphic fear and aggressive behavior in mice. *Neurochem. Res.* 33, 1990–2007. doi:10.1007/s11064-008-9718-5

Pinna, G., Costa, E., and Guidotti, A. (2006). Fluoxetine and norfluoxetine stereospecifically and selectively increase brain neurosteroid content at doses that are inactive on 5-HT reuptake. *Psychopharmacology (Berl.)* 186, 362–372. doi:10.1007/s00213-005-0213-2

Pintér, O., Domokos, Á, Mergl, Z., Mikics, É, and Zelena, D. (2011). Do stress hormones connect environmental effects with behavior in the forced swim test? *Endocr. J.* 58, 395–407. doi:10.1507/endocrj.K10E-375

Pistovcakova, J., Makatsori, A., Sulcova, A., and Jezova, D. (2005). Felbamate reduces hormone release and locomotor hypoactivity induced by repeated stress of social defeat in mice. *Eur. Neuropsychopharmacol.* 15, 153–158. doi:10.1016/j.euroneuro.2004.08.007

Popik, P., Mamczarz, J., Fraczek, M., Widła, M., Hesselink, M., and Danysz, W. (1998). Inhibition of reinforcing effects of morphine and naloxone-precipitated opioid withdrawal by novel glycine site and uncompetitive NMDA receptor antagonists. *Neuropharmacology* 37, 1033–1042. doi:10.1016/S0028-3908(98)00105-1

Porsolt, R. D., Anton, G., Blavet, N., and Jalfre, M. (1978). Behavioural despair in rats: a new model sensitive to antidepressant treatments. *Eur. J. Pharmacol.* 47, 379–391. doi:10.1016/0014-2999(78)90118-8

Pringle, A. K., Schmidt, W., Deans, J. K., Wulfert, E., Reymann, K. G., and Sundstrom, L. E. (2003). 7-Hydroxylated epiandrosterone (7-OH-EPIA) reduces ischaemia-induced neuronal damage both in vivo and in vitro. *Eur. J. Neurosci.* 18, 117–124. doi:10.1046/j.1460-9568.2003.02734.x

Rambousek, L., Bubenikova-Valesova, V., Kacer, P., Syslova, K., Kenney, J., Holubova, K., et al. (2011). Cellular and behavioural effects of a new steroidal inhibitor of the N-methyl-D-aspartate receptor 3α5β-pregnanolone glutamate. *Neuropharmacology* 61, 61–68. doi:10.1016/j.neuropharm.2011.02.018

Razzoli, M., Carboni, L., and Arban, R. (2009). Alterations of behavioral and endocrinological reactivity induced by 3 brief social defeats in rats: relevance to human psychopathology. *Psychoneuroendocrinology* 34, 1405–1416. doi:10.1016/j.psyneuen.2009.04.018

Rodgers, R. J., and Johnson, N. J. (1998). Behaviorally selective effects of neuroactive steroids on plus-maze anxiety in mice. *Pharmacol. Biochem. Behav.* 59, 221–232. doi:10.1016/S0091-3057(97)00339-0

Rodríguez-Landa, J. F., Contreras, C. M., and García-Ríos, R. I. (2009). Allopregnanolone microinjected into the lateral septum or dorsal hippocampus reduces immobility in the forced swim test: participation of the GABAA receptor. *Behav. Pharmacol.* 20, 614–622. doi:10.1097/FBP.0b013e328331b9f2

Rogóz, Z., Skuza, G., Maj, J., and Danysz, W. (2002). Synergistic effect of uncompetitive NMDA receptor antagonists and antidepressant drugs in the forced swimming test in rats. *Neuropharmacology* 42, 1024–1030. doi:10.1016/S0028-3908(02)00055-2

Romeo, E., Ströhle, A., Spalletta, G., di Michele, F., Hermann, B., Holsboer, F., et al. (1998). Effects of antidepressant treatment on neuroactive steroids in major depression. *Am. J. Psychiatry* 155, 910–913.

Rygula, R., Abumaria, N., Flügge, G., Fuchs, E., Rüther, E., and Havemann-Reinecke, U. (2005). Anhedonia and motivational deficits in rats: impact of chronic social stress. *Behav. Brain Res.* 162, 127–134. doi:10.1016/j.bbr.2005.03.009

Schüle, C., Eser, D., Baghai, T. C., Nothdurfter, C., Kessler, J. S., and Rupprecht, R. (2011). Neuroactive steroids in affective disorders: target for novel antidepressant or anxiolytic drugs? *Neuroscience* 191, 55–77. doi:10.1016/j.neuroscience.2011.03.025

Schüle, C., Nothdurfter, C., and Rupprecht, R. (2014). The role of allopregnanolone in depression and anxiety. *Prog. Neurobiol.* 113, 79–87. doi:10.1016/j.pneurobio.2013.09.003

Sequeira-Cordero, A., Mora-Gallegos, A., Cuenca-Berger, P., and Fornaguera-Trías, J. (2013). Individual differences in the immobility behavior in juvenile and adult rats are associated with monoaminergic neurotransmission and with the expression of corticotropin-releasing factor receptor 1 in the nucleus accumbens. *Behav. Brain Res.* 252, 77–87. doi:10.1016/j.bbr.2013.05.046

Serra, M., Pisu, M. G., Littera, M., Papi, G., Sanna, E., Tuveri, F., et al. (2000). Social isolation-induced decreases in both the abundance of neuroactive steroids and GABA(A) receptor function in rat brain. *J. Neurochem.* 75, 732–740. doi:10.1046/j.1471-4159.2000.0750732.x

Sorwell, K. G., and Urbanski, H. F. (2010). Dehydroepiandrosterone and age-related cognitive decline. *Age (Dordr).* 32, 61–67. doi:10.1007/s11357-009-9113-4

Sulcova, A., and Krsiak, M. (1987). Differences among nine 1,4-benzodiazepines: an ethopharmacological evaluation in mice. *Psychopharmacology (Berl.)* 97, 157–159. doi:10.1007/BF00442240

Thase, M. E., Haight, B. R., Richard, N., Rockett, C. B., Mitton, M., and Modell, J. G. (2005). Remission rates following antidepressant therapy with bupropion or selective serotonin reuptake inhibitors: a meta-analysis of original data from 7 randomized controlled trials. *J. Clin. Psychiatry* 66, 974–981. doi:10.4088/JCP.v66n0803

Trullas, R., and Skolnick, P. (1990). Functional antagonists at the NMDA receptor complex exhibit antidepressant actions. *Eur. J. Pharmacol.* 185, 1–10. doi:10.1016/0014-2999(90)90204-J

Urani, A., Roman, F. J., Phan, V. L., Su, T. P., and Maurice, T. (2001). The antidepressant-like effect induced by sigma(1)-receptor agonists and neuroactive steroids in mice submitted to the forced swimming test. *J. Pharmacol. Exp. Ther.* 298, 1269–1279.

Uzunov, D. P., Cooper, T. B., Costa, E., and Guidotti, A. (1996). Fluoxetine-elicited changes in brain neurosteroid content measured by negative ion mass fragmentography. *Proc. Natl. Acad. Sci. U.S.A.* 93, 12599–12604. doi:10.1073/pnas.93.22.12599

Uzunova, V., Sheline, Y., Davis, J. M., Rasmusson, A., Uzunov, D. P., Costa, E., et al. (1998). Increase in the cerebrospinal fluid content of neurosteroids in patients with unipolar major depression who are receiving fluoxetine or fluvoxamine. *Proc. Natl. Acad. Sci. U.S.A.* 95, 3239–3244. doi:10.1073/pnas.95.6.3239

Vales, K., Rambousek, L., Holubova, K., Svoboda, J., Bubenikova-Valesova, V., Chodounska, H., et al. (2012). 3α5β-Pregnanolone glutamate, a use-dependent NMDA antagonist, reversed spatial learning deficit in an animal model of schizophrenia. *Behav. Brain Res.* 235, 82–88. doi:10.1016/j.bbr.2012.07.020

Vallée, M., Mayo, W., Darnaudéry, M., Corpéchot, C., Young, J., Koehl, M., et al. (1997). Neurosteroids: deficient cognitive performance in aged rats depends on low pregnenolone sulfate levels in the hippocampus. *Proc. Natl. Acad. Sci. U.S.A.* 94, 14865–14870. doi:10.1073/pnas.94.26.14865

van Bokhoven, P., Oomen, C. A., Hoogendijk, W. J., Smit, A. B., Lucassen, P. J., and Spijker, S. (2011). Reduction in hippocampal neurogenesis after social defeat is long-lasting and responsive to late antidepressant treatment. *Eur. J. Neurosci.* 33, 1833–1840. doi:10.1111/j.1460-9568.2011.07668.x

Veiga, S., Garcia-Segura, L. M., and Azcoitia, I. (2003). Neuroprotection by the steroids pregnenolone and dehydroepiandrosterone is mediated by the enzyme aromatase. *J. Neurobiol.* 56, 398–406. doi:10.1002/neu.10249

Venzala, E., García-García, A. L., Elizalde, N., Delagrange, P., and Tordera, R. M. (2012). Chronic social defeat stress model: behavioral features, antidepressant action, and interaction with biological risk factors. *Psychopharmacology (Berl.)* 224, 313–325. doi:10.1007/s00213-012-2754-5

Venzala, E., García-García, A. L., Elizalde, N., and Tordera, R. M. (2013). Social vs. environmental stress models of depression from a behavioural and neurochemical approach. *Eur. Neuropsychopharmacol.* 23, 697–708. doi:10.1016/j.euroneuro.2012.05.010

Weaver, C. E., Land, M. B., Purdy, R. H., Richards, K. G., Gibbs, T. T., and Farb, D. H. (2000). Geometry and charge determine pharmacological effects of steroids on N-methyl-D-aspartate receptor-induced Ca(2+) accumulation and cell death. *J. Pharmacol. Exp. Ther.* 293, 747–754.

Wolkowitz, O. M., Reus, V. I., Keebler, A., Nelson, N., Friedland, M., Brizendine, L., et al. (1999). Double-blind treatment of major depression with dehydroepiandrosterone. *Am. J. Psychiatry* 156, 646–649.

Wolkowitz, O. M., Reus, V. I., Roberts, E., Manfredi, F., Chan, T., Raum, W. J., et al. (1997). Dehydroepiandrosterone (DHEA) treatment of depression. *Biol. Psychiatry* 41, 311–318. doi:10.1016/S0006-3223(96)00043-1

Zarate, C. A. Jr., Brutsche, N. E., Ibrahim, L., Franco-Chaves, J., Diazgranados, N., Cravchik, A., et al. (2012). Replication of ketamine's antidepressant efficacy in bipolar depression: a randomized controlled add-on trial. *Biol. Psychiatry* 71, 939–946. doi:10.1016/j.biopsych.2011.12.010

Zarate, C. A. Jr., Singh, J. B., Carlson, P. J., Brutsche, N. E., Ameli, R., Luckenbaugh, D. A., et al. (2006). A randomized trial of an N-methyl-D-aspartate antagonist in treatment-resistant major depression. *Arch. Gen. Psychiatry* 63, 856–864. doi:10.1001/archpsyc.63.8.856

17

Common mechanisms of pain and depression: are antidepressants also analgesics?

Tereza Nekovarova[1,2], Anna Yamamotova[3]*, Karel Vales[1], Ales Stuchlik[1], Jitka Fricova[4] and Richard Rokyta[3]

[1] *Institute of Physiology, Academy of Sciences of the Czech Republic, Prague, Czech Republic*
[2] *Department of Zoology, Ecology and Ethology Research Group, Faculty of Natural Science, Charles University in Prague, Prague, Czech Republic*
[3] *Department of Normal, Pathological and Clinical Physiology, Third Faculty of Medicine, Charles University in Prague, Prague, Czech Republic*
[4] *Department of Anesthesiology and Intensive Care Medicine, Pain Management Center, First Faculty of Medicine and General University Hospital, Charles University in Prague, Prague, Czech Republic*

Edited by:
Tomiki Sumiyoshi, National Center of Neurology and Psychiatry, Japan

****Correspondence:***
Anna Yamamotova, Department of Normal, Pathological and Clinical Physiology, Third Faculty of Medicine, Charles University in Prague, Ke Karlovu 4, 120 00 Prague, Czech Republic
e-mail: yamamoto@lf3.cuni.cz

Neither pain, nor depression exist as independent phenomena *per se*, they are highly subjective inner states, formed by our brain and built on the bases of our experiences, cognition and emotions. Chronic pain is associated with changes in brain physiology and anatomy. It has been suggested that the neuronal activity underlying subjective perception of chronic pain may be divergent from the activity associated with acute pain. We will discuss the possible common pathophysiological mechanism of chronic pain and depression with respect to the default mode network of the brain, neuroplasticity and the effect of antidepressants on these two pathological conditions. The default mode network of the brain has an important role in the representation of introspective mental activities and therefore can be considered as a nodal point, common for both chronic pain and depression. Neuroplasticity which involves molecular, cellular and synaptic processes modifying connectivity between neurons and neuronal circuits can also be affected by pathological states such as chronic pain or depression. We suppose that pathogenesis of depression and chronic pain shares common negative neuroplastic changes in the central nervous system (CNS). The positive impact of antidepressants would result in a reduction of these pathological cellular/molecular processes and in the amelioration of symptoms, but it may also increase survival times and quality of life of patients with chronic cancer pain.

Keywords: chronic pain, depression, antidepressants, default mode network, neuroplasticity, stress, cytokines

INTRODUCTION

Chronic pain is a complex syndrome which affects thinking, mood and behavior, and it can gradually lead to complete psychological and social isolation of the patient; therefore it can have a significant impact on everyday human activities, limiting independence and significantly interfering with interpersonal relationships. Mechanisms underlying chronic pain are different from those of acute pain. Chronic pain could lead to permanent changes of brain structures and functions and these changes could affect also brain processes not directly connected with pain itself (Baliki et al., 2008).

Depression is a psychiatric disorder with various symptoms and is often accompanied by unexplained painful somatic symptoms. In patients with somatic symptoms, especially in primary care, depression is frequently overlooked. On the other hand, psychiatrists do not pay enough attention to somatic or pain symptoms in patients with depression. Depression can precede pain or pain can precede depression, forming a linked dyad sharing common mechanisms (Blackburn-Munro and Blackburn-Munro, 2001; Chou, 2007). As argued by Torta and Munari (2010), depression may reduce the pain threshold and sensitize pain perception. Conversely, chronic pain may lead to an altered emotional state and finally to depression.

The concept of pain has changed dramatically over the last 30 years. As knowledge and understanding of pain have increased, the concept has gradually morphed from a one-dimensional concept to a multi-dimensional concept. In 90th Melzack (1999, 2001) postulated the existence of a pain neuromatrix, which can be thought of as a genetically determined neural network that is significantly modulated by stress, affective and cognitive processes (Iannetti and Mouraux, 2010). The pain neuromatrix is an integration of sensory, interoceptive, affective, and cognitive components and the resulting experience of pain is always dependent on their interactions (Klossika et al., 2006; Wiech et al., 2008; Simons et al., 2014). Various studies particularly emphasize the relationship between pain and emotions (Rhudy, 2009; Kamping et al., 2013). In addition, pain is affected by endogenous opioids, and the endocrine, immune and autonomic systems (Blackburn-Munro and Blackburn-Munro, 2003; Chapman et al., 2008).

This network is constantly under the control of many other factors including the state of attention, anxiety, and expectation; previous experience, learning, personality traits, cultural effects, etc., play important roles. Therefore, we can rationally assume that neuroplastic and cognitive processes have critical roles as links to emotional processes associated with patient suffering.

We will summarize intersections between chronic pain and depression mechanisms at different levels of complexity, i.e., brain networks (default mode network), neurotransmitter systems and neuronal plasticity. We will demonstrate that both chronic pain and depression can lead to stable changes in brain structure and function and that these changes are manifested in the patient's experience, emotion and cognition. There is high comorbidity between chronic pain and depression in severe disorders and there is also a clear link between chronic pain and depression at the level of experience. Chronic pain can induce depression and depression can manifest as pain. In this study we suggest that the association between depression and chronic pain is not just at the level of experience, there may also be a common neural substrate, which could be therapeutically manipulated to improve overall quality of life for patients with both conditions.

DEFAULT MODE NETWORK AS A MECHANISM OF SELF-REFERENCE, NODAL POINT OF DEPRESSION AND CHRONIC PAIN

Neither pain, nor depression exists as an independent phenomenon *per se*; they are highly subjective inner states, created by our brain and formed by our experience, cognition and emotional arousal. The default mode network is a network of interacting brain regions and subsystems that show consistently greater activation during "resting" states compared to external, directed tasks (often referred as "task-induced deactivation") (Shulman et al., 1997). The brain regions involved in these self-referential processes are inversely correlated with the fronto-parietal regions that are typically associated with cognition (Fox et al., 2005).

The default mode network consists of a set of regions in the cerebral cortex—medial prefrontal cortex, posterior cingulate cortex and connected ventral precuneus, medial temporal lobes, and the superior frontal and parietal cortices. The default mode network has an important role in the representation of a person's mental state and "internal mentation", i.e., the introspective mental activities spontaneously emanated by the human brain (Andrews-Hanna, 2012). Such "self-referential thoughts" are necessary to perceive the inner bodily or mental states—including pain and depression.

Self-referential processes have been repeatedly shown to be abnormal, and self-focus is increased in people suffering from depression (Lemogne et al., 2012). Moreover, it has been shown that increased self-focus in depressed individuals may be a predictor of major depressive episodes and chronic depression (Nolen-Hoeksema, 2000). Grimm and her colleagues demonstrated that abnormally increased negative self-attribution, as a hallmark of increased self-focus in major depressive disorders, might be mediated by abnormal neural activity in subcortical-cortical midline structures linked to the default mode network (Grimm et al., 2009, 2011).

There is increasing evidence that the default mode network has a pivotal role in neuronal activity underlying major depressive disorders (Greicius et al., 2007; Xueling et al., 2012; Zhu et al., 2012; Guo et al., 2013; Wenbin et al., 2013) and also in late-life depression (Alexopoulos et al., 2012; Andreescu et al., 2013) and therefore it could serve as a potential biomarker of depressive disorders. Considering the very high relapse rates of patients after a major depressive episode, Li et al. (2013) hypothesized that abnormal default mode network connectivity might persist even after recovery. They have suggested that default mode network functionally dissociates into two subsystems—connectivity in the posterior sub-network is normalized after antidepressant treatment, whereas there was persistent abnormal connectivity in the anterior sub-network.

The above mentioned observations are in accordance with the findings of Marchetti et al. (2012) who propose specific imbalances in the default mode system which could represent a residual neural "depressive scar" that was affected by the severity of previous depressive episodes; it was also suggested that it could be used as a predictor of future depressive episodes.

Chronic pain is associated with changes in brain physiology and anatomy. It has been suggested that neuronal activity underlying subjective perception of chronic pain may be divergent from the activity associated with acute pain. Some studies have indicated that chronic pain can also affect cortical areas unrelated to pain (Apkarian, 2008; Cauda et al., 2012; Hashmi et al., 2013).

Prolonged experience with chronic pain represents a form of emotional learning, shifting from sensory to hedonic neuronal circuits (Farmer et al., 2012). Chronic pain is often accompanied by cognitive and behavioral impairment and decreased quality of life. Increased anxiety, depression and sleep disruption are manifested as an affective association of chronic pain. Moreover, clinicians often observe that these additional effects deepen the patient's suffering and the effects persist even after the pain is reduced by therapy and the source of nociceptive activity has disappeared (Mansour et al., 2013).

Various studies emphasize the complexity of chronic-pain processes that affect large circuits and stimulate extensive reorganization of cortical function and structure (Apkarian et al., 2009; Apkarian, 2011).

Some authors propose that the structural impairments that accompany chronic pain can also influence functions of the default mode network. Baliki and his colleagues demonstrated that patients suffering from chronic back pain displayed reduced deactivation of various default mode network regions during a simple visual attention task, even though the performance of the patient group and control were the same (Baliki et al., 2008). Similar results were obtained in studies by Tagliazucchi et al. (2010). It is important to point out that these studies demonstrated that alterations of the default mode system, in chronic-pain patients, might influence brain mechanisms responsible for processing information unrelated to pain.

Napadow et al. (2010) demonstrated alternating levels of intrinsic connectivity within multiple brain networks in fibromyalgia, which is a central chronic pain syndrome associated with widespread and spontaneously fluctuating pain. This study showed greater connectivity in the default mode network and in the right executive attention network (in contrast to the default mode network, in which the fronto-parietal executive attention network is involved in cognitive processing associated with working memory and attention). It suggests that fibromyalgia pain might be mediated by alternating activity levels in the central nervous system (CNS) (hyperexcitability) more than by peripheral pathological sensations.

A study by Loggia et al. (2013) revealed that greater clinical pain in patients with chronic low back pain at baseline was associated with greater connectivity between the default mode network and insula (brain region involved in pain processing) and decreased connectivity between the default mode system and the pregenual anterior cingulate cortex (involved in brain inhibition). Moreover, baseline pain correlates positively with the level of connectivity between the default mode network and the right insula; while increased clinical pain, induced by physical maneuvers, is correlated with changes in this connectivity. These results suggest that resting default mode connectivity may also encode the severity of clinical pain.

More and more evidence indicates that chronic pain can, at some point, become a sensation that is spontaneous and independent on any external stimuli. Therefore, the default-mode-network perspective could offer fresh insights into the study of chronic pain. Moreover, since the default mode network is deeply involved in self-referential processes and subjective experience, it could represent a nodal point that is common for both chronic pain and depression.

NEUROPLASTICITY

Neuroplasticity involves molecular, cellular and synaptic processes that modify connectivity between neurons and neuronal circuits. They are modulated by behavioral, sensory, cognitive and emotional experience, and are also influenced by pathological states and chronic pain or depression. It is important to stress that transient, but repetitive functional changes induced by pain or depression can lead to more permanent changes. Accordingly, long-lasting interference with the normal activity of the default mode network could initiate plastic changes that could lead to irreversible structural and functional changes of the default mode network.

Patients suffering from serious disorders are under chronic stress, associated with a loss or change in social status, loss of positive expectations, feelings of discomfort, etc. This emotional situation induces a spiral of complaints and stresses mediated by neuronal changes which in turn can lead to alterations in other brain functions and structure. Stress is a common biological denominator connecting patient suffering on the one hand, and emotion, cognition and neuroplastic substrates on the other hand. Stress profoundly affects synaptic form and function (Popoli et al., 2011; Sandi, 2011). Stress is also a well-accepted etiological factor in depression.

Stress induces the release of glucocorticoids (GC) that significantly impact hippocampal functions with the potential to enhance or suppress neuroplastic processes. Stress gives rise, by means of the limbic system and activation of the reticular formation, to increased production of corticotropin-releasing hormone (CRH). A feedback loop from the periphery is maintained by the inhibitory effects of GC on CRH production. This feedback involves several types of glucocorticoid receptors, located mostly inside the hippocampus. Overproduction of CRH leads to overproduction of ACTH and, later on, to overproduction of GC. Such a situation occurs after a hippocampal lesion or during chronic stress. Stress also leads to a reduction in brain derived neurotrophic factor (BDNF)—one of the most predominant neurotrophic factors in the adult brain—in the hippocampus and increases it in the amygdala (Höschl and Hajek, 2001; Finsterwald and Alberini, 2013; Hayley and Litteljohn, 2013). While there is strong evidence linking BDNF to stress and depression, other neuronal growth factors are also involved, most notably glial cell-line derived neurotrophic factor (GDNF) and nerve growth factor (NGF; Hayley and Litteljohn, 2013).

Stress modulation of synaptic plasticity is mediated via activation of mineralocorticoids and GC receptors and exert direct effects on neurons and glia cells and also increase glutamate release in the prefrontal cortex, hippocampus and amygdala (Sandi, 2011). It has been shown that elevated levels of corticoids influence learning processes (Bodnoff et al., 1995). Stress events also disrupt long term potentiation in the hippocampus (Shors et al., 1997), which is a key structure for declarative memory (Hölscher, 1999). Pre-clinical and clinical studies have demonstrated that stress and depression can lead to reductions in the total volume of the adult hippocampus. These structural changes may not necessarily be permanent. The degree of volume reduction can provide information regarding treatment effectiveness or response to treatment (Arnone et al., 2013; Hayley and Litteljohn, 2013).

Repeated stress also produces alterations in brain plasticity in animal models; however, the relevance of hippocampal changes to behavioral changes is still matter of debate. For example, the granule cells of the dentate gyrus are significantly affected via a decreased rate of neurogenesis following prolonged stress (Radley and Morrison, 2005). In contrast, chronic antidepressant treatment up-regulates hippocampal neurogenesis, and therefore could block or reverse the atrophy and damage caused by stress. Some studies have also demonstrated that neurogenesis is required for the actions of antidepressants in behavioral models of depression (Warner-Schmidt and Duman, 2006).

The hippocampus is a target for the effects of GCs and stress, which in turn, could influence its ability to regulate the HPA axis. Chronic GC administration at artificially high levels induces apical dendritic retraction and debranching in rat CA3c pyramidal neurons (Woolley et al., 1990; Watanabe et al., 1992), while longer exposure to GC results in more substantial hippocampal damage, such as neuron death, gliosis, and atrophied perikarya in the principal layers, most notably in the CA3c region (Sapolsky, 1985). Repeated stress exerts effects similar to GCs on dendritic remodeling in the CA3. One key feature of prolonged stress is the change in dendritic spine number and morphology of hippocampal formation (medial prefrontal cortex). Such structural synaptic changes may be compensatory in response to glutamatergic and calcium-induced toxicity in these neurons during prolonged periods of stress. Since repeated stress also induces apical dendritic retraction in the CA3, this could have significant consequences for the total synaptic population. In contrast, antidepressants oppose dendrite atrophy and increase apoptosis markers induced by stress in the hippocampus (Silva et al., 2008).

Corticoids affect various neurotransmission systems. They potentiate efflux and inhibit re-uptake of glutamate and increase N-methyl-D-aspartate (NMDA) receptor expression.

Furthermore, they decrease expression of neurotrophic factors (Smith et al., 1995) and decrease activity of the GABA-ergic system. Glutamate influenced activity of NMDA receptors and the concomitant decrease in GABA-ergic inhibition leads to calcium influx, followed by depolymerization of cytoskeletal proteins, autolysis and eventually neuronal death (Höschl and Hajek, 2001).

With regard to stress induced structural and functional changes in the hippocampus, in particular reduced hippocampal volume, recent studies have indicated reductions in neurogenesis as well as changes in glial density and reductions in the complexity of dendritic arbors that participate in the volumetric decrease (Hayley and Litteljohn, 2013). Alterations in neurobiological properties can result in faulty communication between the hippocampus, amygdala and cortex, which gives rise to disturbed processes of emotionality (Carballedo et al., 2011). However, future studies are needed to assess the potential contribution of volumetric changes in default mode.

The negative effects of stress on hippocampal synaptic plasticity can be reversed by GC antagonists and monoamine antidepressants (Holderbach et al., 2007). Chronic stress can also affect the expression of AMPA and NMDA subunits and various synaptic proteins (Silva et al., 2008), while antidepressant treatment opposes these changes (Martínez-Turrillas et al., 2007; Barbon et al., 2011). Chronic stress promotes pyramidal dendrite retraction in the medial prefrontal cortex by the mechanism of NMDA receptors (Martin and Wellman, 2011). Additionally, tianeptine, an selective serotonin reuptake inhibitor (SSRI) drug with unexplained antidepressive effects, modulates NMDA receptor function in the hippocampus (Kole et al., 2002). Similarly, some studies point to the antidepressive effects of NMDA antagonists (Berman et al., 2000; Zarate et al., 2006; Li et al., 2010). In addition, monoamine systems that represent typical targets for antidepressants are also required for plasticity modulation under stress.

While an obvious logical link between synaptic plasticity and cognition exists, less well understood is the potential for altered synaptic plasticity to disrupt emotional memory, which may be relevant regarding mood disorders. Regardless, the prefrontal cortex-hippocampus-amygdala circuits are likely dysfunctional in depression (Marsden, 2013). It has been suggested that this leads to decreased cognitive control of emotion, resulting in persistent negative emotional reactivity (Murrough et al., 2011).

Stress-induced neurobiological cascades could represent a critical common pathway underlying the biological and psychological characteristics of the default mode of patients suffering from serious disorders. The neuroplasticity hypothesis of depression shows decreased synaptic plasticity in hippocampal circuits and elevated synaptic plasticity in emotional networks including the amygdala (Nissen et al., 2010). Moreover, reduced hippocampal volume may correlate with impairment of cognitive functions in patients with a major depressive disorder (Frodl et al., 2006). There is a huge body of evidence demonstrating the neuropsychological and cognitive deficits associated with depressive disorders. Such deficits have been found in various areas including attention, information processing, memory, verbal fluency, executive functions and psychomotor speed (for review see Austin et al., 2001; Castaneda et al., 2008; Lee et al., 2012).

Although the clinically beneficial effects of antidepressants are well known their direct impact on cognitive (intellectual and psychomotor) functions in less understood. The clinical effects of antidepressants on cognitive functions, both in healthy volunteers and in patients, were reviewed in papers by Amado-Boccara et al. (1995) and Gorenstein et al. (2006). In 2008, Monleon et al. extensively reviewed the effect of antidepressants on memory in animal models. When assessing the cognitive effect of antidepressants in subjects suffering from depression, it is, in theory, necessary to separate the specific effects on cognition from overall clinical improvement. Another methodological difficulty may be discrepancies between subjective assessments of one's own state and results from neuropsychological testing (Amado-Boccara et al., 1995).

Monleón et al. (2008) proposed that memory traces should be understood not only as an individual experiences, but also as genetic and epigenetic phenomena. From this point of view, each neural system has its own memory and antidepressants can affect each of these systems. Antidepressants may promote new memories (new neuronal patterns) at the same time that they impair older ones (Monleón et al., 2008).

Strong arguments for the role of antidepressants in promotion of new "memory" traces, through neurogenesis, suggest the role of neurotrophic factors in the etiology of depression and its treatment. Both acute and chronic stress decrease levels of BDNF expression in the hippocampus and conversely, chronic (but not acute) administration of most classes of antidepressants increase BDNF expression in the hippocampus (Nestler et al., 2002).

The pathophysiology of major depressive disorders could also involve GDNF, which plays a role in the development and function of hippocampal cells. GDNF is a neurotrophic factor in the transforming growth factor-b-family (Michel et al., 2008; Wang et al., 2011).

Increasing numbers of studies have demonstrated the significant role of neurotrophic factors in the transmission of both of physiologic and pathologic pain. Neurotrophins (including BDNF and NGF) can act as a pathogenic pain mediator and are known to be increased in several painful conditions. When administered, they lead to pronounced mechanical and thermal hyperalgesia (Obata and Noguchi, 2006; Siniscalco et al., 2011). BDNF is part of synaptic plasticity and central sensitization in a spinal cord. It contributes to the development and continuation of neuropathic pain by activation of NMDA receptors (NR2B-containing NMDA) in the dorsal horn (Geng et al., 2010). Melemedjian et al. (2013) emphasized the role of protein kinases as essential mediators of the maintenance of a centralized chronic pain state. Molecular mechanisms of chronic pain, as with neuronal changes in depressive states, parallel memory engram encoding in the CNS.

However, the above mentioned role of BDNF in depression and chronic pain is even more complicated by the fact that BDNF may have antidepressive or pro-depressive functions, depending on the brain area and circuits (Racagni and Popoli, 2008). Berton et al. (2006) have shown that infusion of BDNF into the nucleus accumbens exerts a pro-depressive-like effect in rodent stress models and blockade of BDNF function in the nucleus accumbens exerts antidepressant-like effects.

A more integrated approach to chronic pain and depression could facilitate a more efficient therapy. For example the animal model of antidepressant activity supports the hypothesis that impaired cognition is an element of depression and treatment with drugs enhancing cognitive performance can help alleviate depression (Knapp et al., 2002). Therapeutic strategies focused on modulation of synaptic plasticity and biological pathways common for stress and pain might prove useful for developing novel treatments for those suffering from cancer pain and associated diseases such as depression.

Emotional distress is significantly higher in patients with chronic pain. Pain and depression, especially associated with tumors, can lead to serious mental and physical stress in patients (Rokyta et al., 2009). Pain is conceptualized as chronic stress and coping strategies play an important role in those experiencing cancer pain. Poor coping strategies may lead to a worsening of pain which will lead to an increase in depression. A recent study, among patients with metastatic breast cancer, found that both pain and obsessing over pain exacerbated depression (Badr and Shen, 2014). On the other hand, patients with lung cancer using a repressive coping style (an effort to inhibit negative feelings through an overly positive view of life) reported lower pain intensity and lower levels of depression (Prasertsri et al., 2011). In the short-term point, this technique may represent a convenient strategy, but for the long-term, repressive coping is not an efficient mood-regulation strategy since it can intensify anxiety dysfunction (Geraerts et al., 2012).

Pain suffering is closely related to psycho-neuro-immunological changes (Rittner et al., 2008); treatment with antidepressants has been shown to normalize immune parameters (Neveu and Castanon, 1999; Rokyta et al., 2009). This integrated treatment could also help increase the patient's overall quality of life, going beyond the specific clinical target.

COMMON NEUROBIOLOGICAL MECHANISMS OF PAIN AND DEPRESSION

Pro-inflammatory cytokines such as IL-6, IL-1β and TNF-α may directly modulate neuronal activity in the peripheral and CNS (Ozaktay et al., 2006). Proinflammatory cytokines modulate hippocampal neurogenesis and therefore they can affect the mood. An increased production of proinflammatory cytokines has repeatedly been described in depressive patients (Maes et al., 1997; Connor and Leonard, 1998; Müller, 2013; Bai et al., 2014). Cytokines such as IL-1β, TNF-α and IFN-γ seem to contribute to the pathophysiology of depression by stimulating the hypothalamic-pituitary-adrenocortical axis (Rosenblat et al., 2014), thus activating monoamine reuptake (Raison et al., 2009), and decreasing production of serotonin through increased activity of indoleamine-2,3-dioxygenase (IDO; Müller and Schwarz, 2007).

A meta-analysis performed on patients meeting the DSM criteria for major depression has shown higher concentrations of the proinflammatory cytokines TNF-α and IL-6 in depressed subjects compared to control subjects (Dowlati et al., 2010). Similar associations between depression and C-reactive protein (CRP), IL-6, and, to a lesser extent, IL-1 have been found in patients with cardiac disease or cancer (Howren et al., 2009). A recent study by Breitbart et al. (2014) demonstrated an association between depression and IL-6, but not with other cytokines, in patients with pancreatic cancer. Moreover, IL-6 was not significantly associated with other measures of psychological distress (anxiety and hopelessness) or with symptoms of distress (pain, fatigue, and sleep quality).

Evidence supports the possibility that peripheral inflammatory responses manifest themselves in the CNS in a process known as neuro-inflammation. Therefore the treatment of depression with anti-inflammatory drugs looks like a promising way of targeting more mechanisms. Two individual studies (Müller et al., 2006; Nery et al., 2008) and one meta-analysis (Na et al., 2014) have shown that adjunctive celecoxib combined with antidepressants produced a rapid-onset antidepressant effect and was more effective than placebo combined with antidepressants.

In the pathophysiology of pain, cytokines cause hyperalgesia, reduce the pain threshold, sensitize afferent nociceptive neurons and increase the frequency of discharges in nociceptive A-delta and C fibers. All these factors contribute to central sensitization, which is manifested by secondary hyperalgesia and/or allodynia (Zhang and An, 2007).

In inflammatory pain, IL-1β increases the cyclooxygenase-2 (COX-2) dependent production of prostaglandin E_2 (PGE_2), calcitonin gene-related peptide (CGRP; Samad et al., 2001; Neeb et al., 2011) and substance P (Jeanjean et al., 1995), all are factors that induce hypersensitivity. On the other hand, experimental results demonstrate that the neuropeptides substance P and CGRP induce nociceptive sensitization by enhancing IL-1β production in keratinocytes (Shi et al., 2011; Wei et al., 2012).

Celecoxib was the first COX inhibitor with well-defined COX-2 specificity (Tindall, 1999). In animal studies it has been shown that inhibition of spinal COX-2 not only reduces prostaglandin production but also endocannabinoid breakdown (Telleria-Diaz et al., 2010) and expression of purinergic $P2X_3$ receptors in the dorsal root ganglia (Wang et al., 2010). These results provide evidence that the pain suppressive effects of COX-2 inhibitors may be mediated either by the endocannabinoid system or by down-regulation of receptors for ATP or both.

Neurotransmitter systems that are used to control pain overlap with those which are considered to be the main pathophysiological mechanisms in depressive disorders, i.e., serotonergic, noradrenergic, and glutamatergic systems.

It has been repeatedly demonstrated, in depressive patients, that there are decreased levels of serotonin metabolites in the cerebrospinal fluid, particularly in patients after suicide attempts (Asberg et al., 1976; Jokinen et al., 2009; Chatzittofis et al., 2013). Tryptophan depletion (a method of lowering brain serotonin, used as a model of depressive disorders) not only worsens depressive symptoms (Fields et al., 1991; Booij et al., 2005; van Steenbergen et al., 2012) and also can increase the sensation of pain (Schwarz et al., 2003; Supornsilpchai et al., 2006; Wei et al., 2010). The system of antinociception operates primarily through serotonin 5-HT1A and 5-HT2 receptors; the stimulation of 5-HT3 receptors, which are found in the periphery, has pronociceptive effects (Campbell et al., 2003).

However, conflicting results follow from both experimental and clinical observations after identical intravenous routes of application of similar doses of 5-HT3 antagonists. While tropisetron, studied in a human model of acute pain induced by intracutaneous electrical stimulation, led to significant analgesic effects (Bandschapp et al., 2011); ondansetron was ineffective in suppression of mechanical allodynia and spontaneous ongoing pain in peripheral neuropathy (Scott et al., 2006; Tuveson et al., 2011).

The SSRI, fluoxetine, which is widely used in the treatment of depression, also has anti-inflammatory properties. Experimental data have shown that fluoxetine inhibits lipopolysaccharide-induced release of nitric oxide (NO) and PGE_2 in murine serum (Su et al., 2012) and NO and PGE_2 production by connective tissue cells (Yaron et al., 1999).

Although SSRIs are less potent for treatment of chronic pain, paroxetine, due to its inhibitory effect on $P2X_4$ receptors, was found to be effective in suppressing tactile allodynia in a neuropathic pain model in rats (Nagata et al., 2009).

Dysfunction of the noradrenergic system is another pathophysiological characteristic of depression. Noradrenaline levels are decreased, especially in patients who react positively to treatment with noradrenaline reuptake inhibitors (Booij et al., 2003). Conversely, depletion of noradrenaline can cause a relapse of the disease (Delgado and Moreno, 2000; Ruhé et al., 2007). In connection with pain, the mechanism proposed for the analgesic effect of antidepressants is the strengthening of descending serotonergic and noradrenergic systems of antinociception by inhibiting the re-uptake of serotonin and noradrenalin and increasing their availability in the spinal cord. Many experimental and clinical studies with clonidine or medetomidine have demonstrated that the antinociceptive effects of noradrenaline are mediated by α2–adrenoceptors (Kawasaki et al., 2003; Grosu and Lavand'homme, 2010; Blaudszun et al., 2012).

The effect of some antidepressants, especially in neuropathic pain, can also be mediated via the opioidergic system, however, the opioid system appears to be involved in the mechanism of action of antidepressants that only have anti-hyperalgesic action (clomipramine and milnacipran), but not in those with stronger antinociceptive effects such as duloxetine (Wattiez et al., 2011). In a recent study by Bohren et al. (2013), a novel mechanism of antidepressant action was described. They demonstrated that the peripheral nervous system was essential for the anti-allodynic effects of nortriptyline in animal models of neuropathic pain, and acted peripheral β2-adrenoceptors and local inhibition of TNFα production.

Beside these neurotransmitters, substance P is another molecule which participates in the modulation of pain. Substance P is a mediator of C fibers and contributes to central sensitization, depending on the activity of the noradrenergic system. If noradrenergic neuronal activity or the levels of noradrenaline decrease, the increased release of substance P is expressed as hyperalgesia (Jasmin et al., 2002). Depressed patients also had elevated levels of substance P and its level correlated with the severity of clinical symptoms (Bondy et al., 2003).

The dopaminergic system, in terms of pain, has received much less attention, although stimulants like amphetamine or methamphetamine are highly effective analgesics (Yamamotová et al., 2011; Yamamotová and Šlamberová, 2012). Pain is modulated by D2 receptors, particularly within the mesolimbic dopaminergic system and the nucleus accumbens, hence in the "reward system" of the brain (Franklin, 1998; Altier and Stewart, 1999; Wood, 2006).

Both in chronic pain and depression hyperalgesia can results from central sensitization as a consequence of plastic changes in the nervous system. Activation of glutamate NMDA receptors is an essential step in both initiating and maintaining central sensitization, also called the "wind-up" phenomenon (Latremoliere and Woolf, 2009). A study by Klauenberg et al. (2008) demonstrated, for the first time, a considerably enhanced wind-up ratio in depressive patients that was independent of ongoing pain. Wind-up is a physiological process in the spinal cord mainly caused by temporal summation of C-fiber evoked responses that generate a progressive increase in activity of second-order neurons. Consequently, wind-up is increased in some processes with enhanced spinal cord excitability. Ketamine, the non-competitive NMDA receptor antagonist, prevents the wind-up phenomenon and suppresses not only pain but also depression. It acts rapidly and is effective for treatment-resistant patients (Dowben et al., 2013). A recent study showed that a single intravenous dose of ketamine improved depression in 64% of patients within 24 h of administration (Murrough et al., 2013). However, evaluation of antidepressant response showed that not all patients respond to ketamine treatment and that the duration of the antidepressant effect varies across studies (Browne and Lucki, 2013; Sos et al., 2013; Gálvez et al., 2014).

Although the precise mechanisms underlying its antidepressant effects are not fully known, acute administration of ketamine increases BDNF levels in the rat hippocampus. The increase of hippocampal BDNF levels induced by ketamine might also be necessary to produce a rapid onset of antidepressant action in rats (Hayley and Litteljohn, 2013). It should be noted that ketamine also induces rapid and potent anti-inflammatory effects that can be relevant to its antidepressant potential (Hayley and Litteljohn, 2013).

ARE ANTIDEPRESSANTS MORE THAN ADJUVANT ANALGESICS?

A number of studies have demonstrated frequent co-occurrences of depression and pain, as well as their additive effects in several domains of quality of life in oncological patients (Kroenke et al., 2010). However, the question remains: How do antidepressants affect chronic pain and what is the mechanism of action? Over the last few years we have performed two pilot studies concerning the efficacy of antidepressant treatment in patients with chronic cancer pain and non-cancer pain (Rokyta et al., 2009). Antidepressants were indicated in both groups of patients either for psychiatric comorbidity (depression) and/or neuropathic pain. None of the patients had been treated with antidepressants before entering the study.

The investigation started with 40 patients; 20 non-oncological patients and 20 oncological patients. The most frequent diagnosis

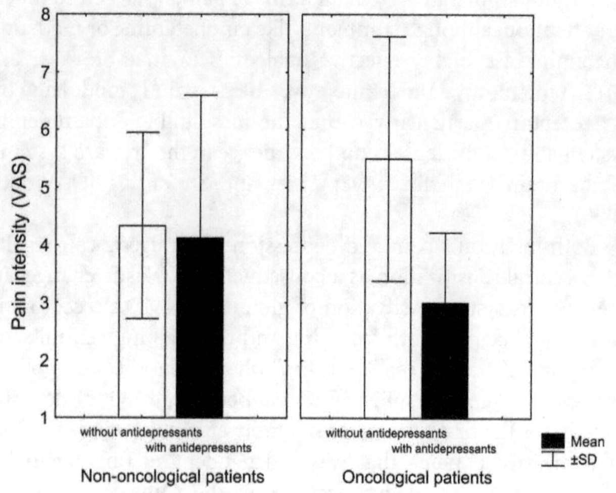

FIGURE 1 | Pain intensity (visual analogue scale) at the end of treatment of patients with chronic nonmalignant and malignant pain treated with antidepressants (black columns) and patients treated without antidepressants (white columns). Antidepressants marginally reduced pain in cancer patients Kruskal-Wallis non-parametric test ($KW\text{-}H_{(1,11)} = 2.9$, $p = 0.08$; *KW-H*: Kruskal-Wallis non-parametric test) (Adopted from Rokyta et al., 2009).

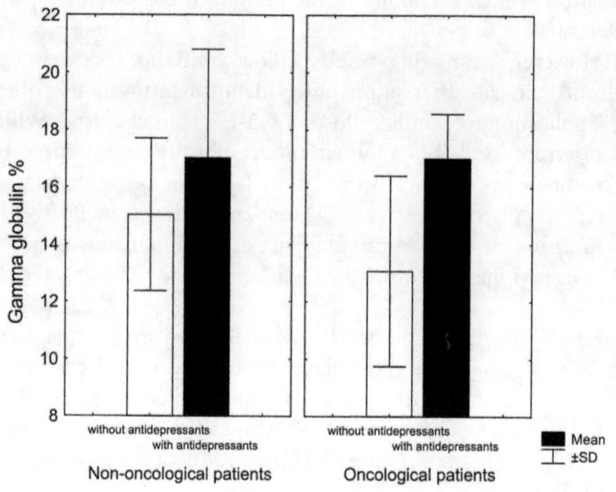

FIGURE 2 | Gamma globulin levels in patients with chronic nonmalignant and malignant pain associated with antidepressant treatment. In both groups, patients treated with antidepressants had higher levels of gamma globulin: in non-oncological patients only marginally ($KW\text{-}H_{(1,20)} = 2.7$, $p = 0.09$), in oncological patients significantly higher ($KW\text{-}H_{(1,18)} = 7.0$, $p = 0.008$) (Adopted from Rokyta et al., 2009).

in the non-oncological group was low back pain and failed back surgery syndrome. Oncological patients were diagnosed as follows: breast carcinoma, carcinoma of the prostate gland, urinary bladder and kidneys, orofacial cavity and larynx, uterus, gastrointestinal tract and pancreas, lung cancer and leukemia.

Therapy for both groups of patients consisted, most often, of administration of non-steroidal anti-inflammatory drugs and tramadol. As necessary, the above mentioned drugs were used in combination with: opioids, anti-epileptics, antidepressants (fluoxetine and tricyclic antidepressants).

Although there was no difference in the intensity of pain in non-oncological patients with respect to adjuvant therapy with antidepressants, the surviving oncological patients that used antidepressants reported lower pain intensity than oncological patients not taking antidepressants (**Figure 1**). Despite the small number of patients, it is interesting that out of 10 patients treated with antidepressants, survived seven, while out of 10 patients not treated with antidepressants, only three patients survived. However, further research with homogeneous diagnostic groups is needed to establish and confirm the observed relationships.

Another our finding was that chronic pain patients taking antidepressants had, regardless of diagnosis, higher levels of gamma globulin compared to patients not treated with antidepressants (Rokyta et al., 2009; **Figure 2**). A similar observation was described by Van Hunsel et al. (1996) who followed patients with depression and found, as we did, that depressive patients have low levels of gamma globulin, which rose significantly, after antidepressant treatment. The fact that immune and endocrine systems are closely related in patients with cancer even at the time when patients were informed about their diagnosis was confirmed by a negative correlation between cortisol and CD4 lymphocytes and a positive correlation between cortisol and CD3 lymphocytes. Moreover, patients with a malignant diagnosis had lower cortisol level than patients with a benign diagnosis (Křikava et al., 2007).

Some research observations indicate that depressed patients treated with antidepressants undergo a normalization of immune parameters (Neveu and Castanon, 1999). Normalization of serum cortisol was shown in patients with severe chronic pain treated with opioids (Tenant and Hermann, 2002). From these clinical studies, it is not possible to conclude whether antidepressants and/or opioids have a direct effect on the immune and endocrine system or whether their supposed effects resulted from improved mood.

Opioid peptides are found in many leukocyte subpopulations including lymphocytes, monocytes, and granulocytes circulating in the peripheral blood. Neurokinin substance P is one of many factors that influence migration of opioid-containing leukocytes. NK1 receptor antagonists seem to act peripherally by directly inhibiting the recruitment of opioid containing leukocytes to sites of inflammation (Rittner et al., 2008). Although opioids are frequently used for the treatment of severe pain in patients with cancer, chronic morphine treatment can also have serious negative effects on tumor growth. Morphine stimulates angiogenesis-dependent tumor growth via stimulation of endothelial NO and COX-2 production (Gupta et al., 2002). Administration of celecoxib together with morphine in murine breast cancer model not only prevented promotion of angiogenesis, tumor growth, metastasis and mortality but also led to better analgesia than with morphine or celecoxib alone (Farooqui et al., 2007). Similar potential therapeutic effects were observed for lumiracoxib by Fox et al. (2004) in a model of bone cancer pain in rats, which were attributed to its anti-hyperalgesic activity.

Other antidepressants have also been studied in animal models of cancer. For example, Fang et al. (2012) found that *in vivo* chronic mirtazapine treatment inhibited tumor growth and prolonged the survival of colon carcinoma-bearing mice. The IFN-γ levels in tumors of mice treated with mirtazapine were significantly higher, while TNF-α expression was lower than in untreated mice.

On the other hand, antidepressant pretreatment with desipramine or fluoxetine increased metastasis formation in mice with melanoma, shortened survival, decreased splenocyte anti-tumor natural killer cell cytotoxicity (*in vitro*), and IFN-γ production (Kubera et al., 2011).

One question arising from our study concerns whether the higher mortality seen in the tumor pain patients without antidepressants was a coincidence or whether it suggested some protective function associated with antidepressants. Meta-analyses from human and animal studies have concluded that several antidepressants have a significant positive association with cancer protection, while others have shown a negative association; the effect seems to be dependent on the type of cancer and the type of antidepressant (Steingart and Cotterchio, 1995; Lussier et al., 2004; Walker et al., 2011, 2012; Bielecka and Obuchowicz, 2013; Jahchan et al., 2013).

Knowledge regarding the role of antidepressants in cancer progression or suppression is essential for choosing the proper treatment and clinicians who wish to use antidepressants in cancer treatment need to take into consideration the type of antidepressant, type of tumor, type of anticancer therapy, as well as the patient's age, phase of cancer and others factors (Bielecka and Obuchowicz, 2013).

It is not possible to unambiguously declare that only one source of the depressive state in oncological patient has a direct relation between depression and pain. There are many different aspects to oncological diseases and their treatment. Depressive states may be caused not only by pain, but also by decreased quality of life, worsening of cognitive functions (Baudino et al., 2012), difficulties accompanying oncological treatment such as gastrointestinal distress and fatigue, and poor life perspectives.

However, we assume that both depression and pain, even though they are experienced in highly subjective ways, are deeply grounded in the neuronal and physiological substrate and therefore can, even if only indirectly, interact on this basis. Chronic pain may alter different systems, including the emotional state and gradually lead to depression, conversely depression affected cognition and perception and may lead to pain sensitization (Torta and Munari, 2010).

CONCLUSION

Our working hypothesis supposes that depression and chronic pain produce common negative neuroplastic changes in the CNS. The positive impact of antidepressants would result in a reduction of these pathological cellular/molecular processes and in the amelioration of symptoms, but it may also increase survival times and quality of life of patients with chronic cancer pain. The benefits go beyond prolongation of lifespan because they are also linked to an improvement in the quality of life of treated patients. These effects represent the most important aspects of antidepressant treatment. After careful validation of both experimental and clinical results, this approach could be ready for clinical practice in a relatively short time, especially in oncology, algesiology and psychiatry.

AUTHOR CONTRIBUTIONS

Richard Rokyta, Karel Vales, Anna Yamamotova and Tereza Nekovarova made substantial contributions to the conception of the paper and are co-responsible for formulation of the hypothesis. Karel Vales contributed mainly to the part of the manuscript concerning neuroplasticity, Anna Yamamotova, Richard Rokyta and Jitka Fricova contributed mainly to the part of the manuscript concerning neurobiological substrate of pain and depression and to the part concerning mechanisms of antidepressants. Tereza Nekovarova contributed mainly to the part focusing on default mode network. Ales Stuchlik critically reviewed the manuscript.

ACKNOWLEDGMENTS

This work was supported by institutional support RVO: 67985823, Project Prvouk P34, project CSM7/CRP/2014, grants IGA MZ CR NT/1448, NT13386, NT13403-4/2012, GACR P304/12/G069 and P303/12/1464 and by AV CR M200111204.

REFERENCES

Alexopoulos, G. S., Hoptman, M. J., Kanellopoulos, D., Murphy, C. F., Lim, K. O., and Gunning, F. M. (2012). Functional connectivity in the cognitive control network and the default mode network in late-life depression. *J. Affect. Disord.* 139, 56–65. doi: 10.1016/j.jad.2011.12.002

Altier, N., and Stewart, J. (1999). The role of dopamine in the nucleus accumbens in analgesia. *Life Sci.* 65, 2269–2287. doi: 10.1016/s0024-3205(99)00298-2

Amado-Boccara, I., Gougoulis, N., Poirier Littré, M. F., Galinowski, A., and Lôo, H. (1995). Effects of antidepressants on cognitive functions: a review. *Neurosci. Biobehav. Rev.* 19, 479–493. doi: 10.1016/0149-7634(94)00068-c

Andreescu, C., Tudorascu, D. L., Butters, M. A., Tamburo, E., Patel, M., Price, J., et al. (2013). Resting state functional connectivity and treatment response in late-life depression. *Psychiatry Res.* 214, 313–321. doi: 10.1016/j.pscychresns.2013.08.007

Andrews-Hanna, J. R. (2012). The brain's default network and its adaptive role in internal mentation. *Neuroscientist* 18, 251–270. doi: 10.1177/1073858411403316

Apkarian, A. V. (2008). Pain perception in relation to emotional learning. *Curr. Opin. Neurobiol.* 18, 464–468. doi: 10.1016/j.conb.2008.09.012

Apkarian, A. V. (2011). The brain in chronic pain: clinical implications. *Pain Manag.* 1, 577–586. doi: 10.2217/pmt.11.53

Apkarian, A. V., Baliki, M. N., and Geha, P. Y. (2009). Towards a theory of chronic pain. *Prog. Neurobiol.* 87, 81–97. doi: 10.1016/j.pneurobio.2008.09.018

Arnone, D., McKie, S., Elliott, R., Juhasz, G., Thomas, E. J., Downey, D., et al. (2013). State-dependent changes in hippocampal grey matter in depression. *Mol. Psychiatry* 18, 1265–1272. doi: 10.1038/mp.2012.150

Asberg, M., Träskman, L., and Thorén, P. (1976). 5-HIAA in the cerebrospinal fluid. A biochemical suicide predictor? *Arch. Gen. Psychiatry* 33, 1193–1197. doi: 10.1001/archpsyc.1976.01770100055005

Austin, M. P., Mitchell, P., and Goodwin, G. M. (2001). Cognitive deficits in depression: possible implications for functional neuropathology. *Br. J. Psychiatry* 178, 200–206. doi: 10.1192/bjp.178.3.200

Badr, H., and Shen, M. J. (2014). Pain catastrophizing, pain intensity and dyadic adjustment influence patient and partner depression in metastatic breast cancer. *Clin. J. Pain* doi: 10.1097/ajp.0000000000000058. [Epub ahead of print].

Bai, Y. M., Chiou, W. F., Su, T. P., Li, C. T., and Chen, M. H. (2014). Pro-inflammatory cytokine associated with somatic and pain symptoms in depression. *J. Affect. Disord.* 155, 28–34. doi: 10.1016/j.jad.2013.10.019

Baliki, M. N., Geha, P. Y., Apkarian, A. V., and Chialvo, D. R. (2008). Beyond feeling: chronic pain hurts the brain, disrupting the default-mode network dynamics. *J. Neurosci.* 28, 1398–1403. doi: 10.1523/jneurosci.4123-07.2008

Bandschapp, O., Filitz, J., Urwyler, A., Koppert, W., and Ruppen, W. (2011). Tropisetron blocks analgesic action of acetaminophen: a human pain model study. *Pain* 152, 1304–1310. doi: 10.1016/j.pain.2011.02.003

Barbon, A., Caracciolo, L., Orlandi, C., Musazzi, L., Mallei, A., La Via, L., et al. (2011). Chronic antidepressant treatments induce a time-dependent up-regulation of AMPA receptor subunit protein levels. *Neurochem. Int.* 59, 896–905. doi: 10.1016/j.neuint.2011.07.013

Baudino, B., D'agata, F., Caroppo, P., Castellano, G., Cauda, S., Manfredi, M., et al. (2012). The chemotherapy long-term effect on cognitive functions and brain metabolism in lymphoma patients. *Q. J. Nucl. Med. Mol. Imaging* 56, 559–568.

Berman, R. M., Cappiello, A., Anand, A., Oren, D. A., Heninger, G. R., Charney, D. S., et al. (2000). Antidepressant effects of ketamine in depressed patients. *Biol. Psychiatry* 47, 351–354. doi: 10.1016/s0006-3223(99)00230-9

Berton, O., McClung, C. A., Dileone, R. J., Krishnan, V., Renthal, W., Russo, S. J., et al. (2006). Essential role of BDNF in the mesolimbic dopamine pathway in social defeat stress. *Science* 311, 864–868. doi: 10.1126/science.1120972

Bielecka, A. M., and Obuchowicz, E. (2013). Antidepressant drugs as a complementary therapeutic strategy in cancer. *Exp. Biol. Med. (Maywood)* 238, 849–858. doi: 10.1177/1535370213493721

Blackburn-Munro, G., and Blackburn-Munro, R. (2003). Pain in the brain: are hormones to blame? *Trends Endocrinol. Metab.* 14, 20–27. doi: 10.1016/s1043-2760(02)00004-8

Blackburn-Munro, G., and Blackburn-Munro, R. E. (2001). Chronic pain, chronic stress and depression: coincidence or consequence? *J. Neuroendocrinol.* 13, 1009–1023. doi: 10.1046/j.0007-1331.2001.00727.x

Blaudszun, G., Lysakowski, C., Elia, N., and Tramèr, M. R. (2012). Effect of perioperative systemic α2 agonists on postoperative morphine consumption and pain intensity: systematic review and meta-analysis of randomized controlled trials. *Anesthesiology* 116, 1312–1322. doi: 10.1097/ALN.0b013e31825681cb

Bodnoff, S. R., Humphreys, A. G., Lehman, J. C., Diamond, D. M., Rose, G. M., and Meaney, M. J. (1995). Enduring effects of chronic corticosterone treatment on spatial learning, synaptic plasticity and hippocampal neuropathology in young and mid-aged rats. *J. Neurosci.* 15, 61–69.

Bohren, Y., Tessier, L. H., Megat, S., Petitjean, H., Hugel, S., Daniel, D., et al. (2013). Antidepressants suppress neuropathic pain by a peripheral β2-adrenoceptor mediated anti-TNFα mechanism. *Neurobiol. Dis.* 60, 39–50. doi: 10.1016/j.nbd.2013.08.012

Bondy, B., Baghai, T. C., Minov, C., Schüle, C., Schwarz, M. J., Zwanzger, P., et al. (2003). Substance P serum levels are increased in major depression: preliminary results. *Biol. Psychiatry* 53, 538–542. doi: 10.1016/s0006-3223(02)01544-5

Booij, L., Van der Does, A. J. W., and Riedel, W. J. (2003). Monoamine depletion in psychiatric and healthy populations: review. *Mol. Psychiatry* 8, 951–973. doi: 10.1038/sj.mp.4001423

Booij, L., Van der Does, A. J., Haffmans, P. M., Riedel, W. J., Fekkes, D., and Blom, M. J. (2005). The effects of high-dose and low-dose tryptophan depletion on mood and cognitive functions of remitted depressed patients. *J. Psychopharmacol.* 19, 267–275. doi: 10.1177/0269881105051538

Breitbart, W., Rosenfeld, B., Tobias, K., Pessin, H., Ku, G. Y., Yuan, J., et al. (2014). Depression, cytokines, and pancreatic cancer. *Psychooncology* 23, 339–345. doi: 10.1002/pon.3422

Browne, C. A., and Lucki, I. (2013). Antidepressant effects of ketamine: mechanisms underlying fast-acting novel antidepressants. *Front. Pharmacol.* 4:161. doi: 10.3389/fphar.2013.00161

Campbell, L. C., Clauw, D. J., and Keefe, F. J. (2003). Persistent pain and depression: a biopsychosocial perspective. *Biol. Psychiatry* 54, 399–409. doi: 10.1016/s0006-3223(03)00545-6

Carballedo, A., Scheuerecker, J., Meisenzahl, E., Schoepf, V., Bokde, A., Möller, H. J., et al. (2011). Functional connectivity of emotional processing in depression. *J. Affect. Disord.* 134, 272–279. doi: 10.1016/j.jad.2011.06.021

Castaneda, A. E., Tuulio-Henriksson, A., Marttunen, M., Suvisaari, J., and Lönnqvist, J. (2008). A review on cognitive impairments in depressive and anxiety disorders with a focus on young adults. *J. Affect. Disord.* 106, 1–27. doi: 10.1016/j.jad.2007.06.006

Cauda, F., Torta, D. M. E., Sacco, K., Geda, E., D'Agata, F., Costa, T., et al. (2012). Shared "core" areas between the pain and other task- related networks. *PLoS One* 7:e41929. doi: 10.1371/journal.pone.0041929

Chapman, C. R., Tuckett, R. P., and Song, C. W. (2008). Pain and stress in a systems perspective: reciprocal neural, endocrine and immune interactions. *J. Pain* 9, 122–145. doi: 10.1016/j.jpain.2007.09.006

Chatzittofis, A., Nordström, P., Hellström, C., Arver, S., Åsberg, M., and Jokinen, J. (2013). CSF 5-HIAA, cortisol and DHEAS levels in suicide attempters. *Eur. Neuropsychopharmacol.* 23, 1280–1287. doi: 10.1016/j.euroneuro.2013.02.002

Chou, K. L. (2007). Reciprocal relationship between pain and depression in older adults: evidence from the English longitudinal study of ageing. *J. Affect. Disord.* 102, 115–123. doi: 10.1016/j.jad.2006.12.013

Connor, T. J., and Leonard, B. E. (1998). Depression, stress and immunological activation: the role of cytokines in depressive disorders. *Life Sci.* 62, 583–606. doi: 10.1016/s0024-3205(97)00990-9

Delgado, P. L., and Moreno, F. A. (2000). Role of norepinephrine in depression. *J. Clin. Psychiatry* 61(Suppl. 1), 5–12.

Dowben, J. S., Grant, J. S., and Keltner, N. L. (2013). Ketamine as an alternative treatment for treatment-resistant depression. *Perspect. Psychiatr. Care* 49, 2–4. doi: 10.1111/ppc.12006

Dowlati, Y., Herrmann, N., Swardfager, W., Liu, H., Sham, L., Reim, E. K., et al. (2010). A meta-analysis of cytokines in major depression. *Biol. Psychiatry* 67, 446–457. doi: 10.1016/j.biopsych.2009.09.033

Fang, C. K., Chen, H. W., Chiang, I. T., Chen, C. C., Liao, J. F., Su, T. P., et al. (2012). Mirtazapine inhibits tumor growth via immune response and serotonergic system. *PLoS One* 7:e38886. doi: 10.1371/journal.pone.0038886

Farmer, M. A., Baliki, M. N., and Apkarian, A. V. (2012). A dynamic network perspective of chronic pain. *Neurosci. Lett.* 520, 197–203. doi: 10.1016/j.neulet.2012.05.001

Farooqui, M., Li, Y., Rogers, T., Poonawala, T., Griffin, R. J., Song, C. W., et al. (2007). COX-2 inhibitor celecoxib prevents chronic morphine-induced promotion of angiogenesis, tumour growth, metastasis and mortality, without compromising analgesia. *Br. J. Cancer* 97, 1523–1531. doi: 10.1038/sj.bjc.6604057

Fields, H. L., Heinricher, M. M., and Mason, P. (1991). Neurotransmitters in nociceptive modulatory circuits. *Annu. Rev. Neurosci.* 14, 219–245. doi: 10.1146/annurev.ne.14.030191.001251

Finsterwald, C., and Alberini, C. M. (2013). Stress and glucocorticoid receptor-dependent mechanisms in long-term memory: from adaptive responses to psychopathologies. *Neurobiol. Learn. Mem.* doi: 10.1016/j.nlm.2013.09.017. [Epub ahead of print].

Fox, A., Medhurst, S., Courade, J. P., Glatt, M., Dawson, J., Urban, L., et al. (2004). Anti-hyperalgesic activity of the cox-2 inhibitor lumiracoxib in a model of bone cancer pain in the rat. *Pain* 107, 33–40. doi: 10.1016/j.pain.2003.09.003

Fox, M. D., Snyder, A. Z., Vincent, J. L., Corbetta, M., Van Essen, D. C., and Raichle, M. E. (2005). The human brain is intrinsically organized into dynamic, anticorrelated functional networks. *Proc. Natl. Acad. Sci. U S A* 102, 9673–9678. doi: 10.1073/pnas.0504136102

Franklin, K. B. J. (1998). Analgesia and abuse potential: an accidental association or a common substrate? *Pharmacol. Biochem. Behav.* 59, 993–1002. doi: 10.1016/s0091-3057(97)00535-2

Frodl, T., Schaub, A., Banac, S., Charypar, M., Jäger, M., Kümmler, P., et al. (2006). Reduced hippocampal volume correlates with executive dysfunctioning in major depression. *J. Psychiatry Neurosci.* 31, 316–323.

Gálvez, V., O'Keefe, E., Cotiga, L., Leyden, J., Harper, S., Glue, P., et al. (2014). Long-lasting effects of a single subcutaneous dose of ketamine for treating melancholic depression: a case report. *Biol. Psychiatry* doi: 10.1016/j.biopsych.2013.12.010. [Epub ahead of print].

Geng, S. J., Liao, F. F., Dang, W. H., Ding, X., Liu, X. D., Cai, J., et al. (2010). Contribution of the spinal cord BDNF to the development of neuropathic pain by activation of the NR2B-containing NMDA receptors in rats with spinal nerve ligation. *Exp. Neurol.* 222, 256–266. doi: 10.1016/j.expneurol.2010.01.003

Geraerts, E., Dritschel, B., Kreplin, U., Miyagawa, L., and Waddington, J. (2012). Reduced specificity of negative autobiographical memories in repressive coping. *J. Behav. Ther. Exp. Psychiatry* 43(Suppl. 1), S32–S36. doi: 10.1016/j.jbtep.2011.05.007

Gorenstein, C., de Carvalho, S. C., Artes, R., Moreno, R. A., and Marcourakis, T. (2006). Cognitive performance in depressed patients after chronic use of antidepressants. *Psychopharmacology (Berl)* 185, 84–92. doi: 10.1007/s00213-005-0274-2

Greicius, M. D., Flores, B. H., Menon, V., Glover, G. H., Solvason, H. B., Kenna, H., et al. (2007). Resting-state functional connectivity in major depression: abnormally increased contributions from subgenual cingulate cortex and thalamus. *Biol. Psychiatry* 62, 429–437. doi: 10.1016/j.biopsych.2006.09.020

Grimm, S., Ernst, J., Boesiger, P., Schuepbach, D., Boeker, H., and Northoff, G. (2011). Reduced negative BOLD responses in the default-mode network and increased self-focus in depression. *World J. Biol. Psychiatry* 12, 627–637. doi: 10.3109/15622975.2010.545145

Grimm, S., Ernst, J., Boesiger, P., Schuepbach, D., Hell, D., Boeker, H., et al. (2009). Increased self-focus in major depressive disorder is related to neural abnormalities in subcortical-cortical midline structures. *Hum. Brain Mapp.* 30, 2617–2627. doi: 10.1002/hbm.20693

Grosu, I., and Lavand'homme, P. (2010). Use of dexmedetomidine for pain control. *F1000 Med. Rep.* 2:90. doi: 10.3410/m2-90

Guo, W., Liu, F., Zhang, J., Zhang, Z., Yu, L., Liu, J., et al. (2013). Dissociation of regional activity in the default mode network in first-episode, drug-naive major depressive disorder at rest. *J. Affect. Disord.* 151, 1097–1101. doi: 10.1016/j.jad.2013.09.003

Gupta, K., Kshirsagar, S., Chang, L., Schwartz, R., Law, P. Y., Yee, D., et al. (2002). Morphine stimulates angiogenesis by activating proangiogenic and survival-promoting signaling and promotes breast tumor growth. *Cancer Res.* 62, 4491–4498.

Hashmi, J. A., Baliki, M. N., Huang, L., Baria, A. T., Torbey, S., Hermann, K. M., et al. (2013). Shape shifting pain: chronification of back pain shifts brain representation from nociceptive to emotional circuits. *Brain* 136, 2751–2768. doi: 10.1093/brain/awt211

Hayley, S., and Litteljohn, D. (2013). Neuroplasticity and the next wave of antidepressant strategies. *Front. Cell. Neurosci.* 7:218. doi: 10.3389/fncel.2013.00218

Holderbach, R., Clark, K., Moreau, J. L., Bischofberger, J., and Normann, C. (2007). Enhanced long-term synaptic depression in an animal model of depression. *Biol. Psychiatry* 62, 92–100. doi: 10.1016/j.biopsych.2006.07.007

Hölscher, C. (1999). Stress impairs performance in spatial water maze learning tasks. *Behav. Brain Res.* 100, 225–235. doi: 10.1016/s0166-4328(98)00134-x

Höschl, C., and Hajek, T. (2001). Hippocampal damage mediated by corticosteroids –a neuropsychiatric research challenge. *Eur. Arch. Psychiatry Clin. Neurosci.* 251(Suppl. 2), S81–S88. doi: 10.1007/bf03035134

Howren, M. B., Lamkin, D. M., and Suls, J. (2009). Associations of depression with C-reactive protein, IL-1 and IL-6: a meta-analysis. *Psychosom. Med.* 71, 171–186. doi: 10.1097/psy.0b013e3181907c1b

Iannetti, G. D., and Mouraux, A. (2010). From the neuromatrix to the pain matrix (and back). *Exp. Brain Res.* 205, 1–12. doi: 10.1007/s00221-010-2340-1

Jahchan, N. S., Dudley, J. T., Mazur, P. K., Flores, N., Yang, D., Palmerton, A., et al. (2013). A drug repositioning approach identifies tricyclic antidepressants as inhibitors of small cell lung cancer and other neuroendocrine tumors. *Cancer Discov.* 3, 1364–1377. doi: 10.1158/2159-8290.cd-13-0183

Jasmin, L., Tien, D., Weishenker, D., Palmiter, R. D., Green, P. G., Janni, G., et al. (2002). The NK1 receptor mediates both the hyperalgesia and resistance to morphine in mice lacking noradrenaline. *Proc. Natl. Acad. Sci. U S A* 99, 1029–1034. doi: 10.1073/pnas.012598599

Jeanjean, A. P., Moussaoui, S. M., Maloteaux, J. M., and Laduron, P. M. (1995). Interleukin-1 beta induces long-term increase of axonally transported opiate receptors and substance P. *Neuroscience* 68, 151–157. doi: 10.1016/0306-4522(95)00106-s

Jokinen, J., Nordström, A-L., and Nordström, P. (2009). CSF 5-HIAA and DST non-suppression–orthogonal biologic risk factors for suicide in male mood disorder inpatients. *Psychiatry Res.* 165, 96–102. doi: 10.1016/j.psychres.2007.10.007

Kamping, S., Bomba, I. C., Kanske, P., Diesch, E., and Flor, H. (2013). Deficient modulation of pain by a positive emotional context in fibromyalgia patients. *Pain* 154, 1846–1855. doi: 10.1016/j.pain.2013.06.003

Kawasaki, Y., Kumamoto, E., Furue, H., and Yoshimura, M. (2003). Alpha 2 adrenoceptor-mediated presynaptic inhibition of primary afferent glutamatergic transmission in rat substantia gelatinosa neurons. *Anesthesiology* 98, 682–689. doi: 10.1097/00000542-200303000-00016

Klauenberg, S., Maier, C., Assion, H.-J., Hoffmann, A., Krumova, E. K., Magerl, W., et al. (2008). Depression and changed pain perception: hints for a central disinhibition mechanism. *Pain* 140, 332–343. doi: 10.1016/j.pain.2008.09.003

Klossika, I., Flor, H., Kamping, S., Bleichhardt, G., Trautmann, N., Treede, R. D., et al. (2006). Emotional modulation of pain: a clinical perspective. *Pain* 124, 264–268. doi: 10.1016/j.pain.2006.08.007

Knapp, R. J., Goldenberg, R., Shuck, C., Cecil, A., Watkins, J., Miller, C., et al. (2002). Antidepressant activity of memory-enhancing drugs in the reduction of submissive behavior model. *Eur. J. Pharmacol.* 440, 27–35. doi: 10.1016/s0014-2999(02)01338-9

Kole, M. H., Swan, L., and Fuchs, E. (2002). The antidepressant tianeptine persistently modulates glutamate receptor currents of the hippocampal CA3 commissural associational synapse in chronically stressed rats. *Eur. J. Neurosci.* 16, 807–816. doi: 10.1046/j.1460-9568.2002.02136.x

Křikava, K., Dostal, M., Balcar, K., Yamamotova, A., and Rokyta, R. (2007). Clinical stress, emotions and lymphocyte subsets in peripheral blood. *Cesk. Psychol.* 51, 12–21.

Kroenke, K., Theobald, D., Wu, J., Loza, J. K., Carpenter, J. S., and Tu, W. (2010). The association of depression and pain with health-related quality of life, disability and health care use in cancer patients. *J. Pain Symptom Manage.* 40, 327–341. doi: 10.1016/j.jpainsymman.2009.12.023

Kubera, M., Grygier, B., Wrona, D., Rogóż, Z., Roman, A., Basta-Kaim, A., et al. (2011). Stimulatory effect of antidepressant drug pretreatment on progression of B16F10 melanoma in high-active male and female C57BL/6J mice. *J. Neuroimmunol.* 240–241, 34–44. doi: 10.1016/j.jneuroim.2011.09.006

Latremoliere, A., and Woolf, C. J. (2009). Central sensitization: a generator of pain hypersensitivity by central neural plasticity. *J. Pain* 10, 895–926. doi: 10.1016/j.jpain.2009.06.012

Lee, R. S. C., Hermens, D. F., Porter, M. A., and Redoblado-Hodge, M. A. (2012). A meta-analysis of cognitive deficits in first-episode major depressive disorder. *J. Affect. Disord.* 140, 113–124. doi: 10.1016/j.jad.2011.10.023

Lemogne, C., Delaveau, P., Freton, M., Guionnet, S., and Fossati, P. (2012). Medial prefrontal cortex and the self in major depression. *J. Affect. Disord.* 136, e1–e11. doi: 10.1016/j.jad.2010.11.034

Li, B., Liu, L., Friston, K. J., Shen, H., Wang, L., Zeng, L., et al. (2013). A treatment-resistant default mode subnetwork in major depression. *Biol. Psychiatry* 74, 48–54. doi: 10.1016/j.biopsych.2012.11.007

Li, N., Lee, B., Liu, R. J., Banasr, M., Dwyer, J. M., Iwata, M., et al. (2010). mTOR-dependent synapse formation underlies the rapid antidepressant effects of NMDA antagonists. *Science* 329, 959–964. doi: 10.1126/science.1190287

Loggia, M. L., Kim, J., Gollub, R. L., Vangel, M. G., Kirsch, I., Kong, J., et al. (2013). Default mode network connectivity encodes clinical pain: an arterial spin labeling study. *Pain* 154, 24–33. doi: 10.1016/j.pain.2012.07.029

Lussier, D., Huskey, A. G., and Portenoy, R. K. (2004). Adjuvant analgesics in cancer pain management. *Oncologist* 9, 571–591. doi: 10.1634/theoncologist.9-5-571

Maes, M., Bosmans, E., De Jongh, R., Kenis, G., Vandoolaeghe, E., and Neels, H. (1997). Increased serum IL-6 and IL-1 receptor antagonist concentrations in major depression and treatment resistant depression. *Cytokines* 9, 853–858. doi: 10.1006/cyto.1997.0238

Mansour, A. R., Farmer, M. A., Baliki, M. N., and Apkarian, A. V. (2013). Chronic pain: the role of learning and brain plasticity. *Restor. Neurol. Neurosci.* doi: 10.3233/RNN-139003. [Epub ahead of print].

Marchetti, I., Koster, E. H. W., Sonuga-Barke, E. J., and De Raedt, R. (2012). The default mode network and recurrent depression: a neurobiological model of cognitive risk factors. *Neuropsychol. Rev.* 22, 229–251. doi: 10.1007/s11065-012-9199-9

Marsden, W. N. (2013). Synaptic plasticity in depression: molecular, cellular and functional correlates. *Prog. Neuropsychopharmacol. Biol. Psychiatry* 43, 168–184. doi: 10.1016/j.pnpbp.2012.12.012

Martin, K. P., and Wellman, C. L. (2011). NMDA receptor blockade alters stress-induced dendritic remodeling in medial prefrontal cortex. *Cereb. Cortex* 21, 2366–2373. doi: 10.1093/cercor/bhr021

Martínez-Turrillas, R., Del Río, J., and Frechilla, D. (2007). Neuronal proteins involved in synaptic targeting of AMPA receptors in rat hippocampus by antidepressant drugs. *Biochem. Biophys. Res. Commun.* 353, 750–755. doi: 10.1016/j.bbrc.2006.12.078

Melemedjian, O. K., Tillu, D. V., Asiedu, M. N., Mandell, E. K., Moy, J. K., Blute, V. M., et al. (2013). BDNF regulates atypical PKC at spinal synapses to initiate and maintain a centralized chronic pain state. *Mol. Pain* 9:12. doi: 10.1186/1744-8069-9-12

Melzack, R. (1999). From the gate to the neuromatrix. *Pain* 82(Suppl. 6), S121–S126. doi: 10.1016/s0304-3959(99)00145-1

Melzack, R. (2001). Pain and the neuromatrix in the brain. *J. Dent. Educ.* 65, 1378–1382.

Michel, T. M., Frangou, S., Camara, S., Thiemeyer, D., Jecel, J., Tatschner, T., et al. (2008). Altered glial cell line-derived neurotrophic factor (GDNF) concentrations in the brain of patients with depressive disorder: a comparative post-mortem study. *Eur. Psychiatry* 23, 413–420. doi: 10.1016/j.eurpsy.2008.06.001

Monleón, S., Vinader-Caerols, C., Arenas, M. C., and Parra, A. (2008). Antidepressant drugs and memory: insights from animal studies. *Eur. Neuropsychopharmacol.* 18, 235–248. doi: 10.1016/j.euroneuro.2007.07.001

Müller, N. (2013). The role of anti-inflammatory treatment in psychiatric disorders. *Psychiatr. Danub.* 25, 292–298.

Müller, N., and Schwarz, M. J. (2007). The immune-mediated alteration of serotonin and glutamate: towards an integrated view of depression. *Mol. Psychiatry* 12, 988–1000. doi: 10.1038/sj.mp.4002006

Müller, N., Schwarz, M. J., Dehning, S., Douhe, A., Cerovecki, A., Goldstein-Müller, B., et al. (2006). The cyclooxygenase-2 inhibitor celecoxib has therapeutic effects in major depression: results of a double-blind, randomized, placebo controlled, add-on pilot study to reboxetine. *Mol. Psychiatry* 11, 680–684. doi: 10.1038/sj.mp.4001805

Murrough, J. W., Iacoviello, B., Neumeister, A., Charney, D. S., and Iosifescu, D. V. (2011). Cognitive dysfunction in depression: neurocircuitry and new therapeutic strategies. *Neurobiol. Learn. Mem.* 96, 553–563. doi: 10.1016/j.nlm.2011.06.006

Murrough, J. W., Iosifescu, D. V., Chang, L. C., Al Jurdi, R. K., Green, C. E., Perez, A. M., et al. (2013). Antidepressant efficacy of ketamine in treatment-resistant major depression: a two-site randomized controlled trial. *Am. J. Psychiatry* 170, 1134–1142. doi: 10.1176/appi.ajp.2013.13030392

Na, K. S., Lee, K. J., Lee, J. S., Cho, Y. S., and Jung, H. Y. (2014). Efficacy of adjunctive celecoxib treatment for patients with major depressive disorder: a meta-analysis. *Prog. Neuropsychopharmacol. Biol. Psychiatry* 48, 79–85. doi: 10.1016/j.pnpbp.2013.09.006

Nagata, K., Imai, T., Yamashita, T., Tsuda, M., Tozaki-Saitoh, H., and Inoue, K. (2009). Antidepressants inhibit P2X4 receptor function: a possible involvement in neuropathic pain relief. *Mol. Pain* 5:20. doi: 10.1186/1744-8069-5-20

Napadow, V., LaCount, L., Park, K., As-Sanie, S., Clauw, D. J., and Harris, R. E. (2010). Intrinsic brain connectivity in fibromyalgia is associated with chronic pain intensity. *Arthritis Rheum.* 62, 2545–2555. doi: 10.1002/art.27497

Neeb, L., Hellen, P., Boehnke, C., Hoffmann, J., Schuh-Hofer, S., Dirnagl, U., et al. (2011). IL-1β stimulates COX-2 dependent PGE_2 synthesis and CGRP release in rat trigeminal ganglia cells. *PLoS One* 6:e17360. doi: 10.1371/journal.pone.0017360

Nery, F. G., Monkul, E. S., Hatch, J. P., Fonseca, M., Zunta-Soares, G. B., Frey, B. N., et al. (2008). Celecoxib as an adjunct in the treatment of depressive or mixed episodes of bipolar disorder: a double-blind, randomized, placebo-controlled study. *Hum. Psychopharmacol.* 23, 87–94. doi: 10.1002/hup.912

Nestler, E. J., Barrot, M., DiLeone, R. J., Eisch, A. J., Gold, S. J., and Monteggia, L. M. (2002). Neurobiology of depression. *Neuron* 34, 13–25. doi: 10.1016/S0896-6273(02)00653-0

Neveu, P. J., and Castanon, N. (1999). "Is there evidence for an effect of antidepressant drugs on immune function," in *Cytokines, Stress and Depression*, eds R. Dantzer, E. E. Wollman and R. Yirmiya (New York: Plenum Publishers, Kluwer Academic), 267–228.

Nissen, C., Holz, J., Blechert, J., Feige, B., Riemann, D., Voderholzer, U., et al. (2010). Learning as a model for neural plasticity in major depression. *Biol. Psychiatry* 68, 544–552. doi: 10.1016/j.biopsych.2010.05.026

Nolen-Hoeksema, S. (2000). The role of rumination in depressive disorders and mixed anxiety/depressive symptoms. *J. Abnorm. Psychol.* 109, 504–511. doi: 10.1037//0021-843x.109.3.504

Obata, K., and Noguchi, K. (2006). BDNF in sensory neurons and chronic pain. *Neurosci. Res.* 55, 1–10. doi: 10.1016/j.neures.2006.01.005

Ozaktay, A. C., Kallakuri, S., Takebayashi, T., Cavanaugh, J. M., Asik, I., DeLeo, J. A., et al. (2006). Effects of interleukin-1 beta, interleukin-6 and tumor necrosis factor on sensitivity of dorsal root ganglion and peripheral receptive fields in rats. *Eur. Spine J.* 15, 1529–1537. doi: 10.1007/s00586-005-0058-8

Popoli, M., Yan, Z., McEwen, B. S., and Sanacora, G. (2011). The stressed synapse: the impact of stress and glucocorticoids on glutamate transmission. *Nat. Rev. Neurosci.* 13, 22–37. doi: 10.1038/nrn3138

Prasertsri, N., Holden, J., Keefe, F. J., and Wilkie, D. J. (2011). Repressive coping style: relationships with depression, pain and pain coping strategies in lung cancer outpatients. *Lung Cancer* 71, 235–240. doi: 10.1016/j.lungcan.2010.05.009

Racagni, R., and Popoli, M. (2008). Cellular and molecular mechanisms in the long-term action of antidepressants. *Dialogues Clin. Neurosci.* 10, 385–400.

Radley, J. J., and Morrison, J. H. (2005). Repeated stress and structural plasticity in the brain. *Ageing Res. Rev.* 4, 271–287. doi: 10.1016/j.arr.2005.03.004

Raison, C. L., Borisov, A. S., Majer, M., Drake, D. F., Pagnoni, G., Woolwine, B. J., et al. (2009). Activation of central nervous system inflammatory pathways by interferon-alpha: relationship to monoamines and depression. *Biol. Psychiatry* 65, 296–303. doi: 10.1016/j.biopsych.2008.08.010

Rhudy, J. L. (2009). The importance of emotional processes in the modulation of pain. *Pain* 146, 233–234. doi: 10.1016/j.pain.2009.07.003

Rittner, H. L., Brack, A., and Stein, C. (2008). Pain and the immune system. *Br. J. Anaesth.* 101, 40–44. doi: 10.1093/bja/aen078

Rokyta, R., Haklova, O., and Yamamotova, A. (2009). Assessment of chronic benign and cancer pain using blood plasma biomarkers. *Neuroendocrinol. Lett.* 30, 637–642.

Rosenblat, J. D., Cha, D. S., Mansur, R. B., and McIntyre, R. S. (2014). Inflamed moods: a review of the interactions between inflammation and mood disorders. *Prog. Neuropsychopharmacol. Biol. Psychiatry* doi: 10.1016/j.pnpbp.2014.01.013. [Epub ahead of print].

Ruhé, H. G., Mason, N. S., and Schene, A. H. (2007). Mood is indirectly related to serotonin, norepinephrine and dopamine levels in humans: a meta-analysis of monoamine depletion studies. *Mol. Psychiatry* 12, 331–359. doi: 10.1038/sj.mp.4001949

Samad, T. A., Moore, K. A., Sapirstein, A., Billet, S., Allchorne, A., Poole, S., et al. (2001). Interleukin-1beta-mediated induction of Cox-2 in the CNS contributes to inflammatory pain hypersensitivity. *Nature* 410, 471–475. doi: 10.1038/35068566

Sandi, C. (2011). Glucocorticoids act on glutamatergic pathways to affect memory processes. *Trends Neurosci.* 34, 165–176. doi: 10.1016/j.tins.2011.01.006

Sapolsky, R. M. (1985). Glucocorticoid toxicity in the hippocampus: temporal aspects of neuronal vulnerability. *Brain Res.* 359, 300–305. doi: 10.1016/0006-8993(85)91440-4

Schwarz, M. J., Offenbaecher, M., Neumeister, A., and Ackenheil, M. (2003). Experimental evaluation of an altered tryptophan metabolism in fibromyalgia. *Adv. Exp. Med. Biol.* 527, 265–275. doi: 10.1007/978-1-4615-0135-0_30

Scott, J. A., Wood, M., and Flood, P. (2006). The pronociceptive effect of ondansetron in the setting of P-glycoprotein inhibition. *Anesth. Analg.* 103, 742–746. doi: 10.1213/01.ane.0000228861.80314.22

Shi, X., Wang, L., Li, X., Sahbaie, P., Kingery, W. S., and Clark, J. D. (2011). Neuropeptides contribute to peripheral nociceptive sensitization by regulating interleukin-1β production in keratinocytes. *Anesth. Analg.* 113, 175–183. doi: 10.1213/ane.0b013e31821a0258

Shors, T. J., Gallegos, R. A., and Breindl, A. (1997). Transient and persistent consequences of acute stress on long-term potentiation (LTP), synaptic efficacy, theta rhythms and bursts in area CA1 of the hippocampus. *Synapse* 26, 209–217. doi: 10.1002/(sici)1098-2396(199707)26:3<209::aid-syn2>3.0.co;2-b

Shulman, G. L., Fiez, J. A., Corbetta, M., Buckner, R. L., Miezen, F. M., and Raichle, M. E. (1997). Common blood flow changes across visual tasks: II. Decreases in cerebral cortex. *J. Cog. Neurosci.* 9, 648–663. doi: 10.1162/jocn.1997.9.5.648

Silva, R., Mesquita, A. R., Bessa, J., Sousa, J. C., Sotiropoulos, I., Leão, P., et al. (2008). Lithium blocks stress-induced changes in depressive-like behavior and hippocampal cell fate: the role of glycogen-synthase-kinase-3beta. *Neuroscience* 152, 656–669. doi: 10.1016/j.neuroscience.2007.12.026

Simons, L. E., Elman, I., and Borsook, D. (2014). Psychological processing in chronic pain: a neural systems approach. *Neurosci. Biobehav. Rev.* doi: 10.1016/j.neubiorev.2013.12.006. [Epub ahead print].

Siniscalco, D., Giordano, C., Rossi, F., Maione, S., and de Novellis, V. (2011). Role of neurotrophins in neuropathic pain. *Curr. Neuropharmacol.* 9, 523–529. doi: 10.2174/157015911798376208

Smith, M. A., Makino, S., Kvetnansky, R., and Post, R. M. (1995). Stress and glucocorticoids affect the expression of brain-derived neurotrophic factor and neurotrophin-3 mRNAs in the hippocampus. *J. Neurosci.* 15, 1768–1777.

Sos, P., Klirova, M., Novak, T., Kohutova, B., Horacek, J., and Palenicek, T. (2013). Relationship of ketamine's antidepressant and psychotomimetic effects in unipolar depression. *Neuro. Endocrinol. Lett.* 34, 287–293.

Steingart, A. B., and Cotterchio, M. (1995). Do antidepressants cause, promote, or inhibit cancers? *J. Clin. Epidemiol.* 48, 1407–1412. doi: 10.1016/0895-4356(95)00545-5

Su, H. C., Ma, C. T., Yu, B. C., Chien, Y. C., Tsai, C. C., Huang, W. C., et al. (2012). Glycogen synthase kinase-3β regulates anti-inflammatory property of fluoxetine. *Int. Immunopharmacol.* 14, 150–156. doi: 10.1016/j.intimp.2012.06.015

Supornsilpchai, W., Sanguanrangsirikul, S., Maneesri, S., and Srikiatkhachorn, A. (2006). Serotonin depletion, cortical spreading depression and trigeminal nociception. *Headache* 46, 34–39. doi: 10.1111/j.1526-4610.2006.00310.x

Tagliazucchi, E., Balenzuela, P., Fraiman, D., and Chialvo, D. R. (2010). Brain resting state is disrupted in chronic back pain patients. *Neurosci. Lett.* 485, 26–31. doi: 10.1016/j.neulet.2010.08.053

Telleria-Diaz, A., Schmidt, M., Kreusch, S., Neubert, A. K., Schache, F., Vazquez, E., et al. (2010). Spinal antinociceptive effects of cyclooxygenase inhibition during inflammation: involvement of prostaglandins and endocannabinoids. *Pain* 148, 26–35. doi: 10.1016/j.pain.2009.08.013

Tenant, F., and Hermann, L. (2002). Normalization of serum cortisol concentration with opioid treatment of severe chronic pain. *Pain Med.* 3, 132–134. doi: 10.1046/j.1526-4637.2002.02019.x

Tindall, E. (1999). Celecoxib for the treatment of pain and inflammation: the preclinical and clinical results. *J. Am. Osteopath. Assoc.* 99(Suppl. 11), S13–S17.

Torta, R. G., and Munari, J. (2010). Symptom cluster: depression and pain. *Surg. Oncol.* 19, 155–159. doi: 10.1016/j.suronc.2009.11.007

Tuveson, B., Leffler, A. S., and Hansson, P. (2011). Ondansetron, a 5HT3-antagonist, does not alter dynamic mechanical allodynia or spontaneous ongoing pain in peripheral neuropathy. *Clin. J. Pain* 27, 323–329. doi: 10.1097/ajp.0b013e31820215c5

Van Hunsel, F., Wauters, A., Vandoolaeghe, E., Neels, H., Demedts, P., and Maes, M. (1996). Lower total serum protein, albumin and beta- and gamma-globulin in major and treatment-resistant depression: effects of antidepressant treatments. *Psychiatry Res.* 65, 159–169. doi: 10.1016/s0165-1781(96)03010-7

van Steenbergen, H., Booij, L., Band, G. P., Hommel, B., and van der Does, A. J. (2012). Affective regulation of cognitive-control adjustments in remitted depressive patients after acute tryptophan depletion. *Cogn. Affect. Behav. Neurosci.* 12, 280–286. doi: 10.3758/s13415-011-0078-2

Walker, A. J., Card, T., Bates, T. E., and Muir, K. (2011). Tricyclic antidepressants and the incidence of certain cancers: a study using the GPRD. *Br. J. Cancer* 104, 193–197. doi: 10.1038/sj.bjc.6605996

Walker, A. J., Grainge, M., Bates, T. E., and Card, T. R. (2012). Survival of glioma and colorectal cancer patients using tricyclic antidepressants post-diagnosis. *Cancer Causes Control* 23, 1959–1964. doi: 10.1007/s10552-012-0073-0

Wang, X., Hou, Z., Yuan, Y., Hou, G., Liu, Y., Li, H., et al. (2011). Association study between plasma GDNF and cognitive function in late-onset depression. *J. Affect. Disord.* 132, 418–421. doi: 10.1016/j.jad.2011.03.043

Wang, Y., Zhang, X., Guo, Q. L., Zou, W. Y., Huang, C. S., and Yan, J. Q. (2010). Cyclooxygenase inhibitors suppress the expression of P2X(3) receptors in the DRG and attenuate hyperalgesia following chronic constriction injury in rats. *Neurosci. Lett.* 478, 77–81. doi: 10.1016/j.neulet.2010.04.069

Warner-Schmidt, J. L., and Duman, R. S. (2006). Hippocampal neurogenesis: opposing effects of stress and antidepressant treatment. *Hippocampus* 16, 239–249. doi: 10.1002/hipo.20156

Watanabe, Y., Gould, E., Cameron, H. A., Daniels, D. C., and McEwen, B. S. (1992). Phenytoin prevents stress - and corticosterone - induced atrophy of CA3 pyramidal neurons. *Hippocampus* 2, 431–435. doi: 10.1002/hipo.450020410

Wattiez, A. S., Libert, F., Privat, A. M., Loiodice, S., Fialip, J., Eschalier, A., et al. (2011). Evidence for a differential opioidergic involvement in the analgesic effect of antidepressants: prediction for efficacy in animal models of neuropathic pain? *Br. J. Pharmacol.* 163, 792–803. doi: 10.1111/j.1476-5381.2011.01297.x

Wei, F., Dubner, R., Zou, S., Ren, K., Bai, G., Wei, D., et al. (2010). Molecular depletion of descending serotonin unmasks its novel facilitatory role in the development of persistent pain. *J. Neurosci.* 30, 8624–8636. doi: 10.1523/jneurosci.5389-09.2010

Wei, T., Guo, T. Z., Li, W. W., Hou, S., Kingery, W. S., and Clark, J. D. (2012). Keratinocyte expression of inflammatory mediators plays a crucial role in substance P-induced acute and chronic pain. *J. Neuroinflammation* 9:181. doi: 10.1186/1742-2094-9-181

Wenbin, G., Feng, L., Zhimin, X., Keming, G., Zhening, L., Changqing, X., et al. (2013). Abnormal resting-state cerebellar-cerebral functional connectivity in treatment-resistant depression and treatment sensitive depression. *Prog. Neuropsychopharmacol. Biol. Psychiatry* 44, 51–57. doi: 10.1016/j.pnpbp.2013.01.010

Wiech, K., Ploner, M., and Tracey, I. (2008). Neurocognitive aspects of pain perception. *Trends Cogn. Sci.* 12, 306–313. doi: 10.1016/j.tics.2008.05.005

Wood, P. B. (2006). Mesolimbic dopaminergic mechanisms and pain control. *Pain* 120, 230–234. doi: 10.1016/j.pain.2005.12.014

Woolley, C. S., Gould, E., and McEwen, B. S. (1990). Exposure to excess glucocorticoids alters dendritic morphology of adult hippocampal pyramidal neurons. *Brain Res.* 531, 225–231. doi: 10.1016/0006-8993(90)90778-a

Xueling, Z., Xiang, W., Jin, X., Jian, L., Mingtian, Z., Wei, W., et al. (2012). Evidence of a dissociation pattern in resting-state default mode network connectivity in first-episode, treatment-naive major depression patients. *Biol. Psychiatry* 71, 611–617. doi: 10.1016/j.biopsych.2011.10.035

Yamamotová, A., Hrubá, L., Schutová, B., Rokyta, R., and Šlamberová, R. (2011). Perinatal effect of methamphetamine on nociception in adult Wistar rats. *Int. J. Dev. Neurosci.* 29, 85–92. doi: 10.1016/j.ijdevneu.2010.08.004

Yamamotová, A., and Šlamberová, R. (2012). Behavioral and antinociceptive effects of different psychostimulant drugs in prenatally methamphetamine-exposed rats. *Physiol. Res.* 61(Suppl. 2), S139–S147.

Yaron, I., Shirazi, I., Judovich, R., Levartovsky, D., Caspi, D., and Yaron, M. (1999). Fluoxetine and amitriptyline inhibit nitric oxide, prostaglandin E2 and hyaluronic acid production in human synovial cells and synovial tissue cultures. *Arthritis Rheum.* 42, 2561–2568. doi: 10.1002/1529-0131(199912)42:12<2561::AID-ANR8>3.0.CO;2-U

Zarate, C. A. Jr., Singh, J. B., Quiroz, J. A., De Jesus, G., Denicoff, K. K., Luckenbaugh, D. A., et al. (2006). A double-blind, placebo-controlled study of memantine in the treatment of major depression. *Am. J. Psychiatry* 163, 153–155. doi: 10.1176/appi.ajp.163.1.153

Zhang, J.-M., and An, J. (2007). Cytokines, inflammation and pain. *Int. Anesthesiol. Clin.* 45, 27–37. doi: 10.1097/AIA.0b013e318034194e

Zhu, X., Wang, X., Xiao, J., Liao, J., Zhong, M., Wang, W., et al. (2012). Evidence of a dissociation pattern in resting-state default mode network connectivity in first-episode, treatment-naive major depression patients. *Biol. Psychiatry* 71, 611–617. doi: 10.1016/j.biopsych.2011.10.035

18

Spatial reversal learning in chronically sensitized rats and in undrugged sensitized rats with dopamine D2-like receptor agonist quinpirole

Hana Hatalova*, Dominika Radostova, Adela Pistikova, Karel Vales and Ales Stuchlik*

Institute of Physiology, Academy of Sciences of the Czech Republic, Prague, Czech Republic

Edited by:
Tomiki Sumiyoshi, National Center of Neurology and Psychiatry, Japan

****Correspondence:***
Hana Hatalova and Ales Stuchlik, Institute of Physiology, Academy of Sciences of the Czech Republic, Videnska 1083, Prague 142 20, Czech Republic
e-mail: hanulienka@gmail.com; stuchlik@biomed.cas.cz

Dopamine plays a role in generating flexible adaptive responses in changing environments. Chronic administration of D2-like agonist quinpirole (QNP) induces behavioral sensitization and stereotypical behaviors reminiscent of obsessive–compulsive disorder (OCD). Some of these symptoms persist even after QNP discontinuation. In QNP-sensitization, perseverative behavior has often been implicated. To test the effect of QNP-sensitization on reversal learning and its association with perseveration we selected an aversively motivated hippocampus-dependent task, active place avoidance on a Carousel. Performance was measured as the number of entrances into a to-be-avoided sector (errors). We tested separately QNP-sensitized rats in QNP-drugged and QNP-undrugged state in acquisition and reversal tasks on the Carousel. In acquisition learning there were no significant differences between groups and their respective controls. In reversal, QNP-sensitized drugged rats showed a robust but transient increase in number of errors compared to controls. QNP-sensitized rats in an undrugged state were not overtly different from the control animals but displayed an altered learning manifested by more errors at the beginning compensated by quicker learning in the second session compared to control animals. Importantly, performance was not associated with perseveration in neither QNP-sensitized drugged nor QNP-sensitized undrugged animals. The present results show that chronic QNP treatment induces robust reversal learning deficit only when the substance is continuously administered, and suggest that QNP animal model of OCD is also feasible model of cognitive alterations in this disorder.

Keywords: reversal, flexibility, cognitive coordination, quinpirole, behavior, rat, obsessive–compulsive disorder

INTRODUCTION

Cognitive flexibility is an ability to detect a shift in stimulus–feedback contingencies. It requires the recognition of the irrelevance of a response and response to a new stimulus/reward contingency. Due to its relevance to many psychiatric conditions including schizophrenia (Pantelis et al., 1999; Morris, 2013), obsessive–compulsive spectrum disorders (OCD) (Chamberlain et al., 2005), substance abuse (Jentsch et al., 2002; Ersche et al., 2008, 2011), autism (Yerys et al., 2009), and due to its necessity for successful functioning of every organism in a changing environment – cognitive flexibility is an intensively studied cognitive domain. One common task to assess cognitive flexibility is reversal learning (Klanker et al., 2013). Reversal learning has also been recently proposed to mimic some aspects of compulsivity (Homberg, 2013).

It has been proposed that dopamine plays an important role in reversal learning via dopamine D2-like receptor signaling. Systemic D2/D3 antagonist raclopride impaired reversal learning, while D1/D5 antagonist SCH 23390 did not (Lee et al., 2007). A blockade of D2-like receptors in the prefrontal cortex (PFC) was associated with a pronounced perseverative deficit in a set-shifting task (Floresco and Grace, 2003) and an activation of D2-like receptors in the nucleus accumbens impeded maintaining novel stimulus–reward contingencies (Haluk and Floresco, 2009). There is compelling evidence of D2-like signaling in striatal regions being essentially involved in reversal learning (Haluk and Floresco, 2009; Clarke et al., 2011; Groman et al., 2011); yet compared to antagonizing D2-like receptors very few studies have focused on effect of selective stimulation of D2-like receptors. For example, only one study has focused on the effect of systemic application of quinpirole (QNP), a D2-like agonist on reversal learning (Boulougouris et al., 2009). Boulougouris and colleagues showed that QNP produces a perseverative reversal learning deficit after acute systemic administration without a deficit in acquisition learning. This effect was attributed to D2-like receptor stimulation because concurrent antagonizing of D3 receptors by nafadotride did not ameliorate the effect, while D2/D3 antagonist raclopride did have this effect.

Repeated QNP administration produces escalated behavioral effects of acute QNP administration. Similarly to other stimulants it produces hyperlocomotion (Mattingly et al., 1993). In addition, QNP-treated rats also display environment-dependent perseveration in a spontaneous alternation task (Einat and Szechtman, 1995). QNP-sensitization is not associated with stereotypy of body movements such as after application of amphetamine (Wolgin, 2012), but only with path stereotypy and checking in an enriched open-field (Szechtman et al., 1998). Based on the striking similarity between QNP-sensitized behavior in rats and obsessive–compulsive symptoms in humans, it was proposed that sensitization with QNP may serve as a useful rat model of OCD. Co-administration of the tricyclic antidepressant clomipramine, effective in ameliorating symptoms in the treatment of OCD (Piccinelli et al., 1995), adds to the predictive validity of QNP-sensitization as a rat model of OCD (Szechtman et al., 1998). Additionally, the behavioral effects of chronic QNP administration are considered also to mimic some of behavioral characteristics of schizophrenia, specifically psychotic polydipsia (Goldman et al., 1988; De Carolis et al., 2010, 2011; Milella et al., 2010).

Prolonged QNP treatment was associated with changes in CNS but very little is known about the behavioral effects after QNP treatment is terminated. Sensitization by QNP alters dopamine levels in the *substantia nigra*, *striatum*, and the PFC (Sullivan et al., 1998) and alters D2 and D3 receptor binding in the *nucleus accumbens*, ventral *pallidum*, and *substantia nigra* (Stanwood et al., 2000). Based on these wide scale alterations in the dopamine system, we expect that these alterations manifest themselves on a behavioral level as well. Indeed, some QNP-specific behaviors of sensitized drugged rats such as perseveration and conservativeness of travel routes are also observed in sensitized undrugged rats, albeit to a lesser extent (Einat and Szechtman, 1993). No change in reversal learning performance or locomotion – alterations, which are observed in drugged rats – was detected in this study.

The present study employed active place avoidance on a Carousel [also known as active allothetic place avoidance; AAPA; (Bures et al., 1997; Petrasek et al., 2013; for review, see Stuchlík et al., 2013)]. This task is a hippocampus-dependent spatial task originally developed in our laboratory to study higher-order spatial navigation and cognitive coordination and was shown to be sensitive in the detection of cognitive impairments (Wesierska et al., 2005). Cognitive coordination is the ability to manage multiple conflicting information streams and selectively pay attention to relevant information while ignoring irrelevant information. A recent study (Lobellova et al., 2013) showed that active place avoidance on a Carousel in its reversal modification was more sensitive to cognitive impairment by acute dizocilpine administration than was the Morris water maze (MWM) (but for opposite cases for acquisition, see Stuchlik et al., 2004 or Vales et al., 2006). Active place avoidance with reversal is an aversively motivated dynamic-environment-task with high demands for "perceptual segregation" (cognitive coordination) and "mnemonic" segregation. Perceptual segregation is the continuous segregation of multiple frames of reference, i.e., information streams where arena- and room-frames of reference are in continuous conflict (Abdel Baki et al., 2010). Mnemonic segregation has been tested in reversal modification with the need to segregate previous irrelevant memory for to-be-avoided zone from the new one (Perera et al., 2013). As mentioned before, the role of D2-like receptors in the flexibility of spatial avoidance behavior is an understudied phenomenon, which makes this task less comparable to other studies, but at the same time is capable of providing new insights into dopamine function in learning.

Specifically, in this experiment reversal learning in QNP-sensitized drugged and undrugged rats was examined from the viewpoint of a rat model of OCD. Since acute QNP treatment induced a reversal learning deficit (Boulougouris et al., 2009), we expected to confirm such deficit would be seen after repeated QNP treatment under the drug's effect in first experiment. In the second experiment, reversal learning was tested in sensitized but undrugged rats. Since undrugged behavior appears to mimic aspects of the behavior of sensitized drugged rats we hypothesized a reversal learning deficit would be apparent due to high sensitivity of the reversal part of the task (Lobellova et al., 2013).

MATERIALS AND METHODS

EXPERIMENTAL DESIGN

Two consecutive experiments were conducted. Experiment 1 tested acquisition and reversal in QNP-sensitized rats in a drugged state during the acquisition and reversal sessions on a Carousel. Experiment 2 had the same experimental design and tested acquisition and reversal in QNP-sensitized but undrugged rats. Since these two experiments were conducted at different time periods, pooling experiments together would not be statistically correct, so they are reported separately. Experiment 1 compared learning between QNP-sensitized drugged rats with QNP ($n = 10$) and saline-treated rats ($n = 11$). Experiment 2 compared learning between QNP-sensitized undrugged rats ($n = 10$) and saline-treated rats ($n = 9$).

RATS

Adult male Long–Evans rats from the breeding colony of the Institute of Physiology AS CR were used. All rats weighed 300–400 g at the start of experiment and were 12–15 weeks of age. Rats were housed 3–4 rats per cage in an air-conditioned rat room with a stable temperature of 22°C, constant humidity, and 12/12 light/dark cycle. Both experiments were conducted in the light phase of the day. Food and water were freely available. Prior to the experiments, rats were handled for 2 min daily for 3 days. Rats were also gently implanted with a subcutaneous needle connector, which pierced the skin between rat's shoulders. The needle had a blunted and swirled tip for the attachment of an alligator clip connecting a shock-delivering wire. This procedure is analogous to a hypodermic injection in humans and does not require anesthesia. All rat manipulations were conducted in accordance with the Animal Protection Code of the Czech Republic and a corresponding directive of the European Community Council on the use of laboratory animals (2010/63/EC).

DRUGS

Quinpirole hydrochloride (Sigma-Aldrich, Czech Republic, Cat. No. Q102) was dissolved in saline solution (0.9% NaCl) to achieve a concentration of 0.5 mg/mL. When appropriate, each rat was injected with 1 mL/kg of QNP solution or a corresponding volume of saline solution (1 mL/kg).

APPARATUS – CAROUSEL

The apparatus (Carousel, **Figure 1A**) is a circular metallic disk (82-cm diameter) elevated 1 m above the floor with a low rim. The arena is surrounded by 60-cm-high transparent Plexiglas wall. The arena rotated at 1 revolution/min in a clockwise direction. An unmarked 60°-to-be-avoided sector was defined in stable room-frame coordinates on the rotating arena. Whenever a rat

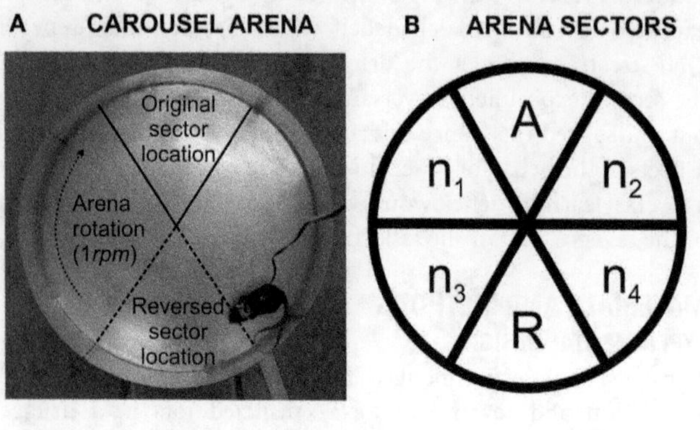

FIGURE 1 | (A) Illustration shows the Carousel arena. The arena is a rotating metallic disk on which is, directly imperceptible by the rat, a 60° sector where it receives a mild electric shock. This sector can be localized only by using extra-maze cues, which are abundant in the experimental room. As not to disturb, the experimenter observes rat's movement on a TV screen from a different room. **(B)** Describes calculation of *percentage of time spent in the former to-be-avoided sector*. The arena was divided into six equal non-overlapping sectors. *A* labels the former shock sector (during ACQ1–ACQ4). *R* is the segment of the arena that is punished in reversal (and was formerly safe) (REV1–REV4). *n1–n4* are sectors that were never punished. Level of perseveration can be inferred from the *percentage of time spent in the former shock sector* (*A*) of time spent in safe sectors during first 10 min of reversal (*A+n1–n4*): $\%A = \left(\frac{A}{A+n1+n2+n3+n4}\right) \times 100$. High perseveration is more likely when a rat is less in the former to-be-avoided sector, while low perseveration is more likely when rat spends a higher fraction of time there. To note, 20% indicates that a rat distributes its time equally between all safe sectors.

entered the sector for more than 300 ms, constant-current regulated electric footshocks (AC, 50 Hz, 200–600 μA) were delivered at 1200-ms intervals until the rat left the sector. The shocks were administrated through the above-described subcutaneous needle connector implanted on the back of the rat standing on the grounded floor. The highest voltage drop of the current passing through the rat was at the high-impedance contact between the paws and grounded metal floor. The appropriate current was individualized for each rat in order to elicit a rapid escape reaction but prevent freezing. This aversive procedure has been shown to be efficient and safe in previous studies (for review, see Stuchlík et al., 2013).

Each rat was allowed to move freely within the arena boundaries. To localize the sector rats had to navigate purely using distant extra-maze landmarks because proximal intra-maze landmarks (such as scents, urine marks, or feces) were made irrelevant by arena rotation. During acquisition (ACQ) sessions the to-be-avoided sector was arbitrarily defined at North. During reversal (REV) sessions the sector was relocated to South – the opposite side of the disk, while the direction of arena rotation remained the same.

The constant-current-regulated source, which carries current for the shock application also contains a unit for powering a light-emitting diode (LED), attached by a latex harness on rat's back signaling the position of the rat to an overhead camera and a computer. The second LED diode is on the arena periphery signaling arena rotation. The analog signal from an overhead infrared camera is digitized by a DT-3155 card (Data Translation, USA) in the Tracker program (Biosignal Group, USA), which samples rat's position at the rate of 25 Hz.

QUINPIROLE SENSITIZATION AND HABITUATION TO CAROUSEL

Prior to avoidance testing, rats were sensitized by repeated administration of a QNP solution (or saline solution for control groups) in the course of 3 weeks. QNP (0.5 mg/kg) was applied on Mondays, Wednesdays, and Fridays up to a total of 10 injections. Sensitization was conducted in the same Carousel apparatus where later avoidance learning was tested. During the sensitization procedure each rat received a QNP or saline injection in its home cage and 30 min later was placed onto the Carousel for 30-min exploration (with no shock). This means that sensitization was conducted together with repeated exposure to the experimental environment. To minimize potential conditioning to the injection schedule, the order of rats during sensitization was varied pseudo-randomly.

PROCEDURE – ACQUISITION AND REVERSAL TESTING

Behavioral testing included two phases – acquisition (ACQ) and reversal (REV). Acquisition preceded reversal. Both acquisition and reversal sessions took place in four 30-min sessions each conducted every other day. The only difference in setup between acquisition and reversal sessions was the location of the sector (180° shift).

In both experiments (1 and 2) testing in the Carousel commenced 2 days after sensitization/habituation sessions ended (10 sessions, see **Figures 2A** and **3A** for experimental scheme illustrations). Rats in experiment 1 received an injection of 0.5 mg/kg QNP or saline 30-min prior to the arena testing. Rats in experiment 2 were not treated at all during the testing and therefore did not require any time delay before placement into the arena. In the beginning of each session, each rat was placed into the arena opposite to the location of the shock sector, facing the experimenter. Carousel rotation and tracking was turned on immediately after an experimenter left the room. Since the arena was rotating independently of the to-be-avoided sector, the best strategy to solve the task was to walk constantly or intermittently in the counterclockwise direction to avoid being transported into the shock sector by arena rotation. Our observations suggest that four acquisition and four reversal sessions are sufficient for rat to acquire a successful learning strategy.

MEASURED PARAMETERS AND STATISTICAL ANALYSIS

Parameters presented here were extracted from an offline analysis program for Tracker (Track Analysis, Biosignal Group, USA) and an open-source Carousel Maze Manager (Bahník, 2013). The output parameters that were assessed in analysis were locomotor activity measured as distance walked throughout a session in meters (movement of arena detected by peripheral LED diode was subtracted from total locomotion), number of entrances into the sector (errors), time to the first error, and *percentage of time spent in the former to-be-avoided sector* during reversal.

First, we assessed a distance animals walked during the session because locomotion between experimental groups was expected to differ due to the stimulant effect of QNP. If the expected locomotor activity difference between control and treatment groups

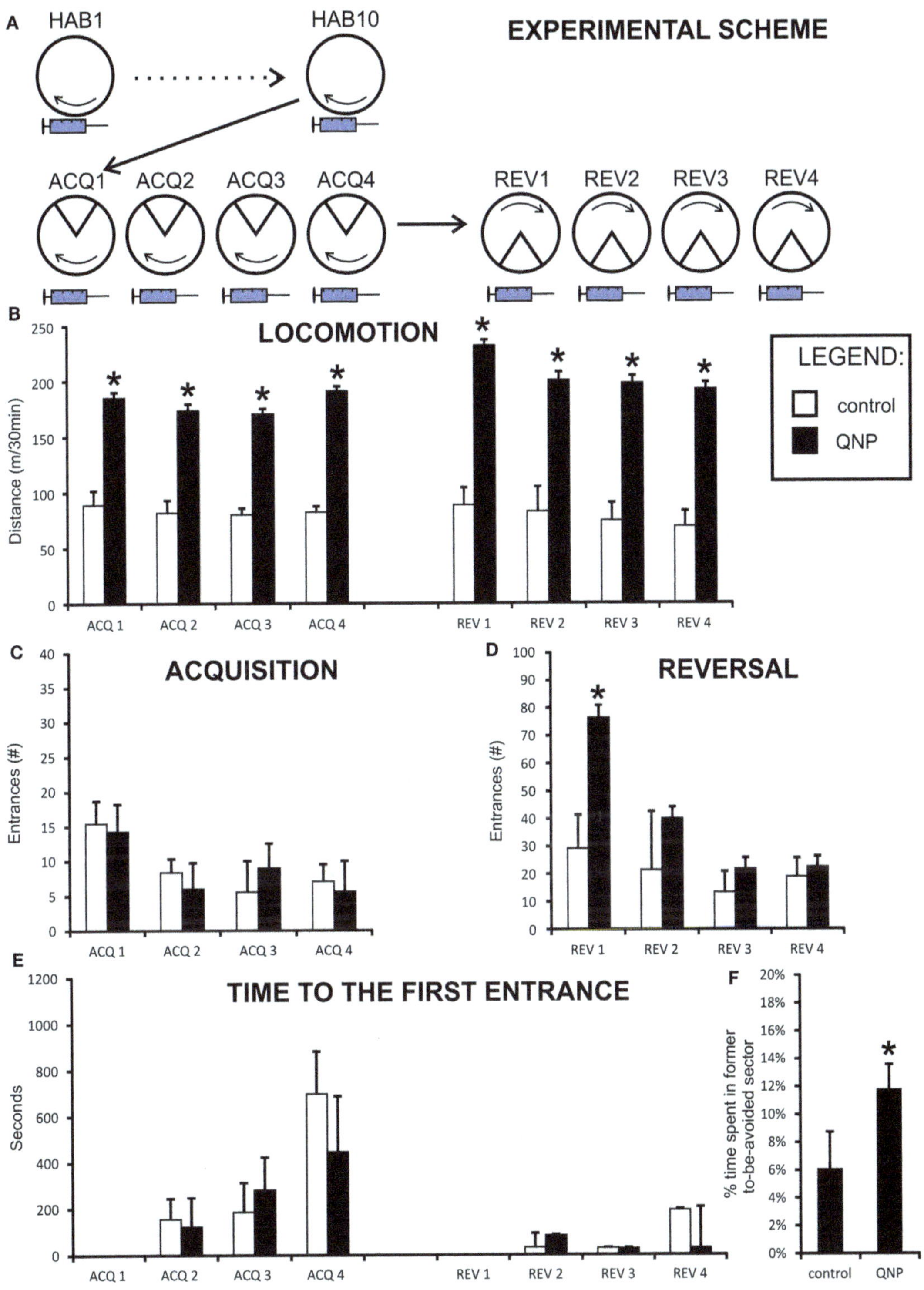

FIGURE 2 | Graph shows results from experiment 1 (QNP-sensitized drugged rats). Data are presented as mean values ± SEM. Asterisks denote significant simple effect analysis that followed significant group effect in ANOVA ($p < 0.05$). **(A)** The scheme of experiment 1. **(B)** Locomotion (meters/30 min) of chronically treated drugged with QNP-rats compared to saline-treated rats. There is significantly higher locomotion in QNP-rats compared to their controls during all sessions (ACQ1–REV4). **(C)** Number of entrances into the to-be-avoided sector (#/30 min) during acquisition sessions (ACQ1–ACQ4) when all rats are included. **(D)** Number of errors (#/30 min) in four reversal sessions (REV1–REV4). Data show a significant difference in number of errors in first day of reversal testing (REV1). **(E)** Time to the first error (mean seconds ± SEM) in experiment 1 (ACQ2–ACQ4; REV2–REV4). There was no significant effect at $p < 0.05$. **(F)** *Percentage of time spent in former shock sector* (*A*) compared to mean time spent in always safe sectors (*A* + *n*1–*n*4) during first 10 min of reversal (REV1). QNP-treated group shows significantly higher percentage of time spent in former to-be-avoided sector, indicating more distributed time spent in all safe sectors, suggesting lower rate of perseveration than control rats.

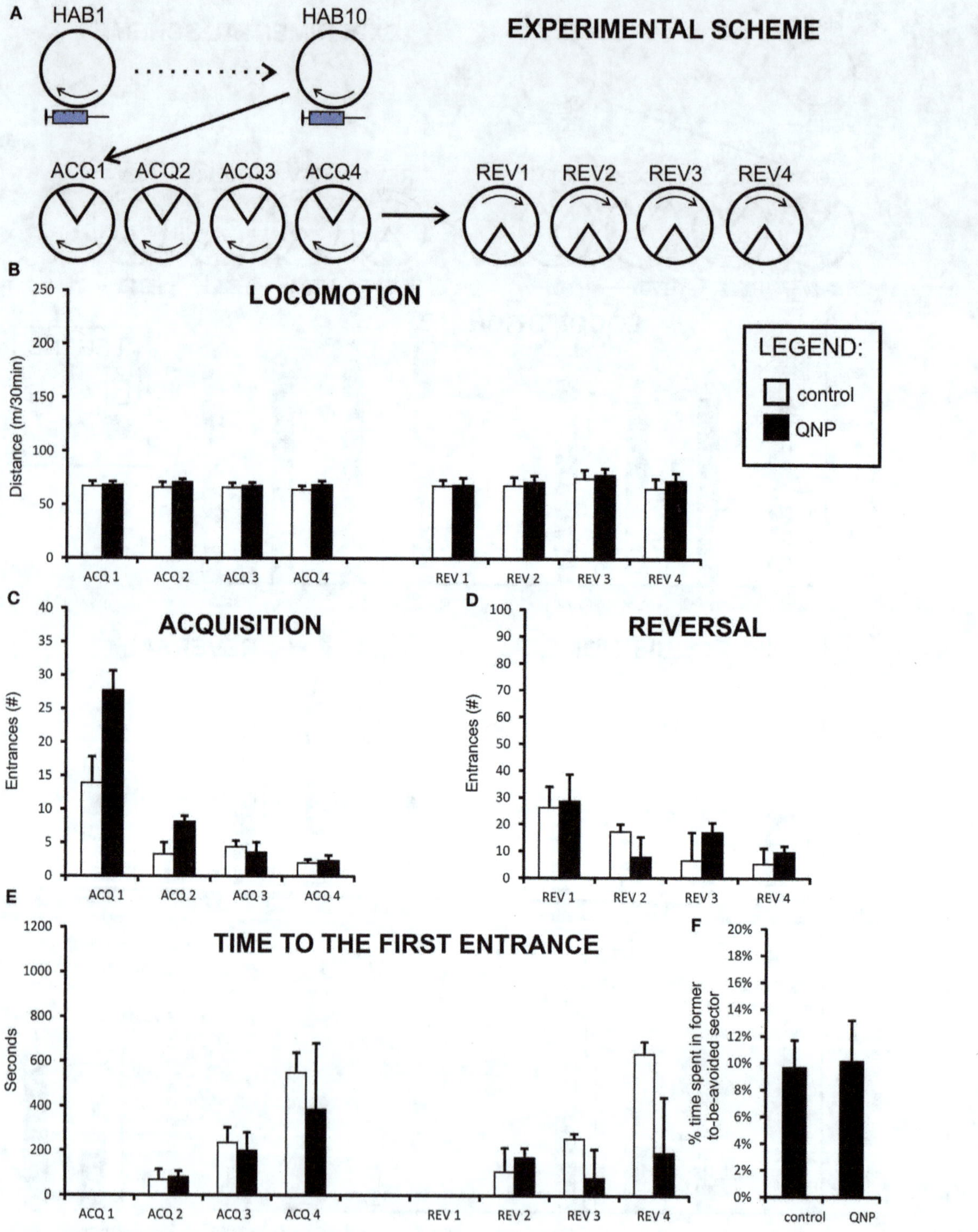

FIGURE 3 | Graphs illustrating results from experiment 2 (QNP-sensitized but undrugged rats). Data are presented as mean values ± SEM. Asterisks denote significant simple effect analysis that followed significant group effect in ANOVA ($p < 0.05$). **(A)** The scheme of experiment 2. **(B)** Locomotion (meters/30 min) of sensitized rats. It is apparent that there is no significant difference in locomotion between QNP-sensitized rats and a non-sensitized control rats. **(C)** Number of errors (#/30 min) during all acquisition sessions (ACQ1–ACQ4). **(D)** Number of errors during four reversal sessions (#/30 min; REV1–REV4). Significant interaction term is not displayed, but data suggest that it is due to higher error rate in QNP-sensitized rats (REV1) compensated by faster learning in a second reversal day (REV2). **(E)** Time to the first error in seconds (mean ± SEM) in experiment 2 (ACQ2–ACQ4; REV2–REV4). There was no significant effect at $p < 0.05$. **(F)** *Percentage of time spent in former shock sector* (*A*) compared to mean time spent in always safe sectors ($A + n1–n4$) during first 10 min of reversal (REV1). QNP-sensitized rats appear not to differ from non-sensitized control rats in distribution of movement in safe sectors of the arena (and avoidance of previously punished sector).

in experiment 1 was present, an issue of hyperlocomotion influencing the number of errors had to be addressed. Hypothetically, if a rat walked randomly into the arena, higher locomotor activity would result in an increased number of errors per unit of time into the shock sector solely by chance. To assure that the variation in number of errors between the groups was not associated with higher locomotion in QNP group; correlations were computed to assess a relationship between these two parameters. For all correlation analyses when data showed normal distribution Pearson's product moment coefficient was used and when data were not normally distributed Spearman's rho was used.

The principal spatial parameter was the *number of errors.* A low number of errors reflect comprehension of the task, well-managed avoidance strategy, and intact cognitive coordination. Additionally, to assess long-term between-session memory, *time-to-first-error* was analyzed. Since a rat was never placed directly into the sector, a solid memory trace enables the rat to avoid receiving a shock from the very beginning of every session with the exception of the first day of acquisition (ACQ1) and first day of reversal (REV1).

To discern types of errors that animals make when the to-be-avoided sector is reversed, *percentage of time spent in former to-be-avoided sector* was assessed for the first day of reversal (REV1). The calculation is similar to one described in detail by Petrasek et al. (2013). In short, the arena was divided into the six 60°-sectors. One of these sectors was the one reinforced in acquisition sessions (now a former to-be-avoided sector; *A*), the second sector was a current (reversed; *R*) sector (opposite to former to-be-avoided sector). The remaining four sectors, *n*1–*n*4, were never punished and were located in pairs between former and currently to-be-avoided sector (illustrated in **Figure 1B**). The percentage was calculated from a ratio of time spent in the former to-be-avoided sector divided by average time spent in always safe sectors $[A/(n1\text{–}n4+A)]$. The reversed (current) to-be-avoided sector was excluded from the calculation because electric shock affects the time spent in this sector. Since perseveration can be quickly overridden by re-learning, the new sector position, the initial 10 min of the first reversal session were analyzed. In the reversal learning task, rats can make two types of errors. One type of mistake can be produced by the inability to shift from the previously relevant strategy – referred to as perseverative errors. Other types of mistakes result from the inability of the rat to learn a new strategy – referred to as memory saturation. A lower percentage indicates, with a high incidence of errors, that the rat failed because it avoided former to-be-avoided sector during reversal learning, while failing to adapt to the new shock location. The higher percentage (ratio) (20% indicates an equal preference of all five safe sectors) suggests that the rat avoided former shock sector less, which could indicate either low perseveration or weak long-term memory. If a high number of errors would accompany high ratio, it can be claimed that these errors were not perseverative in nature but caused by other factors such as memory saturation.

Every batch of rats used in this study included rats which did not learn the paradigm. An inability to achieve effective avoidance can be caused by many factors often unrelated to the experiment itself, such as breeding issues or an unknown stressful event. Specific cases are rats which do not opt for avoidance strategy but instead display prolonged freezing resulting in a complete absence of avoidance behavior and locomotor activity (approximately 10% of all rats, unpublished observations from multiple experiments). These rats and rats which did not find effective learning strategy in acquisition had to be excluded from the reversal learning task (A rat cannot learn to reverse the task if it did not learn it in the first place.). For the exclusion of rats in the reversal a threshold of minimum 10 errors during the last 30-min session was used (ACQ4).

For the assessment of learning differences in acquisition and reversal sessions, a two-way repeated measures ANOVA was conducted using the factor of sessions as a repeated measure (session; ACQ1–ACQ4, REV1–REV4) and groups as a between-subject factor (QNP vs. saline). Significant ANOVA was followed by simple effect analysis when sessions × groups interaction was significant. If necessary, acquisition learning was analyzed twice, once with included and once with the excluded "non-learners." This is to uncover any bias that could be present due to exclusion of non-learning rats (i.e., non-learners had greater impact in one group than in the other). If the data were not normally distributed or did not meet the assumption of homogeneity of variance, appropriate transformations (logarithmic; for acquisition sessions in experiment 1, acquisition and reversal in experiment 2) were conducted. If no transformation was able to transform data into the parametric data sets, differences between the groups were assessed by a non-parametric Mann–Whitney sum ranks test with Bonferroni correction applied to the level of test significance (acquisition with non-learners included in experiment 1). All statistical tests were considered significant at the threshold of $p < 0.05$ (two tailed).

RESULTS

EXPERIMENT 1

This experiment assessed learning in rats sensitized with dopamine D2-like agonist QNP under QNP treatment (**Figure 2A**). Two rats in each group did not reach learning criterion of having <10 errors in the last acquisition session (QNP group: rats with 17 and 21 errors; control group: rats with 30 and 37 errors). These rats were not included in reversal learning. Specifically, in the control group one of these rats froze throughout most of the session and second did not find an effective avoidance strategy. In QNP group neither of the two excluded rats appeared to abide by an effective avoidance strategy (visual observation).

LOCOMOTION

All rats from experiment 1 were included in the assessment of locomotor activity throughout all four acquisition and four reversal sessions by repeated measure two-way ANOVA. Data were normally distributed in both groups, and variances between groups were not significantly different. Because Mauchly's test indicated that the assumption of sphericity had been violated, $[\chi^2(27)=66.99,\ p<0.001]$, degrees of freedom were corrected using the Greenhouse–Geisser estimate of sphericity ($\varepsilon=0.45$) for tests that included a repeated measure. There was a significant main effect of sessions on distance $[F(3.26, 52.15)=2.95,\ p<0.05]$ and significant effect of groups $[F(1,16)=234.05,\ p<0.001]$. Also, analysis showed a significant effect of sessions × groups interaction $[F(3.26, 52.15)=3.78,$

$p < 0.05$]. Planned contrasts for the effect of both sessions and interaction term showed a significant change in locomotion between acquisition day 3 (ACQ3) and day 4 (ACQ4) [session: $F(1,16) = 9.69$, $p < 0.01$; interaction: $F(1,16) = 9.17$, $p < 0.01$] and between acquisition day 4 (ACQ4) and first day of reversal (REV1) [session: $F(1,16) = 11.25$, $p < 0.01$; interaction: $F(1,16) = 9.49$, $p < 0.01$]. Because by visual inspection control group did not show any fluctuations (**Figure 2B**) in locomotor activity, the up-regulation of activity in the QNP group probably accounts for both significant sessions and interaction effect.

DISTANCE-ERRORS CORRELATION

When groups were pooled together, (including excluded rats) data did not show any correlation between distance walked and errors during all acquisition sessions pooled together $rs = -0.04$, ns. However, it is obvious from the graph (**Figure 4A**) that data were sectioned into two distinct populations based on treatment a rat received. When treatment groups were considered separately there was no significant correlation between number of errors and locomotor activity, ($rs = -0.266$, ns), in control group and no statistically significant correlation in the QNP-treated group, ($rs = 0.136$, ns). After exclusion of rats that did not reach the threshold of learning there was still no overall or group specific significant correlation between number of errors and distance walked by a rat (control group: $rs = -0.05$, ns; QNP group: $rs = 0.04$, ns; pooled groups: $rs = 0.12$, ns) (**Figure 4B**). This indicates that in rats which have entered reversal testing, there was no correlation between the distance and number of errors despite the large difference in locomotion between the groups. To visually compare trajectories of hyperlocomotor QNP-treated and control rats, example trajectories of each of these rats are included where individuals did not make any entrance into the to-be-avoided sector. **Figure 4C** depicts an example in ACQ4 of the trajectories of locomotion for a control rat and for a QNP-sensitized rat under QNP.

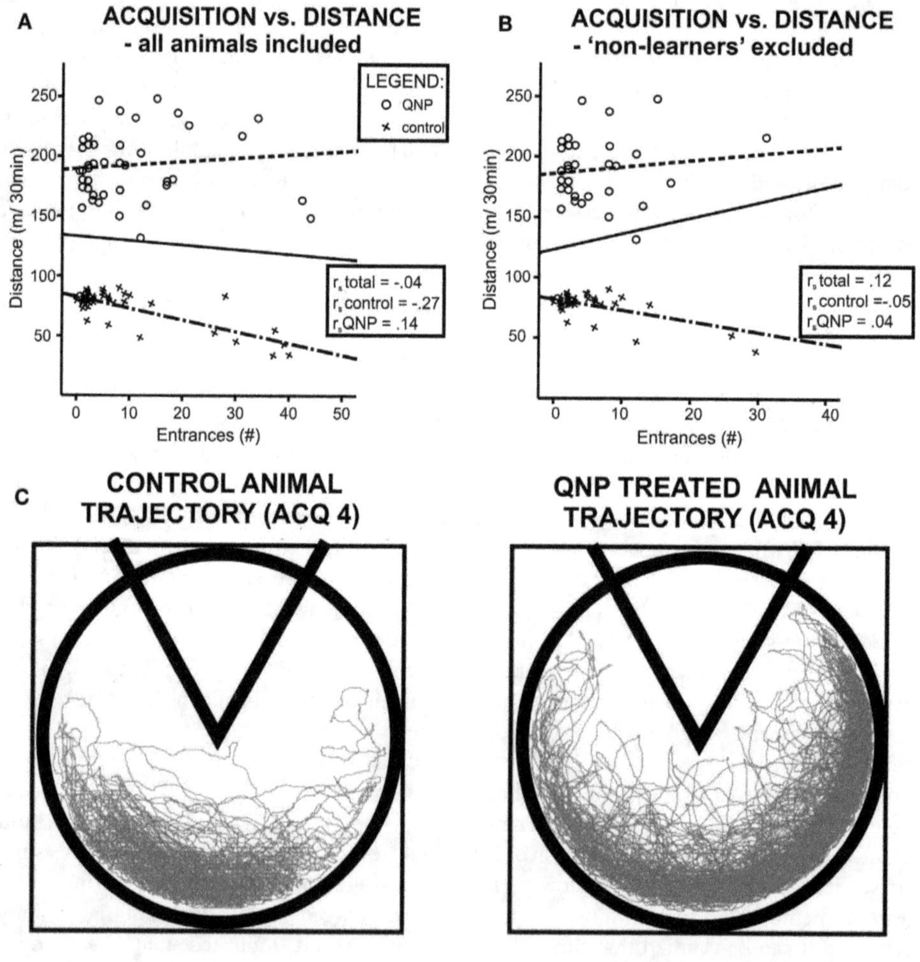

FIGURE 4 | Scatter plots visualizing correlation between number of errors and locomotion in experiment 1. (A) Data when all rats are included. **(B)** Only rats that will enter reversal (non-learners excluded). Blue color denotes QNP-treated rats, green color saline-treated rats. Both groups show different patterns of association between number of errors and distance walked, namely in the QNP group, there is a trend of worsened performance (more errors) with higher locomotion, and in the saline-treated group, there is an opposite trend. Nonetheless, this trend was not significant with or without non-learners included. **(C)** Trajectory of hyperlocomotor QNP-treated and control rat where neither individual made any error into the to-be-avoided sector. Control and QNP-sensitized and drugged rats' trajectories are from last-day of acquisition (ACQ4).

ACQUISITION AND REVERSAL LEARNING

Learning behavior was analyzed for acquisition and reversal learning separately. Acquisition learning (ACQ1–ACQ4) was analyzed with all cases included (to determine if there is a significant difference in overall learning capability between groups) and with "non-learners" excluded from analysis.

In acquisition learning, when all rats were included, the number of errors distributions was not normal and no transformation was able to normalize them. Therefore, the Mann–Whitney test was used to compare two experimental groups in each acquisition learning day. The Bonferroni correction was applied to control for family wise error caused by the high number of comparisons (new significance threshold was calculated to be $p < 0.0125$). No significant differences were detected between groups in any of the acquisition sessions (ACQ1: $U = 42.00$, $z = -0.92$, ns; ACQ2: $U = 54.50$, $z = -0.04$, ns; ACQ3: $U = 41.50$, $z = -0.97$, ns; ACQ4: $U = 42.50$, $z = -0.90$, ns) (**Figure 2C**). The results show there was no difference between QNP and control groups in acquisition learning with all rats included in the study.

After the exclusion of rats which did not meet learning criteria (therefore only rats, which learned acquisition task remained) data showed normal distribution and equal variances after logarithmic transformations, which allowed two-way repeated measure ANOVA to be conducted. Because Mauchly's test indicated that the assumption of sphericity had been violated [$\chi^2(5) = 42.39$, $p < 0.001$], degrees of freedom were corrected using the Greenhouse–Geisser estimate of sphericity ($\varepsilon = 0.40$) for tests that included repeated measure. Session was considered a repeated measure and group was a between-subject factor. The only significant effect was main effect of session [$F(1.19,17.88) = 26.59$, $p < 0.001$]. There was no significant group effect [$F(1,15) = 39.95$, ns] or sessions × groups interaction [$F(1.19,17.88) = 0.93$, ns]. No simple effect *post hoc* analysis was conducted since there were no significant differences between the groups (data not shown).

Two-way repeated measure ANOVA was conducted on the number of errors in four reversal sessions (REV1–REV4, only rats which achieved <10 errors in ACQ4 were included) (**Figure 2D**). Data were normally distributed so no transformation was needed. Assumption of homogeneity of variances was broken and it was not possible to correct it with any transformation. Therefore, the Brown and Forsythe correction was applied during F score calculation. Specifically, effect of session was significant [$F(1.939, 25.204) = 5.444$, $p < 0.05$], even after degrees of freedom were corrected by the Greenhouse–Geisser estimate of sphericity ($\varepsilon = 0.65$) because the assumption of sphericity was significantly violated [$\chi^2(5) = 18.673$, $p < 0.05$]. Sessions × groups interaction was also significant, even after the Greenhouse–Geisser correction to degrees of freedom [$F(1.94, 25.20) = 4.61$, $p < 0.05$]. Effect of groups was also highly significant [$F(1,13) = 31.72$, $p < 0.001$]. To break down an interaction term between QNP-treated and control rats, simple effect analysis was conducted. It showed that a significant difference was observed only on the first day of reversal (REV1) $F(1,13) = 11.18$, $p < 0.01$ [other sessions: REV2 $F(1,13) = 2.14$, ns; REV3 $F(1,13) = 0.73$, ns; REV4 $F(1,13) = 0.02$, ns].

TIME TO THE FIRST ERROR

Between-session long-term memory was measured by time-to-the-first error. Data were non-parametrically distributed and no transformation was capable of normalizing them. Therefore, the non-parametric Mann–Whitney test had to be used to analyze the data. The Bonferroni correction was applied to control for family wise error caused by high number of comparisons (new significance threshold was calculated to be $p < 0.008$). Despite the apparent trend (**Figure 2E**) we did not find the differences in this parameter significant (ACQ2: $U = 53.00$, $z = -0.14$, ns; ACQ3: $U = 37.00$, $z = -1.27$, ns; ACQ4: $U = 27.00$, $z = -1.97$, $p = 0.049$; REV2: $U = 52.00$, $z = -0.21$, ns; REV3: $U = 44.50$, $z = -0.42$, ns; REV4: $U = 49.00$, $z = -0.42$, ns). In summary, after the family wise correction of significance threshold, there was no significant difference in between-session memory between saline-treated rats and rats chronically drugged with QNP.

PERCENTAGE OF TIME SPENT IN FORMER TO-BE-AVOIDED SECTOR DURING REVERSAL

A more detailed look into the differences in reversal learning behavior is offered by analysis of time spent in the former to-be-avoided sector after change of shock location. It is defined by percentage of time spent in the formerly to-be-avoided sector of time spent in always safe sector (all sectors excluding the reversed to-be-avoided sector). Intriguingly, t-test shows that control rats spent only 5.12% (SEM = ±1.7%) of the time in former shock zone while QNP-treated rats spent up to 13.32% (SEM = ±2.5%) in the former shock zone in the first 10 min of first reversal session (REV1) [$t(15) = -2.76$, $p < 0.05$] (**Figure 2F**). On a probability basis it could be argued that with a higher locomotion rate QNP-treated rats enter the former shock zone sooner and more often, an experience which could quickly dis-inhibit the previously learned response. Therefore a correlation analysis was conducted to assess any relationship between distance and measure of perseveration. The correlation analysis showed that there was no significant correlation between the two measures in this study (rs = 0.31, ns). In conclusion, QNP-treated rats entered former-to-be-avoided sector significantly more than control rats. These results do not show perseverative behavior in controls and demonstrate that QNP-sensitization and treatment does not increase perseveration during the reversal task on the Carousel.

EXPERIMENT 2

This experiment aimed to assess an effect of sensitization by dopamine D2-like agonist QNP on acquisition and reversal learning on a Carousel in undrugged rats (for experimental scheme see **Figure 3A**). Three rats were excluded from the analysis due to technical complications (one from QNP-treated group and two control rats). Rats which remained reached a pre-defined threshold of max 10 errors by the fourth acquisition sitting (ACQ4). Thus eight control rats and nine QNP-treated rats were included in all analyses.

LOCOMOTION

Two-way repeated measure ANOVA was conducted to compare the locomotion between group sensitized to QNP (but undrugged during both acquisition and reversal learning sessions) compared to control rats. Data were normally distributed and variances of the groups were not significantly different. Mauchly's test indicated that an assumption of sphericity for repeated measure test had not been met [$\chi^2(27) = 65.56$, $p < 0.001$] and therefore all the degrees of freedom in repeated measure tests (session and sessions × groups interaction) were corrected by a Greenhouse–Geisser estimate of sphericity ($\varepsilon = 0.40$). As can be observed from the graph (**Figure 3B**) there was no group effect in locomotion between sensitized and control rats [$F(1,15) = 0.004$, ns]. The locomotion remained stable throughout sessions for there was no effect of session observed [$F(2.77,41.57) = 0.75$, ns]. Non-significant sessions × groups interaction terms indicate that the two groups did not differ with the regard to locomotor activity [$F(2.77,41.56) = 0.197$, ns.].

ACQUISITION AND REVERSAL LEARNING

Acquisition and reversal learning was analyzed separately and all rats were included in the study. Since locomotion between the groups did not vary, there was no need for correlation analysis testing the relationship between distance and number of errors into the to-be-avoided sector. In both acquisition and reversal learning, the *number of errors* data were not normally distributed and had to be transformed by a logarithmic transformation to correct the issue. Variances between the groups were homogenous.

Two-way ANOVA was conducted to compare acquisition learning between QNP-sensitized and control rats (**Figure 3C**). The effect of session [$F(2.05,30.72) = 50.68$, $p < 0.001$] was significant even after the Greenhouse–Geissler correction, of sphericity ($\varepsilon = 0.68$) which was necessary because the data significantly deviated from the assumption of sphericity [$\chi^2(5) = 13.04$, $p < 0.05$]. There was no significant group effect observed [$F(1,15) = 3.36$, ns], or sessions × group interaction [$F(2.05, 30.72) = 1.59$, ns]. The results suggest that in acquisition learning there were no differences in learning between QNP-sensitized and control groups (**Figure 3B**). Although interaction term was not significant from the inspection of the graph it appears that there is a difference in performance on ACQ1 where QNP-rats performed worse than control rats (more errors).

Reversal session learning measured by number of errors was also analyzed using two-way repeated measure ANOVA. Data were logarithmically transformed to correct for deviation from normal distribution. Since the sphericity assumption was met, no adjustment to degrees of freedom was necessary in results which included repeated measure. The effect of session was highly significant [$F(3,45) = 12.72$, $p < 0.001$], while group effect was shown to be not significant [$F(1,15) = 0.18$, ns]. Significant interaction term sessions × group [$F(3,45) = 3.64$, $p < 0.5$] indicated that there was a difference in learning between the QNP group compared to the control group (**Figure 3D**). Nonetheless, the interpretation of this effect must be very cautious because there was no observable group effect in reversal. We checked if the significant interaction could not have been caused by one or two highly deviating animals. After Grubb's test to detect outliers it was found that one rat in the QNP group was a significant outlier. However, even after removal of this outlying point, the interaction effect remained significant [$F(3,42) = 3.11$, $p < 0.05$] (assumption of sphericity was met). By visual observation, it appears that QNP-treated rats learn significantly faster than control rats between REV1 and REV2. In summary, in experiment 2 there was no effect in acquisition learning between QNP-sensitized and control rats, but a significant interaction term may suggest an initial steeper learning curve in QNP-treated rats in reversal learning.

TIME TO THE FIRST ERROR

Time-to-first-error was analyzed by a non-parametric Mann–Whitney test since no transformation was capable of normalizing the data. A Bonferroni correction was applied to control for family wise error caused by a high number of comparisons (new significance threshold was calculated to be $p < 0.008$). First day of acquisition (ACQ1) and first day of reversal (REV1) were excluded from the analysis since time-to-first-error measures a memory trace could not be present at the beginning of these two sessions. No significant differences were detected between groups in any of the acquisition days (ACQ2: $U = 26.00$, $z = -0.96$, ns; ACQ3: $U = 32.00$, $z = -0.39$, ns; ACQ4: $U = 30.00$, $z = -0.58$, ns; REV2: $U = 31.00$, $z = -0.48$, ns; REV3: $U = 22.00$, $z = -1.35$, ns; REV4: $U = 35.00$, $z = -0.10$, ns) (**Figure 3E**). Thus, our analysis did not find any difference in the long-term between-the-session memory in rats sensitized to QNP.

PERCENTAGE OF TIME SPENT IN FORMER TO-BE-AVOIDED SECTOR DURING REVERSAL

Percentage of time spent in the former to-be-avoided sector was calculated for experiment 2 in the same manner as for experiment 1. A t-test was used to compare the difference in this value between groups. Results showed that there was no difference in percentage of time spent in the former to-be-avoided sector out of all safe sectors between control and QNP-sensitized groups [$t(15) = 0.11$, ns] (**Figure 3F**) with the mean percentage spent in the former shock sector being 9.9% (SEM = ±2.8%) and 9.52% (SEM = ±2.1%), respectively.

DISCUSSION

Quinpirole-sensitized drugged rats during cognitive testing (experiment 1) showed comparable acquisition learning with control rats but displayed impaired reversal learning, which was not associated with perseverative responding. Rats acquired the task at a similar rate as the control group, despite hyperlocomotion in QNP-drugged rats, and the same number of rats per group reached the threshold of 10 errors in 30-min session by the fourth session. This indicated that chronic sensitization of dopamine D2-like receptors by QNP (and their ongoing stimulation) did not affect cognitive coordination (perceptual segregation). Cognitive coordination deficits are consistently observed in schizophrenia patients (Han et al., 2012) and in rat models of schizophrenia (Lobellova et al., 2013). The present lack of effect on cognitive coordination suggests that chronic QNP treatment did not involve such an aspect. It can be speculated that defective acquisition learning due to the effect of impaired cognitive coordination in schizophrenic patients (Phillips and Silverstein, 2003) was not caused by sensitized dopamine D2-like receptors despite clear evidence of dopamine involvement in the pathology of schizophrenia (Carlsson et al., 1999). It is very interesting that despite much higher locomotion rate, these animals managed to avoid to-be-avoided sector with no problem. However, dispersion of locomotion in the safe part of the arena is much wider in QNP-treated animals. This may be related to the hyperlocomotion induced by QNP.

In the reversal learning, QNP-sensitized drugged rats showed a significant, but transient reversal deficit manifested by an increased number of errors during the first session compared to the control group. It should be noted that this deficit was indeed specific only for the beginning of reversal training, since by the third and fourth reversal session the deficit was ameliorated and rats displayed comparable results with the control group.

It was proposed that there are three parallel processes that have to occur during successful reversal: extinction of response that is no longer rewarded, behavioral switch to the new reward, and response maintenance (Klanker et al., 2013). A deficit in extinction would be characterized by a perseverative responding. A defect in behavioral switch would be associated with disorganized behavior while a defect in response maintenance would be associated with the inability to improve in both acquisition and reversal tasks (both between sessions and within one session). Our results suggest that the only defective process in the case of QNP-sensitized drugged rats is the behavioral switch. From the results, it is apparent that in reversal, control rats did not significantly improve their performance, compared to improvement observed in QNP-treated rats. This could indicate that QNP actually improves response maintenance. However, since significant improvement was observed in control group in experiment 2, which received exactly the same treatment, this effect might also be a batch-specific artifact.

Importantly, the observed reversal deficit was not associated with the perseverative behavior as can be deduced from *percentage of time spent in the former to-be-avoided sector*. QNP-treated rats actually spent a higher percent of time in the former to-be-avoided sector than control rats. We hypothesized that QNP-treated rats would perseverate – to keep avoiding the former to-be-avoided sector – more than controls based on studies that had shown that chronic administration of QNP is associated with perseverative behavior in alternation tasks (Einat and Szechtman, 1995; Kontis et al., 2008) and on studies that document enhanced "compulsive" lever pressing after repeated administration of QNP (Joel et al., 2001). Also, the only study that tested reversal in rats treated with systemic acute QNP reported a marked reversal learning deficit associated with high incidence of perseverative responding (Boulougouris et al., 2009). Despite the often observed perseverative behavior, non-perseverative behavior in reversal was also reported following D2-like manipulation. For example, non-perseverative errors in reversal were demonstrated when QNP was infused locally into the nucleus accumbens (Haluk and Floresco, 2009) and after dopamine depletion in the *striatum* (Clarke et al., 2011) or depletion in orbitofrontal cortex (Walker et al., 2009). Non-perseverative errors were observed in reversal learning in humans on spatial tasks after systemic administration of bromocriptine, another D2-like agonist (Mehta et al., 2001). Although not uncommon, a lower perseveration in QNP-treated rats in our study is very intriguing in light of previous studies specifically regarding the effects of systemic QNP administration, which showed high perseverative behavior in QNP-treated rats (Kontis et al., 2008; Boulougouris et al., 2009).

We propose several theories to explain why QNP-treated rats were entering faster into the former to-be-avoided sector than control rats despite often cited increased perseveration during the reversal task. Possibly, drugged rats sensitized to QNP might have exacerbated checking, which would suggest that they might have inspected the previously punished region more frequently. Also, fast entrance into the former to-be-avoided sector may be simply caused by an increased locomotion – as mentioned before, animal that moves more has a higher chance of entering into any location of the arena sooner. Alternatively, QNP-treated animals could simply enter the former to-be-avoided sector because of impaired long-term memory. This hypothesis is supported by the trend we observed in time-to-the-first-error. Although not significant, QNP-treated animals consistently entered to-be-avoided sector very soon after session commencement, suggesting these animals had to be "reminded" where the to-be-avoided sector is located. It is interesting that in our experiments the trend of disruption of between-session learning is observed in QNP-sensitized animals regardless of drugged state (in both experiments 1 and 2). Also, in OCD patients a long-term episodic memory appears to be impaired (Savage et al., 2000; Deckersbach et al., 2004). Despite the results appearing very suggestive, they never reach a significant level presumably due to high variability within the control group. A larger cohort of animals would be necessary to properly address the issue.

In human studies, rather ambiguous evidence of a reversal learning deficit was demonstrated in OCD patients. Alterations in fronto-striatal circuits (without reversal learning deficit *per se*) were observed during reversal in OCD patients (Remijnse et al., 2006) and their unaffected relatives (Chamberlain, 2007). Some studies detected worsened overall performance on the reversal task (Remijnse et al., 2006) but most found only increased time latencies to complete the task possibly indicating increased cognitive demand (Valerius et al., 2008; Remijnse et al., 2009; Ersche et al., 2011). It must be noted that in active place avoidance on a Carousel, time is an important limiting factor. A rat does not have infinite amount of time to make a correct choice due to the rotation of arena. Therefore, a longer latency to make a choice results in punishment (rat would be transported to the sector by arena rotation). In this light increased time latencies to make a choice observed in patients could be viewed as an indiscernible reversal error. Also, it was proposed that currently used reversal tasks are too simple to make gross behavioral abnormalities apparent (Klanker et al., 2013).

How cognitive flexibility is related to repetitive behavior is a relatively unaddressed topic. This is the first study, to our knowledge, to address cognitive coordination and flexibility in a QNP-induced rat model of OCD and a second study that addresses spatial flexibility in any rat model of OCD as well. Previously, only stereotyped jumping was correlated with reversal learning in a T-maze in deer mice, a genetic model of OCD, where a positive relationship between stereotypy and reversal errors was discovered (Tanimura et al., 2008). Still more studies exploring links between OCD-like behavior and reversal deficit are needed to disambiguate these somewhat contradictory findings.

An important limitation of these findings is that even acute administration of QNP is associated with reversal learning deficit;

therefore the reversal learning deficit cannot be attributed solely to the model of OCD. The second limitation is a possibility of QNP-treated animals being less sensitive to electric shock, which was not directly tested. Since acquisition in both QNP and saline-treated animals is similar it can be assumed that sensitivity to electrical stimulation is unchanged by QNP treatment. Scarce literature on the QNP effect on pain sensitivity offers contradictory results with some studies proposing hyper-analgesic (Roane and Paul, 1992) and some hypo-analgesic effects (Magnusson and Fisher, 2000; Munro, 2007). Lastly, a lesion of the *nigrostriatal* dopaminergic projection had no effect on escape learning and response to electric shock suggesting that intact dopaminergic transmission is not necessary for avoidance learning (Price and Fibiger, 1975).

The second experiment (experiment 2) explored the effect of long-term sensitization by D2-like agonist QNP on reversal learning in QNP-sensitized undrugged rats. In both phases of the task rats were improving with each consecutive session. There was no difference between the groups in learning although there was worse performance in the QNP-sensitized group at the beginning of reversal. Significant interaction term in reversal learning was detected, which suggests that QNP-treated rats learn faster compared to control rats once they comprehend the task in the initial reversal session. However, this interaction term should be regarded with a caution, because of the difficulty of its interpretation. With regard to stimulants, it is known that rats remain sensitized to the substance up to a year when presented with a substance challenge (Paulson et al., 1991). As mentioned before, in QNP-treated rats perseverative behavior was observed even 12 weeks after treatment discontinuation (Einat and Szechtman, 1993). In a verification experiment, we re-applied QNP for a month and a half after discontinuation of QNP treatment, which resulted in a heightened locomotor response in these rats compared to the drug-naïve rats (unpublished results). It can be concluded, that the molecular substrate of sensitization was present at the time our experiments were conducted.

To our knowledge only one study has focused on the effect of long-term QNP administration on behavioral flexibility after it was discontinued (Einat and Szechtman, 1993). In our study we have chosen a different and, in some aspects, more demanding cognitive task – active place avoidance on a Carousel. Similarly to the previous study, we did not find any significant difference in acquisition or reversal learning between the groups [despite the time window from the last QNP treatment day was minimized to 2 days compared 10 days in the MWM experiment by Einat and Szechtman (1993)]. Also, we did not find a difference in *the percentage of time spent in the former to-be-avoided sector*, indicating lack of difference in the tendency to perseverate. This is in contrast to previously observed higher perseveration compared to saline-treated rats in MWM (Einat and Szechtman, 1993). The discrepancy could be caused by differences in the task setup, where we assessed perseveration (deduced from *percentage of time spent in the former to-be-avoided sector*) in the reversal phase. In the MWM, task perseveration was measured in the extinction session before reversal. Overall, it appears that QNP-induced sensitization is associated with alterations in reversal learning characterized by a higher error rate in the initial reversal session.

CONCLUSION

We have shown a cognitive flexibility deficit in a rat model of OCD, which was not associated with increased perseveration. This robust deficit is present only when D2-like receptors are directly stimulated with QNP. When D2-like receptors are sensitized, but unstimulated by the agonist, there is no difference in number of errors between the groups in reversal of active place avoidance on a Carousel. Nonetheless, sensitized rats displayed a significantly altered learning style characterized by a higher error rate at the beginning of the reversal and faster learning in the second reversal session compared to control rats.

ACKNOWLEDGMENTS

This work was supported by IGA MZ CR NT13386 and GACR 14-03627S. We thank all colleagues and laboratory assistant for their immense support. We are grateful to P.M. Luketic for proofreading services. Institutional support was provided by RVO: 67985823.

REFERENCES

Abdel Baki, S. G., Schwab, B., Haber, M., Fenton, A. A., and Bergold, P. J. (2010). Minocycline synergizes with N-acetylcysteine and improves cognition and memory following traumatic brain injury in rats. *PLoS ONE* 5:e12490. doi:10.1371/journal.pone.0012490

Bahník, Š. (2013). *Carousel Maze Manager (Version 0.3.5)*. Available at: https://github.com/bahniks/CM_Manager_0_3_5.

Boulougouris, V., Castañé, A., and Robbins, T. W. (2009). Dopamine D2/D3 receptor agonist quinpirole impairs spatial reversal learning in rats: investigation of D3 receptor involvement in persistent behavior. *Psychopharmacology (Berl.)* 202, 611–620. doi:10.1007/s00213-008-1341-2

Bures, J., Fenton, A. A., Kaminsky, Y., and Zinyuk, L. (1997). Place cells and place navigation. *Proc. Natl. Acad. Sci. U.S.A.* 94, 343–350. doi:10.1073/pnas.94.1.343

Carlsson, A., Waters, N., and Carlsson, M. L. (1999). Neurotransmitter interactions in schizophrenia – therapeutic implications. *Biol. Psychiatry* 46, 1388–1395. doi:10.1016/S0006-3223(99)00117-1

Chamberlain, S. (2007). Impaired cognitive flexibility and motor inhibition in unaffected first-degree relatives of patients with obsessive-compulsive disorder. *Am. J. Psychiatry* 164, 335–338. doi:10.1176/appi.ajp.164.2.335

Chamberlain, S. R., Blackwell, A. D., Fineberg, N. A., Robbins, T. W., and Sahakian, B. J. (2005). The neuropsychology of obsessive compulsive disorder: the importance of failures in cognitive and behavioural inhibition as candidate endophenotypic markers. *Neurosci. Biobehav. Rev.* 29, 399–419. doi:10.1016/j.neubiorev.2004.11.006

Clarke, H. F., Hill, G. J., Robbins, T. W., and Roberts, A. C. (2011). Dopamine, but not serotonin, regulates reversal learning in the marmoset caudate nucleus. *J. Neurosci.* 31, 4290–4297. doi:10.1523/JNEUROSCI.5066-10.2011

De Carolis, L., Schepisi, C., Milella, M. S., and Nencini, P. (2011). Clomipramine, but not haloperidol or aripiprazole, inhibits quinpirole-induced water contrafreeloading, a putative rat model of compulsive behavior. *Psychopharmacology (Berl.)* 218, 749–759. doi:10.1007/s00213-011-2372-7

De Carolis, L., Stasi, M. A., Serlupi-Crescenzi, O., Borsini, F., and Nencini, P. (2010). The effects of clozapine on quinpirole-induced non-regulatory drinking and prepulse inhibition disruption in rats. *Psychopharmacology (Berl.)* 212, 105–115. doi:10.1007/s00213-010-1937-1

Deckersbach, T., Savage, C. R., Reilly-Harrington, N., Clark, L., Sachs, G., and Rauch, S. L. (2004). Episodic memory impairment in bipolar disorder and obsessive-compulsive disorder: the role of memory strategies. *Bipolar Disord.* 6, 233–244. doi:10.1111/j.1399-5618.2004.00118.x

Einat, H., and Szechtman, H. (1993). Longlasting consequences of chronic treatment with the dopamine agonist quinpirole for the undrugged behavior of rats. *Behav. Brain Res.* 54, 35–41. doi:10.1016/0166-4328(93)90046-S

Einat, H., and Szechtman, H. (1995). Perseveration without hyperlocomotion in a spontaneous alternation task in rats sensitized to the dopamine agonist quinpirole. *Physiol. Behav.* 57, 55–59. doi:10.1016/0031-9384(94)00209-N

Ersche, K. D., Roiser, J. P., Abbott, S., Craig, K. J., Müller, U., Suckling, J., et al. (2011). Response perseveration in stimulant dependence is associated with striatal dysfunction and can be ameliorated by a D2/3 receptor agonist. *Biol. Psychiatry* 70, 754–762. doi:10.1016/j.biopsych.2011.06.033

Ersche, K. D., Roiser, J. P., Robbins, T. W., and Sahakian, B. J. (2008). Chronic cocaine but not chronic amphetamine use is associated with perseverative responding in humans. *Psychopharmacology (Berl.)* 197, 421–431. doi:10.1007/s00213-007-1051-1

Floresco, S. B., and Grace, A. A. (2003). Gating of hippocampal-evoked activity in prefrontal cortical neurons by inputs from the mediodorsal thalamus and ventral tegmental area. *J. Neurosci.* 23, 3930–3943.

Goldman, M. B., Luchins, D. J., and Robertson, G. L. (1988). Mechanisms of altered water metabolism in psychotic patients with polydipsia and hyponatremia. *N. Engl. J. Med.* 318, 397–403. doi:10.1056/NEJM198802183180702

Groman, S. M., Lee, B., London, E. D., Mandelkern, M. A., James, A. S., Feiler, K., et al. (2011). Dorsal striatal D2-like receptor availability co-varies with sensitivity to positive reinforcement during discrimination learning. *J. Neurosci.* 31, 7291–7299. doi:10.1523/JNEUROSCI.0363-11.2011

Haluk, D. M., and Floresco, S. B. (2009). Ventral striatal dopamine modulation of different forms of behavioral flexibility. *Neuropsychopharmacology* 34, 2041–2052. doi:10.1038/npp.2009.21

Han, K., Young Kim, I., and Kim, J.-J. (2012). Assessment of cognitive flexibility in real life using virtual reality: a comparison of healthy individuals and schizophrenia patients. *Comput. Biol. Med.* 42, 841–847. doi:10.1016/j.compbiomed.2012.06.007

Homberg, J. R. (2013). Measuring behaviour in rodents: towards translational neuropsychiatric research. *Behav. Brain Res.* 236, 295–306. doi:10.1016/j.bbr.2012.09.005

Jentsch, J. D., Olausson, P., De La Garza, R., and Taylor, J. R. (2002). Impairments of reversal learning and response perseveration after repeated, intermittent cocaine administrations to monkeys. *Neuropsychopharmacology* 26, 183–190. doi:10.1016/S0893-133X(01)00355-4

Joel, D., Avisar, A., and Doljansky, J. (2001). Enhancement of excessive lever-pressing after post-training signal attenuation in rats by repeated administration of the D1 antagonist SCH 23390 or the D2 agonist quinpirole, but not the D1 agonist SKF 38393 or the D2 antagonist haloperidol. *Behav. Neurosci.* 115, 1291–1300. doi:10.1037/0735-7044.115.6.1291

Klanker, M., Feenstra, M., and Denys, D. (2013). Dopaminergic control of cognitive flexibility in humans and rats. *Front. Neurosci.* 7:201. doi:10.3389/fnins.2013.00201

Kontis, D., Boulougouris, V., Papakosta, V. M., Kalogerakou, S., Papadopoulos, S., Poulopoulou, C., et al. (2008). Dopaminergic and serotonergic modulation of persistent behaviour in the reinforced spatial alternation model of obsessive-compulsive disorder. *Psychopharmacology (Berl.)* 200, 597–610. doi:10.1007/s00213-008-1241-5

Lee, B., Groman, S., London, E. D., and Jentsch, J. D. (2007). Dopamine D2/D3 receptors play a specific role in the reversal of a learned visual discrimination in monkeys. *Neuropsychopharmacology* 32, 2125–2134. doi:10.1038/sj.npp.1301337

Lobellova, V., Entlerova, M., Svojanovska, B., Hatalova, H., Prokopova, I., Petrasek, T., et al. (2013). Two learning tasks provide evidence for disrupted behavioural flexibility in an rat model of schizophrenia-like behaviour induced by acute MK-801: a dose-response study. *Behav. Brain Res.* 246, 55–62. doi:10.1016/j.bbr.2013.03.006

Magnusson, J. E., and Fisher, K. (2000). The involvement of dopamine in nociception: the role of D1 and D2 receptors in the dorsolateral striatum. *Brain Res.* 855, 260–266. doi:10.1016/S0006-8993(99)02396-3

Mattingly, B. A., Rowlett, J. K., and Lovell, G. (1993). Effects of daily SKF 38393, quinpirole, and SCH 23390 treatments on locomotor activity and subsequent sensitivity to apomorphine. *Psychopharmacology (Berl.)* 110, 320–326. doi:10.1007/BF02251287

Mehta, M. A., Swainson, R., Ogilvie, A. D., Sahakian, J., and Robbins, T. W. (2001). Improved short-term spatial memory but impaired reversal learning following the dopamine D(2) agonist bromocriptine in human volunteers. *Psychopharmacology (Berl.)* 159, 10–20. doi:10.1007/s002130100851

Milella, M., Passarelli, F., Carolis, L., Schepisi, C., Nativio, P., Scaccianoce, S., et al. (2010). Opposite roles of dopamine and orexin in quinpirole-induced excessive drinking: a rat model of psychotic polydipsia. *Psychopharmacology (Berl.)* 211, 355–366. doi:10.1007/s00213-010-1909-5

Morris, R. (2013). "Neurobiology of learning and memory," in *Neuroscience in the 21st Century SE - 81*, ed. D. Pfaff (New York: Springer), 2173–2211.

Munro, G. (2007). Dopamine D1 and D2 receptor agonism enhances antinociception mediated by the serotonin and noradrenaline reuptake inhibitor duloxetine in the rat formalin test. *Eur. J. Pharmacol.* 575, 66–74. doi:10.1016/j.ejphar.2007.07.062

Pantelis, C., Barber, F. Z., Barnes, T. R., Nelson, H. E., Owen, A. M., and Robbins, T. W. (1999). Comparison of set-shifting ability in patients with chronic schizophrenia and frontal lobe damage. *Schizophr. Res.* 37, 251–270. doi:10.1016/S0920-9964(98)00156-X

Paulson, P. E., Camp, D. M., and Robinson, T. E. (1991). transient behavioral depression and persistent behavioral sensitization in relation to regional brain monoamine concentrations during amphetamine withdrawal in rats. *Psychopharmacology (Berl.)* 103, 480–492. doi:10.1007/BF02244248

Perera, T. D., Thirumangalakudi, L., Glennon, E., Park, S., Insanally, M., Persky, M., et al. (2013). Role of hippocampal neurogenesis in mnemonic segregation: implications for human mood disorders. *World J. Biol. Psychiatry* 4, 1–9. doi:10.3109/15622975.2013.768356

Petrasek, T., Prokopova, I., Bahnik, S., Schonig, K., Berger, S., Vales, K., et al. (2013). Nogo-A downregulation impairs place avoidance in the Carousel maze but not spatial memory in the Morris water maze. *Neurobiol. Learn. Mem.* 107, 42–49. doi:10.1016/j.nlm.2013.10.015

Phillips, W. A., and Silverstein, S. M. (2003). Convergence of biological and psychological perspectives on cognitive coordination in schizophrenia. *Behav. Brain Sci.* 26, 65–82. doi:10.1017/S0140525X03000025

Piccinelli, M., Pini, S., Bellantuono, C., and Wilokinson, G. (1995). Efficacy of drug treatment in obsessive-compulsive disorder: a meta-analytic review. *Br. J. Psychiatry* 166, 424–443. doi:10.1192/bjp.166.4.424

Price, M. T. C., and Fibiger, H. C. (1975). Discriminated escape learning and response to electric shock after 6-hydroxydopamine lesions of the nigroneostriatal dopaminergic projection. *Pharmacol. Biochem. Behav.* 3, 285–290. doi:10.1016/0091-3057(75)90159-8

Remijnse, P. L., Nielen, M. M. A., van Balkom, A. J. L. M., Cath, D. C., van Oppen, P., Uylings, H. B. M., et al. (2006). Reduced orbitofrontal-striatal activity on a reversal learning task in obsessive-compulsive disorder. *Arch. Gen. Psychiatry* 63, 1225–1236. doi:10.1001/archpsyc.63.11.1225

Remijnse, P. L., Nielen, M. M. A., van Balkom, A. J. L. M., Hendriks, G. J., Hoogendijk, W. J., Uylings, H. B. M., et al. (2009). Differential frontal-striatal and paralimbic activity during reversal learning in major depressive disorder and obsessive–compulsive disorder. *Psychol. Med.* 39, 1503–1518. doi:10.1017/S0033291708005072

Roane, D. S., and Paul, D. (1992). Evidence of hyperglycemic hyperalgesia by quinpirole. *Pharmacol. Biochem. Behav.* 41, 65–67. doi:10.1016/0091-3057(92)90060-S

Savage, C. R., Deckersbach, T., Wilhelm, S., Rauch, S. L., Baer, L., Reid, T., et al. (2000). Strategic processing and episodic memory impairment in obsessive compulsive disorder. *Neuropsychology* 14, 141–151. doi:10.1037/0894-4105.14.1.141

Stanwood, G. D., Lucki, I., and McGonigle, P. (2000). Differential regulation of dopamine D2 and D3 receptors by chronic drug treatments. *J. Pharmacol. Exp. Ther.* 295, 1232–1240.

Stuchlík, A., Petrásek, T., Prokopová, I., Holubová, K., Hatalová, H., Valeš, K., et al. (2013). Place avoidance tasks as tools in the behavioral neuroscience of learning and memory. *Physiol. Res.* 62, S1–S19.

Stuchlik, A., Rezacova, L., Vales, K., Bubenikova, V., and Kubik, S. (2004). Application of a novel active allothetic place avoidance task (AAPA) in testing a pharmacological model of psychosis in rats: comparison with the Morris water maze. *Neurosci. Lett.* 366, 162–166. doi:10.1016/j.neulet.2004.05.037

Sullivan, R. M., Talangbayan, H., Einat, H., and Szechtman, H. (1998). Effects of quinpirole on central dopamine systems in sensitized and non-sensitized rats. *Neuroscience* 83, 781–789. doi:10.1016/S0306-4522(97)00412-0

Szechtman, H., Sulis, W., and Eilam, D. (1998). Quinpirole induces compulsive checking behavior in rats: a potential rat model of obsessive-compulsive disorder (OCD). *Behav. Neurosci.* 112, 1475–1485. doi:10.1037/0735-7044.112.6.1475

Tanimura, Y., Yang, M. C., and Lewis, M. H. (2008). Procedural learning and cognitive flexibility in a mouse model of restricted, repetitive behaviour. *Behav. Brain Res.* 189, 250–256. doi:10.1016/j.bbr.2008.01.001

Valerius, G., Lumpp, A., Kuelz, A.-K., Freyer, T., and Voderholzer, U. (2008). Reversal learning as a neuropsychological indicator for the neuropathology of obsessive compulsive disorder? A behavioral study. *J. Neuropsychiatry Clin. Neurosci.* 20, 210–218. doi:10.1176/appi.neuropsych.20.2.210

19

Consequences of early postnatal benzodiazepines exposure in rats. I. Cognitive-like behavior

Anna Mikulecká*, Martin Šubrt, Aleš Stuchlík and Hana Kubová

Institute of Physiology, Academy of Sciences of the Czech Republic, Prague, Czech Republic

Edited by:
Tomiki Sumiyoshi, National Center of Neurology and Psychiatry, Japan

***Correspondence:**
Anna Mikulecká, Institute of Physiology, Academy of Sciences of the Czech Republic, Videňská 1083, 142 20 Prague 4, Czech Republic
e-mail: nmikul@epilepsy.biomed.cas.cz

Clinical and experimental studies suggest possible risks associated with the repeated administration of benzodiazepines (BZDs) during the prenatal or early postnatal period on further development and behavior. In the present study, we assess short- and long-term effects of early exposure to clonazepam (CZP) on cognitive tasks. CZP (0.5 or 1.0 mg/kg/day) was administered from postnatal day (P)7 until P11, and animals were exposed to the following behavioral tests at different developmental stages: (1) a homing response (HR) test, which exploits the motivation of a rat pup to reach its home nest, was administered on P12, P15, P18 and P23 rats; (2) passive avoidance was tested in three trials (at 0, 2 and 24 h intervals) on P12, P15, P18, P25 and P32 rats; (3) within- and between-session habituation was tested in an open field (OF) at P70; and (4) a long-term memory (LTM) version of the Morris water maze (MWM) was tested at P80. A 1.0 mg/kg dose of CZP extended latency in the HR and decreased the number of correct responses when tested at P12 and P23. In the first trial of the passive avoidance test, latency to enter a dark compartment was shorter in the CZP-exposed rats. Both treated and control animals older than P15 learned the passive-avoidance response at the same rate. Irrespective of the treatments, all adult animals showed within-session habituation. Between-session habituation, however, was found only in the controls. With respect to the MWM test, all animals learned to reach the platform, but animals exposed to higher doses of CZP spent more time swimming in the first acquisition test. No difference between groups was found in a repeated acquisition test (10 and 40 days after the first acquisition test). The results of the present study show that even short-term exposure to CZP alters behavioral responsiveness in pre-weaning, juvenile and adult animals. Not only were changes observed on conventional cognitive tests in our study, but the changes also seem to be related to emotional/motivational responsiveness.

Keywords: benzodiazepines, clonazepam, cognitive functions, development, rats

INTRODUCTION

Experiences during early life critically affect the development of the brain. The ultimate effect of early life experiences can contribute to either risk or resilience to neuropsychiatric conditions later in life. In rats, the 1st week of life represents a period of intense development of neural systems involved in the processing of non-spatial and spatial memory. Cognitive representation emerges and develops as rat pups first begin to explore their environment, and it continues to develop throughout adolescence (Ainge and Langston, 2012). Published data demonstrate that these hippocampal dependent functions are established between the 2nd and 3rd weeks of life (for review Avishai-Eliner et al., 2002).

Benzodiazepines (BZDs), which are psychoactive drugs commonly used among all age groups of patients, possess marked anxiolytic, sedative, hypnotic, and anticonvulsant properties. Preclinical and clinical studies suggest stable therapeutic effects of BZDs during development (Kubová and Mareš, 1989; Kubová et al., 1993). While cognitive impairment represents one of the most frequent behavioral alterations reported during acute treatment, such impairment usually disappears shortly after therapy withdrawal. Enduring cognitive alterations following the termination of exposure to BZDs is not documented in adult patients (for review Lader, 2011). Nevertheless, sparse developmental studies suggest that exposure of the immature brain to BZDs can result in cognitive alterations lasting long after the cessation of BZD exposure. However, results of these studies are inconsistent. Some studies have documented impairment in cognitive tests, whereas other studies find no difference between exposed animals and controls (for review, see Tucker, 1985). The results are often not directly comparable because of differences in the schedules of drug administration, different ages among those tested, and differences in tests. In addition, in most published studies, animals are exposed to BZDs through several developmental stages, beginning in the prenatal period. In many of these studies, exposure duration is extremely long, lasting through gestation and pre-weaning periods, thus making it impossible to specify a critical period of increased vulnerability of the immature brain to BZD-induced functional deficits later in life.

We designed a series of experiments to answer the following questions. Does short-term exposure to therapeutically relevant doses of clonazepam (CZP) during early postnatal development (1) lead to disturbances of cognitive-like behavior in immature and juvenile rats or (2) impair cognitive-like behavior later in adulthood? To address these questions, rat pups were injected intraperitoneally with CZP in doses of 0.5 and 1.0 mg/kg/day for 5 consecutive days starting at P7. The doses used are in the anticonvulsant dose range in rodent seizure models for these age groups of rats (Kubová and Mareš, 1989; Mikulecká et al., 2011). CZP was selected because it is a classic BZD with pronounced anticonvulsant and anxiolytic effects but with only mild sedative effects (Nardi and Perna, 2006). We used a HR test and a passive-avoidance test in the pre-weaning and juvenile periods, as well as the habituation of exploratory activity within an open-field (OF) arena and the long-term memory (LTM) version of the Morris water maze (MWM) in adults.

METHODS

ANIMALS

Male albino Wistar rats (Institute of Physiology, Academy of Sciences, Prague) were used ($n = 160$). Animals were maintained under controlled temperature (22 ± 1°C) and humidity (50–60%) with a 12/12 h light/dark cycle (lights on at 6:00 AM). Food and water were provided ad libitum (with the exception of the testing period). On day 5 (birth counted as day 0), the pups were randomly fostered, and each litter was adjusted to 10 males. The animals were weaned at postnatal day (P) 28. To exclude the participation of a litter effect, only a limited number of animals from the same litter were used. Experiments were approved by the Animal Care and Use Committee of the Institute of Physiology, Academy of Sciences of the Czech Republic, (v.v.i) and determined to be in agreement with the Animal Protection Law of the Czech Republic, which is fully compatible with the guidelines of the European Community Council directives 86/609/EEC.

DRUG EXPOSURE

CZP (Hoffmann - Switzerland; obtained as a gift) was suspended in one drop of Tween 80 and 1 ml of saline. Subsequently, this solution was diluted in such a way that all used doses of CZP were administered in the same volume of 5 μl/g of body weight. The doses were selected according to our previous studies on anticonvulsant effects of CZP in developing animals (Kubová and Mareš, 1989; Mikulecká et al., 2011). CZP at the doses of 0.5 and/or 1.0 mg/kg was administered intraperitoneally for 5 consecutive days from P7 to P11. Control siblings received the corresponding volume of vehicle. Animals were weighed daily during their exposure to CZP, and their overall health condition was regularly examined.

BEHAVIORAL TESTS

Behavioral tests were performed in a special room with constant temperature (22 ± 2°C) and light conditions (35–45 lx). Before testing, animals were allowed to adapt to the testing room for 30 min. All tests were performed between 9:00 AM and 3:00 PM. The detailed experimental schedule is summarized in **Figure 1**. The same animals (controls $n = 12$; CZP 0.5 mg/kg/day, $n = 12$; CZP 1.0 mg/kg/day, $n = 16$) were used for the homing test, the habituation test and the MWM test, and the order of tests was always the same (homing test → habituation test → MWM). An additional 120 animals were used for the passive avoidance test. For each age group tested (P12, P15, P18, P25, P32), naïve animals were always used (controls $n = 12$; CZP 1.0 mg/kg/day, $n = 12$). The control group and the group exposed to CZP at the dose of 1.0 mg/kg each consisted of 12 animals. Behaviors in the OF and on the MWM were video-recorded and then analyzed using EthoVision (Noldus Information Technology).

HOMING RESPONSE (HR) TEST

The homing response (HR) procedure exploits the motivation of a rat pup to reach its home nest and maintain contact with its dam and siblings. This test is suitable and biologically relevant for examining the spatial learning in immature rodents as remembering the home localization has a high adaptive value

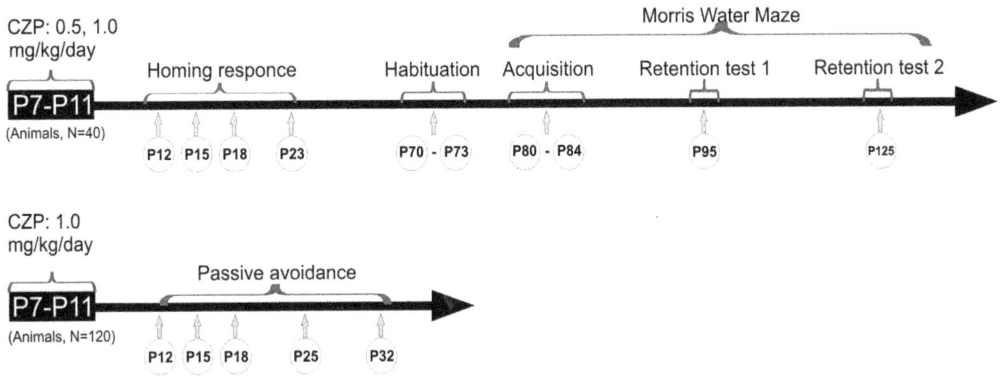

FIGURE 1 | Design/time diagram of CZP experimental procedure. The upper part shows a timeline for behavioral tests such as homing response (HR), habituation, and the Morris water maze (MWM) after exposure to 0.5 and 1.0 mg/kg/day of CZP between P7 and P11. The lower part shows a timeline for passive avoidance after exposure to 1.0 mg/kg/day of CZP.

in pre-weaning animals. Cooperation between olfactory and/or visual cues is considered to be an important factor in mastering the HR (Rossier and Schenk, 2003; Mikulecká and Mareš, 2009). The same procedure as in our previous work was employed (Mikulecká and Mareš, 2009). The same groups of animals were tested repeatedly at four different ages: P12, P15, P18, and P23. The following parameters were quantified: (1) mean latency to homing; (2) ratio of correct responses (latency < 60 s) to the total number of trials (correct/total responses $\times$ 100); and (3) occurrence of five consecutive correct HR (HR acquisition). The number of animals that fulfill these criteria was calculated.

PASSIVE AVOIDANCE RESPONDING

The immature and juvenile animals were subjected to a three-trial step-through passive-avoidance paradigm (Carey et al., 2001). Animals (naive groups for each age group) were tested at P12, P15, P18, P25, and P32. The apparatus (Ugo Basile, Italy) was a rectangular Plexiglas cage (47 $\times$ 18 $\times$ 26) for P12, P15, and P18, and (52 $\times$ 30 $\times$ 35 cm) for P25 and P32 rats, consisting of two compartments of equal size. The animals were tested in three trials (at 0, 2 and 24 h intervals). The 2nd and the 3rd trial were performed without delivery any shock to measure short-term memory (STM) and LTM retention, respectively (Izquierdo et al., 1999).

OPEN FIELD TEST (OF)

Within- and between-session habituations were evaluated in P70 to P73 animals using the method described and validated by Thiel and collaborators in the OF test (Thiel et al., 1999). The OF arena consisted of a square black plastic box (48 $\times$ 48 cm, walls 30 cm). Animals were tested for 4 consecutive days (one 10 min session each day). The following behavioral variables were analyzed automatically. Locomotion (distance moved) was evaluated by analyzing the track record for the distance traveled and center time (i.e., time in the central 30 $\times$ 30 cm section of the OF). Habituation of locomotion was evaluated in two ways. Within-session habituation was measured by comparing the 1st vs. the 2nd 5 min interval of a given testing period (session). As previous studies demonstrated that between-session habituation could most appropriately be described by comparing the 1st session with the 4th session of 4 day consecutive exposure to the OF (Thiel et al., 1999), a comparison between the 1st day (1st session) vs. the 4th day (4th session) was used for the data analysis and presentation.

MORRIS WATER MAZE (MWM)

Place learning and long-term spatial memory were tested in adult animals (P80–P84) using the MWM (Morris, 1981, 1984; D'Hooge and De Deyn, 2001). The MWM consisted of a black circular pool (210 $\times$ 50 cm) filled with clear water (20°C). A circular transparent Plexiglas platform (10 cm in diameter) was submerged 1.5 cm below the surface of the water in the center of an arbitrarily defined quadrant of the pool (northwest) and remained in the same position throughout the testing. In the acquisition test, each rat received one session (8 trials) per day for 5 consecutive days. A trial began by placing the animal into one of the four psuedo-random starting positions (N, W, S, or E). In case the rat failed to locate the platform in 60 s, the experimenter guided the rat to the platform where it was allowed to rest for 30 s. After each session, the rat was dried with a towel and kept in a warmed cage. Escape latency (time to reach the hidden platform) was measured. To test the rat's knowledge of the hidden platform location, a spatial probe trial was run immediately after the completion of the 5th session. The platform was then removed from the maze and rat was allowed to swim freely for 90 s. The time spent in the quadrant that previously contained the platform was measured. A short re-acquisition test (one session) was performed in the same manner as the acquisition, 10 and 40 days after the final acquisition session (at P95 and P125, respectively). Re-acquisition sessions were conducted to determine the ability to retrain as a simple controlled condition compared to acquisition and probe.

STATISTICAL ANALYSYS

Because the data from the HR test did not meet the assumption of equal variance of parametric ANOVA, the Friedman repeated-measures analysis using Student-Newman-Keuls method was applied to compare the individual age groups. The Kruskal-Wallis analysis with *post-hoc* Dunn's method was applied to compare the individual age groups. The differences in HR acquisition between the control and the CZP groups were evaluated by means of the χ^2-test. The data set from the passive avoidance, habituation and MWM tests were analyzed by two-way repeated-measure ANOVA with one between-group factor (treatment) and one within-subject factor (repeated session). During the habituation experiment, as a computer error affecting the data collection occurred in two animals, 14 animals were included in the group exposed to CZP at the dose of 1.0 mg/kg for analysis. The *post-hoc* Holm-Sidak method was used to explore main significant effects or interactions resulting from ANOVA. The level of significance was set at $P < 0.05$ (Sigma Stat®, SPSS Inc., Chicago, IL). To simplify the text, only statistically significant values are provided in the Results section.

RESULTS

BODY WEIGHT

The control animals gained more weight than the CZP-exposed rats during CZP administration. From P8 to P11, the relative body weight was significantly lower in animals treated with CZP at both doses (0.5 and 1.0 mg/kg) than in the controls [drug effect: $F_{(2,148)} = 35.7, p < 0.001$; age $F_{(4,148)} = 1450.8, p < 0.001$; drug $\times$ age interaction $F_{(8,148)} = 22.8, p < 0.001$] (**Figure 2**).

HOMING RESPONSE (HR) TEST

HR improved gradually during development. In the controls, homing latency decreased and the ratio of correct responses increased gradually with age ($p < 0.001$), while exposure to CZP at either dose did not affect this developmental trend ($p < 0.001$). In P12 rats, CZP at the dose of 1.0 mg/kg increased the homing latency and decreased the ratio of correct responses ($H = 16.4, p < 0.001$ and $H = 15.8, p < 0.001$, respectively). No significant differences were found in either evaluated parameters at P15 or P18. In P23, rats the high CZP dose (1.0 mg/kg) prolonged the homing latency and decreased the ratio of correct

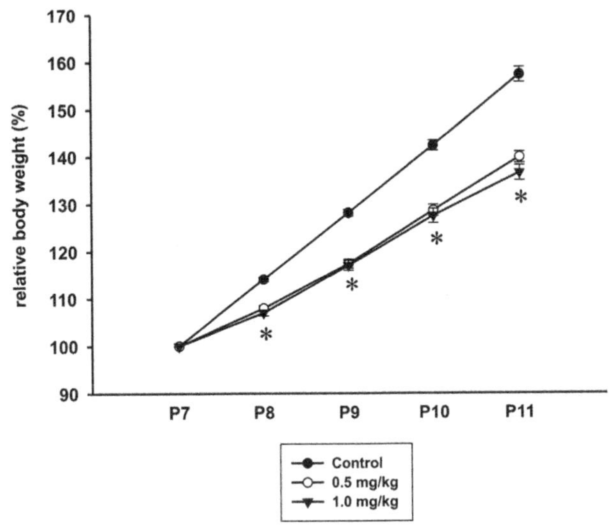

FIGURE 2 | Body weight (mean + SEM) of rats during CZP exposure. Abscissa: age in days. Ordinate: relative weight (body weight was measured on the 1st day of drug administration, 100%). * Significant difference compared to appropriate control group.

responses ($H = 9.6$, $p = 0.008$ and $H = 8.2$, $p = 0.01$, respectively). In controls, the HR learning improved with age. The criteria for correct HRs were achieved in 75% of the P12 and P15 rats, and in 100% of the P18 and P23 animals. Conversely, the CZP worsened the HR in a dose and age dependent manner. In P12, only 50% treated with 0.5 mg/kg and only 6.3% treated with 1.0 mg/kg learned the HR. In P15 rats, 91.6% rats treated with 0.5 mg/kg and 75% treated with 1.0 mg/kg achieved the criteria for the HR. In P18 and P23 rats, all animals treated with the 0.5 mg/kg dose achieved the criteria for correct HRs. In P23, only 56.3% rats treated with the high CZP dose were able to achieve the criteria for five consecutive correct responses (**Figure 3**).

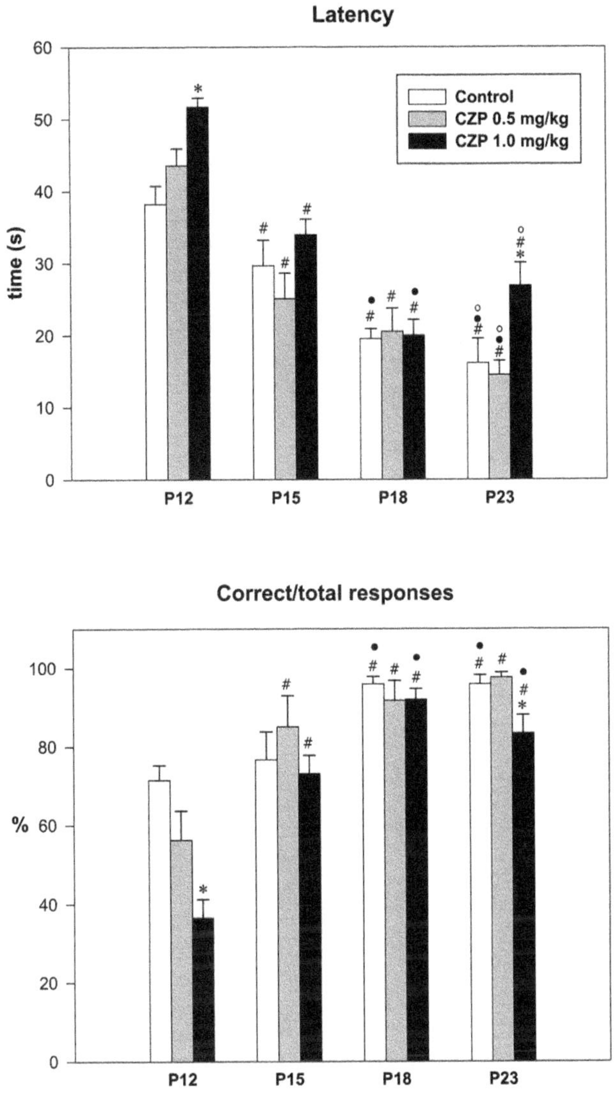

FIGURE 3 | Effects of CZP exposure on HR. Upper graph—latency to reach home part of the cage; lower graph—ratio of correct to total responses. Abscissae: four age groups. Ordinate for the upper graph: time in seconds. Ordinate for the lower graph: percentage of correct responses. For individual doses, see inset. * Significant difference compared to an appropriate control group, # significant difference compared to P12 animals, • significant difference compared to P15 and ° significant difference compared to P18 animals.

PASSIVE AVOIDANCE RESPONDING

In the first trial, step-through latency decreased with maturation. In the retention trials, performed at 2 h and at 24 h, the latency increased continuously as a function of age, indicating the development of avoidance memory. CZP did not affect this developmental trend ($p < 0.001$ for both controls and CZP-exposed animals). Criteria set for full retention was achieved at P25 in both the controls and the CZP-exposed animals ($p < 0.001$). Passive avoidance response was not present in P12 rats in any trial, and CZP had no effect. In the first trial, the CZP-exposed animals tested at P15, P18, and P25 displayed shorter step-through latencies than the controls. This suggested that all CZP animals reacted differently than the controls to a new environment, with low exploration of the light box and suppressed risk-assessment behavior (animals enter the dark box without hesitation), whereas control animals demonstrated caution and risk-assessment behavior before walking into the dark box. This behavior was not observed in P32 animals. In P15, the step-through latency increase was observed only at 24 h after the first trial in both control and CZP-exposed rats [$F_{(2,44)} = 21.9$, $p < 0.001$]. Starting at P18, the step-through latency significantly increased in both retention trials, that is, 2 and 24 h after the first trial [$F_{(2,44)} = 55.9$, $p < 0.001$; $F_{(2,44)} = 289.4$, $p < 0.001$; $F_{(2,44)} = 342.2$, $p < 0.001$, respectively]. There was no difference between the controls and the CZP animals, suggesting that CZP exposure did not impair the retention of memory avoidance (**Figure 4**).

OPEN FIELD (OF)

In the 1st session, distance moved decreases with time in both the control and the CZP-exposed animals [$F_{(1,35)} = 9.6$, $p = 0.004$]. A comparison between the 1st 5 min and 2nd 5 min

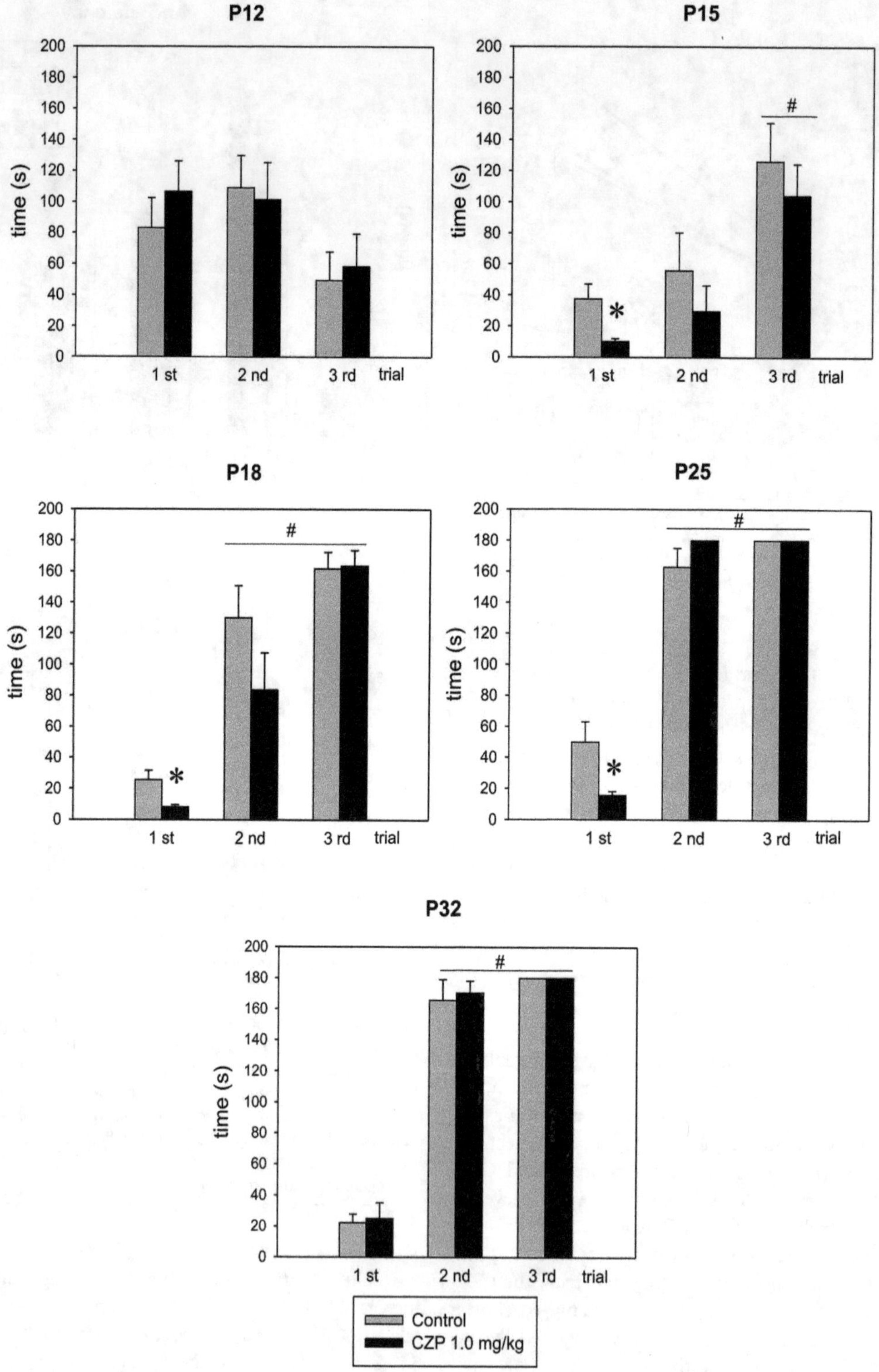

FIGURE 4 | Effect of CZP exposure (1.0 mg/kg) on passive avoidance retention performance. The animals were tested at P12, P15, P18, P25 and at P32. Abscissae: the 1st, the 2nd and the 3rd trials. Ordinate: time of entry latencies in seconds. * Significant differences compared to an appropriate control group; # significant difference between sessions.

interval revealed significant difference only in the 1.0 mg/kg. CZP-exposed animals In the 4th session, both the control and the CZP-exposed animals showed significant decreases in distance moved, which was more expressed within-session habituation with repeated sessions [$F_{(1,35)} = 47.1, p < 0.001$], thus indicating that the animals adapted to the experimental conditions. As for between-session habituation, the comparison of the 1st 5 min interval of a given session showed significant increases in distance moved in CZP-exposed animals with repeated exposure [$F_{(1,35)} = 4.8, p = 0.03$]. Furthermore, the *post-hoc* test revealed significant increases in the distance moved in animals exposed to both doses of CZP in the first 5 min interval of the 4th session, suggesting a lack of between-session habituation in the 1st 5 min interval. A comparison of the 2nd 5 min interval of a given session revealed significant decreases in distance moved with repeated sessions [$F_{(1,35)} = 12.1, p = 0.001$]. However, the *post-hoc* test confirmed decreases in the distance moved only in the control animals, thus suggesting between-session habituation in the controls, but not in the CZP-exposed animals. In addition, the distance moved in the 2nd 5 min interval was significantly shorter in controls than in the CZP-exposed animals, thus indicating hyperactivity of the treated rats (**Figure 5**). Animals exposed to CZP in either dose tended to increase the time spent in the central zone of the OF. In the 1st session, this tendency was dose- and time-dependent [$F_{(2,35)} = 4.1, p = 0.\ 02$; $F_{(1,35)} = 4.6, p = 0.03$, respectively], and in both 5 min intervals, it reached the level of significance only in animals exposed to CZP at the dose of 1.0 mg/kg. A similar dose- and time-dependent trend was observed in the 4th session [$F_{(2,35)} = 6.3, p = 0.005$; $F_{(1,35)} = 10.04, p = 0.003$, respectively]. CZP increased the center time in the 4th session compared to the 1st session in both 5 min intervals. For the 1st interval, there were significant main effects of treatment [$F_{(2,35)} = 0.7, p < 0.001$] and session [$F_{(1,35)} = 11.8, p = 0.001$]. Similarly, there were significant main effects of treatment [$F_{(2,35)} = 7.6, p = 0.002$] and session [$F_{(1,35)} = 5.07, p = 0.03$] for the 2nd interval, thus indicating hyperactivity/excitability of CZP-exposed animals (**Figure 5**).

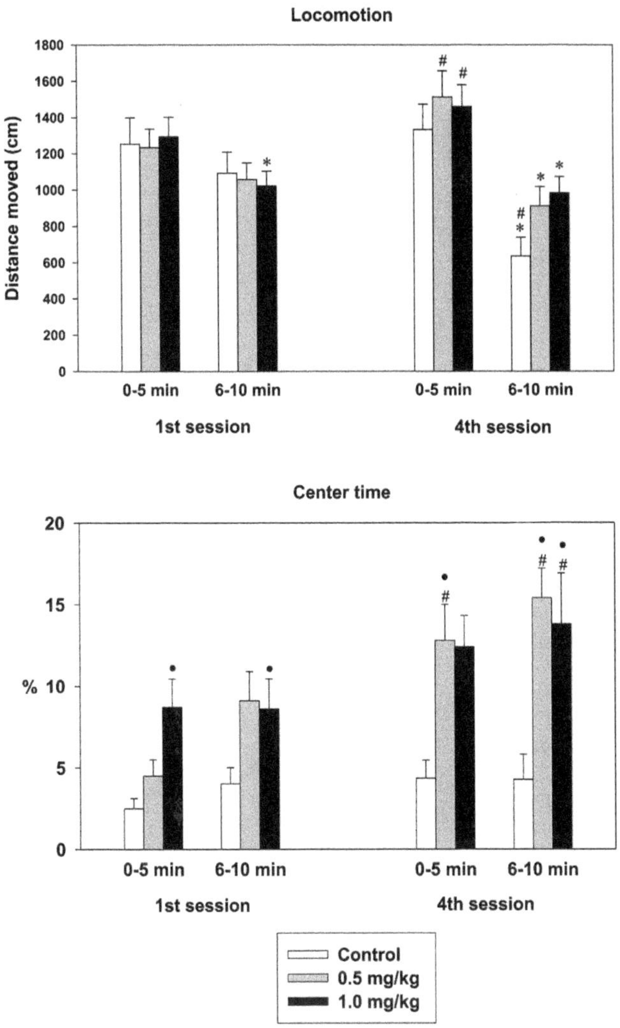

FIGURE 5 | Effect of CZP exposure on habituation in adult animals. Upper graph—locomotor activity measured as the distance moved in the open field. Abscissae: between-session habituation (1st session vs. 2nd session) and within-session habituation (1st session vs. 2nd session, 5 min interval for a given testing period). Ordinate: distance moved in cm. * Significant difference in within-session habituation compared to an appropriate group. # Significant difference in between-session habituation. Lower graph: time spent in the center part of the OF. Abscissae: similar to upper graph. Ordinate: time expressed in percentage. • Significant difference compared to controls.

MORRIS WATER MAZE (MWM)

In both the control and the CZP-exposed animals, the time required to locate the platform decreased over the five successive sessions [$F_{(4,148)} = 82.4, p < 0.001$]. Furthermore, there was no difference between rats exposed to the lower dose of CZP (0.5 mg/kg) and the controls. In contrast, rats exposed to CZP at the dose of 1.0 mg/kg had significantly longer latencies in the 2nd, 3rd, and 4th sessions [$F_{(2,148)} = 4.5, p < 0.01$]. In the probe trial, which immediately followed the final acquisition session, the controls and the animals exposed to CZP at the dose of 0.5 mg/kg spent more time in the quadrant where the platform was placed during training (50.8%, 49.3% of 90 s, respectively) compared to the animals exposed to the 1.0 mg/kg dose of CZP (36.4%) [$F_{(2,35)} = 5.0, p = 0.01$]. On the contrary, no difference was found between the 5th session of the acquisition test and the 1st re-acquisition test for both the control and the CZP-treated rats. In addition, there was no difference between the 1st and the 2nd re-acquisition sessions. These data may suggest that in the reference memory version of the MWM, the high dose of CZP impaired acquisition and memory strength in the probe, but did not affect the re-acquisition of a previously pre-trained skill in a familiar environment with the same goal position (**Figure 6**). The lower dose was without effect in this test.

DISCUSSION

Results of the present study indicate that even short lasting exposure of postnatal rats to CZP in an anticonvulsant dose range leads to mild alterations of behavioral responsiveness in cognitive-related behavior in immature, juvenile and adult animals. While developing animals were exposed to CZP for only 5 days, the exposure occurred during the brain growth spurt when there is

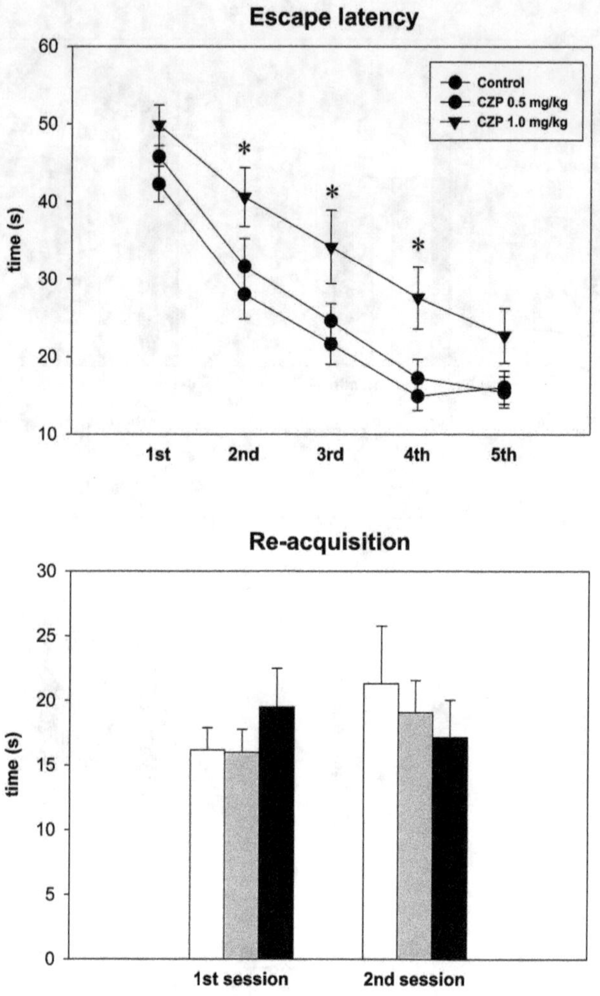

FIGURE 6 | Effect of CZP exposure on long-term memory (LTM) version of the Morris water maze (MWM). Upper graph: escape latencies per daily sessions (each session consists of 8 trials). Lower graph: re-acquisition test. Abscissae: 1st session (10 days after the final acquisition session) and 2nd session (40 days after the final acquisition session). Ordinate: escape latencies (s). * Significant differences compared to controls in the appropriate session.

considerable brain plasticity that is critical for network formation. The newborn rat is equivalent to a 6-month-old human fetus, and P12 rats are equivalent to early infancy in humans (Dobbing and Sands, 1979; Avishai-Eliner et al., 2002; Clancy et al., 2007). Therefore, we assume that the level of maturation of the rat brain during the CZP exposure corresponds with the perinatal development of the human brain. Repeated administration of CZP in doses used for our study had only limited effects on body growth, and mortality was negligible. While the drug caused transient growth retardation during the period of administration, the body weight normalized rapidly after P18.

The measurement of cognitive performance in rats incorporates modulatory functions such as sensory, attentional, motivational, emotional, and motor processes (Myhrer, 2003). Immature animals generally show a good learning capacity in conventional or modified tests, which take into account the ethological characteristics and sensorimotor abilities of animals at a particular developmental stage.

In concordance with previously published results (Sigling et al., 2009), our data show a gradual increase in the preference for the home nest from postnatal P12 with a maximal preference at P23. The performance of pups on this test improved during maturation, while the latency to homing decreased and the percentage of correct responses increased with age. This developmental pattern reflects a gradual maturation of rat sensorimotor systems (Altman and Sudarshan, 1975; Spear, 1990). Exposure to CZP did not affect the developmental trend evidenced in the controls. Nevertheless, the administration of CZP at a dose of 1.0 mg resulted in a latency prolongation and a decrease of correct HRs in P12 rats. We previously showed that after a single administration of CZP at P12, motor abilities were compromised for 4 h, whereas anxiety-like behavior was suppressed for 48 h (Mikulecká et al., 2011). These data suggest that higher plasma levels of CZP are necessary to affect motor behavior. While data on the pharmacokinetics of CZP in rats are sparse (Hoogerkamp et al., 1996) showed that the terminal half-life of CZP in adult rats is approximately 1 h. Given that immature organisms eliminate CZP more slowly than adults (Markowitz et al., 2010), we speculate that factors other than the sedative effects of CZP are responsible for the alteration of the HR in P12 animals. Interestingly, home-response impairment was also observed in P23 animals, the oldest group tested. Exposed animals preferred the exploration of the empty box. The response delay could be related to decreased motivation of exposed pups to reach the home box/nest, a factor that may have accounted for the learning curve shift. Despite the fact that performance in the HR test does not require place navigation in the narrow sense, i.e., navigation to hidden goals, these results suggest an impairment of learning. Nonetheless, such impairment might also be associated with altered emotionality.

The developmental profile of passive-avoidance responses evidenced in our experiments is consistent with results of previously published studies (Stehouwer and Campbell, 1980). While P12 rats failed to remember the passive-avoidance response, P15 animals were able to recall the association between the context and the foot shock 24 h but not 2 h after the first exposure. These data suggest that long-term memories can be formed by P15, and they support previous findings showing that STM and LTM involve separate mechanisms and that both memory types are independently processed (Izquierdo et al., 1999; Vianna et al., 2000). In accordance with previous studies (File, 1986), our results show that early exposure to CZP does not affect performance in the task requiring a passive-avoidance response. Interestingly, compared to controls, step-through latencies in the first exposure to the apparatus were shorter in P15, P18 and P25 animals exposed to CZP. CZP animals reacted differently to the new environment based on their low degree of exploration of the light box and their suppressed risk-assessment due to their disinhibited response (e.g., excitement) to novelty. Control animals demonstrated caution and risk-assessment behavior before stepping into the dark box. This can be interpreted as a result of differences in the variables of emotional domain and strategies in coping with a task requiring passive-avoidance (Morellini and Schachner, 2006).

Habituation is commonly defined as a change in exploratory or locomotor activity over time (within-session) or as a change in exploratory or locomotor activity with repeated exposure (between-session) (for review Leussis and Bolivar, 2006). CZP exposure did not alter the within-session habituation, indicating intact adaptation to novelty in both the controls and in the CZP-exposed animals. In contrast, alteration of between-session habituation evidenced in CZP-exposed animals suggests an impairment of a non-associative form of learning. Alternatively, it is possible that the CZP-treated animals had problems recognizing the context upon repeated exposure to it, which might be in accord with a pattern found in the MWM (see next paragraph). CZP-exposed animals exhibited higher locomotion in the 4th session and spent more time in the central area of the OF, indicating behavioral disinhibition (hyperactivity/excitability) triggered by novelty and/or decreased anxiety. These data support a delay of habituation described previously in animals exposed to BZDs during gestation (Laviola et al., 1992) or during gestation and lactation (Marczynski et al., 1988). This suggests that, together with altered anxiety, developmental CZP exposure also results in corrupted habituation or context recognition.

Only early exposure to a high dose of CZP led to impairment of learning abilities in the MWM. During the acquisition phase of the test, while escape latencies were longer in the animals of the exposed group, the shape of the learning curve did not differ from other groups. We hypothesize that CZP-exposed animals used a combination of visual and egocentric strategies to localize the platform. Perhaps changes in the strategy, together with a cognitive impairment, are responsible for slower learning (Moghaddam and Bureš, 1996). In addition, in the immediate spatial probe trial (without platform), animals exposed to 1.0 mg/kg of CZP spent a shorter time in the target quadrant, suggesting either impaired strategy or memory trace formation. In contrast, an earlier study (Wang and Huang, 1990) found no learning impairment on the MWM in infant mice exposed to CZP. This difference is likely explained, however, by different experimental procedures used in the study. Nonetheless, we propose that the impairment of probe trial performance in the CZP-treated rats (shorter time in the target quadrant) clearly demonstrates impaired spatial representation in the group treated with the higher dose of CZP.

Taken together, the results of the present study show that even short-term exposure to BZDs during the early postnatal period can result in complex behavioral changes detectable later in life as behavioral alterations had already manifested in preweaning animals. These changes were observed both in a domain of emotionality (e.g., time in the OF center) and in measures of learning and memory (e.g., impaired probe trial). Despite the fact that the tests used in the present study do not allow for a clear dissociation between altered affect and cognition, they do suggest that both domains were impaired concurrently. Our results are in concordance with previously published data that demonstrate that changes induced by exposure to BZDs during gestation and infancy are related to changes in emotionality, to changes in levels of hyperactivity/hyperarousal and attention deficit (Frieder et al., 1984; Livezey et al., 1986; Schroeder et al., 1997) and to changes in memory function. This underscores the usefulness of ontogenetic CZP treatment as an animal model of neurodevelopmental disturbance in the GABAergic system, which may manifest in the domain of behavior.

In conclusion, the results of our study demonstrate that in immature rats, even brief exposure to BZDs leads to mild impairment of cognitive abilities and also changes emotional/motivational responsiveness, hyperactivity and attention deficits later in life. Some of these alterations can persist until adulthood. Finally, these results have clinical importance as CZP treatment is routinely used in epileptic children.

ACKNOWLEDGMENTS

This study was supported by grants No. 305/09/086 and No. P304/12/G069 from the Czech Science Foundation and Research Project RVO 67985823.

REFERENCES

Ainge, J. A., and Langston, R. F. (2012). Ontogeny of neural circuits underlying spatial memory in the rat. *Front. Neural Circuits* 6:8. doi: 10.3389/fncir.2012.00008

Altman, J., and Sudarshan, K. (1975). Postnatal development of locomotion in the laboratory rat. *Anim. Behav.* 23, 896–920. doi: 10.1016/0003-3472(75)90114-1

Avishai-Eliner, S., Brunson, K. L., Sandman, C. A., and Baram, T. Z. (2002). Stressed-out, or in (utero)? *Trends Neurosci.* 25, 518–524. doi: 10.1016/s0166-2236(02)02241-5

Carey, G. J., Billard, W., Binch, H. 3rd, Cohen-Williams, M., Crosby, G., Grzelak, M., et al. (2001). SCH 57790, a selective muscarinic M(2) receptor antagonist, releases acetylcholine and produces cognitive enhancement in laboratory animals. *Eur. J. Pharmacol.* 431, 189–200. doi: 10.1016/s0014-2999(01)01440-6

Clancy, B., Finlay, B. L., Darlington, R. B., and Anand, K. J. (2007). Extrapolating brain development from experimental species to humans. *Neurotoxicology* 28, 931–937. doi: 10.1016/j.neuro.2007.01.014

D'Hooge, R., and De Deyn, P. P. (2001). Applications of the Morris water maze in the study of learning and memory. *Brain Res. Brain Res. Rev.* 36, 60–90. doi: 10.1016/s0165-0173(01)00067-4

Dobbing, J., and Sands, J. (1979). Comparative aspects of the brain growth spurt. *Early Hum. Dev.* 3, 79–83. doi: 10.1016/0378-3782(79)90022-7

File, S. E. (1986). The effects of neonatal administration of clonazepam on passive avoidance and on social, aggressive and exploratory behavior of adolescent male rats. *Neurobehav. Toxicol. Teratol.* 8, 447–452.

Frieder, B., Epstein, S., and Grimm, V. E. (1984). The effects of exposure to diazepam during various stages of gestation or during lactation on the development and behavior of rat pups. *Psychopharmacology (Berl)* 83, 51–55. doi: 10.1007/bf00427422

Hoogerkamp, A., Arends, R. H., Bomers, A. M., Mandema, J. W., Voskuyl, R. A., and Danhof, M. (1996). Pharmacokinetic/pharmacodynamic relationship of benzodiazepines in the direct cortical stimulation model of anticonvulsant effect. *J. Pharmacol. Exp. Ther.* 279, 803–812.

Izquierdo, I., Medina, J. H., Vianna, M. R., Izquierdo, L. A., and Barros, D. M. (1999). Separate mechanisms for short- and long-term memory. *Behav. Brain Res.* 103, 1–11. doi: 10.1016/s0166-4328(99)00036-4

Kubová, H., and Mareš, P. (1989). Influence of clonazepam on epileptic afterdischarges induced by perforant path stimulation in rats. *Arch. Int. Pharmacodyn. Ther.* 299, 35–43.

Kubová, H., Mareš, P., and Vorlíček, J. (1993). Stable anticonvulsant action of benzodiazepines during development in rats. *J. Pharm. Pharmacol.* 45, 807–810. doi: 10.1111/j.2042-7158.1993.tb05690.x

Lader, M. (2011). Benzodiazepines revisited–will we ever learn? *Addiction* 106, 2086–2109. doi: 10.1111/j.1360-0443.2011.03563.x

Laviola, G., Pick, C. G., Yanai, J., and Alleva, E. (1992). Eight-arm maze performance, neophobia, and hippocampal cholinergic alterations after prenatal oxazepam in mice. *Brain Res. Bull.* 29, 609–616. doi: 10.1016/0361-9230(92)90130-p

Leussis, M. P., and Bolivar, V. J. (2006). Habituation in rodents: a review of behavior, neurobiology, and genetics. *Neurosci. Biobehav. Rev.* 30, 1045–1064. doi: 10.1016/j.neubiorev.2006.03.006

Livezey, G. T., Marczynski, T. J., and Isaac, L. (1986). Prenatal diazepam: chronic anxiety and deficits in brain receptors in mature rat progeny. *Neurobehav. Toxicol. Teratol.* 8, 425–432.

Marczynski, T. J., Hawkins, M. C., Swann, P. G., Krivograd, A. F., Patel, M. K., and Dugich, M. (1988). Perinatal upregulation of benzodiazepine receptor ontogenesis: "fearless" and more efficient goal-directed behavior of adult rat progenies. *Neurotoxicol. Teratol.* 10, 101–111. doi: 10.1016/0892-0362(88)90073-6

Markowitz, G. J., Kadam, S. D., Boothe, D. M., Irving, N. D., and Comi, A. M. (2010). The pharmacokinetics of commonly used antiepileptic drugs in immature CD1 mice. *Neuroreport* 21, 452–456. doi: 10.1097/wnr.0b013e328338ba18

Mikulecká, A., and Mareš, P. (2009). Effects of mGluR5 and mGluR1 antagonists on anxiety-like behavior and learning in developing rats. *Behav. Brain Res.* 204, 133–139. doi: 10.1016/j.bbr.2009.05.032

Mikulecká, A., Mareš, P., and Kubová, H. (2011). Rebound increase in seizure susceptibility but not isolation-induced calls after single administration of clonazepam and Ro 19-8022 in infant rats. *Epilepsy Behav.* 20, 12–19. doi: 10.1016/j.yebeh.2010.10.021

Moghaddam, M., and Bureš, J. (1996). Contribution of egocentric spatial memory to place navigation of rats in the Morris water maze. *Behav. Brain Res.* 78, 121–129. doi: 10.1016/0166-4328(95)00240-5

Morellini, F., and Schachner, M. (2006). Enhanced novelty-induced activity, reduced anxiety, delayed resynchronization to daylight reversal and weaker muscle strength in tenascin-C-deficient mice. *Eur. J. Neurosci.* 23, 1255–1268. doi: 10.1111/j.1460-9568.2006.04657.x

Morris, R. (1981). Spatial localization does not require the presence of local cues. *Learn. Motiv.* 12, 239–260. doi: 10.1016/0023-9690(81)90020-5

Myhrer, T. (2003). Neurotransmitter systems involved in learning and memory in the rat: a meta-analysis based on studies of four behavioral tasks. *Brain Res. Brain Res. Rev.* 41, 268–287. doi: 10.1016/s0165-0173(02)00268-0

Nardi, A. E., and Perna, G. (2006). Clonazepam in the treatment of psychiatric disorders: an update. *Int. Clin. Psychopharmacol.* 21, 131–142. doi: 10.1097/01.yic.0000194379.65460.a6

Rossier, J., and Schenk, F. (2003). Olfactory and/or visual cues for spatial navigation through ontogeny: olfactory cues enable the use of visual cues. *Behav. Neurosci.* 117, 412–425. doi: 10.1037/0735-7044.117.3.412

Schroeder, H., Humbert, A. C., Desor, D., and Nehlig, A. (1997). Long-term consequences of neonatal exposure to diazepam on cerebral glucose utilization, learning, memory and anxiety. *Brain Res.* 766, 142–152. doi: 10.1016/s0006-8993(97)00538-6

Sigling, H. O., Wolterink-Donselaar, I. G., and Spruijt, B. M. (2009). Home seeking behavior in rat pups: attachment vs. kin selection, oxytocin vs. vasopressin. *Eur. J. Pharmacol.* 612, 48–53. doi: 10.1016/j.ejphar.2009.03.070

Spear, L. P. (1990). Neurobehavioral assessment during the early postnatal period. *Neurotoxicol. Teratol.* 12, 489–495. doi: 10.1016/0892-0362(90)90012-2

Stehouwer, D. J., and Campbell, B. A. (1980). Ontogeny of passive avoidance: role of task demands and development of species-typical behaviors. *Dev. Psychobiol.* 13, 385–398. doi: 10.1002/dev.420130405

Thiel, C. M., Muller, C. P., Huston, J. P., and Schwarting, R. K. (1999). High versus low reactivity to a novel environment: behavioural, pharmacological and neurochemical assessments. *Neuroscience* 93, 243–251. doi: 10.1016/s0306-4522(99)00158-x

Tucker, J. C. (1985). Benzodiazepines and the developing rat: a critical review. *Neurosci. Biobehav. Rev.* 9, 101–111. doi: 10.1016/0149-7634(85)90036-3

Vianna, M. R., Izquierdo, L. A., Barros, D. M., Walz, R., Medina, J. H., and Izquierdo, I. (2000). Short- and long-term memory: differential involvement of neurotransmitter systems and signal transduction cascades. *An. Acad. Bras. Cienc.* 72, 353–364. doi: 10.1590/s0001-37652000000300009

Wang, L., and Huang, Z. (1990). Effect of clonazepam on brain development of mice. *Dev. Pharmacol. Ther.* 15, 21–25.

20

Dynamic learning and memory, synaptic plasticity and neurogenesis: an update

Ales Stuchlik*

Institute of Physiology, Academy of Sciences of the Czech Republic, Prague, Czech Republic

Edited by:
Tomiki Sumiyoshi, National Center of Neurology and Psychiatry, Japan

****Correspondence:***
Ales Stuchlik, Institute of Physiology, Academy of Sciences of the Czech Republic, Videnska 1803, 142 20 Prague, Czech Republic
e-mail: stuchlik@biomed.cas.cz

Mammalian memory is the result of the interaction of millions of neurons in the brain and their coordinated activity. Candidate mechanisms for memory are synaptic plasticity changes, such as long-term potentiation (LTP). LTP is essentially an electrophysiological phenomenon manifested in hours-lasting increase on postsynaptic potentials after synapse tetanization. It is thought to ensure long-term changes in synaptic efficacy in distributed networks, leading to persistent changes in the behavioral patterns, actions and choices, which are often interpreted as the retention of information, i.e., memory. Interestingly, new neurons are born in the mammalian brain and adult hippocampal neurogenesis is proposed to provide a substrate for dynamic and flexible aspects of behavior such as pattern separation, prevention of interference, flexibility of behavior and memory resolution. This work provides a brief review on the memory and involvement of LTP and adult neurogenesis in memory phenomena.

Keywords: learning, memory, behavior, synaptic plasticity, adult neurogenesis, hippocampus

INTRODUCTION

The brain, with billions of cells' connections and plethora of cell types in mutual interactions, is one of the most complicated organs in the human body and attracts attention of both scientific researchers and the public. This is underlined by the fact that we do not know the pathophysiology of many devastating brain disorders, which often affect memory and cognition (such as schizophrenia, Alzheimer's disease etc.). Notably, the brain definitely does not work as an "elevated supervisor"; indeed, researchers working in neuroscience have now started to appreciate the "systems-level" understanding of the human body function in health and disease (Qureshi and Mehler, 2013).

Studying detailed physiology of any living system without evaluating its output (behavior), cannot give us enough information for understanding the function of the system. *Vice versa*, studying behavior without looking at the proximate mechanisms cannot provide sufficient insight, although striking exceptions from physiology exist such as ant navigation (e.g., Wohlgemuth et al., 2001), when scientists proceeded from studying behavioral outputs downstream to physiological mechanisms. Many scientists concerned with the integration of molecular and cellular views with systems-level and behavioral studies focus on the learning and memory. This particular function of nervous system in animals is well accessible by methods with different resolution (from spikes to molecules and cells to the whole organism).

In this review, I will try to provide a short update on integration of memory formation with a concept of synaptic plasticity (Hebb, 1949) (mainly long-term potentiation (LTP; Bliss and Lomo, 1973)) and adult neurogenesis in the dentate gyrus (DG) of the hippocampus (Altman, 1963; Altman and Das, 1965). My selection must obviously be subjective; there are excellent reviews on other issues related to this topic, such as the role of transcriptional factors and various kinases (Kandel, 2012; Xia and Storm, 2012). The rationale for selecting these subtopics settles on prevailing view on synaptic plasticity processes as a "hotspot" of current research into basic mechanisms of learning and memory (Glanzman, 2013). Focus on neurogenesis is based on the fact that despite many memory studies involve static settings, our world is endlessly dynamic and learning should be considered a highly dynamic process; neurogenesis may provide these flexible aspects of memory. These fields open ways for searching mechanisms of deficits in many neuropsychiatric disorders with enormous human and socioeconomic impact and suggest ways of novel causal therapies for depression, PTSD, Alzheimer's disease or schizophrenia (Voineskos et al., 2013). Scientists relate both LTP and neurogenesis to memory (Brown et al., 1990; Snyder et al., 2001), LTP as a candidate mechanism for long-term retention of information and hippocampal neurogenesis as a candidate mechanism for specific dynamic and flexible aspects of learning.

LEARNING AND MEMORY

Memory refers to a capability of virtually any animal to encode, store and retrieve information, to guide behavioral output. Learning is viewed as acquisition or encoding the information to memory. It is an excellent example of model system allowing for multi-level analysis (again, note close relation of memory deficits to these pathological conditions). Absence/presence of a memory trace (engram) is often presented or even defined as a change of a particular behavior (such as a rat with lesions to the hippocampus may get lost in a spatial maze), or then, as a change of ability to learn/remember. The term engram was first coined by Richard Semon, a German biologist (Semon, 1921). It usually refers to mechanisms (or tags) by which the memories are stored. The prevailing view today is that memory should leave physical (e.g., molecular) and often rather distributed changes in neuronal tissue (Moser and Moser, 1998; Frey and Frey, 2008).

Another well-accepted opinion is that there is nothing like "universal memory"; instead, multiple memory systems exist (Doeller et al., 2008; Lee et al., 2008; Schwabe, 2013) having their specific (partially competing but also shared) brain resources to fulfill their tasks (Squire, 2004). Temptating is a concept that memory may be stored (at least in mammals) in distributed changes in synaptic weights, which may modulate synchronization and grouping of firing of neuronal assemblies (Hebb, 1949; Harris et al., 2003). Further introspection of the engram and its nature also provokes many questions about stability, localization, time course of possible changes, and consolidation and transformation of a memory trace (reviewed in Dudai, 2004).

Importantly, complex and vulnerable mammalian memory types, i.e., declarative and spatial memory, depend on the medial temporal lobes (MTL) of the brain (reviewed in Eichenbaum, 2001). These are the hippocampus, subiculum and neighboring cortical areas such as entorhinal, perirhinal and postrhinal cortices (Amaral and Witter, 1989). Many scientist today are convinced that the hottest candidates for neural correlate of a long-term memory trace are long-term changes in synaptic strengths (Hebb, 1949), i.e., LTP and long-term depression (LTD). For the sake of simplicity, this minireview selects LTP out of the synaptic plasticity mechanisms, although there is a great evidence for LTD role in learning and memory as well (reviewed in Kemp and Manahan-Vaughan, 2007).

LTP, PROTEIN KINASE Mzeta AND MEMORY

Already in 1973, Terje Lomo a Timothy Bliss published a seminal study (Bliss and Lomo, 1973) showing that tetanization of specific pathway in the hippocampal formation of anesthetized rabbit resulted in significant increase in the excitatory postsynaptic potentials in postsynaptic cells, which further supported Hebb's theories (Hebb, 1949). Later on, this phenomenon was demonstrated in anesthetized and freely moving rats and mice. Today, LTP attracts many scientists, because it represents an intriguing but artificial model of long-term changes of the CNS function (more than 12,000 hits in PubMed on the term search). However, causal link between LTP and memory has been suspected but not settled for a long time, although supportive studies were provided earlier, in which interference with LTP affected learning and memory.

Multiple studies have demonstrated that interference with NMDA and AMPA receptor function (e.g., Steele and Morris, 1999; Bast et al., 2005) blocks certain phases of LTP and memory. Importance of NMDA receptors was documented especially in one-trial learning, such as in the delayed-matching to place version of the Morris water maze (MWM), a classical spatial task (Steele and Morris, 1999). Other studies used a different approach, i.e., tetanization of the majority of hippocampal synapses and subsequent testing in hippocampus-dependent task. Initially, it was shown that such LTP saturation disrupts subsequent spatial memory in the MWM probe trials (Moser and Moser, 1999), but this effect has been found to be eliminated by non-spatial pretraining (Otnæss et al., 1999), suggesting that LTP induction may provide a mechanism for capturing the proper strategy in the task. Despite controversies, all these studies corroborated the hypothesis that LTP has some relation to learning and memory.

In 2006, two studies convincingly reported the link between LTP and learning and memory. Whitlock et al. (2006) examined the hypothesis that not only tetanization but also memory encoding *per se* may induce long-term plastic changes. The study showed that training rats to solve inhibitory avoidance, in which animal learns to avoid a preferred dark compartment punished by mild footshocks led to induction of the LTP in a subset of hippocampal synapses. Some synapses were unaffected, again supporting the concept of distributed memory trace. It is interesting to note that inhibitory avoidance learning, despite a simple paradigm, contains both operant and contextual fear conditioning component and involves highly coordinated recruitment of molecular and cellular machinery in the hippocampal formation (Izquierdo et al., 2002). The paper by Whitlock and colleagues contributed much to the notion that memory encoding may produce LTP in some synapses and that memory acquisition could be analogized to electrical tetanization of the synapse. Other studies have strongly corroborated this view (Cohen et al., 2011; Rodríguez-Durán et al., 2011; Kenney and Manahan-Vaughan, 2013).

Another paper in the same issue of Science (Pastalkova et al., 2006) focused on the maintenance phase of LTP as a candidate mechanism for memory storage, based on previous robust evidence from the laboratory of Todd Sacktor that an atypical form of protein kinase C (PKMzeta) is necessary and sufficient for maintenance phase of the LTP (Ling et al., 2002). The study employed so-called zeta-inhibiting peptide (ZIP), which was injected into hippocampi of rats that previously acquired the spatial active place avoidance task. Subsequently, memory retention was tested and it was found selectively impaired by ZIP injection. Interestingly, such microinjection failed to abolish novel learning in the same task, suggesting that PKMzeta erased previous memory trace but did not block encoding of novel information.

Subsequently, Shema et al. (2007) have shown that injection of ZIP into the insular cortex of the rat erased conditioned taste aversion, an evolutionary advantageous type of conditioning. This memory is traditionally measured by avoidance of ingestion of a food, the flavor of which had been associated previously with sickness (Buresová et al., 1979). Another study has corroborated these findings by extension to erasure of other types of memory, such as classical or instrumental conditioning (Serrano et al., 2008). Injection of ZIP also reduced the precision of the MWM representation in the probe trial, despite the rough localization of the goal was still present. Additional evidence on PKMzeta and memory storage came from a recent study (Shema et al., 2011), which showed that overexpression of PKMzeta in the insular region enhanced the conditioned taste aversion memory. Moreover, Pauli et al. (2012) has revealed that blockade of PKMzeta also has an effect in the striatum, affecting instrumental response selection and habits.

However, Volk et al. (2013) have recently generated constitutive and conditional PKMzeta-knockout mice and detected no impairment of either LTP maintenance or hippocampus-dependent memory (Volk et al., 2013). Since the previous reports sometimes used pharmacological blockade of enzyme by ZIP, Volk et al. also applied ZIP to their transgenic mice lacking PKMzeta and detected LTP suppression. This suggests ZIP targets other enzymes required for LTP. Analogous results have been found by Lee et al. (2013) in PKMzeta-null mice. The role of PKMzeta has therefore been questioned (Kwapis and Helmstetter, 2013).

Interestingly, another form of PKC named iota (Selbie et al., 1993) was suggested to compensate for deficient PKMzeta in these experiments, suggesting that more diverse cascade can provide basis for memory maintenance rather than a single "memory molecule" (Glanzman, 2013). In any case, scientists appear to be on the track of interesting discovery of how our vivid everyday memories relate to molecular and cellular brain processes.

ADULT NEUROGENESIS IN THE DENTATE GYRUS AND MEMORY

Importantly, the hippocampus, specifically the subgranular zone of the DG, is one of two sites of neurogenesis in the adult brain (Altman, 1963; Altman and Das, 1965). Some of the dividing neural progenitor cells survive, differentiate into neurons and incorporate into the hippocampal network. The physiological, especially the behavioral role of adult neurogenesis is a subject of controversies until today. Newly born neurons in the DG are proposed to facilitate learning in the hippocampus by separating overlapping patterns in hippocampal inputs, thus ensuring formation of distinct representations.

Enhancing adult neurogenesis in the DG was found to suffice for improvement of pattern separation (Sahay et al., 2011) and another recent study (Nakashiba et al., 2012) suggested that newly-born hyper-excitable neurons may participate preferentially in pattern separation, while older adult granule neurons provide mainly pattern completion (a complementary process which allows adding missing features into incomplete hippocampal representations). This study did not focus directly on the autoassociative network in CA3, but in light of paper by Rolls (2013), I propose that strong, "consolidated" synapses between older granule neurons via mossy fibers to CA3 may provide a significant contribution to pattern completion. It should be noted that a precise balance between pattern completion and pattern separation is probably one if the functions of CA3 upstream region innervated by mossy fibers from dentate granule cells, which mediates a proper hippocampus function and such interplay may be disrupted in memory disorders (Hanson and Madison, 2010).

Another branch of research on the functional role of adult neurogenesis has proposed that adult neurogenesis in the hippocampus may also ensure prevention of interference of new memories with old ones (Wiskott et al., 2006). A study using olfactory memory task demanding interference resolution has also supported such role for new granule neurons in the DG (Luu et al., 2012). A recent study by Gordon Winocur et al. have strongly supported this prediction (Winocur et al., 2012) using a visual discrimination task under conditions of low or high interference. A very recent study by Déry et al. (2013) confirmed such role of neurogenesis even in humans and shown a positive impact of voluntary exercise and adverse effects of depression. Recently, the role of DG adult neurogenesis has been extended to increase "memory resolution" so that cooperation between newly born, hyperexcitable granule cells and older neurons that code sparsely for salient features increases the amount of detail encoded in hippocampal memories (Aimone et al., 2011).

Studies also showed that hippocampal neurogenesis promotes behavioral flexibility in mice. A study by Garthe et al. (2009) demonstrated the subtle but significant effects of neurogenesis ablation. Using chronic treatment with a cytostatic temozolomide and efficient recovery protocol, the memory differences between mice with and without adult neuronal proliferation were revealed in the MWM not by traditional measures such as distance to reach the platform, but by evaluating spatial/non-spatial strategies possessed in the maze. Robust evidence on behavioral flexibility account of neurogenesis has been provided by Burghardt et al. (2012), who showed that neurogenesis ablation in mice led to impairments of reversal learning in active place avoidance task (reviewed by Stuchlik et al., 2013). It also disrupted flexible incorporation of second reference frame (second to-be-avoided place, i.e., two-frame place avoidance; reviewed in Stuchlik et al., 2013). The deficit could not be explained by alteration of memory extinction, or with inability to acquire new memory in a novel environment; these functions were spared in both groups. Interestingly, the flexibility impairment was accompanied by immediate-early gene *Arc* up-regulation, suggesting effects on excitability and plasticity of the hippocampal network (Pevzner et al., 2012).

Recently, time-limited role of new, hyper-excitable granule neurons in the DG in hippocampus-dependent memory has been shown by optogenetic approach (Gu et al., 2012). This study showed that newly born cells form functional synapses on pyramidal neurons of CA3 region from 2 weeks after their birth reaching a stable state at 4 weeks. Newborn neurons at this age were more plastic than neurons at other stages. The study also showed that switching off this cell type of 4-week-old cells after encoding disrupted retrieval of hippocampal memory. This suggests that these 4 weeks represent a functional time window for adult-born neurons in hippocampus-dependent memory retrieval (Gu et al., 2012). Using multiple high-resolution methods, a study of Ikrar et al. (2013) clearly documented that blocking adult neurogenesis increased excitability in the DG networks while its enhancement has reduced it, and also pointed to an important role of inhibitory GABAergic interneurons (Ikrar et al., 2013).

Based on this, we propose that neurogenesis in the hippocampus might underlie so-called behavioral separation, which we define as selective recruitment of distinct and dissociable hippocampus-functions such as spatial representation and cognitive coordination (Kubík and Fenton, 2005; Wesierska et al., 2005). Such role might be shown by selective neurogenesis ablation and testing in massed/alternate protocols using the specific behavioral tasks (MWM, Morris, 1981) and active place avoidance on Carousel (Stuchlik et al., 2013). Additionally, newly born neurons may contribute to coping with dynamic, changing aspects of memory (such as with moving goals) in accordance with the evolutionary hypothesis of neurogenesis role (Kempermann, 2012).

SHORT NOTES ON SOME OTHER FACTORS AFFECTING LTP, NEUROGENESIS AND MEMORY

There are additional factors affecting memory, LTP, and neurogenesis. For instance, a recent study on human glial cells implanted into mouse hippocampus documented enhanced LTP, suggesting strong functional role of this cell type in the brain (Zhang and Barres, 2013). Neurogenesis is also significantly affected by ageing, stress and disease but contrarily enhanced e.g., by enriched environment (Kempermann et al., 1997) and physical exercise (van Praag et al., 1999). Generally, all these phenomena in parallel affect memory as well (Nilsson et al., 1999; Lithfous et al., 2013). An intriguing study by Van der Borght et al. (2007) showed beneficial effects of physical exercise and dietary restriction on spatial T-maze performance and surprisingly, T-maze learning and reversal training actually led to reduced neurogenesis, suggesting optimal balance of these processes for proper memory maintenance.

Of high importance is the role of sleep in memory (McCoy et al., 2013). It has been shown that during both non-REM and REM sleep cellular processes may take part, subserving memory (Benington and Frank, 2003). A factual necessity of sleep for forming and consolidation of memories has emerged recently (Prince et al., 2014). Sleep is also related to neurogenesis (Mueller et al., 2013) as well as to LTP (Kim et al., 2005). From a pharmacological point of view, a recent study have shown that anti-diabetes drug metformin might offer a promising way of increasing adult neurogenesis and memory function (Wang et al., 2012) that is impaired in several neuropsychiatric disorders.

CONCLUSIONS

Much evidence converges on the view that learning and memory, synaptic plasticity and neurogenesis are inter-related phenomena. Specifically, the latter two are considered to provide substrate for specific aspects of learning and memory function. LTP maintenance probably underlies memory retention and its inhibition erases memory. Encoding of a memory trace induces LTP in subset of hippocampal synapses. Neurogenesis underlies specific dynamic and flexible features of learning and memory phenomena in the precisely regulated and time-restricted manner. Nowadays and in the future, collaborative and multidisciplinary efforts involving optogenetics, transgenes, *in vivo* patch-clamp etc. will bring significant insight into mechanisms of memory.

ACKNOWLEDGMENTS

This work was supported by GACR grant 14-03627S, Academic project M200111204, and institutional support RVO67985823. We thank all colleagues from the laboratory for their support, to Prof. P. Mares for critical reading and comments on the manuscript and to T. Hua and P. Luketic for proofreading.

REFERENCES

Aimone, J. B., Deng, W., and Gage, F. H. (2011). Resolving new memories: a critical look at the dentate gyrus, adult neurogenesis and pattern separation. *Neuron* 70, 589–596. doi: 10.1016/j.neuron.2011.05.010

Altman, J. (1963). Autoradiographic investigation of cell proliferation in the brains of rats and cats. *Anat. Rec.* 145, 573–591. doi: 10.1002/ar.1091450409

Altman, J., and Das, G. D. (1965). Autoradiographic and histological evidence of postnatal hippocampal neurogenesis in rats. *J. Comp. Neurol.* 124, 319–335. doi: 10.1002/cne.901240303

Amaral, D. G., and Witter, M. P. (1989). The three-dimensional organization of the hippocampal formation: a review of anatomical data. *Neuroscience* 31, 571–591. doi: 10.1016/0306-4522(89)90424-7

Bast, T., da Silva, B. M., and Morris, R. G. M. (2005). Distinct contributions of hippocampal NMDA and AMPA receptors to encoding and retrieval of one-trial place memory. *J. Neurosci.* 25, 5845–5856. doi: 10.1523/jneurosci.0698-05.2005

Benington, J. H., and Frank, M. G. (2003). Cellular and molecular connections between sleep and synaptic plasticity. *Prog. Neurobiol.* 69, 71–101. doi: 10.1016/S0301-0082(03)00018-2

Bliss, T. V., and Lomo, T. (1973). Long-lasting potentiation of synaptic transmission in the dentate area of the anaesthetized rabbit following stimulation of the perforant path. *J. Physiol.* 232, 331–356.

Brown, T. H., Kairiss, E. W., and Keenan, C. L. (1990). Hebbian synapses: biophysical mechanisms and algorithms. *Annu. Rev. Neurosci.* 13, 475–511. doi: 10.1146/annurev.neuro.13.1.475

Buresová, O., Aleksanyan, Z. A., and Bures, J. (1979). Electrophysiological analysis of retrieval of conditioned taste aversion in rats. Unit activity changes in critical brain regions. *Physiol. Bohemoslov.* 28, 525–536.

Burghardt, N. S., Park, E. H., Hen, R., and Fenton, A. A. (2012). Adult-born hippocampal neurons promote cognitive flexibility in mice. *Hippocampus* 22, 1795–1808. doi: 10.1002/hipo.22013

Cohen, Y., Avramoav, S., Barkai, E., and Maroun, M. (2011). Olfactory learning-induced enhancement of the predisposition for LTP induction. *Learn. Mem.* 18, 594–597. doi: 10.1101/lm.2231911

Déry, N., Pilgrim, M., Gibala, M., Gillen, J., Wojtowicz, J. M., Macqueen, G., et al. (2013). Adult hippocampal neurogenesis reduces memory interference in humans: opposing effects of aerobic exercise and depression. *Front. Neurosci.* 7:66. doi: 10.3389/fnins.2013.00066

Doeller, C. F., King, J. A., and Burgess, N. (2008). Parallel striatal and hippocampal systems for landmarks and boundaries in spatial memory. *Proc. Natl. Acad. Sci. U S A* 105, 5915–5920. doi: 10.1073/pnas.0801489105

Dudai, Y. (2004). The neurobiology of consolidations, or, how stable is the engram? *Annu. Rev. Psychol.* 55, 51–86. doi: 10.1146/annurev.psych.55.090902.142050

Eichenbaum, H. (2001). The hippocampus and declarative memory: cognitive mechanisms and neural codes. *Behav. Brain Res.* 127, 199–207. doi: 10.1016/s0166-4328(01)00365-5

Frey, S., and Frey, J. U. (2008). 'Synaptic tagging' and 'cross-tagging' and related associative reinforcement processes of functional plasticity as the cellular basis for memory formation. *Prog. Brain Res.* 169, 117–143. doi: 10.1016/s0079-6123(07)00007-6

Garthe, A., Behr, J., and Kempermann, G. (2009). Adult-generated hippocampal neurons allow the flexible use of spatially precise learning strategies. *PLoS One* 4:e5464. doi: 10.1371/journal.pone.0005464

Glanzman, D. L. (2013). PKM and the maintenance of memory. *F1000 Biol. Rep.* 5:4. doi: 10.3410/B5-4

Gu, Y., Arruda-Carvalho, M., Wang, J., Janoschka, S. R., Josselyn, S. A., Frankland, P. W., et al. (2012). Optical controlling reveals time-dependent roles for adult-born dentate granule cells. *Nat. Neurosci.* 15, 1700–1706. doi: 10.1038/nn.3260

Hanson, J. E., and Madison, D. V. (2010). Imbalanced pattern completion vs. separation in cognitive disease: network simulations of synaptic pathologies predict a personalized therapeutics strategy. *BMC Neurosci.* 11:96. doi: 10.1186/1471-2202-11-96

Harris, K. D., Csicsvari, J., Hirase, H., and Dragoi, G. (2003). Organization of cell assemblies in the hippocampus. *Nature* 424, 552–556. doi: 10.1038/nature01834

Hebb, D. (1949). *The Organization of Behavior.* New York: Wiley.

Ikrar, T., Guo, N., He, K., Besnard, A., Levinson, S., Hill, A., et al. (2013). Adult neurogenesis modifies excitability of the dentate gyrus. *Front. Neural Circuits* 7:204. doi: 10.3389/fncir.2013.00204

Izquierdo, L. A., Barros, D. M., Vianna, M. R., Coitinho, A., deDavid e Silva, T., Choi, H., et al. (2002). Molecular pharmacological dissection of short- and long-term memory. *Cell. Mol. Neurobiol.* 22, 269–287. doi: 10.1023/A:1020715800956

Kandel, E. R. (2012). The molecular biology of memory: cAMP, PKA, CRE, CREB-1, CREB-2 and CPEB. *Mol. Brain* 5:14. doi: 10.1186/1756-6606-5-14

Kemp, A., and Manahan-Vaughan, D. (2007). Hippocampal long-term depression: master or minion in declarative memory processes? *Trends Neurosci.* 30, 111–118. doi: 10.1016/j.tins.2007.01.002

Kempermann, G. (2012). New neurons for 'survival of the fittest'. *Nat. Rev. Neurosci.* 13, 727–736. doi: 10.1038/nrn3319

Kempermann, G., Kuhn, H. G., and Gage, F. H. (1997). More hippocampal neurons in adult mice living in an enriched environment. *Nature* 386, 493–495. doi: 10.1038/386493a0

Kenney, J., and Manahan-Vaughan, D. (2013). Learning-facilitated synaptic plasticity occurs in the intermediate hippocampus in association with spatial learning. *Front. Synaptic Neurosci.* 29:10. doi: 10.3389/fnsyn.2013.00010

Kim, E. Y., Mahmoud, G. S., and Grover, L. M. (2005). REM sleep deprivation inhibits LTP in vivo in area CA1 of rat hippocampus. *Neurosci. Lett.* 388, 163–167. doi: 10.1016/j.neulet.2005.06.057

Kubík, S., and Fenton, A. A. (2005). Behavioral evidence that segregation and representation are dissociable hippocampal functions. *J. Neurosci.* 25, 9205–9212. doi: 10.1523/jneurosci.1707-05.2005

Kwapis, J. L., and Helmstetter, F. J. (2013). Does PKM(zeta) maintain memory? *Brain Res. Bull.* doi: 10.1016/j.brainresbull.2013.09.005. [Epub ahead of print].

Lee, A. M., Kanter, B. R., Wang, D., Lim, J. P., Zou, M. E., Qiu, C., et al. (2013). Prkcz null mice show normal learning and memory. *Nature* 493, 416–419. doi: 10.1038/nature11803

Lee, A. S., Duman, R. S., and Pittenger, C. (2008). A double dissociation revealing bidirectional competition between striatum and hippocampus during learning. *Proc. Natl. Acad. Sci. U S A* 105, 17163–17168. doi: 10.1073/pnas.0807749105

Ling, D. S. F., Benardo, L. S., Serrano, P. A., Blace, N., Kelly, M. T., Crary, J. F., et al. (2002). Protein kinase Mzeta is necessary and sufficient for LTP maintenance. *Nat. Neurosci.* 5, 295–296. doi: 10.1038/nn829

Lithfous, S., Dufour, A., and Despres, O. (2013). Spatial navigation in normal aging and the prodromal stage of Alzheimer's disease: insights from imaging and behavioral studies. *Ageing Res. Rev.* 12, 201–213. doi: 10.1016/j.arr.2012.04.007

Luu, P., Sill, O. C., Gao, L., Becker, S., Wojtowicz, J. M., and Smith, D. M. (2012). The role of adult hippocampal neurogenesis in reducing interference. *Behav. Neurosci.* 126, 381–391. doi: 10.1037/a0028252

McCoy, J. G., Christie, M. A., Kim, Y., Brennan, R., Poeta, D. L., McCarley, R. W., et al. (2013). Chronic sleep restriction impairs spatial memory in rats. *Neuroreport* 24, 91–95. doi: 10.1097/wnr.0b013e32835cd97a

Morris, R. G. M. (1981). Spatial localization does not require presence of local cues. *Learn. Mot.* 260, 239–260. doi: 10.1016/0023-9690(81)90020-5

Moser, E. I., and Moser, M. B. (1999). Is learning blocked by saturation of synaptic weights in the hippocampus? *Neurosci. Biobehav. Rev.* 23, 661–672. doi: 10.1016/s0149-7634(98)00060-8

Moser, M., and Moser, E. I. (1998). Distributed encoding and retrieval of spatial memory in the hippocampus. *J. Neurosci.* 18, 7535–7542.

Mueller, A. D., Meerlo, P., McGinty, D., and Mistlberger, R. E. (2013). Sleep and adult neurogenesis: implications for cognition and mood. *Curr. Top. Behav. Neurosci.* doi: 10.1007/7854_2013_251. [Epub ahead of Print].

Nakashiba, T., Cushman, J. D., Pelkeym, K. A., Renaudineau, S., Buhl, D. L., McHugh, T. J., et al. (2012). Young dentate granule cells mediate pattern separation, whereas old granule cells facilitate pattern completion. *Cell* 149, 188–201. doi: 10.1016/j.cell.2012.01.046

Nilsson, M., Perfilieva, E., Johansson, U., Orwar, O., and Eriksson, P. S. (1999). Enriched environment increases neurogenesis in the adult rat dentate gyrus and improves spatial memory. *J. Neurobiol.* 39, 569–578. doi: 10.1002/(sici)1097-4695(19990615)39:4<569::aid-neu10>3.0.co;2-f

Otnæss, M. K., Brun, V. H., Moser, M. B., and Moser, E. I. (1999). Pretraining prevents spatial learning impairment after saturation of hippocampal long-term potentiation. *J. Neurosci.* 19, RC49.

Pastalkova, E., Serrano, P., Pinkhasova, D., Wallace, E., Fenton, A., and Sacktor, T. C. (2006). Storage of spatial information by the maintenance mechanism of LTP. *Science* 313, 1141–1144. doi: 10.1126/science.1128657

Pauli, W. M., Clark, A. D., Guenther, H. J., O'Reilly, R. C., and Rudy, J. W. (2012). Inhibiting PKMζ reveals dorsal lateral and dorsal medial striatum store the different memories needed to support adaptive behavior. *Learn. Mem.* 19, 307–314. doi: 10.1101/lm.025148.111

Pevzner, A., Miyashita, T., Schiffman, A. J., and Guzowski, J. F. (2012). Temporal dynamics of Arc gene induction in hippocampus: relationship to context memory formation. *Neurobiol. Learn. Mem.* 97, 313–320. doi: 10.1016/j.nlm.2012.02.004

Prince, T. M., Wimmer, M., Choi, J., Havekes, R., Aton, S., and Abel, T. (2014). Sleep deprivation during a specific 3-hour time window post-training impairs hippocampal synaptic plasticity and memory. *Neurobiol. Learn. Mem.* 109, 122–130. doi: 10.1016/j.nlm.2013.11.021

Qureshi, I. A., and Mehler, M. F. (2013). Towards a "systems"-level understanding of the nervous system and its disorders. *Trends Neurosci.* 36, 674–684. doi: 10.1016/j.tins.2013.07.003

Rodríguez-Durán, L. F., Castillo, D. V., Moguel-González, M., and Escobar, M. L. (2011). Conditioned taste aversion modifies persistently the subsequent induction of neocortical long-term potentiation in vivo. *Neurobiol. Learn. Mem.* 95, 519–526. doi: 10.1016/j.nlm.2011.03.003

Rolls, E. T. (2013). The mechanisms for pattern completion and pattern separation in the hippocampus. *Front. Syst. Neurosci.* 7:74. doi: 10.3389/fnsys.2013.00074

Sahay, A., Scobie, K. N., Hill, A. S., O'Carroll, C. M., Kheirbek, M. A., Burghardt, N. S., et al. (2011). Increasing adult hippocampal neurogenesis is sufficient to improve pattern separation. *Nature* 472, 466–470. doi: 10.1038/nature09817

Schwabe, L. (2013). Stress and the engagement of multiple memory systems: integration of animal and human studies. *Hippocampus* 23, 1035–1043. doi: 10.1002/hipo.22175

Selbie, L. A., Schmitz-Peiffer, C., Sheng, Y., and Biden, T. J. (1993). Molecular cloning and characterization of PKC iota, an atypical isoform of protein kinase C derived from insulin-secreting cells. *J. Biol. Chem.* 268, 24296–24302.

Semon, R. (1921). *The Mneme.* London: Allen and Unwin.

Serrano, P., Friedman, E. L., Kenney, J., Taubenfeld, S. M., Zimmerman, J. M., Hanna, J., et al. (2008). PKMzeta maintains spatial, instrumental, and classically conditioned long-term memories. *PLoS Biol.* 6:60318. doi: 10.1371/journal.pbio.0060318

Shema, R., Haramati, S., Ron, S., Hazvi, S., Chen, A., Sacktor, T. C., et al. (2011). Enhancement of consolidated long-term memory by overexpression of protein kinase Mzeta in the neocortex. *Science* 331, 1207–1210. doi: 10.1126/science.1200215

Shema, R., Sacktor, T. C., and Dudai, Y. (2007). Rapid erasure of long-term memory associations in the cortex by an inhibitor of PKM zeta. *Science* 317, 951–953. doi: 10.1126/science.1144334

Snyder, J. S., Kee, N., and Wojtowicz, J. M. (2001). Effects of adult neurogenesis on synaptic plasticity in the rat dentate gyrus. *J. Neurophysiol.* 85, 2423–2431.

Squire, L. R. (2004). Memory systems of the brain: a brief history and current perspective. *Neurobiol. Learn. Mem.* 82, 171–177. doi: 10.1016/j.nlm.2004.06.005

Steele, R. J., and Morris, R. G. (1999). Delay-dependent impairment of a matching-to-place task with chronic and intrahippocampal infusion of the NMDA-antagonist D-AP5. *Hippocampus* 9, 118–136. doi: 10.1002/(sici)1098-1063(1999)9:2<118::aid-hipo4>3.0.co;2-8

Stuchlik, A., Petrasek, T., Prokopova, I., Holubova, K., Hatalova, H., Vales, K., et al. (2013). Place avoidance tasks as tools in the behavioral neuroscience of learning and memory. *Physiol. Res.* 62, S1–S19.

Van der Borght, K., Havekes, R., Bos, T., Eggen, B. J., and Van der Zee, E. A. (2007). Exercise improves memory acquisition and retrieval in the Y-maze task: relationship with hippocampal neurogenesis. *Behav. Neurosci.* 121, 324–334. doi: 10.1037/0735-7044.121.2.324

van Praag, H., Christie, B. R., Sejnowski, T. J., and Gage, F. H. (1999). Running enhances neurogenesis, learning, and long-term potentiation in mice. *Proc. Natl. Acad. Sci. U S A* 96, 13427–13431. doi: 10.1073/pnas.96.23.13427

Voineskos, D., Rogasch, N. C., Rajji, T. K., Fitzgerald, P. B., and Daskalakis, Z. J. (2013). A review of evidence linking disrupted neural plasticity to schizophrenia. *Can. J. Psychiatry* 58, 86–92.

Volk, L. J., Bachman, J. L., Johnson, R., Yu, Y., and Huganir, R. L. (2013). PKM-ζ is not required for hippocampal synaptic plasticity, learning, and memory. *Nature* 493, 420–423. doi: 10.1038/nature11802

Wang, J., Gallagher, D., DeVito, L. M., Cancino, G. I., Tsui, D., He, L., et al. (2012). Metformin activates an atypical PKC-CBP pathway to promote neurogenesis and enhance spatial memory formation. *Cell Stem Cell* 11, 23–35. doi: 10.1016/j.stem.2012.03.016

Wesierska, M., Dockery, C., and Fenton, A. A. (2005). Beyond memory, navigation, and inhibition: behavioral evidence for hippocampus-dependent cognitive coordination in the rat. *J. Neurosci.* 25, 2413–2419. doi: 10.1523/jneurosci.3962-04.2005

Whitlock, J. R., Heynen, A. J., Shuler, M. G., and Bear, M. F. (2006). Learning induces long-term potentiation in the hippocampus. *Science* 313, 1093–1097. doi: 10.1126/science.1128134

Wiskott, L., Rasch, M. J., and Kempermann, G. (2006). A functional hypothesis for adult hippocampal neurogenesis: avoidance of catastrophic interference in the dentate gyrus. *Hippocampus* 16, 329–343. doi: 10.1002/hipo.20167

Wohlgemuth, S., Ronacher, B., and Wehner, R. (2001). Ant odometry in the third dimension. *Nature* 411, 795–798. doi: 10.1038/35081069

Xia, Z., and Storm, D. R. (2012). Role of signal transduction crosstalk between adenylyl cyclase and MAP kinase in hippocampus-dependent memory. *Learn. Mem.* 19, 369–374. doi: 10.1101/lm.027128.112

Zhang, Y., and Barres, B. A. (2013). A smarter mouse with human astrocytes. *Bioessays* 35, 876–880. doi: 10.1002/bies.201300070

21

Consequences of early postnatal benzodiazepines exposure in rats. II. Social behavior

Anna Mikulecká *, Martin Šubrt, Martina Pařízková, Pavel Mareš and Hana Kubová

Institute of Physiology, Academy of Sciences of the Czech Republic, Prague, Czech Republic

Edited by:
Tomiki Sumiyoshi, National Center of Neurology and Psychiatry, Japan

***Correspondence:**
Anna Mikulecká, Institute of Physiology, Academy of Sciences of the Czech Republic, Videňská 1083, 142 20 Prague 4, Czech Republic
e-mail: nmikul@epilepsy.biomed.cas.cz

Social behavior represents an integral part of behavioral repertoire of rats particularly sensitive to pharmacological and environmental influences. The aim of the present study was to investigate whether early postnatal clonazepam (CZP) exposure can induce age-dependent changes related to expression of social behavior. The drug was administered from postnatal day (P) 7 until P11 at daily doses of 0.1, 0.5 and 1.0 mg/kg i.p. We designed three experiments to assess whether exposure to CZP affects social behavior in respect to the age of rats and the test circumstances, specifically their familiarity with test conditions during adolescence (P32), social behavior in juveniles and adolescents (P18–P42) and social behavior in a resident-intruder paradigm. The frequency and duration of a various patterns of social behavior related to play and social investigation not related to play were evaluated. The results showed that CZP postnatal exposure decreased social play behavior regardless of age and familiarity or unfamiliarity of experimental environment but did not affect the social investigation *per se*. When rats were confronted with an intruder in their home cages intense wrestling and inhibition of genital investigation were found. In conclusion, these findings show that short-term CZP postnatal exposure inhibits social play behavior and alters specific patterns of social behavior in an age and environment related manner.

Keywords: benzodiazepines, clonazepam, social behavior, development, rats

INTRODUCTION

Benzodiazepine (BZD) exposure during brain development can result in persistent modification of brain functions, behavioral alterations and cognitive deficits (for rev. Gai and Grimm, 1982; Tucker, 1985; Kellogg, 1988). Enduring behavioral, biochemical and molecular effects can also occur when drugs are administered after neuronal differentiation, but before complete maturation of the central system, i.e., during the first three weeks of life in rats (Avishai-Eliner et al., 2002) or later during adolescence (Hulin et al., 2012). In spite of possible risk of adverse effects, BZDs are widely prescribed to treat anxiety, depression and insomnia, to control epileptic seizures, promote anesthesia or to induce muscle relaxation in all age groups of patients including neonate and children (for rev. Lader, 1994; Lalive et al., 2011).

Effects of BZDs are specifically mediated by their interaction with BZD receptor binding site, which modulates the efficacy of the major inhibitory neurotransmitter, γ-aminobutyric acid (GABA), at the BZD-sensitive $GABA_A$ (BZD/$GABA_A$) receptors. In rats, BZD/$GABA_A$ receptors can be detected during the last week of gestation and they reach the adult level by the third-fourth week of life (Lippa et al., 1981). Changes of BZD/$GABA_A$ receptor features were detected in animals exposed to BZDs prenatally as well as postnatally (for rev. Tucker, 1985). A recent study documented that early treatment with BZDs induces selective alteration of subunit expression. Changes at receptor level were observed also after administration of other $GABA_A$ receptor ligands as barbiturates (Raol et al., 2005). In addition, administration of GABAergic drugs including BZDs during the 1st week of life increases apoptosis (Bittigau et al., 2002; Forcelli et al., 2012). Therefore changes at both molecular and cellular level can result in alteration of neuronal circuitry in the immature brain and induce functional impairment.

Despite high clinical importance, possible long-term risks of early postnatal exposure to BZDs are only rarely investigated. Some changes of behavior related to anxiety, aggression, emotional state and cognitive abilities were reported in animals exposed to BZDs from birth until weaning (P1–P21) and tested during adolescence or adulthood (File, 1986a,b,c; Schroeder et al., 1997). In these studies exposure to BZDs lasted for long time and affected several critical developmental periods including switch in BZDs receptor structure and maturation of the hippocampal formation (Garrett et al., 1990; Avishai-Eliner et al., 2002). Due to sedation and myorelexation (for rev. Tucker, 1985), long lasting administration of BZDs was found to cause undernutrition and significant growth retardation, which can negatively impact future functional abilities of exposed individuals (Smart et al., 1973). Even though adverse effects of long lasting BZD exposure can substantially affect results of developmental studies, chronic consequences of short lasting BZD exposure are sparse. File (1987) demonstrated changes of exploratory activity and emotional state (e.g., increased aggression) in adolescent animals exposed to diazepam at P1–P7 (File, 1987). Recently, studies with another modulator of $GABA_A$ receptors, allopregnanolone, showed long-lasting emotional and cognitive impairment in adult animals exposed to this neurosteroid between P5 and P9 (Darbra and Pallarès, 2009; Mòdol et al., 2013). Thus available data clearly document that early modulation of $GABA_A$ receptors can modify behavior at later stages of development and relate to a susceptibility to psychopathology in adulthood.

Studies on functional cosequences of early BZD exposure have focused mostly on cognitive abilities and emotional state. Alterations of social behavior are examined only sporadically despite an importance of normal social interactions for further development and life in highly organized groups. Only File's studies have documented impairment of social interactions in animals exposed to BZDs early in the life and suggested that alteration depends on the time-course of drug exposure, dose and experimental approach (File, 1986b,c, 1987). Data are however still fragmentary.

Present study was designed to determine whether exposure to BZDs at early postnatal stage (P7–P11) which corresponds with perinatal period in humans (Dobbing and Sands, 1979; Avishai-Eliner et al., 2002; Clancy et al., 2007), affects: (1) social behavior during adolescence (P32); (2) social behavior in juveniles and adolescents (P18–P42); and (3) social behavior of rats in their homing environment at three developmental stages: middle adolescence (P32), sexual maturity (P60), and adulthood (P80). The general design of used behavioral tests was adapted from the literature (Meaney and Stewart, 1981; Fraňková and Mikulecká, 1990; Vanderschuren et al., 1995b; Mitchell and Redfern, 2005).

As a model BZD, we chose clonazepam (CZP), a partial BZD agonist, first used for treatment of certain types of seizures (Morishita, 2009). Safety and negligible adverse effects of CZP in immature rats were demonstrated before (Mikulecká et al., 2011). Data on pharmacokinetics of CZP in rats are sparse, but Hoogerkamp et al. (1996) showed that terminal half-life of CZP in adult rats is approximately 1 h. Immature organisms eliminate CZP more slowly than adults (André et al., 1986). Our previous studies demonstrated duration of both anticonvulsive and anxiolytic effects in rat pups. After single administration of CZP in a dose of 1.0 mg/kg both P7 and P12, animals were partially protected against pentylenetetrazole (PTZ)-induced seizures for 24 h (Kubová and Mareš, 1989). CZP in the same dose exhibited anxiolytic effects in P12 rats for 48 h whereas motor impairment was observed for only 3 h (Mikulecká et al., 2011). Also repeated CZP administration only minimally affected body growth and did not affect maternal attention and care (Mikulecká et al., 2014).

MATERIAL AND METHODS

ANIMALS

Male Wistar albino rats (Institute of Physiology, Academy of Sciences, Prague, $n = 190$) were used and maintained under controlled temperature (22 ± 1°C) and humidity (50 to 60%) with a 12/12 h light/dark cycle (lights on at 6:00 AM). Food and water were provided ad libitum (with the exception of the testing period). On day 5, (birth counted as day 0) the pups were randomly fostered and each litter was adjusted to ten males. At P7 the animals were marked for identification and mixed by treatment. To exclude the participation of a litter effect, only a limited number of animals from the same litter were used. They were weaned at postnatal day (P) 28. After weaning, the animals were housed in groups of 3–4 per cage. Experiments were approved by the animal Care and Use Committee of the Institute of Physiology, Academy of Sciences of the Czech Republic (v.v.i), and determined to be in agreement with the Animal Protection Law of the Czech Republic, which is fully compatible with the guidelines of the European Community Council directives 86/609/EEC.

DRUG EXPOSURE

CZP (Hoffmann–Switzerland; obtained as a gift) was suspended in one drop of Tween 80 and 1 ml of saline. Subsequently, this solution was diluted in such a way that all used doses of CZP were administered in the same volume of 5 μl/g of body weight. The doses were selected according to our previous studies on anticonvulsant effects of CZP in developing animals (Kubová and Mareš, 1989; Mikulecká et al., 2011). The doses were optimized according to results obtained in the first experiment, *social behavior in adolescence* (Experiment 1). In this experiment CZP at the doses of 0.1, 0.5 and/or 1.0 mg/kg were administered intraperitoneally for 5 consecutive days, starting from P7 to P11. In other experiments only doses of 0.5 or 1.0 mg/kg were used. Control animals received the corresponding volume of vehicle. Animals were weighted daily during the CZP exposure, on P12 and P15, and at the beginning of each experiment. Overall health condition was regularly examined.

EXPERIMENTAL DESIGN

The experimental procedures are depicted in **Figure 1**. All experiments were performed in a room with constant temperature (22 ± 1°C), under low-light conditions (35–45 lx), between 9:00 AM and 3:00 PM. Animals behavior was video recorded and then analyzed using Observer, and locomotion was assessed using

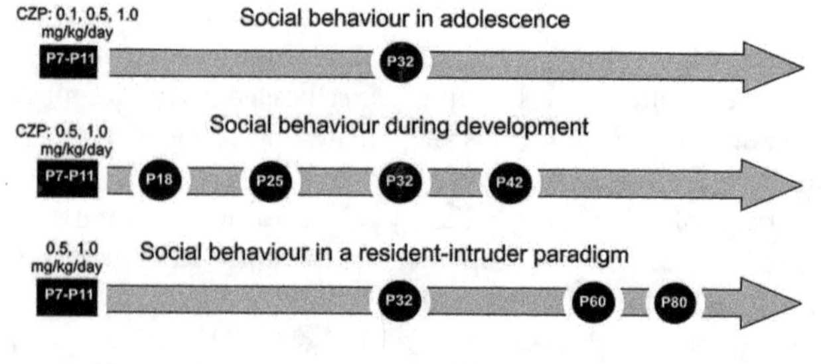

FIGURE 1 | Design/time diagram of experimental procedure: *social behavior in adolescence, social behavior during development and social behavior in a resident-intruder paradigm*. The upper part shows a timeline for the Experiment 1: *social behavior in adolescence* after 0.1, 0.5 and 1.0 mg/kg/day of CZP exposure between P7 and P11. The middle part shows a timeline for the Experiment 2: *social behavior during development* after 0.5 and 1.0 mg/kg/day of CZP exposure. The lower part shows a timeline for the Experiment 3: *social behavior in a resident-intruder paradigm*.

EthoVision (both software Noldus Information Technology). Two experimenters analyzed the video recordings simultaneously and repeatedly until both of them were able to recognize the same patterns. The patterns with duration of one second or more were counted. Then, both observers performed evaluation of recordings separately, and between-reliability was calculated (between-reliability >0.9).

Experiment 1: Social behavior in adolescence

Animals were tested at the age of 32 days (P32). The control group consisted of nine pairs of rats. The group exposed to CZP at a dose of 0.1 mg/kg consisted of eight pairs and those exposed to CZP at a dose of 0.5 mg/kg and 1.0 mg/kg both consisted of nine pairs. Two consecutive days before social interaction, the animals were familiarized to the experimental condition by placing them individually into the open field arena (OF) (45 × 45 × 30 cm) for 5 min. On the day of social interaction test, the rats were weighted, marked and individually isolated into small cages (21 × 27 cm) for three hours. Two rats from different litters with identical treatment (C vs. C, CZP vs. CZP) were placed into the OF arena at opposite corners and their behavior was recorded for 10 min. To reduce any lingering olfactory cues, OF was thoroughly wiped with water-moistened tissue paper after each pair tested. The frequency and the duration of the following patterns per pair of rats were observed: following/chasing (moving in the direction of or pursuing the partner that is moving away); climbing over/under; mutual sniffing; boxing (the animals stand upright facing one another and pawing toward each other); wrestling (the animals rolled over each other in rough-and-tumble play) and pinning (one of the animals is lying in supine position and the other is laying over it). These behavioral patterns were divided into *Behavior related to play* (pinning, boxing/wrestling, following/chasing) and *Behavior unrelated to play* (climbing over/under and mutual sniffing) and then analyzed separately.

Experiment 2: social behavior during development

Social behavior during development was studied in 10 pairs of controls and two groups of 10 pairs of animals exposed to CZP. Animals were tested for the first time at P18 and then repeatedly at P25, P32 and P42. At the beginning of each test, animals were weighted, marked and individually isolated into small cages (21 × 27 cm) for 30 min. Similar to Experiment 1, two rats from different litters with identical treatment (C vs. C, CZP vs. CZP) were placed into the OF arena at opposite corners and their behavior was recorded for 10 min. The duration of following behavioral patterns per pair was evaluated: passive contact (pups in close contact, resting, with no movement), active contacts (crawling over/under, mutual sniffing), following (one pup followed the other pup rapidly so that it almost touched it) and play fighting (the animals rolled over each other in rough-and-tumble play). Locomotion expressed as the distance travelled was assessed for both animals in the pair.

Experiment 3: social behavior in a resident-intruder paradigm

Three groups of rats each consisting of 10 animals were used. Two groups were exposed to CZP at doses of 0.5 or 1.0 mg/kg and one control group was injected with saline. The animals were housed in cages containing three to four rats. Twenty four hours before testing, the animals designated as resident rats were housed individually in standard cages in order to provide territorial advantage. The rats serving as social stimuli (intruder rats), were not isolated. On the experimental day (P32), the animals in their home cages were transferred to the experimental room for an acclimatization period of 30 min before testing. Each resident was paired with an unfamiliar untreated intruder. The test started by placing an intruder in the resident home cage and their social interaction was video recorded for 10 min. After the test was completed, both resident and intruder rats were returned to their respective group cages (to re-establish each group member's rank position within the social hierarchy). The same pairs of animals were tested at P60 and P80 following the same procedure as at P32. The following behavioral patterns were observed: pouncing (one rat soliciting the other, by attempting to nose or rub the nape of its neck); following (the pursuit of one animal by another); wrestling (rough and tumble play); pinning (the one animal stands over the exposed ventral area of the other pressing it down); genital investigation (sniffing anogenital area). Behavioral patterns were observed separately for each member of a pair (resident and intruder) except for wrestling because this pattern involved two animals concurrently performing the same behavior (**Figure 2**). The day following the social interaction test, locomotion of residents was assessed in the OF (see below).

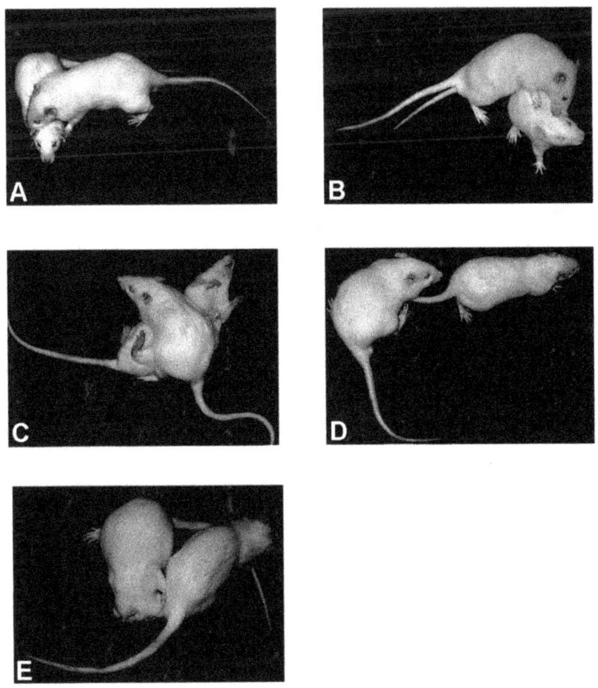

FIGURE 2 | Social behavioral patterns displayed by rats in a resident-intruder paradigm. **(A)** pouncing, **(B)** wrestling, **(C)** pinning, **(D)** following, and **(E)** genital investigation.

LOCOMOTION

After 30 min of adaptation to the experimental room, a rat was placed into the left corner of the arena to explore the new environment for 5 min. Locomotion was evaluated by analyzing the track record for the distance travelled. In both Experiment 1 (*social behavior in adolescence*) and Experiment 2 (*social behavior during development*) locomotion for each rat in the pair was calculated. In Experiment 3 (*social behavior in a resident-intruder paradigm*) locomotion was assessed only for resident rats one day after social behavior test.

STATISTICAL ANALYSIS

The frequency and duration of social interaction patterns were evaluated. All data were presented as mean ± standard error of mean. One-way ANOVA was used to analyze data from Experiment 1 (*social behavior in adolescence*). Data from Experiment 2 (*social behavior during development*) and from Experiment 3 (*social behavior in a resident-intruder paradigm*) were analyzed with two-way ANOVA (one treatment factor and age as a repeated-measures factor). Further, *post hoc* Holm-Sidak method was used to explore significant main effects or interactions resulting from the ANOVA (SigmaStat® SPSS Inc., Chicago, IL). The level of statistical significance was set at $P < 0.05$. In Experiment 1, only seven pairs of animals exposed to 0.1 mg/kg CZP dose were included in the analysis, as one animal died during the CZP exposure. Due to technical problem during the collection data in Experiment 3, only nine pairs of rats per group were included in the analysis. ANOVA analysis yielded highly similar results for both frequency and duration of behavioral patterns in both Experiment 2 (*social behavior during development*) and 3 (*social behavior in a resident-intruder paradigm*), therefore only data on duration were reported. In addition, we calculated the time in percentage of the occurrence of individual patterns relative to total time spent in social interaction; the values of the most expressed social patterns are given in the results section.

RESULTS

BODY WEIGHT

There was no difference in average body weight (BW) between litters or between animals selected for individual treatments. BW of P7 animals was 17.8 ± 0.3 g in controls vs. 18.2 ± 0.2 g in CZP 0.5 mg/kg and 18.0 ± 0.3 g in CZP 1.0 mg/kg. CZP exposure had only limited effects on body growth. Controls gained more weight than the CZP exposed rats. Further analysis revealed that from P9 to P12 relative body weight was lower in animals receiving CZP with both doses (0.5 and 1.0 mg/kg) than in controls. In animals exposed to higher dose of CZP (1.0 mg/kg/day) relative body weights were still lower at P15 and P18. No significant differences were found in subsequent days of behavioral testing (i.e., at P25, P32 and P42) [drug effect: $F_{(2,570)} = 13.34, p < 0.001$; age $F_{(10,570)} = 6057.9, p < 0.001$; drug × age interaction $F_{(20,570)} = 0.64, p = 0.88$] (**Figure 3**).

Experiment 1: social behavior during adolescence

Behavior related to play. The analysis revealed significant effect of CZP exposure in both the duration $F_{(3,30)} = 6.50, P = 0.002$ and

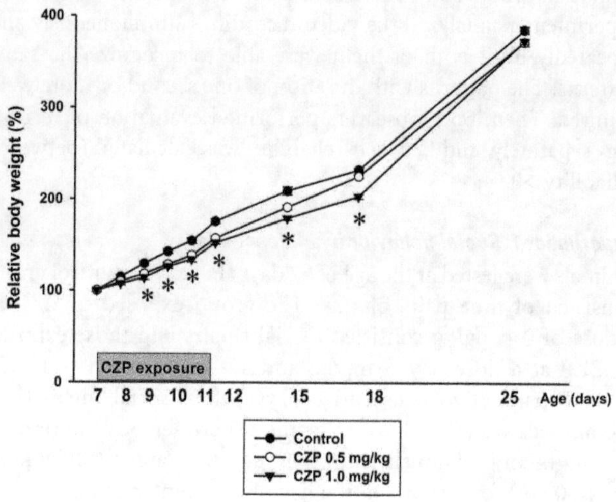

FIGURE 3 | Body weight (mean +SEM) of rats during CZP exposure and at P12, P15, P18 and P25. Abscissa: age in days, ordinate: relative weight (body weight on the first day of the drug administration was taken as 100%). * Significant difference compared to appropriate control groups.

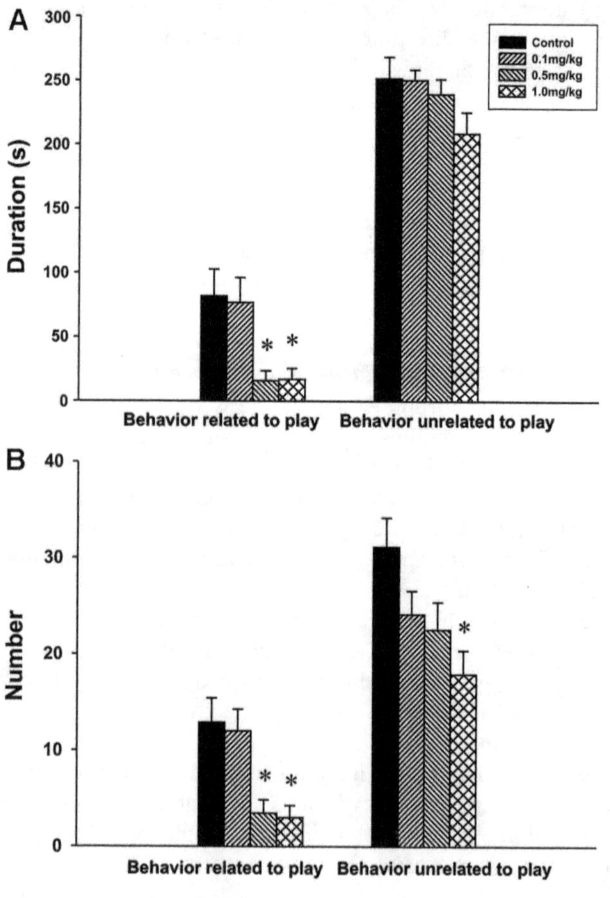

FIGURE 4 | Duration (A) and number (B) of social behavior related and unrelated to play in P32 animals exposed to CZP from P7 to P11 postnatal day. * Significant difference compared to control group.

the number $F_{(3,30)} = 7.89$, $P < 0.001$ of behavior related to play. At doses of 0.5 and 1.0 mg/kg CZP, *post hoc* comparison showed a significant decrease in the duration and the number of behavior related to play.

Behavior unrelated to play. There was no significant main effect of CZP exposure in the duration of behavior unrelated to play $F_{(3,30)} = 1.75$, $P = 0.17$ but a significant effect was found in the number of behavior unrelated to play $F_{(3,30)} = 4.11$, $P = 0.01$. *Post hoc* test showed that CZP exposure at the dose of 1.0 mg/kg decreased the number of behavior unrelated to play (**Figures 4A, B**).

Experiment 2: social behavior during development

Passive contacts. There was a significant effect of age in the duration of passive contacts [$F_{(3,81)} = 99.04$, $p < 0.001$]. Both controls and CZP exposed animals spent less time in passive contact at P25, P32 and P42 compared to those at P18. The overall analysis revealed significant effect of CZP exposure [$F_{(2,27)} = 9.60$, $p < 0.001$], and drug × age interaction [$F_{(6,81)} = 4.33$, $p < 0.001$]. *Post hoc* comparison showed that both doses of CZP increased passive contact in animals at P18 compared to controls. Further, the animals exposed to CZP at P32 and P42 spent a shorter time in passive contact compared to animals at P25 (**Figure 5A**).

Active contacts. The analysis revealed significant effects of age [$F_{(3,81)} = 10.78$, $p < 0.001$], CZP exposure [$F_{(2,27)} = 6.79$, $P = 0.004$], and drug × age interaction [$F_{(6,81)} = 4.13$, $p = 0.001$]. Control animals at P18 spent significantly less time in active contacts than controls at all subsequent developmental stages. In addition, both controls at P32 and P42 spent more time in active contact compared to those at P25. Furthermore, subsequent analysis showed that P32 animals at the dose of 1.0 mg/kg CZP decreased the time spent in active contact compared to controls. At P42, both doses of CZP decreased the time spent in active contact (**Figure 5B**).

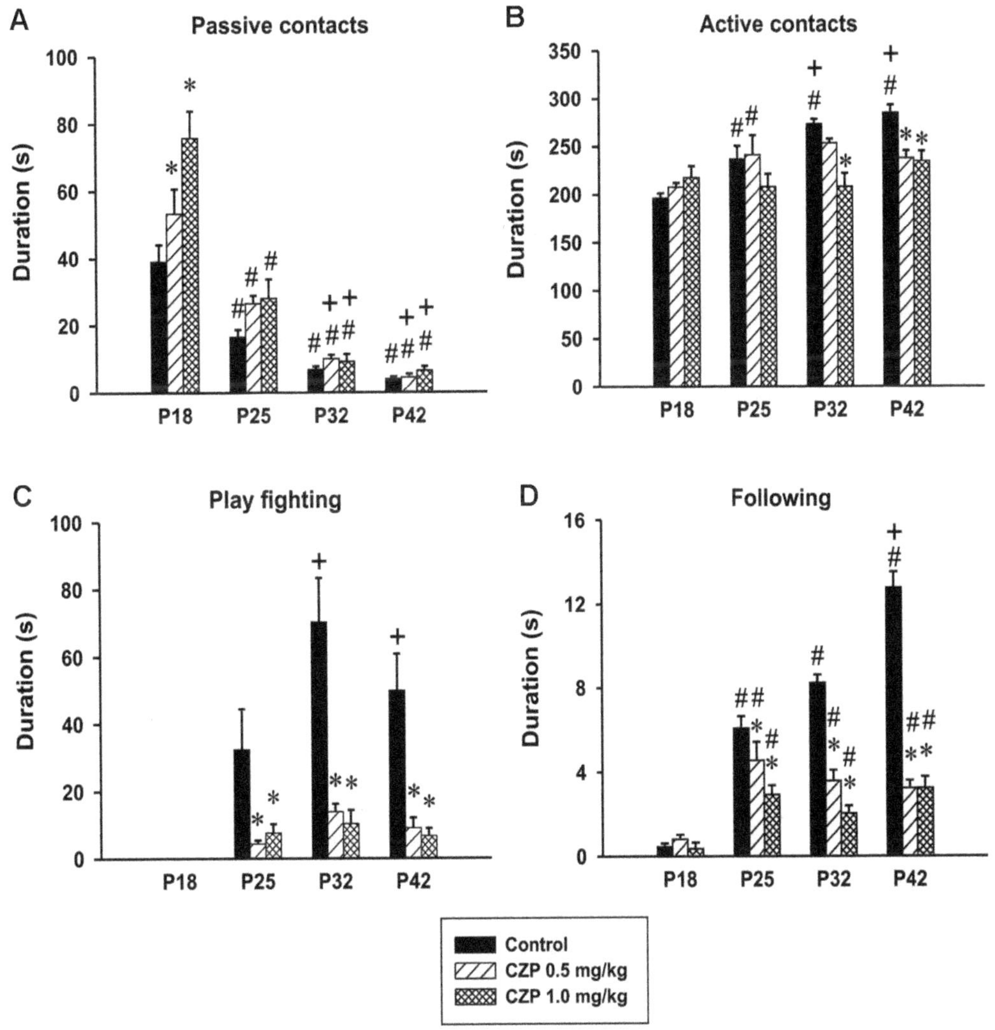

FIGURE 5 | Effects of CZP exposure (P7–P11) on *social behavior during development*. Illustrated here are the means + SEM for the total duration of passive contacts **(A)**, total duration of active contacts **(B)**, total duration of play fighting **(C)**, and total duration of following **(D)**. * Significant difference compared to appropriate control groups. # Significant difference compared to P18, + Significant difference compared to P25.

Play fighting. The animals at P18 did not display fighting. Repeated measures of ANOVA revealed significant effects of age [$F_{(3,81)} = 15.26$, $p < 0.001$], drug exposure [$F_{(2,27)} = 23.31$, $p < 0.001$], and drug × age interaction [$F_{(6,81)} = 6.00$, $p < 0.001$]. Control rats at P32 and P42 spent more time fighting compared to those at P25. Both doses of CZP significantly decreased fighting in all age groups (**Figure 5C**). In addition, the percentage evaluation of the time spent in individual behavioral patterns revealed that CZP exposure irrespective of the dose (0.5 and 1.0 mg) markedly suppressed play fighting at P25 (0.65% and 3.07%), P32 (1.24%

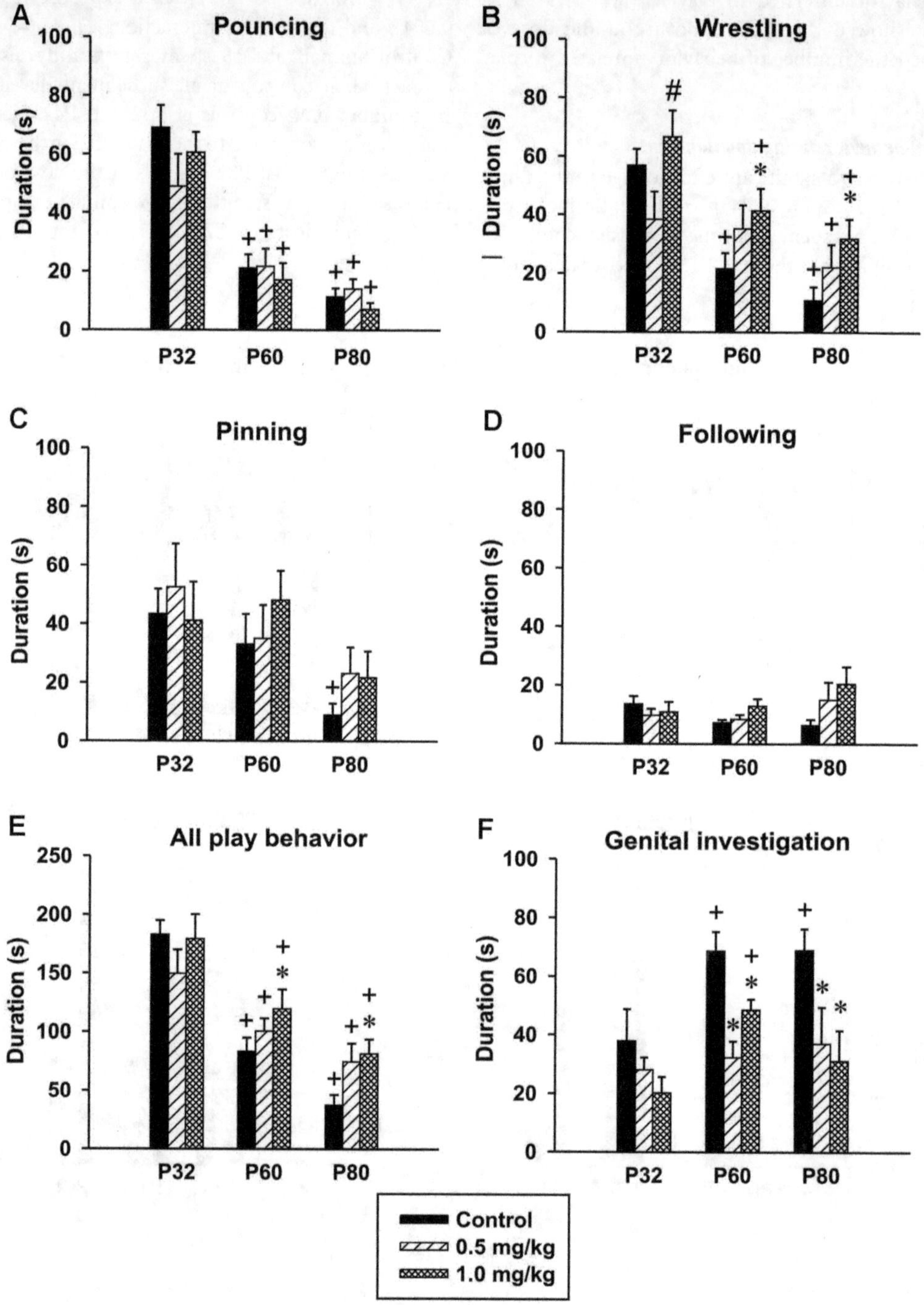

FIGURE 6 | Effect of CZP exposure (P7–P11) on resident social behavior in a *resident-intruder paradigm*. Illustrated here are the means+SEM for total duration of pouncing **(A)**, total duration of wrestling **(B)**, total duration of pinning **(C)**, total duration of following **(D)**, total duration of (all play behavior) **(E)** and total duration of genital investigation **(F)**. * Significant difference compared to corresponding control groups. + Significant difference compared to P32. # Significant difference compared to 0.5 mg/kg dose of CZP.

and 4.48%) and at P42 (1.23% and 2.65%). The percentage values in the control group are as follows: P25 = 11.09%, P32 = 19.59% and P42 = 14.18%.

Following. Finally, the analysis revealed significant effects of age [$F_{(3,81)}$=67.99, $p < 0.001$], CZP exposure [$F_{(2,27)} = 133.62$, $p < 0.001$], and drug × age interaction [$F_{(6,81)} = 22.01$, $p < 0.001$] in the time spent following. At P18, a very short duration of following behavior was observed. Subsequent analysis showed that all animals at P25, P32 and P42 irrespective of treatment spent more time following compared to those at P18. In addition, control animals at P42 spent more time following compared to animals at P 25. Moreover, both CZP doses decreased time spent in following behavior at P25, P32 and P42 compared to the appropriate controls (**Figure 5D**). In addition, both CZP doses suppressed the percentage of time spent in following, above all, at P32 (1.30% and 0.88%) and P42 (1.29% and 1.28%) relative to the control group P32 = 2.30% and P42 = 3.63%.

Experiment 3: social behavior of residents in a resident-intruder paradigm

Pouncing. There was significant effect of age in the time spent pouncing [$F_{(2,48)} = 55.40$, $p < 0.001$]. The animals at both P60 and P80 spent less time pouncing compared to animals at P32. No significant effect of CZP exposure [$F_{(2,24)} = 0.73$, $p = 0.48$] or drug × age interaction was found [$F_{(4,48)} = 1.24$, $p < 0.30$] (**Figure 6A**).

Wrestling. The analysis revealed significant effects of age [$F_{(2,48)} = 24.93$, $p < 0.001$], CZP exposure [$F_{(2,24)} = 4.97$, $p = 0.01$], but not of drug × age interaction [$F_{(4,48)} = 1.78$, $p = 0.14$]. Controls as well as CZP exposed animals spent less time wrestling at P60 and P80 compared to animals at P32. Further, *post hoc* comparison showed that at a dose of 1.0 mg/kg, CZP increased wrestling time in P60 and P80 animals (**Figure 6B**). The higher dose of CZP increased the percentage of time spent wrestling at P60 = 24.6% and P80 = 28.3% relative to their control groups P60 = 14.3% and P80 = 10.2%.

Pinning. There was a significant effect of age [$F_{(2,48)} = 6.62$, $p < 0.003$], but no significant effect of CZP exposure [$F_{(2,24)} = 0.54$, $p = 0.58$], or drug × age interaction $F_{(4,48)} = 0.49$, $p = 0.73$. The *post hoc* analysis showed that only control animals at P80 spent less time pinning compared to those at P32 (**Figure 6C**).

Following. ANOVA failed to identify any significant effect of age [$F_{(2,48)} = 1.55$, $p = 0.22$], CZP exposure [$F_{(2,24)} = 1.85$, $p = 0.18$], and drug × age interaction [$F_{(4,48)} = 1.98$, $p = 0.1$](**Figure 6D**).

All play behavior. Analysis of behavior related to play (pouncing, wrestling, pinning and following) revealed significant age effect [$F_{(2,48)} = 39.40$, $p < 0.001$]. Both controls and CZP exposed animals at P60 and P80 spent less time playing compared to those at P32. ANOVA did not revealed any significant effects of CZP exposure [$F_{(2,24)} = 2.31$, $p = 0.12$], as well as drug × age interaction [$F_{(4,48)} = 1.58$, $p = 0.19$]. Nevertheless, *post hoc* comparison showed that animals exposed to CZP at a dose of 1.0 mg/kg spent more time playing compared to their respective controls (**Figure 6E**).

Genital investigation. There was significant effect of age in the time spent investigating genitals [$F_{(2,48)} = 6.13$, $p = 0.004$]. Control animals at P60 and P80 spent more time investigating genitals compared to those at P32. Both doses of CZP affected genital investigation [$F_{(2,24)} = 11.41$, $p < 0.001$]. *Post hoc* test revealed that at both P60 and P80 the animals spent less time investigating genitals than the corresponding controls. Animals exposed to 1.0 mg/kg CZP at P60 spent more time investigating, compared to those at P32. No drug × age interaction effect was found [$F_{(2,48)} = 1.37$, $p = 0.26$] (**Figure 6F**). As for the percentage of time spent in genital investigation, both CZP doses markedly suppressed this behavior at P60 (24.3% and 24.3%) and P80 (33.2% and 27.7%) relative to control groups (P60 = 45.2% and P80 = 64.7%).

LOCOMOTION

In Experiment 1 (*social behavior during adolescence*) ANOVA did not reveal significant difference in the distance moved between

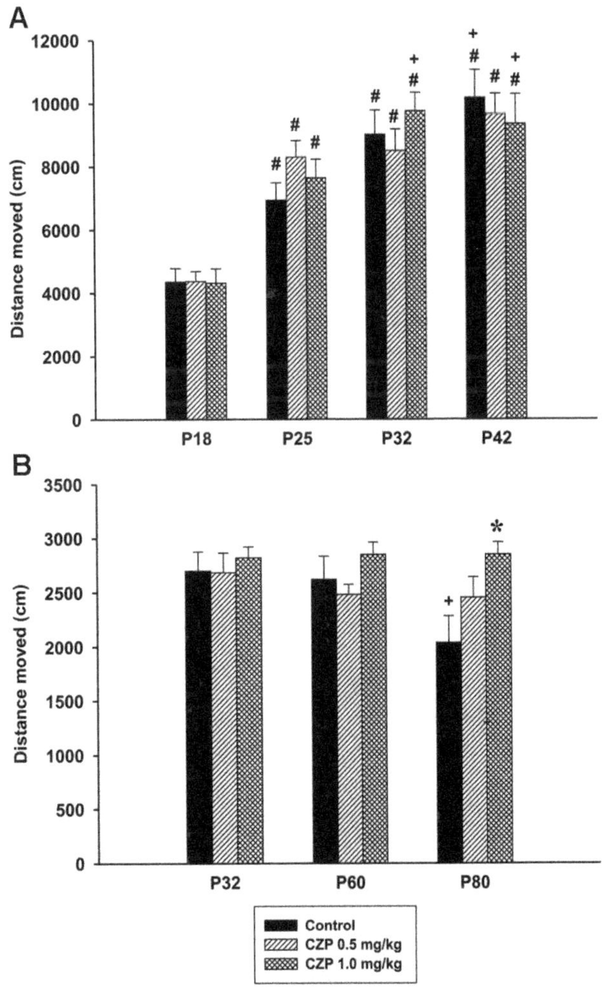

FIGURE 7 | Effect of CZP exposure (P7–P11) on locomotion. Illustrated here are the data from Experiment 2 (*social behavior during development*, **A**) and Experiment 3 (*social behavior in a resident-intruder paradigm*, **B**). # Significant difference compared to P18. + Significant difference compared to P25. * Significant difference compared to control group.

the control and CZP animals, aged 32 days (control: mean = 8215.56, SEM = 445.50, CZP 0.1 mg/kg: mean = 8128.01, SEM = 787.61, CZP 0.5 mg/kg: mean = 7560.67, SEM = 737.79, CZP 1.0 mg/kg: mean = 8123.96, SEM = 445.557). During development (Experiment 2), there was a significant effect of age [$F_{(3,81)} = 71.71$, $p < 0.001$], but not of CZP exposure [$F_{(2,27)} = 0.24$, $p = 0.97$], nor of drug × age interaction [$F_{(6,81)} = 1.40$, $p = 0.22$]. *Post hoc* test revealed that animals in all age groups walked a longer distance than those at P18. The dose of 1.0 mg/kg CZP significantly prolonged the distance moved at P32 and P42 compared to those of animals at P25 (**Figure 7A**). As for locomotion of resident rats, ANOVA revealed a significant effect of age [$F_{(2,48)} = 4.20$, $p = 0.021$] and drug × age interaction [$F_{(4,48)} = 2.57$ $p = 0.04$]. No significant effect of CZP exposure [$F_{(2,24)} = 2.38$, $p = 0.11$] was observed in the distance moved. *Post hoc* test showed a significant decline in locomotion in control animals at P80 compared to those at P32 and P60. Moreover, the animals at P80 exposed to a higher CZP dose, walked for a longer distance compared to respective controls (**Figure 7B**).

DISCUSSION

In the present study, we evaluated the effects of early life exposure to clonazepam on the social behavior of rats in respect to their familiarity with test conditions. The results of this study have shown that short-lasting exposure to CZP during early postnatal period affects social play and social interaction differentially, depending on age and environment.

Social behavior represents a relevant category of behavior essential for the acquisition of motor, social, sexual and cognitive skills (Vanderschuren et al., 1997; Pellis and Pellis, 1998; Auger and Olesen, 2009; Trezza et al., 2010). In rats, social behavior is a complex dynamic interaction that begins with social play behavior at about P18, peaks between P32 and P40 and gradually declines thereafter (Panksepp, 1981; Pellis and Pellis, 1997; Terranova et al., 1999) but never disappears completely (Vanderschuren et al., 1995a; Pellis and Pellis, 1997). Social interactions and play behavior especially are highly dependent not only on the age of rats, but also on test circumstances, primarily on the familiarity or unfamiliarity of the environment (Vanderschuren et al., 1995b; Varlinskaya and Spear, 2008). Novel environment represents a highly anxiogenic condition and novelty was found to suppress social interaction in pubescent and young adult animals (P35 and P60) but not in younger animals (P28) (Primus and Kellogg, 1989, 1990).

Many experimental studies already documented that social behavior is particularly sensitive to pharmacological influences (Varlinskaya and Spear, 2002; File and Seth, 2003; Schneider and Koch, 2005; Homberg et al., 2007; Koros et al., 2007; Trezza et al., 2009; Mooney and Varlinskaya, 2011). Also early pharmacological intervention was found to modify social behavior long time after treatment cessation. File (1986b) reported minor increase of social interactions between control adolescent rats and rats treated with diazepam or lorazepam throughout preweaning period, but no difference in animals treated with CZP according to the same treatment protocol (File, 1986c). In both studies, animals spent more time in active social interaction when being in familiar than in unfamiliar environment. On the contrary, in our study CZP exposure suppressed play behavior in adolescence, but not other forms of social interaction irrespective of environmental context. Discrepancy between these studies probably relates to differences in experimental protocol and way of evaluation. In our study, we differentiated between "*social behavior related to play*" and "*social behavior unrelated to play*" and these two categories were evaluated separately, whereas File evaluated all social contacts in one category. Thus we hypothesize that early CZP exposure leads to increased social anxiety and/or decreased motivation for play behavior and that the lack of familiarity effects is due to impaired adaptation to novelty. The adolescent animals were familiarized to OF before social test. In contrast, in developmental study animals were not habituated to environment. Pre-weaning rats do not display intra-session habituation and even older rats are not able to remember the environment if exposure is repeated after seven days from the first exposure (Leussis and Bolivar, 2006).

In present study, adolescent animals were isolated for three hours before the social interaction took place in order to promote social behavior (Vanderschuren et al., 1995b). It has been shown that social deprivation, especially during the acquisition period of social play, leads to social disturbances independent of subsequent social stimulation (Hol et al., 1999) and may induce a predisposition to either anxiety or depressive-like behavior (Tsoory et al., 2007). Developing animals were repeatedly tested thus the time period of isolation was cut to 30 min. Therefore we assume that the inhibition of social play in CZP-exposed animals cannot be attributed to a long-term or repeated isolation.

When allowed to establish a territory, a male rat defends his territory if an unfamiliar conspecific intruder is introduced. Such behavior is indicative of the territorial advantage of resident animal, and it is apparent after the resident has been singly housed for only a few days (for rev. Mitchell and Redfern, 2005). In concordance with previous studies on the role of territoriality on social behavior in a resident-intruder paradigm, our data show that play behavior gradually decreases with age but never disappear completely and even adult rats continue to play (Pellis and Pellis, 1987, 1990). Early exposure to CZP modified social interaction in resident-intruder test. Exposure to CZP in a dose of 1.0 mg/kg increased the duration of wrestling which was always initiated by the resident rat reflecting a high degree of dominance for his territory. This social activity never changed to an aggressive form of fighting characterized by a threat posture, serious attacks to partner's rump, and biting (Pellis and Pellis, 1987; Blanchard et al., 2001). This finding is in agreement with results of previous study showing that if a male intruder is weight-matched to resident, the aggressive form of interaction does not emerge (Robinson et al., 2011). In earlier studies, File reported that the administration of CZP from birth until weaning enhances offensive behavior when adolescent rats were resident in their home cage (File, 1986c). Similarly, the same author showed that neonatal treatment (P1–P7) with a high dose of diazepam (10 mg/kg) increases aggression in adolescent resident rats (File, 1987). Taken together, these findings indicate that BZDs exposure during postnatal period affects the specific forms of social behavior that reflect dominance for an established territory. Our data in addition revealed a remarkable inhibition of genital investigation in the adults exposed to CZP early in life. This component of social behavior represents a natural propensity of laboratory rats to investigate and olfactory discriminate conspecifics (Engelmann et al., 1995, 2011). Thus present findings suggest that postnatal CZP exposure shifts the behavior from social investigation to a higher motivation pattern, such as play wrestling. Opposite effects of early CZP exposure on social play and other forms of social behavior are consistent with recent studies demonstrating that social play and social behaviors represent separate behavioral categories with different pharmacological sensitivity (Varlinskaya et al., 1999; Varlinskaya and Spear, 2008; Trezza et al., 2009).

Early CZP exposure did not result in substantial changes of locomotion in any social test. Therefore we consider it unlikely that the differences in social behavior are related to locomotor alteration. Exposure to the high dose of CZP however resulted in decrease of capability to adapt to environmental condition. In contrast to controls, in CZP exposed animals distance moved did not decrease with repeated exposure. As previously reported animals exposed to CZP exhibited higher locomotion, spent more time in the central part of the OF, suggesting decresed anxiety, and had impaired between-session habituation in (Mikulecká et al., 2014).

The expression of social behavior and specifically play behavior involves a wide variety of neuronal systems. The various aspects of social play are evidently regulated and/or modulated by different neurotransmitters and can be influenced differently by environmental and social factors (Varlinskaya et al., 1999; Trezza et al., 2009). The recent progress in the neuropharmacology of play behavior have pointed to neurotransmitter systems, such as opioids, cannabinoids, cholinergic and dopaminergic that modulate the rewarding, motivational and cognitive aspects of play behavior, and to the nonspecific effects of serotonin and norepinephrine (Vanderschuren et al., 1997; Homberg et al., 2007; Trezza et al., 2010; Siviy and Panksepp, 2011; Siviy et al., 2011). In addition, GABAergic and dopaminergic transmission play a major role in the pharmacology, neurochemistry and physiopathology of the emotional states. For example, $GABA_A$ receptor substrate which controls bidirectional reward signaling between dopaminergic and non-dopaminergic reward systems, play a role in positive emotional processes such as social play (Laviolette and van der Kooy, 2001; Burgdorf and Panksepp, 2006).

Interactive social play represents a separate and characteristic form of social behavior expressed predominantly between weaning and adolescence. This form of social behavior is highly rewarding and indispensable for the development of social competence and cognitive skills (Panksepp, 1981; Pellis and Mckenna, 1995). Social play during a juvenile period prepares the motor system of animals for engagement in adult behavior. In addition, the experience of positive social interaction during key developmental ages has profound and long-lasting effects on brain function and behavior in emotional, motivational and cognitive domain (Trezza et al., 2011). When available, play can also facilitate and refine brain areas that are involved in the very social skills, and serves for training animals to cope with unpredictable events. Play deprivation during juvenile and adolescence can lead to incompetence in sexual performance in adulthood and produce long-term cognitive, behavioral and emotional deficits (for rev. Pellis and Pellis, 2006; Trezza et al., 2011). Short-term CZP exposure in the critical period of neurobehavioral development may interfere with the formation of social motivation or positive emotional processes, thereby altering the emotional reactivity and expression of social behavior. Inadequate social behavior is the main hallmark of psychiatric disorders (DMS IV, American Psychiatric Association, 1994) and to some extent, the disturbances shown in animal studies are comparable to symptomatological as well as etiological aspects of neurodevelopmental disorders (Schneider and Koch, 2005). The data from animal experiments have to be translated to human situation with extreme caution. In concordance with previous studies, our results however indicate that the exposure to benzodiazepines during the critical developmental period may alter the responsiveness in social relationship.

ACKNOWLEDGMENTS

This study was supported by grants No.305/09/086 and No. P304/12/G069 from the Czech Science Foundation and Research Project RVO 67985823.

REFERENCES

American Psychiatric Association. (1994). *Diagnostic and Statistical Manual of Mental Disorders.* Washington, DC: American Psychiatric Press.

André, M., Boutroy, M. J., Dubruc, C., Thenot, J. P., Bianchetti, G., Sola, L., et al. (1986). Clonazepam pharmacokinetics and therapeutic efficacy in neonatal seizures. *Eur. J. Clin. Pharmacol.* 30, 585–589. doi: 10.1007/bf00542419

Auger, A. P., and Olesen, K. M. (2009). Brain sex differences and the organisation of juvenile social play behaviour. *J. Neuroendocrinol.* 21, 519–525. doi: 10.1111/j.1365-2826.2009.01871.x

Avishai-Eliner, S., Brunson, K. L., Sandman, C. A., and Baram, T. Z. (2002). Stressed-out, or in (utero)? *Trends Neurosci.* 25, 518–524. doi: 10.1016/s0166-2236(02)02241-5

Bittigau, P., Sifringer, M., Genz, K., Reith, E., Pospischil, D., Govindarajalu, S., et al. (2002). Antiepileptic drugs and apoptotic neurodegeneration in the developing brain. *Proc. Natl. Acad. Sci. U S A* 99, 15089–15094. doi: 10.1073/pnas.222550499

Blanchard, R. J., Yudko, E., Dulloog, L., and Blanchard, D. C. (2001). Defense changes in stress nonresponsive subordinate males in a visible burrow system. *Physiol. Behav.* 72, 635–642. doi: 10.1016/s0031-9384(00)00449-2

Burgdorf, J., and Panksepp, J. (2006). The neurobiology of positive emotions. *Neurosci. Biobehav. Rev.* 30, 173–187. doi: 10.1016/j.neubiorev.2005.06.001

Clancy, B., Finlay, B. L., Darlington, R. B., and Anand, K. J. (2007). Extrapolating brain development from experimental species to humans. *Neurotoxicology* 28, 931–937. doi: 10.1016/j.neuro.2007.01.014

Darbra, S., and Pallarès, M. (2009). Neonatal allopregnanolone increases novelty-directed locomotion and disrupts behavioural responses to GABA(A) receptor modulators in adulthood. *Int. J. Dev. Neurosci.* 27, 617–625. doi: 10.1016/j.ijdevneu.2009.05.008

Dobbing, J., and Sands, J. (1979). Comparative aspects of the brain growth spurt. *Early. Hum. Dev.* 3, 79–83. doi: 10.1016/0378-3782(79)90022-7

Engelmann, M., Hadicke, J., and Noack, J. (2011). Testing declarative memory in laboratory rats and mice using the nonconditioned social discrimination procedure. *Nat. Protoc.* 6, 1152–1162. doi: 10.1038/nprot.2011.353

Engelmann, M., Wotjak, C. T., and Landgraf, R. (1995). Social discrimination procedure: an alternative method to investigate juvenile recognition abilities in rats. *Physiol. Behav.* 58, 315–321. doi: 10.1016/0031-9384(95)00053-l

File, S. E. (1986a). Behavioral changes persisting into adulthood after neonatal benzodiazepine administration in the rat. *Neurobehav. Toxicol. Teratol.* 8, 453–461.

File, S. E. (1986b). Effects of neonatal administration of diazepam and lorazepam on performance of adolescent rats in tests of anxiety, aggression, learning and convulsions. *Neurobehav. Toxicol. Teratol.* 8, 301–306.

File, S. E. (1986c). The effects of neonatal administration of clonazepam on passive avoidance and on social, aggressive and exploratory behavior of adolescent male rats. *Neurobehav. Toxicol. Teratol.* 8, 447–452.

File, S. E. (1987). Diazepam and caffeine administration during the first week of life: changes in neonatal and adolescent behavior. *Neurotoxicol. Teratol.* 9, 9–16. doi: 10.1016/0892-0362(87)90063-8

File, S. E., and Seth, P. (2003). A review of 25 years of the social interaction test. *Eur. J. Pharmacol.* 463, 35–53. doi: 10.1016/s0014-2999(03)01273-1

Forcelli, P. A., Kozlowski, R., Snyder, C., Kondratyev, A., and Gale, K. (2012). Effects of neonatal antiepileptic drug exposure on cognitive, emotional and motor function in adult rats. *J. Pharmacol. Exp. Ther.* 340, 558–566. doi: 10.1124/jpet.111.188862

Fraňková, S., and Mikulecká, A. (1990). Ontogeny of social behavior of pups of laboratory rats genetically selected for activity level. *Act. Nerv. Super. (Praha)* 32, 167–173.

Gai, N., and Grimm, V. E. (1982). The effect of prenatal exposure to diazepam on aspects of postnatal development and behavior in rats. *Psychopharmacology (Berl)* 78, 225–229. doi: 10.1007/bf00428155

Garrett, K. M., Saito, N., Duman, R. S., Abel, M. S., Ashton, R. A., Fujimori, S., et al. (1990). Differential expression of gamma-aminobutyric acidA receptor subunits. *Mol. Pharmacol.* 37, 652–657.

Hol, T., Van den Berg, C. L., Van Ree, J. M., and Spruijt, B. M. (1999). Isolation during the play period in infancy decreases adult social interactions in rats. *Behav. Brain Res.* 100, 91–97. doi: 10.1016/s0166-4328(98)00116-8

Homberg, J. R., Schiepers, O. J., Schoffelmeer, A. N., Cuppen, E., and Vanderschuren, L. J. (2007). Acute and constitutive increases in central serotonin levels reduce social play behaviour in peri-adolescent rats. *Psychopharmacology (Berl)* 195, 175–182. doi: 10.1007/s00213-007-0895-8

Hoogerkamp, A., Arends, R. H., Bomers, A. M., Mandema, J. W., Voskuyl, R. A., and Danhof, M. (1996). Pharmacokinetic/pharmacodynamic relationship of benzodiazepines in the direct cortical stimulation model of anticonvulsant effect. *J. Pharmacol. Exp. Ther.* 279, 803–812.

Hulin, M. W., Amato, R. J., and Winsauer, P. J. (2012). GABA(A) receptor modulation during adolescence alters adult ethanol intake and preference in rats. *Alcohol. Clin. Exp. Res.* 36, 223–233. doi: 10.1111/j.1530-0277.2011.01622.x

Kellogg, C. K. (1988). Benzodiazepines: influence on the developing brain. *Prog. Brain Res.* 73, 207–228. doi: 10.1016/s0079-6123(08)60506-3

Koros, E., Rosenbrock, H., Birk, G., Weiss, C., and Sams-Dodd, F. (2007). The selective mGlu5 receptor antagonist MTEP, similar to NMDA receptor antagonists, induces social isolation in rats. *Neuropsychopharmacology* 32, 562–576. doi: 10.1038/sj.npp.1301133

Kubová, H., and Mareš, P. (1989). Time course of the anticonvulsant action of clonazepam during ontogenesis in the rat. *Arch. Int. Pharmacodyn. Ther.* 298, 15–24.

Lader, M. (1994). Biological processes in benzodiazepine dependence. *Addiction* 89, 1413–1418. doi: 10.1111/j.1360-0443.1994.tb03737.x

Lalive, A. L., Rudolph, U., Luscher, C., and Tan, K. R. (2011). Is there a way to curb benzodiazepine addiction? *Swiss Med. Wkly.* 141:w13277. doi: 10.4414/smw.2011.13277

Laviolette, S. R., and van der Kooy, D. (2001). GABA(A) receptors in the ventral tegmental area control bidirectional reward signalling between dopaminergic and non-dopaminergic neural motivational systems. *Eur. J. Neurosci.* 13, 1009–1015. doi: 10.1046/j.1460-9568.2001.01458.x

Leussis, M. P., and Bolivar, V. J. (2006). Habituation in rodents: a review of behavior, neurobiology, and genetics. *Neurosci. Biobehav. Rev.* 30, 1045–1064. doi: 10.1016/j.neubiorev.2006.03.006

Lippa, A. S., Beer, B., Sano, M. C., Vogel, R. A., and Meyerson, L. R. (1981). Differential ontogeny of type 1 and type 2 benzodiazepine receptors. *Life Sci.* 28, 2343–2347. doi: 10.1016/0024-3205(81)90498-7

Meaney, M., and Stewart, J. (1981). A descriptive study of social development in the rat (*Rattus norvegicus*). *Anim. Behav.* 29, 34–45. doi: 10.1016/s0003-3472(81)80149-2

Mikulecká, A., Mareš, P., and Kubová, H. (2011). Rebound increase in seizure susceptibility but not isolation-induced calls after single administration of clonazepam and Ro 19–8022 in infant rats. *Epilepsy Behav.* 20, 12–19. doi: 10.1016/j.yebeh.2010.10.021

Mikulecká, A., Šubrt, M., Stuchlík, A., and Kubová, H. (2014). Consequences of early postnatal benzodiazepines exposure in rats. I. Cognitive-like behavior. *Front. Behav. Neurosci.* 8:101. doi: 10.3389/fnbeh.2014.00101

Mitchell, P. J., and Redfern, P. H. (2005). Animal models of depressive illness: the importance of chronic drug treatment. *Curr. Pharm. Des.* 11, 171–203. doi: 10.2174/1381612053382250

Mòdol, L., Darbra, S., Vallèe, M., and Pallarès, M. (2013). Alteration of neonatal Allopregnanolone levels affects exploration, anxiety, aversive learning and adult behavioural response to intrahippocampal neurosteroids. *Behav. Brain Res.* 241, 96–104. doi: 10.1016/j.bbr.2012.11.043

Mooney, S. M., and Varlinskaya, E. I. (2011). Acute prenatal exposure to ethanol and social behavior: effects of age, sex and timing of exposure. *Behav. Brain Res.* 216, 358–364. doi: 10.1016/j.bbr.2010.08.014

Morishita, S. (2009). Clonazepam as a therapeutic adjunct to improve the management of depression: a brief review. *Hum. Psychopharmacol.* 24, 191–198. doi: 10.1002/hup.1015

Panksepp, J. (1981). The ontogeny of play in rats. *Dev. Psychobiol.* 14, 327–332. doi: 10.1002/dev.420140405

Pellis, S. M., and Mckenna, M. (1995). What do rats find rewarding in play fighting—an analysis using drug-induced non-playful partners. *Behav. Brain Res.* 68, 65–73. doi: 10.1016/0166-4328(94)00161-8

Pellis, S. M., and Pellis, V. C. (1987). Play fighting differs from serious fighting in both target of attack and tactics of fighting in the laboratory rat (*Rattus norvegicus*). *Aggress. Behav.* 13, 227–242. doi: 10.1002/1098-2337(1987)13:4<227::aid-ab2480130406>3.0.co;2-c

Pellis, S. M., and Pellis, V. C. (1990). Differential rates of attack, defense and counterattack during the developmental decrease in play fighting by male and female rats. *Dev. Psychobiol.* 23, 215–231. doi: 10.1002/dev.420230303

Pellis, S. M., and Pellis, V. C. (1997). The prejuvenile onset of play fighting in laboratory rats (*Rattus norvegicus*). *Dev. Psychobiol.* 31, 193–205. doi: 10.1002/(sici)1098-2302(199711)31:3<193::aid-dev4>3.3.co;2-#

Pellis, S. M., and Pellis, V. C. (1998). Play fighting of rats in comparative perspective: a schema for neurobehavioral analyses. *Neurosci. Biobehav. Rev.* 23, 87–101. doi: 10.1016/s0149-7634(97)00071-7

Pellis, S. M., and Pellis, V. C. (2006). "Play and the development of social engagement: a comparative perspective," in *The Development of Social Engagement: Neurobiological Perspectives*, eds P. J. Marshall and N. A. Fox (New York: Oxford University Press), 247–274.

Primus, R. J., and Kellogg, C. K. (1989). Pubertal-related changes influence the development of environment-related social interaction in the male rat. *Dev. Psychobiol.* 22, 633–643. doi: 10.1002/dev.420220608

Primus, R. J., and Kellogg, C. K. (1990). Developmental influence of gonadal function on the anxiolytic effect of diazepam on environment-related social interaction in the male rat. *Behav. Pharmacol.* 1, 437–446. doi: 10.1097/00008877-199000150-00005

Raol, Y. H., Zhang, G., Budreck, E. C., and Brooks-Kayal, A. R. (2005). Long-term effects of diazepam and phenobarbital treatment during development on GABA receptors, transporters and glutamic acid decarboxylase. *Neuroscience* 132, 399–407. doi: 10.1016/j.neuroscience.2005.01.005

Robinson, D. L., Zitzman, D. L., Smith, K. J., and Spear, L. P. (2011). Fast dopamine release events in the nucleus accumbens of early adolescent rats. *Neuroscience* 176, 296–307. doi: 10.1016/j.neuroscience.2010.12.016

Schneider, M., and Koch, M. (2005). Deficient social and play behavior in juvenile and adult rats after neonatal cortical lesion: effects of chronic pubertal cannabinoid treatment. *Neuropsychopharmacology* 30, 944–957. doi: 10.1038/sj.npp.1300634

Schroeder, H., Humbert, A. C., Desor, D., and Nehlig, A. (1997). Long-term consequences of neonatal exposure to diazepam on cerebral glucose utilization, learning, memory and anxiety. *Brain Res.* 766, 142–152. doi: 10.1016/s0006-8993(97)00538-6

Siviy, S. M., Crawford, C. A., Akopian, G., and Walsh, J. P. (2011). Dysfunctional play and dopamine physiology in the Fischer 344 rat. *Behav. Brain Res.* 220, 294–304. doi: 10.1016/j.bbr.2011.02.009

Siviy, S. M., and Panksepp, J. (2011). In search of the neurobiological substrates for social playfulness in mammalian brains. *Neurosci. Biobehav. Rev.* 35, 1821–1830. doi: 10.1016/j.neubiorev.2011.03.006

Smart, J. L., Dobbing, J., Adlard, B. P., Lynch, A., and Sands, J. (1973). Vulnerability of developing brain: relative effects of growth restriction during the fetal and suckling periods on behavior and brain composition of adult rats. *J. Nutr.* 9, 1327–1338.

Terranova, M. L., Cirulli, F., and Laviola, G. (1999). Behavioral and hormonal effects of partner familiarity in periadolescent rat pairs upon novelty exposure. *Psychoneuroendocrinology* 24, 639–656. doi: 10.1016/s0306-4530(99)00019-0

Trezza, V., Baarendse, P. J., and Vanderschuren, L. J. (2009). Prosocial effects of nicotine and ethanol in adolescent rats through partially dissociable neurobehavioral mechanisms. *Neuropsychopharmacology* 34, 2560–2573. doi: 10.1038/npp.2009.85

Trezza, V., Baarendse, P. J., and Vanderschuren, L. J. (2010). The pleasures of play: pharmacological insights into social reward mechanisms. *Trends Pharmacol. Sci.* 31, 463–469. doi: 10.1016/j.tips.2010.06.008

Trezza, V., Campolongo, P., and Vanderschuren, L. J. (2011). Evaluating the rewarding nature of social interactions in laboratory animals. *Dev. Cogn. Neurosci.* 1, 444–458. doi: 10.1016/j.dcn.2011.05.007

Tsoory, M., Cohen, H., and Richter-Levin, G. (2007). Juvenile stress induces a predisposition to either anxiety or depressive-like symptoms following stress in adulthood. *Eur. Neuropsychopharmacol.* 17, 245–256. doi: 10.1016/j.euroneuro.2006.06.007

Tucker, J. C. (1985). Benzodiazepines and the developing rat: a critical review. *Neurosci. Biobehav. Rev.* 9, 101–111. doi: 10.1016/0149-7634(85)90036-3

Vanderschuren, L. J., Niesink, R. J., Spruijt, B. M., and van Ree, J. M. (1995a). Effects of morphine on different aspects of social play in juvenile rats. *Psychopharmacology (Berl)* 117, 225–231. doi: 10.1007/bf02245191

Vanderschuren, L. J., Niesink, R. J., Spruijt, B. M., and van Ree, J. M. (1995b). Influence of environmental factors on social play behavior of juvenile rats. *Physiol. Behav.* 58, 119–123. doi: 10.1016/0031-9384(94)00385-i

Vanderschuren, L. J., Niesink, R. J., and van Ree, J. M. (1997). The neurobiology of social play behavior in rats. *Neurosci. Biobehav. Rev.* 21, 309–326. doi: 10.1016/s0149-7634(96)00020-6

Varlinskaya, E. I., and Spear, L. P. (2002). Acute effects of ethanol on social behavior of adolescent and adult rats: role of familiarity of the test situation. *Alcohol. Clin. Exp. Res.* 26, 1502–1511. doi: 10.1111/j.1530-0277.2002.tb02449.x

Varlinskaya, E. I., and Spear, L. P. (2008). Social interactions in adolescent and adult Sprague-Dawley rats: impact of social deprivation and test context familiarity. *Behav. Brain Res.* 188, 398–405. doi: 10.1016/j.bbr.2007.11.024

Varlinskaya, E. I., Spear, L. P., and Spear, N. E. (1999). Social behaviour and social motivation in adolescent rats: role of housing conditions and partner's activity. *Physiol. Behav.* 67, 475–482. doi: 10.1016/s0031-9384(98)00285-6

22

Links between circadian rhythms and psychiatric disease

Ilia N. Karatsoreos*

Department of Integrative Physiology and Neuroscience, Washington State University, Pullman, WA, USA

Edited by:
Ales Stuchlik, Institute of Physiology Academy of Sciences of the Czech Republic, Czech Republic

****Correspondence:***
Ilia N. Karatsoreos, Department of Integrative Physiology and Neuroscience, Washington State University, Pullman, WA 99164, USA
e-mail: iliak@vetmed.wsu.edu

Determining the cause of psychiatric disorders is a goal of modern neuroscience, and will hopefully lead to the discovery of treatments to either prevent or alleviate the suffering caused by these diseases. One roadblock to attaining this goal is the realization that neuropsychiatric diseases are rarely due to a single gene polymorphism, environmental exposure, or developmental insult. Rather, it is a complex interaction between these various influences that likely leads to the development of clinically relevant syndromes. Our lab is exploring the links between environmental exposures and neurobehavioral function by investigating how disruption of the circadian (daily) clock alters the structure and function of neural circuits, with the hypothesis that disrupting this crucial homeostatic system can directly contribute to altered vulnerability of the organism to other factors that interact to produce psychiatric illness. This review explores some historical and more recent findings that link disrupted circadian clocks to neuropsychiatric disorders, particularly depression, mania, and schizophrenia. We take a comparative approach by exploring the effects observed in human populations, as well as some experimental models used in the laboratory to unravel mechanistic and causal relationships between disruption of the circadian clock and behavioral abnormalities. This is a rich area of research that we predict will contribute greatly to our understanding of how genes, environment, and development interact to modulate an individual's vulnerability to psychiatric disorders.

Keywords: biological rhythms, schizophrenia, depression, anxiety, bipolar disorder

INTRODUCTION

A significant problem that modern neuroscience aims to solve is the distress caused by neuropsychiatric disorders. The fundamental challenge is that these disorders are far from the unitary constructs we sometimes imagine, and almost certainly not caused by a single event, gene mutation, or neurotransmitter abnormality. Instead, these disorders are multifaceted neurobehavioral dysfunctions that in many cases also include symptoms outside the central nervous system. As such, neuroscience needs to address these challenges in an integrated fashion, leveraging the advances made using genetic, molecular, and physiological approaches. Several research groups are tackling the puzzle of neuropsychiatric disorders by exploring the hypothesis that homeostatic perturbations are at the root of such disease states. Understanding the mechanisms that maintain homeostasis and respond to environmental challenges that threaten homeostasis is of crucial importance. One such system is the circadian (daily) timing system, and studying how circadian rhythms are perturbed in psychiatric disorders may provide insight into their contribution to neurobehavioral changes in some mental disease.

This review will describe the function of the circadian timing system, discuss how various neuropsychiatric disorders such as depression, anxiety, and schizophrenia display disruptions in circadian timing, and present the hypothesis that in some cases these disorders may be triggered or exacerbated by a dysfunction in this crucial homeostatic system.

CIRCADIAN RHYTHMS: A BRIEF REVIEW

One of the most salient environmental signals available to organisms is the rotation of the Earth about its axis. The reliable and predicable circadian (daily) changes in light and temperature (to mention only a few variables) have provided organisms – from single-celled organisms to humans – a framework on which to temporally organize physiology. This framework allows organisms to accomplish two major tasks. The first task is predicting regularly repeating changes in the environment. Anticipating such changes in the environment can aid even the simplest single-celled photosynthetic organism in the prediction of daylight hours to optimize energy collection by allowing different biochemical pathways to become active at appropriate times. This then allows potentially incompatible biochemical processes to exist in their own temporal compartments, ensuring they do not interfere with each other. Equally as important is the adaptation to unanticipated or less periodic changes in the environment. The circadian system allows for stimuli in the environment to "phase shift" the endogenous clock, pushing it forward or backward, in order to adapt to changes in the outside world. Unfortunately, modern industrialized society can regularly produce light at the wrong times of day (e.g., light at night from electronics) that then can activate phase shifting processes inappropriately. This problem is exacerbated when individuals are chronically living "out of time" with their circadian clocks, such as shift workers, airline pilots, and medical workers to name a few. Growing evidence suggests that chronic circadian disruption can result in significant mental and physical health problems. However, the mechanisms by which disrupted circadian clocks lead to these health problems remain unknown. To determine potential pathways by which disrupted clocks can contribute to neuropsychiatric disease, we need to explore the processes that underlie circadian timing at the molecular and cellular levels.

Almost all biological processes in organisms with lifespans longer than 24 h display circadian rhythms. In more complex animals, the most obvious of these is the regulation of the rest–activity cycle. In mammals, the master circadian clock regulating nearly all circadian rhythms in the organism is located in the suprachiasmatic nucleus (SCN) of the hypothalamus. This neural structure contains a self-sustaining oscillator that synchronizes local clocks throughout the brain and body (Moore-Ede et al., 1984; Butler et al., 2009). These "peripheral" clocks are thought to set local time in many body tissues, and are hypothesized to allow optimal functioning by temporally organizing biochemical and cellular processes throughout the organism. Animal studies have shown that shifting the SCN clock by light causes an almost instant resetting of oscillators there, but oscillators in the rest of the body take numerous cycles to fully resynchronize to the SCN and the external environment (Yamazaki et al., 2000), the root cause of the general malaise associated with jet lag. The mechanisms by which this resynchronization occurs remain unclear, although numerous candidates have been suggested (Cheng et al., 2002, 2006; Buhr et al., 2010).

HOW DOES CIRCADIAN DISRUPTION AFFECT NEUROBEHAVIORAL FUNCTION?

Anecdotally, most of us are aware that disruptions in circadian timing through shift work, jet lag, or other processes can lead to neurobehavioral deficits. Such changes can manifest as alterations in mood, affect, or cognitive function. It should be noted that several of the most notorious industrial accidents in the past few decades, including the Bhopal disaster in India, the Chernobyl nuclear accident in Ukraine, and the Exxon Valdez oil spill in Alaska occurred during the night, with the individuals involved being shift workers of one sort or another. It is thought that several factors, including fatigue, interacted in each of these cases to cause or exacerbate the chain of events that lead to catastrophe (Colten and Altevogt, 2006). Thus, particularly in occupations with high cognitive loads, disrupted circadian clocks and sleep cycles could lead to significant degradation in cognitive function. An intriguing study in flight crews demonstrated that short recovery crews (those that are traveling mostly on transmeridian flights requiring repeated resynchronizations) showed decreased reaction times, increased error rates, and marked temporal lobe atrophy (Cho, 2001).

Animal models have also been applied to probe the connection between disrupted circadian clocks and neural and behavioral deficits. Gibson et al. (2010) used a repeated jet lag model in Syrian hamsters to explore the effects of chronic experimental "jet lag" on behavioral outcomes and neurogenesis in the hippocampus, since hippocampal neurogenesis is related to both cognitive and affective regulation, and may underlie depression (Samuels and Hen, 2011). They demonstrated that chronic jet lag by repeated phase shifting of the light–dark cycle results in learning and memory deficits accompanied by reductions in hippocampal neurogenesis. An important contribution of this study was the finding that deficits in hippocampal-dependent learning and memory persisted after cessation of the experimental jet lag (Gibson et al., 2010), suggesting that there may be long-lasting negative consequences of circadian disruption on brain function, even after the disrupting stimulus has been removed. In mice, Karatsoreos et al. (2011) demonstrated profound effects of circadian misalignment on the structure and function of prefrontal cortical neurons (Karatsoreos et al., 2011). Chronic (12 weeks) exposure to a shortened 20-h day (10 h light, 10 h dark) resulted in morphological changes in neurons in the medial prefrontal cortex (mPFC). Specifically, following circadian disruption neurons in layer II/III of the prelimbic mPFC had significant shrinkage of the apical dendrite, without observed changes in the basal dendrites. These gross changes were accompanied by simplification of the apical dendritic tree (Karatsoreos et al., 2011). Although the neural effects of the circadian disruption were stark, the behavioral effects were equally clear. Using a modified Morris Water Maze task that is sensitive to damage in the mPFC, circadian disrupted mice showed marked decreases in cognitive flexibility. In addition to the cognitive impairments, circadian disrupted mice demonstrated an "impulsive"-like phenotype, evidenced by entering a novel environment more quickly than controls. These findings were some of the first to experimentally link chronic circadian disruption to a reduction in the complexity of neurons that are important for attention, cognitive flexibility, and executive function. Although the mechanisms are still unknown, accumulating evidence supports a role for circadian disruption as a causative contributor to neurocognitive deficits.

LINKS BETWEEN CIRCADIAN DISRUPTION AND PSYCHIATRIC DISORDERS: UNFORTUNATE SIDE EFFECT OR CONTRIBUTING FACTOR?

One of the most common, and highly disruptive co-morbid problems in many psychiatric conditions, including depression, obsessive–compulsive disorder, and schizophrenia, is disruption in the sleep–wake cycle. However, there is ample debate if these effects are merely *symptoms* of these disorders, or in fact, if they may be contributing causes.

Depressive disorders are characterized by multiple physiological and psychological symptoms, and present with circadian disruption in both behavior and in physiology. The disruption of the circadian clock can manifest as changes in sleep–wake cycles (Van Cauter and Turek, 1986; Turek, 2007), but growing evidence also shows circadian disruption at the level of the molecular circadian clock (Mendlewicz, 2009). Recent findings show that intensity of major depressive symptoms in humans is correlated with the misalignment of circadian rhythms (Emens et al., 2009), in that more severe depressive states are associated with the circadian pacemaker being more delayed relative to the timing of sleep onset. Whether this is a causal change is still unclear, but shift workers often suffer from mood disturbances and an increased risk for depression (Scott et al., 1997; Asaoka et al., 2013). It is important to consider that links between circadian function and depression might occur at many levels (Wirz-Justice, 2009). An interesting example of this multi-level interaction is evident in the development and use of agomelatine, a melatonin agonist that also has serotonergic activity. This drug is actively being used for its antidepressant actions, with significant results (de Bodinat et al., 2010). It is thought that agomelatine can also act as a circadian "resynchronizer" in models of depression (Morley-Fletcher et al., 2011; Koresh et al., 2012; Mairesse et al., 2013). In human studies, it has been demonstrated that agomelatine can increase the relative amplitude of circadian rhythms in the rest–activity cycle, including effects on sleep, which was accompanied by parallel improvement in depressive symptoms (Kasper et al., 2010). When taken as a whole, these findings suggest that circadian disruption may contribute to depression, though unraveling the etiology from symptomology can be difficult. Given that changes in hippocampal neurogenesis are observed following chronic circadian disruption, and that cell birth and proliferation in the hippocampus is related to mood and antidepressant efficacy (Gibson et al., 2010), it is evident that circadian disruption may contribute to the development or exacerbation of depressive disorders. As yet, how these various pathways interact and synergize is unknown, though changes in multiple interacting physiological systems induced by chronic circadian dysfunction are likely to be a precipitating factor. Although it is clear that there is a strong relationship between circadian disruption and depression, these effects are likely bidirectional.

In addition to cognitive deficits and depression, circadian rhythm abnormalities have also been explored in mania. It is well established that during manic episodes, sleep patterns are significantly altered (Wehr et al., 1983; Plante and Winkelman, 2008; Robillard et al., 2013), and circadian patterns of several physiological functions are attenuated (Goetze and Tolle, 1987; Souetre et al., 1988; McClung, 2007). To probe potential causative links between disrupted circadian clocks and mania, animal models must be leveraged. Several lines of evidence demonstrate that treating hamsters with lithium chloride (a potent pharmacological agent used to treat manic depressive disorders) significantly lengthens the period of their circadian clock (Terao, 1992; LeSauter and Silver, 1993; Klemfuss and Kripke, 1995; Iwahana et al., 2007). Detailed molecular work has shown that lithium treatment can alter several intracellular signaling cascades, including glycogen synthase kinase-3beta, a link to the circadian molecular clockworks (Iwahana et al., 2004; Padiath et al., 2004; Iitaka et al., 2005; Ko et al., 2010; Lamont et al., 2010; Osland et al., 2011). These studies suggest that this pharmacological treatment can reduce the symptoms of mania while also having direct effects on the circadian clock at both the cell/molecular level and the behavioral level. More recent work has begun to explore how defects in several key clock genes affect behaviors in mouse (McClung, 2011, 2013). Mutations in the core clock gene *Clock* can lead to mania-like behaviors (Roybal et al., 2007), and site-specific knockdown of *Clock* in the VTA can induce similar manic-like behaviors (Mukherjee et al., 2010). Together, the human and non-human animal models provide strong evidence that circadian dysfunction is not only a component of some forms of mania, but that altering the function of the molecular circadian clock can mimic many of these effects.

While pathways linking disrupted circadian clocks to cognitive function, depression, and perhaps even mania are being more clearly elucidated, links between circadian abnormalities and schizophrenia are less clear, both at the epidemiological and mechanistic levels. One reason for this lack of clarity is that the cause of schizophrenia remains elusive, and is likely a result of a combination of genetic and experiential factors. However, there are lines of evidence that point to strong links between disrupted circadian clocks and schizophrenia (reviewed in Jamadar et al., 2013; Monti et al., 2013). Epidemiological studies show that fragmented circadian rhythms, as measured by changes in rest–activity cycles or in sleep regulation, are observed in schizophrenic patients (Wirz-Justice et al., 1997, 2001; Wulff et al., 2006, 2012; Pritchett et al., 2012). This includes both sleep onset and sleep maintenance insomnia. Correlations have also been observed between the phasing of the melatonin rhythm and sleep in schizophrenia, and are commonly observed in many schizophrenic patients (Mills et al., 1977; Rao et al., 1994; Wirz-Justice et al., 1997). It is interesting to note that in most cases, the sleep/circadian effects observed in schizophrenia are *independent* of either the course of the disease or the pharmacological status of the patient (Monti et al., 2013). Several animal models are now being applied to attempt to gain a mechanistic handle on the interaction between circadian timing and schizophrenia. The "blind-drunk" (Bdr) mouse line, which presents schizophrenic-like symptoms (Jeans et al., 2007), has been shown to have phase-advanced (i.e., earlier starting) rest–activity cycles while also showing a fragmentation of their circadian cycles (Oliver et al., 2012). The Bdr mouse carries a mutation in the gene for synaptosomal-associated protein (Snap)-25 that leads to disruption of exocytosis. This points to an association between altered synaptic activity and neurobehavioral function observed in schizophrenia-like models and circadian rhythms. However, this work should be interpreted cautiously, as the effects of this mutation on circadian rhythms may have little to do with the effects of the mutation on schizophrenia-like behavior. It is more likely that rather than directly causing schizophrenia, disruption of the circadian clock may somehow alter susceptibility in individuals at risk of developing schizophrenia. Work by Vacic et al. (2011) shows that in humans, a copy number variant in the gene encoding for the receptor for vasoactive intestinal polypeptide that is found in the SCN (i.e., *Vipr2*) can result in an increase risk of developing schizophrenia (Vacic et al., 2011). As such, there is compelling and somewhat provocative evidence that disruption of the circadian clock may not only be a symptom of schizophrenia, but perhaps a contributing cause.

CONCLUSION AND FUTURE DIRECTIONS

The circadian timing system controls all physiological and behavioral rhythms, synchronizes them to the external environment, and ensures temporal isolation of incompatible physiological or behavioral processes (Kalsbeek et al., 2007; Karatsoreos and Silver, 2007; Butler et al., 2009). Thus, the circadian system sits at the center of a "web," and can modulate the function of myriad physiological systems, both peripherally and centrally (Reppert and Weaver, 2002; Hastings et al., 2003). Since circadian rhythms are phylogenetically ancient, with many molecular components conserved between diverse species, from *Drosophila* to mouse to human (Bell-Pedersen et al., 2005), understanding how optimal functioning of this system contributes to fitness or vulnerability could have significant impact. That disrupted rhythms are observed in psychiatric conditions as diverse as depression, bipolar disorder, and schizophrenia (Mansour et al., 2005; Roybal et al., 2007; Mendlewicz, 2009; Cortesi et al., 2010; Sacco et al., 2010; Karatsoreos, 2012), makes it intriguing to hypothesize that they may play a role in their etiology. However, as this and many other reviews indicate, whether circadian disruption represents a symptom or an etiology is unclear, and the specific contributions of disrupted circadian rhythms to mental disease are poorly understood.

This review has presented several findings from both the human and non-human animal literature that support a role for disrupted circadian clocks in the etiology of mental disease. Since the causes of many of these neuropsychiatric disorders are multifaceted, it is unlikely that a single circadian mutation, or single instance of circadian disruption, would directly cause the development of a mental disorder. It is also important to note that while there is ample and growing evidence of a circadian contribution to many of the disorders discussed in this review, some of the evidence is indirect, and none of the evidence specifically obviates other causes for these neuropsychiatric diseases. It is our hope that this review provides an additional context to the already rich work on the genetic, developmental, and environmental etiologies of mental disorders. We hypothesize that disrupted circadian clocks may instead make individuals more *susceptible* to the development of neuropsychiatric disorders (Karatsoreos and McEwen, 2011, 2013). This effect may be in a manner similar to the stress-diathesis model, whereby environmental challenges have more severe outcomes due to underlying genetic or experiential differences (Morley, 1983). Thus, chronic circadian disruption through genetic abnormalities or environmental perturbation could make neural systems less able to cope with insults. This failure in resilience could lead to the onset of neuropsychiatric conditions in those individuals who are made more vulnerable because of other factors such as genetics, developmental experiences, or environmental exposures. While still conjecture, we feel that this is an exciting area for future research that will hopefully lead to great strides being made in understanding the complex causes of mental disorders.

ACKNOWLEDGMENTS

I would like to thank my laboratory members for their hard work, and comments on a previous version of this manuscript. I would also like to thank the two reviewers who helped to significantly strengthen this manuscript. This work was supported in part by a Brain Research Foundation NARSAD Young Investigator Award to INK.

REFERENCES

Asaoka, S., Aritake, S., Komada, Y., Ozaki, A., Odagiri, Y., Inoue, S., et al. (2013). Factors associated with shift work disorder in nurses working with rapid-rotation schedules in Japan: the nurses' sleep health project. *Chronobiol. Int.* 30, 628–636. doi:10.3109/07420528.2012.762010

Bell-Pedersen, D., Cassone, V. M., Earnest, D. J., Golden, S. S., Hardin, P. E., Thomas, T. L., et al. (2005). Circadian rhythms from multiple oscillators: lessons from diverse organisms. *Nat. Rev. Genet.* 6, 544–556. doi:10.1038/nrg1633

Buhr, E. D., Yoo, S. H., and Takahashi, J. S. (2010). Temperature as a universal resetting cue for mammalian circadian oscillators. *Science* 330, 379–385. doi:10.1126/science.1195262

Butler, M. P., Kriegsfeld, L. J., and Silver, R. (2009). "Circadian regualtion of endocrine functions," in *Hormones, Brain and Behavior*, eds D. Pfaff, A. Arnold, A. Etgen, S. Fahrbach, and R. Rubin (San Diego, CA: Academic Press), 473–505.

Cheng, M. Y., Bullock, C. M., Li, C., Lee, A. G., Bermak, J. C., Belluzzi, J., et al. (2002). Prokineticin 2 transmits the behavioural circadian rhythm of the suprachiasmatic nucleus. *Nature* 417, 405–410. doi:10.1038/417405a

Cheng, M. Y., Leslie, F. M., and Zhou, Q. Y. (2006). Expression of prokineticins and their receptors in the adult mouse brain. *J. Comp. Neurol.* 498, 796–809. doi:10.1002/cne.21087

Cho, K. (2001). Chronic "jet lag" produces temporal lobe atrophy and spatial cognitive deficits. *Nat. Neurosci.* 4, 567–568. doi:10.1038/88384

Colten, H. R., and Altevogt, B. M. (eds). (2006). *Sleep Disorders and Sleep Deprivation: An Unmet Public Health Problem.* Washington, DC: The National Academies Press.

Cortesi, F., Giannotti, F., Ivanenko, A., and Johnson, K. (2010). Sleep in children with autistic spectrum disorder. *Sleep Med.* 11, 659–664. doi:10.1016/j.sleep.2010.01.010

de Bodinat, C., Guardiola-Lemaitre, B., Mocaer, E., Renard, P., Munoz, C., and Millan, M. J. (2010). Agomelatine, the first melatonergic antidepressant: discovery, characterization and development. *Nat. Rev. Drug Discov.* 9, 628–642. doi:10.1038/nrd3140

Emens, J., Lewy, A., Kinzie, J. M., Arntz, D., and Rough, J. (2009). Circadian misalignment in major depressive disorder. *Psychiatry Res.* 168, 259–261. doi:10.1016/j.psychres.2009.04.009

Gibson, E. M., Wang, C., Tjho, S., Khattar, N., and Kriegsfeld, L. J. (2010). Experimental "jet lag" inhibits adult neurogenesis and produces long-term cognitive deficits in female hamsters. *PLoS ONE* 5:e15267. doi:10.1371/journal.pone.0015267

Goetze, U., and Tolle, R. (1987). Circadian rhythm of free urinary cortisol, temperature and heart rate in endogenous depressives and under antidepressant therapy. *Neuropsychobiology* 18, 175–184. doi:10.1159/000118414

Hastings, M. H., Reddy, A. B., and Maywood, E. S. (2003). A clockwork web: circadian timing in brain and periphery, in health and disease. *Nat. Rev. Neurosci.* 4, 649–661. doi:10.1038/nrn1177

Iitaka, C., Miyazaki, K., Akaike, T., and Ishida, N. (2005). A role for glycogen synthase kinase-3beta in the mammalian circadian clock. *J. Biol. Chem.* 280, 29397–29402. doi:10.1074/jbc.M503526200

Iwahana, E., Akiyama, M., Miyakawa, K., Uchida, A., Kasahara, J., Fukunaga, K., et al. (2004). Effect of lithium on the circadian rhythms of locomotor activity and glycogen synthase kinase-3 protein expression in the mouse suprachiasmatic nuclei. *Eur. J. Neurosci.* 19, 2281–2287. doi:10.1111/j.0953-816X.2004.03322.x

Iwahana, E., Hamada, T., Uchida, A., and Shibata, S. (2007). Differential effect of lithium on the circadian oscillator in young and old hamsters. *Biochem. Biophys. Res. Commun.* 354, 752–756. doi:10.1016/j.bbrc.2007.01.042

Jamadar, S., O'Neil, K. M., Pearlson, G. D., Ansari, M., Gill, A., Jagannathan, K., et al. (2013). Impairment in semantic retrieval is associated with symptoms in schizophrenia but not bipolar disorder. *Biol. Psychiatry* 73, 555–564. doi:10.1016/j.biopsych.2012.07.027

Jeans, A. F., Oliver, P. L., Johnson, R., Capogna, M., Vikman, J., Molnar, Z., et al. (2007). A dominant mutation in Snap25 causes impaired vesicle trafficking, sensorimotor gating, and ataxia in the blind-drunk mouse. *Proc. Natl. Acad. Sci. U.S.A.* 104, 2431–2436. doi:10.1073/pnas.0610222104

Kalsbeek, A., Kreier, F., Fliers, E., Sauerwein, H. P., Romijn, J. A., and Buijs, R. M. (2007). Circadian control of metabolism by the SCN. *Endocrinology* 148, 5635–5639. doi:10.1210/en.2007-0776

Karatsoreos, I. N. (2012). Effects of circadian disruption on mental and physical health. *Curr. Neurol. Neurosci. Rep.* 12, 218–225. doi:10.1007/s11910-012-0252-0

Karatsoreos, I. N., Bhagat, S., Bloss, E. B., Morrison, J. H., and McEwen, B. S. (2011). Disruption of circadian clocks has ramifications for metabolism, brain, and behavior. *Proc. Natl. Acad. Sci. U.S.A.* 108, 1657–1662. doi:10.1073/pnas.1018375108

Karatsoreos, I. N., and McEwen, B. S. (2011). Psychobiological allostasis: resistance, resilience and vulnerability. *Trends Cogn. Sci.* 15, 576–584. doi:10.1016/j.tics.2011.10.005

Karatsoreos, I. N., and McEwen, B. S. (2013). Resilience and vulnerability: a neurobiological perspective. *F1000Prime Rep.* 5, 13. doi:10.12703/P5-13

Karatsoreos, I. N., and Silver, R. (2007). Minireview: the neuroendocrinology of the suprachiasmatic nucleus as a conductor of body time in mammals. *Endocrinology* 148, 5640–5647. doi:10.1210/en.2007-1083

Kasper, S., Hajak, G., Wulff, K., Hoogendijk, W. J., Montejo, A. L., Smeraldi, E., et al. (2010). Efficacy of the novel antidepressant agomelatine on the circadian rest–activity cycle and depressive and anxiety symptoms in patients with major depressive disorder: a randomized, double-blind comparison with sertraline. *J. Clin. Psychiatry* 71, 109–120. doi:10.4088/JCP.09m05347blu

Klemfuss, H., and Kripke, D. F. (1995). Antimanic drugs stabilize hamster circadian rhythms. *Psychiatry Res.* 57, 215–222. doi:10.1016/0165-1781(95)02687-R

Ko, H. W., Kim, E. Y., Chiu, J., Vanselow, J. T., Kramer, A., and Edery, I. (2010). A hierarchical phosphorylation cascade that regulates the timing of PERIOD nuclear entry reveals novel roles for proline-directed kinases and GSK-3beta/SGG in circadian clocks. *J. Neurosci.* 30, 12664–12675. doi:10.1523/JNEUROSCI.1586-10.2010

Koresh, O., Kozlovsky, N., Kaplan, Z., Zohar, J., Matar, M. A., and Cohen, H. (2012). The long-term abnormalities in circadian expression of period 1 and period 2 genes in response to stress is normalized by agomelatine administered immediately after exposure. *Eur. Neuropsychopharmacol.* 22, 205–221. doi:10.1016/j.euroneuro.2011.07.012

Lamont, E. W., Coutu, D. L., Cermakian, N., and Boivin, D. B. (2010). Circadian rhythms and clock genes in psychotic disorders. *Isr. J. Psychiatry Relat. Sci.* 47, 27–35.

LeSauter, J., and Silver, R. (1993). Lithium lengthens the period of circadian rhythms in lesioned hamsters bearing SCN grafts. *Biol. Psychiatry* 34, 75–83. doi:10.1016/0006-3223(93)90259-G

Mairesse, J., Silletti, V., Laloux, C., Zuena, A. R., Giovine, A., Consolazione, M., et al. (2013). Chronic agomelatine treatment corrects the abnormalities in the circadian rhythm of motor activity and sleep/wake cycle induced by prenatal restraint stress in adult rats. *Int. J. Neuropsychopharmacol.* 16, 323–338. doi:10.1017/S1461145711001970

Mansour, H. A., Monk, T. H., and Nimgaonkar, V. L. (2005). Circadian genes and bipolar disorder. *Ann. Med.* 37, 196–205. doi:10.1080/07853890510007377

McClung, C. A. (2007). Circadian genes, rhythms and the biology of mood disorders. *Pharmacol. Ther.* 114, 222–232. doi:10.1016/j.pharmthera.2007.02.003

McClung, C. A. (2011). Circadian rhythms and mood regulation: insights from pre-clinical models. *Eur. Neuropsychopharmacol.* 21(Suppl. 4), S683–S693. doi:10.1016/j.euroneuro.2011.07.008

McClung, C. A. (2013). How might circadian rhythms control mood? Let me count the ways. *Biol. Psychiatry* 74, 242–249. doi:10.1016/j.biopsych.2013.02.019

Mendlewicz, J. (2009). Disruption of the circadian timing systems: molecular mechanisms in mood disorders. *CNS Drugs* 23(Suppl. 2), 15–26. doi:10.2165/11318630-000000000-00000

Mills, J. N., Morgan, R., Minors, D. S., and Waterhouse, J. M. (1977). The free-running circadian rhythms of two schizophrenics. *Chronobiologia* 4, 353–360.

Monti, J. M., BaHammam, A. S., Pandi-Perumal, S. R., Bromundt, V., Spence, D. W., Cardinali, D. P., et al. (2013). Sleep and circadian rhythm dysregulation in schizophrenia. *Prog. Neuropsychopharmacol. Biol. Psychiatry* 43, 209–216. doi:10.1016/j.pnpbp.2012.12.021

Moore-Ede, M. C., Sulzman, F. M., and Fuller, C. A. (1984). *The Clocks that Time Us: Physiology of the Circadian Timing System.* Cambridge, MA: Harvard University Press.

Morley, S. (1983). The stress-diathesis model of illness. *J. Psychosom. Res.* 27, 86–87. doi:10.1016/0022-3999(83)90115-0

Morley-Fletcher, S., Mairesse, J., Soumier, A., Banasr, M., Fagioli, F., Gabriel, C., et al. (2011). Chronic agomelatine treatment corrects behavioral, cellular, and biochemical abnormalities induced by prenatal stress in rats. *Psychopharmacology (Berl.)* 217, 301–313. doi:10.1007/s00213-011-2280-x

Mukherjee, S., Coque, L., Cao, J. L., Kumar, J., Chakravarty, S., Asaithamby, A., et al. (2010). Knockdown of Clock in the ventral tegmental area through RNA interference results in a mixed state of mania and depression-like behavior. *Biol. Psychiatry* 68, 503–511. doi:10.1016/j.biopsych.2010.04.031

Oliver, P. L., Sobczyk, M. V., Maywood, E. S., Edwards, B., Lee, S., Livieratos, A., et al. (2012). Disrupted circadian rhythms in a mouse model of schizophrenia. *Curr. Biol.* 22, 314–319. doi:10.1016/j.cub.2011.12.051

Osland, T. M., Ferno, J., Havik, B., Heuch, I., Ruoff, P., Laerum, O. D., et al. (2011). Lithium differentially affects clock gene expression in serum-shocked NIH-3T3 cells. *J. Psychopharmacol.* 25, 924–933. doi:10.1177/0269881110379508

Padiath, Q. S., Paranjpe, D., Jain, S., and Sharma, V. K. (2004). Glycogen synthase kinase 3beta as a likely target for the action of lithium on circadian clocks. *Chronobiol. Int.* 21, 43–55. doi:10.1081/CBI-120027981

Plante, D. T., and Winkelman, J. W. (2008). Sleep disturbance in bipolar disorder: therapeutic implications. *Am. J. Psychiatry* 165, 830–843. doi:10.1176/appi.ajp.2008.08010077

Pritchett, D., Wulff, K., Oliver, P. L., Bannerman, D. M., Davies, K. E., Harrison, P. J., et al. (2012). Evaluating the links between schizophrenia and sleep and circadian rhythm disruption. *J. Neural Transm.* 119, 1061–1075. doi:10.1007/s00702-012-0817-8

Rao, M. L., Gross, G., Strebel, B., Halaris, A., Huber, G., Braunig, P., et al. (1994). Circadian rhythm of tryptophan, serotonin, melatonin, and pituitary hormones in schizophrenia. *Biol. Psychiatry* 35, 151–163. doi:10.1016/0006-3223(94)91147-9

Reppert, S. M., and Weaver, D. R. (2002). Coordination of circadian timing in mammals. *Nature* 418, 935–941. doi:10.1038/nature00965

Robillard, R., Naismith, S. L., and Hickie, I. B. (2013). Recent advances in sleep–wake cycle and biological rhythms in bipolar disorder. *Curr. Psychiatry Rep.* 15, 402. doi:10.1007/s11920-013-0402-3

Roybal, K., Theobold, D., Graham, A., DiNieri, J. A., Russo, S. J., Krishnan, V., et al. (2007). Mania-like behavior induced by disruption of CLOCK. *Proc. Natl. Acad. Sci. U.S.A.* 104, 6406–6411. doi:10.1073/pnas.0609625104

Sacco, R., Curatolo, P., Manzi, B., Militerni, R., Bravaccio, C., Frolli, A., et al. (2010). Principal pathogenetic components and biological endophenotypes in autism spectrum disorders. *Autism Res.* 3, 237–252. doi:10.1002/aur.151

Samuels, B. A., and Hen, R. (2011). Neurogenesis and affective disorders. *Eur. J. Neurosci.* 33, 1152–1159. doi:10.1111/j.1460-9568.2011.07614.x

Scott, A. J., Monk, T. H., and Brink, L. L. (1997). Shiftwork as a risk factor for depression: a pilot study. *Int. J. Occup. Environ. Health* 3, S2–S9.

Souetre, E., Salvati, E., Wehr, T. A., Sack, D. A., Krebs, B., and Darcourt, G. (1988). Twenty-four-hour profiles of body temperature and plasma TSH in bipolar patients during depression and during remission and in normal control subjects. *Am. J. Psychiatry* 145, 1133–1137.

Terao, T. (1992). Calcium, lithium, and circadian rhythms. *Biol. Psychiatry* 32, 105–106. doi:10.1016/0006-3223(92)90149-T

Turek, F. W. (2007). From circadian rhythms to clock genes in depression. *Int. Clin. Psychopharmacol.* 22(Suppl. 2), S1–S8. doi:10.1097/01.yic.0000277956.93777.6a

Vacic, V., McCarthy, S., Malhotra, D., Murray, F., Chou, H. H., Peoples, A., et al. (2011). Duplications of the neuropeptide receptor gene VIPR2 confer significant risk for schizophrenia. *Nature* 471, 499–503. doi:10.1038/nature09884

Van Cauter, E., and Turek, F. W. (1986). Depression: a disorder of timekeeping? *Perspect. Biol. Med.* 29, 510–519.

Wehr, T. A., Sack, D., Rosenthal, N., Duncan, W., and Gillin, J. C. (1983). Circadian rhythm disturbances in manic-depressive illness. *Fed. Proc.* 42, 2809–2814.

Wirz-Justice, A. (2009). From the basic neuroscience of circadian clock function to light therapy for depression: on the emergence of chronotherapeutics. *J. Affect. Disord.* 116, 159–160. doi:10.1016/j.jad.2009.04.024

Wirz-Justice, A., Cajochen, C., and Nussbaum, P. (1997). A schizophrenic patient with an arrhythmic circadian restactivity cycle. *Psychiatry Res.* 73, 83–90. doi:10.1016/S0165-1781(97)00117-0

Wirz-Justice, A., Krauchi, K., and Graw, P. (2001). An underlying circannual rhythm in seasonal affective disorder? *Chronobiol. Int.* 18, 309–313. doi:10.1081/CBI-100103193

Wulff, K., Dijk, D. J., Middleton, B., Foster, R. G., and Joyce, E. M. (2012). Sleep and circadian rhythm disruption in schizophrenia. *Br. J. Psychiatry* 200, 308–316. doi:10.1192/bjp.bp.111.096321

Wulff, K., Joyce, E., Middleton, B., Dijk, D. J., and Foster, R. G. (2006). The suitability of actigraphy, diary data, and urinary melatonin profiles for quantitative assessment of sleep disturbances in schizophrenia: a case report. *Chronobiol. Int.* 23, 485–495. doi:10.1080/07420520500545987

Yamazaki, S., Numano, R., Abe, M., Hida, A., Takahashi, R., Ueda, M., et al. (2000). Resetting central and peripheral circadian oscillators in transgenic rats. *Science* 288, 682–685. doi:10.1126/science.288.5466.682

23

Does sleep improve memory organization?

Masashi Takeuchi[1,2], Hisakazu Furuta[3], Tomiki Sumiyoshi[4]*, Michio Suzuki[1], Yoko Ochiai[3], Munehito Hosokawa[3], Mie Matsui[5] and Masayoshi Kurachi[1]

[1] *Department of Neuropsychiatry, University of Toyama Graduate School of Medicine and Pharmaceutical Sciences, Toyama, Japan*
[2] *Kamiichi General Hospital, Kamiichi-machi, Japan*
[3] *Sleep Disorders Center, Hokuriku National Hospital, Nanto-shi, Japan*
[4] *Department of Clinical Research Promotion, National Center Hospital, National Center of Neurology and Psychiatry, Tokyo, Japan*
[5] *Department of Psychology, University of Toyama Graduate School of Medicine and Pharmaceutical Sciences, Toyama, Japan*

Edited by:
Ales Stuchlik, Academy of Sciences of the Czech Republic, Czech Republic

***Correspondence:**
Tomiki Sumiyoshi, Department of Clinical Research Promotion, National Center of Neurology and Psychiatry, 4-1-1 Ogawa-Higashi, Kodaira, Tokyo 187-8551, Japan
e-mail: sumiyot@ncnp.go.jp

Sleep can integrate information into existing memory networks, look for common patterns and distil overarching rules, or simply stabilize and strengthen the memory exactly as it was learned. Recent research has shown that sleep facilitates abstraction of gist information as well as integration across multiple memories, insight into hidden solutions, and even the ability to make creative connections between distantly related ideas and concepts. To investigate the effect of sleep on memory organization, 35 normal volunteers were randomly assigned either to the sleep ($n = 17$) or wake group ($n = 18$). The sleep subjects performed the Japanese Verbal Learning Test (JVLT), a measure of learning and memory, three times in the evening, and slept. On the following morning (9 h later), they were asked to recall the words on the list. The wake subjects took the same test in the morning, and were asked to recall the words in the same time interval as in the sleep group. The semantic clustering ratio (SCR), divided by the total number of words recalled, was used as an index of memory organization. Our main interest was whether the sleep subjects elicit a greater increase in this measure from the third to the fourth assessments. Time × Group interaction effect on SCR was not significant between the sleep group and wake group as a whole. Meanwhile, the change in the SCR between the third and fourth trials was negatively correlated with duration of nocturnal waking in the sleep group, but not other sleep indices. Based on this observation, further analysis was conducted for subjects in the sleep group who awoke nocturnally for <60 min for comparison with the wake group. A significant Time × Group interaction was noted; these "good-sleepers" showed a significantly greater improvement in the memory index compared with the wake subjects. These results provide the first suggestion that sleep may enhance memory organization, which requires further study.

Keywords: sleep, memory organization, Japanese Verbal Learning Test, wake after sleep onset, polysomnographic recordings

INTRODUCTION

Sleep is important for a variety of physiological functions, e.g., homeostatic maintenance (Achermann and Borbély, 2005). Recently, sleep has been shown to enhance processing of information obtained during wakefulness, and consolidate it in the form of memory (Peigneux et al., 2001; Smith, 2001).

Memory is generally classified into short-term memory and long-term memory; the latter divided into episodic memory, semantic memory, and procedural memory (Tulving and Fergus, 2000). The concepts of memory organization refer to the possibility that the internal representation of a given perceptual input may assume different forms depending upon certain operation on the input, or on its representation in the memory store. Memory organization carries the implication of changes in the memory trace of an event that are influenced by the presence of certain other traces in the episodic memory store. Temporal encoding of an input implies the registration of the date of an episode without regard to other episodes, and it may not represent the way the system works, and the temporal date of a stored event may be determined by its organization in relation to other events with their temporal dates. Semantic encoding of a verbal item in episodic memory implies that the trace of the item is influenced by the information already available about its referent concept in semantic memory, while semantic organization refers to the grouping of items in a given set that reflects the semantic relations among the corresponding concepts. Memory organization refers to the collection and associations of memorized items and their recall (Kirimura, 1999), and implicitly serves as a strategy for facilitating memory itself. With memory organization, it is defined as "the method of summarizing, arranging, and memorizing related information." Since other information which is related to it can be remembered as nature if more information can be memorized efficiently and certain information is remembered if information can be systematized by systematization, the burden in the case of search also decreases.

From the view point of cognitive psychology, primary aspects of memory organization are already integrated in long-term memory. Generally, we unconsciously categorize items from the materials being learned, and judge novel items if they fall into a certain category. Memory organization is assessed by several ways, e.g., verbal fluency (Sumiyoshi et al., 2005), story memory (Sumiyoshi et al., 2001), and word memory (Nohara et al., 2000; Yamashita et al., 2000) tests. Accordingly, the Japanese Verbal Learning Test (JVLT), a word list test, was developed as a measure of memory organization (Yamashita et al., 2000). JVLT is a learning task and consists of a word list of 16 words. This test was developed based on previous reports (Gold, 1992) that employed three word lists (random, blocked, and unblocked lists), with a differential degree of semantic organization. The unblocked list is constituted by four semantic categories (animals, countries, musical instruments, and vegetables) with four words in each category. The unblocked list is organized in a manner that the words in the same category do not appear one after another. Thus, this list has an implicit category structure. JVLT uses a 16-word unblocked list involves four semantic categories with four words in each category. The words in the list are selected from everyday Japanese vocabulary; they are used approximately in the same frequency (Nohara et al., 2000; Yamashita et al., 2000). The number of semantic categories (semantic clustering ratio, SCR) is counted when a separate word belonging to the same semantic category is recalled consequently. Thus, the SCR implicitly reflects the degree of memory organization. However, this index by itself can be affected by the total number of words recalled. Therefore, this study used the ratio of SCR vs. the total number of recalled words (SCR ratio) as an index of memory organization (Matsui et al., 2006) (**Figure 1**). Further, this cognitive domain is impaired in patients with psychiatric diseases such as schizophrenia (Nohara et al., 2000).

A relationship between memory and sleep has been reported (Stickgold, 2005). For example, a facilitative effect of sleep on declarative memory has been demonstrated in humans (Stickgold and Walker, 2007). Specifically, performance on paired-association task has been associated with slow-wave sleep (Plihal and Born, 1997; Gais et al., 2002; Gais and Born, 2004), REM sleep (Koninck et al., 1989), stage 2 sleep (Walker et al., 2002), and spindles (Fogel et al., 2007). In particular, subjects with sleep apnea syndrome perform worse on tests of memory consolidation compared with healthy individuals (Kloepfer et al., 2009). Further, sleep deprivation has been shown to impair attention span (Hsieh et al., 2010). These lines of evidence suggest an importance of an appropriate amount of sleep in general and the maintenance, and, possibly, enhancement of memory.

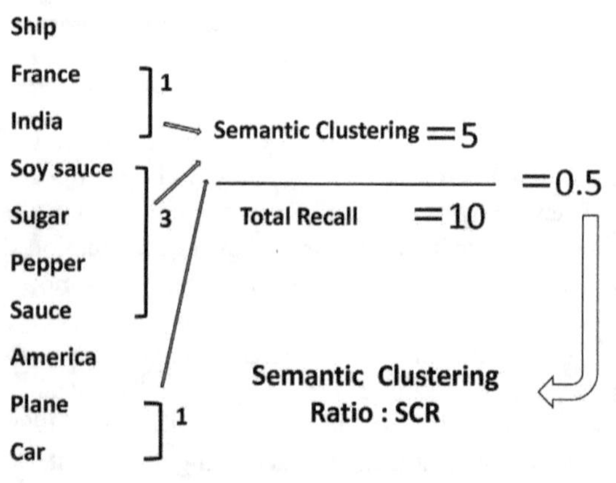

FIGURE 1 | An example of memory organization as assessed by the Japanese Verbal Learning Test. The number of semantic categories (SCR) is counted when a separate word belonging to the same semantic category is recalled consequently. Thus, the SCR implicitly reflects the degree of memory organization. However, this index by itself can be affected by the total number of words recalled. Therefore, this study used the ratio of SCR vs. the total number of recalled words (SCR ratio) as an index of memory organization (see Materials and Methods).

The over lapping replay of related memories selectively strengthens shared elements (Lewis and Durrant, 2011). Repeated reactivation of memories in different combinations progressively builds schematic representations of the relationships between stimuli. Sleep can integrate information into existing memory networks, look for common patterns and distil overarching rules, or simply stabilize and strengthen the memory exactly as it was learned (Stickgold and Walker, 2013).

The above considerations led us to hypothesize that sleep would improve memory organization. To date, however, there is little information on the link between this domain of cognitive ability and sleep. Therefore, the present study was performed to determine whether organization of memory, as evaluated word list learning, would be enhanced during sleep in healthy subjects.

MATERIALS AND METHODS

SUBJECTS

Thirty-five healthy female subjects (university students; average age: 20.9 ± 1.9 years) participated in the study. They were randomly assigned into either the sleep group ($n = 17$) or wake group ($n = 18$) (**Table 1**). All participants were right-handed, had an academic history of 12 years, and were without physical problems (head trauma) or mental health problems (schizophrenia, mood disorder, dependency syndrome). No subjects were receiving medical treatment or suspected of having sleep disorders as determined by the International Classification of Sleep Disorders, Second Edition (American Academy of Sleep Medicine, 2005). All subjects were given an explanation of the research, including the instruction that they can withdraw from the study at any time. Subjects were paid for their participation in this study, and written informed consent was obtained.

Table 1 | Demographic data.

	Sleep group ($n = 17$)	Wake group ($n = 18$)
Age (years)	20.4 ± 0.5	21.3 ± 2.5
Education (years)	12.0 ± 0.0	12.0 ± 0.0
IQ	99.6 ± 8.0	99.5 ± 8.6
JVLT1 total reproduction	11.4 ± 2.1	10.9 ± 1.7
SCR(1) ratio	0.31 ± 0.2	0.42 ± 0.2

JVLT, Japanese Verbal Learning Test; SCR, semantic clustering ratio. Mean ± SD.

JAPANESE VERBAL LEARNING TEST

Japanese Verbal Learning Test is a learning task and consists of a word list of 16 words (Matsui et al., 2007a). The list is constituted by four semantic categories (animals, countries, musical instruments, and vegetables) with four words in each category. The list is organized in a manner that the words in the same category do not appear one after another. Thus, this list has an implicit category structure. JVLT uses a 16-word unblocked list involves four semantic categories with four words in each category. The words in the list are selected from everyday Japanese vocabulary; they are used approximately in the same frequency (Nohara et al., 2000; Yamashita et al., 2000).

The number of semantic categories (SCR) is counted when a separate word belonging to the same semantic category is recalled consequently. Thus, the SCR implicitly reflects the degree of memory organization. However, this index by itself can be affected by the total number of words recalled. Therefore, this study used the ratio of SCR vs. the total number of recalled words (SCR ratio) as an index of memory organization (Matsui et al., 2006) (**Figure 1**).

The Japanese Adult Reading Test (JART) was used to measure IQ. Subjects are required to read aloud 100 *kanji* (Chinese character) idioms (Matsuoka et al., 2002). IQ is calculated as follows; estimated $IQ = 126.5 - 0.72x$ (the number of wrong answers).

POLYSOMNOGRAPHIC RECORDINGS

Polysomnography was performed based on standardized techniques (Rechtschaffen and Kales, 1968). Digital electroencephalography (EEG), electromyography (EMG), and electrooculography (EOG) signals were acquired by Polymate system (DIGITEX LAB.CO., LTD, Tokyo, Japan). EEG electrodes (Fp1, Fp2, C3, C4, P3, P4, O1, O2) were placed on the subject's head according to the International 10-20 system. Parameters for EEG recordings were as follows: sampling rate – 200 Hz, low- and high-pass filter – 0.3 and 60 Hz, and notch filter – 50 Hz. Polysomnography (PSG) data were scored automatically by Night Owl Professional (NoruPro Light Systems, Inc., Tokyo, Japan), and were rescored visually every 30-s epoch, according to standardized techniques (Rechtschaffen and Kales, 1968).

PROCEDURE

Figure 2 shows the experiment procedure. The sleep group was instructed to report to the laboratory at 18:00. They took the JVLT. In the JVLT, subjects were instructed to remember as many words as possible without knowing the existence of any category. JVLT was consecutively performed three times before subjects were allowed to sleep. Each word was orally presented by the examiner with 1-s intervals. After all words had been presented, subjects were asked to recall them immediately. They were instructed to sleep. At the following morning, the fourth JVLT was performed. For this trial, subjects were asked to recall the words once without presentation of the stimulus words. This testing had not been notified to the subjects at the time of completion of the third JVLT. After took the fourth JVLT, subjects took the JART.

The wake group performed the same examination during waking hours with the same 9-h interval between the third and fourth trials of the JVLT as in the sleep group (08:00 and 17:00). These subjects were instructed not to perform excessive exercise or sleep during the interval. Adherence to these directions was confirmed with an Actigraph.

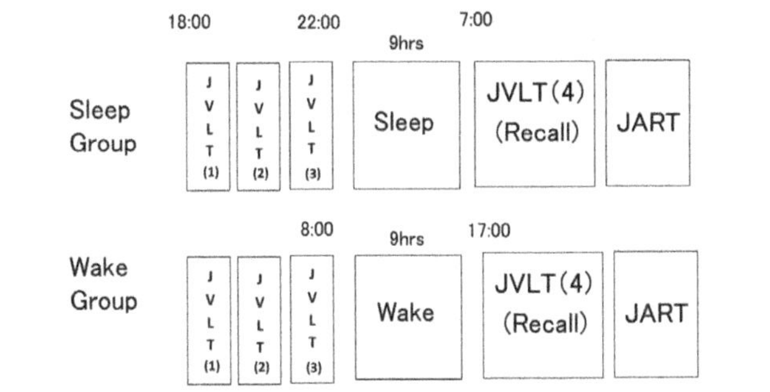

FIGURE 2 | Experimental procedure. The sleep group received a learning session by means of three consecutive administrations of the Japanese Verbal Learning Test (JVLT) before initiation of sleep. On the morning of the following day, subjects were asked to recall as many words as possible without presentation of words. The wake group underwent the same examination procedure, as described in the figure (below).

STATISTICAL ANALYSIS

Mann–Whitney test was used to compare age, academic background (year), estimated IQ, and the change of SCR ratio between the sleep and wake groups. Data from the total number of words recalled and SCR ratio were examined using repeated measures analysis of variance (ANOVA) with Group (wake group vs. sleep group) or (wake group vs. good sleep group) as between subject variable, and time (time points for the third and fourth JVLT administrations) as within-subject variable.

A t-test whether the two groups (wake group and good sleep group) indeed significantly differed before the retention interval between time point 3 and 4. A repeated measures analysis of covariance (ANCOVA) was performed for the memory organization parameter at time point 3 as covariate in the analysis of the change in memory organization between time point 3 and 4. Correlations between the change in the SCR ratio and sleep variables [total sleep time (TST), time in stage 1, time in stage 2, time in stage 3, time in stage 4, time in stage 3 and 4, time in REM sleep, time in non-REM sleep, and wake after sleep onset (WASO)] and wake variables were analyzed using Spearman's rank correlation coefficient test.

RESULTS

Data from one subject in the sleep group were excluded from the analysis due to considerable artifacts in the polysomnography data. There were no significant differences between the sleep and wake groups in terms of age, academic background, and IQ (**Table 1**). The quality of sleep for the current subjects was the following results: stage 1 (67.8 ± 16.3 min), stage 2 (250.8 ± 22.6 min), slow-wave sleep (stage 3 + stage 4) (82.9 ± 14.3 min), REM sleep (74.2 ± 17.4 min), WASO (52.1 ± 23.4 min), and TST (480.3 ± 19.2 min).

The total number of words recalled and SCR ratio are shown in **Table 2** and **Figure 3**.

Time × Group interaction effect was not significant for the total number of words recalled [$F(1, 32) = 0.26$, $p = 0.61$], and a significant main effect of time was not observed [$F(1, 32) = 0.82$, $p = 0.78$]. Time × Group interaction was not significant for the SCR ratio [$F(1, 32) = 2.77$, $p = 0.11$], although a significant main effect of time was observed [$F(1, 32) = 13.2$, $p = 0.01$].

On the other hand, a significant negative correlation was observed between the change of SCR ratio from the third to fourth trials and nocturnal waking, as represented by WASO ($p = 0.023$, $r_s = -0.53$) (**Figure 4**), but no correlation was observed between the change of total number of recall (TNR) from the third to fourth trials and nocturnal waking ($p = 0.31$, $r_s = -0.27$) (**Figure 5**).

In view of these results, further analysis was conducted to determine if subjects with a small amount of nocturnal waking (WASO ≤ 60 min) would elicit a greater improvement of memory organization compared with awake subjects. It is said that wake after sleep onset is 75–80% of total sleep time (Hori, 2006). In our subjects, 75–80% of total sleep time is about 30 min. So we distinguished wake after sleep onset by being twice of 30 min.

Repeated measures ANOVA was conducted to see the effect of sleep on the SCR ratio with Group [sleepers showing WASO ≤60 min ($n = 11$) vs. awake subjects] as between subject variable, and time as within-subject variable. A significant Group × Time

Table 2 | Demographic data.

	Sleep group		Wake group	
	Total number of recall	SCR ratio	Total number of recall	SCR ratio
JVLT1	11.4 ± 0.5	0.31 ± 0.05	10.9 ± 0.4	0.42 ± 0.03
JVLT2	13.9 ± 0.4	0.41 ± 0.05	13.4 ± 0.6	0.37 ± 0.04
JVLT3	15.1 ± 0.3	0.47 ± 0.06	13.9 ± 0.6	0.57 ± 0.04
JVLT4	15.2 ± 0.2	0.66 ± 0.03	13.7 ± 0.5	0.64 ± 0.04

Mean ± SE.

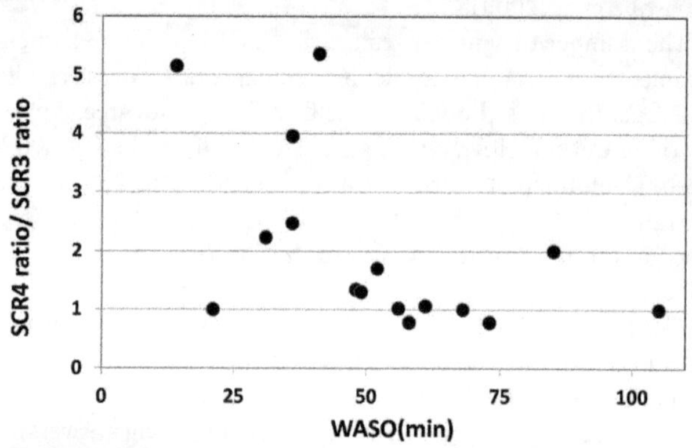

FIGURE 4 | Correlation between the change in the SCR ratio and the amount of nocturnal waking, as represented by WASO (wake after sleep onset) in the sleep group ($r_s = 0.53$, $p < 0.05$).

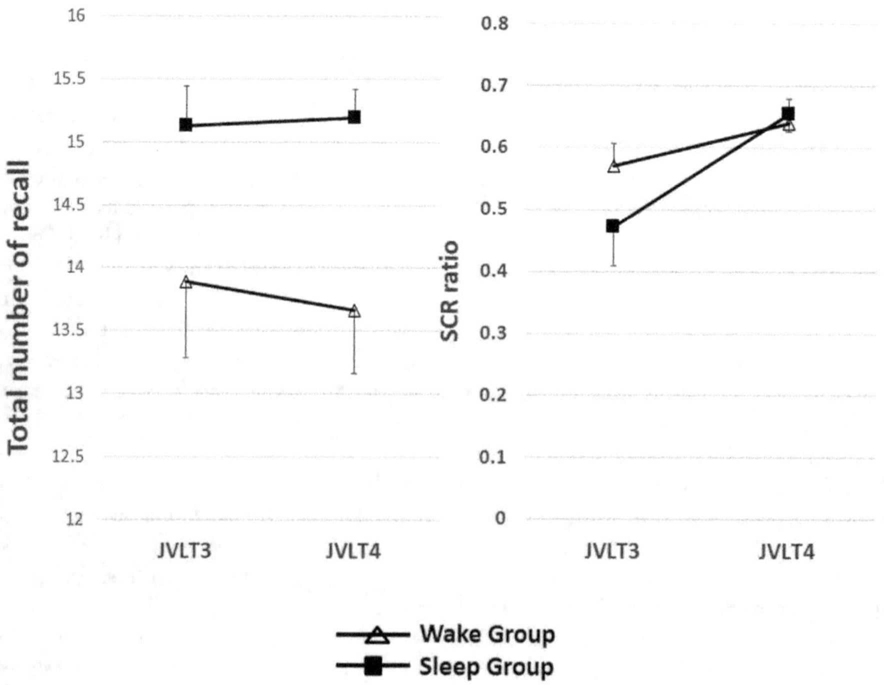

FIGURE 3 | The total number of words recalled (left) and the SCR ratio (right) from the JVLT test in awake ($n = 18$) and sleep ($n = 17$) groups. Time × Group interaction effect was not significant for the total number of words recalled [$F(1, 32) = 0.26$, $p = 0.61$], and a significant main effect of time was not observed [$F(1, 32) = 0.82$, $p = 0.78$]. Time × Group interaction was not significant for the SCR ratio [$F(1, 32) = 2.77$, $p = 0.11$], although a significant main effect of Time was observed [$F(1, 32) = 13.2$, $p = 0.01$]. The error bars represent standard error of the mean.

interaction was observed in the SCR ratio [$F(1, 27)=6.23$, $p=0.019$] (**Figure 6**).

On the other hand, repeated measures ANOVA was conducted to see the effect of sleep on the TNR with Group [sleepers showing WASO $\leq$60 min ($n=11$) vs. awake subjects] as between subject variable, and time as within-subject variable. Time × Group interaction effect was not significant for the total number of words recalled [$F(1, 27)=0.57$, $p=0.46$], and a significant main effect of time was not observed [$F(1, 27)=0.06$, $p=0.94$].

Subsequent analysis indicated a significant increase in the SCR ratio from the third to fourth JVLT trials only in the sleep group ($p<0.01$). In fact, the change in the SCR ratio was significantly greater for these "good-sleepers" compared to wake subjects (Mann–Whitney test, $U=53$, $p=0.04$) (**Figure 7**).

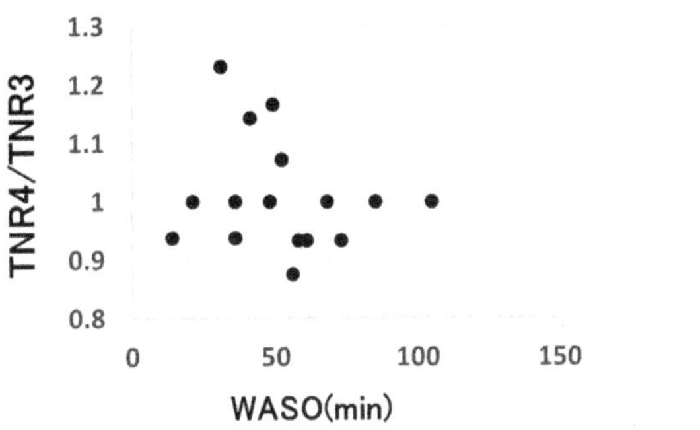

FIGURE 5 | Correlation between the change in the total number of recall and the amount of nocturnal waking, as represented by WASO (wake after sleep onset) in the sleep group ($p=0.31$).

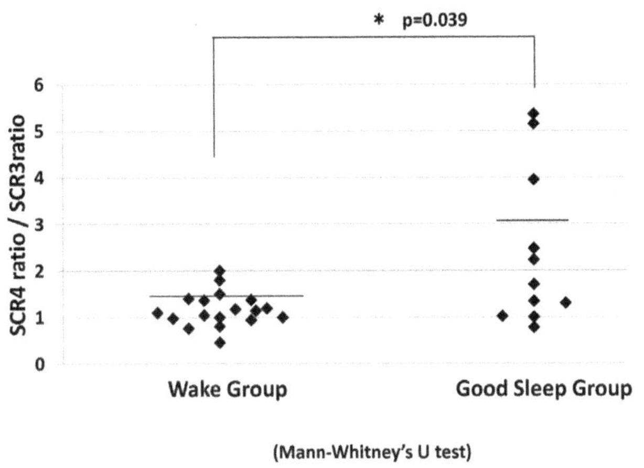

FIGURE 7 | SCR ratio for the fourth JVLT trial/SCR ratio for the third trial for the wake group and good sleep groups. *$p<0.05$ by Mann–Whitney U-test.

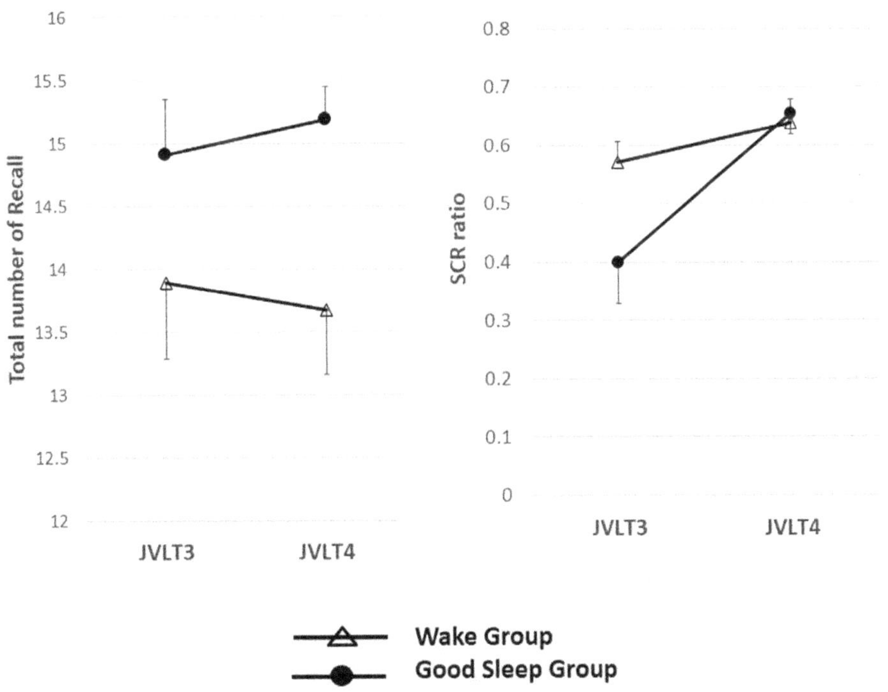

FIGURE 6 | The total number of words recalled (left) and the SCR ratio (right) from the JVLT in the good sleeper group ($n=11$) and control subjects ($n=15$). Left; repeated measures ANOVA was conducted to see the effect of sleep on the total number of recall with Group [sleepers showing WASO $\leq$60 min ($n=11$) vs. awake subjects] as between subject variable, and time as within-subject variable. Time × Group interaction effect was not significant for the total number of words recalled [$F(1, 27)=0.57$, $p=0.46$], and a significant main effect of Time was not observed [$F(1, 27)=0.06$, $p=0.94$]. The error bars represent standard error of the mean. Repeated measures ANOVA was conducted to see the effect of sleep on the SCR ratio with Group [sleepers showing WASO $\leq$60 min ($n=11$) vs. awake subjects] as between subject variable, and time as within-subject variable. A significant Group × Time interaction was observed in the SCR ratio [$F(1, 27)=6.23$, $p=0.019$].

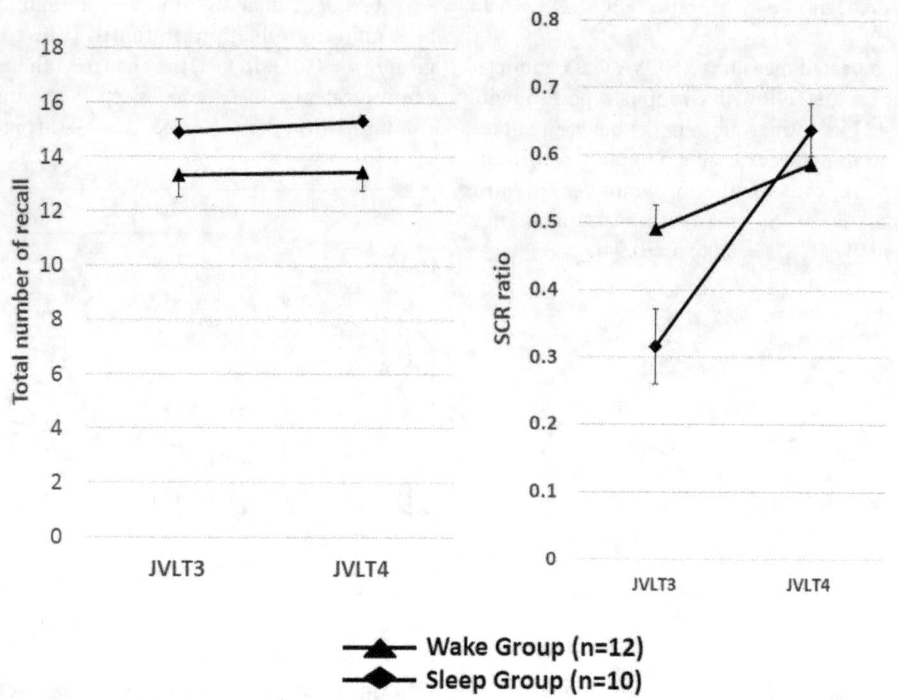

FIGURE 8 | The total number of words recalled (left) and the SCR ratio (right) from the JVLT in the SCR ratio in the third JVLT under 0.65 ($n = 10$) and awake subjects showing the SCR ratio in the third JVLT under 0.65 ($n = 12$). A significant Group × Time interaction was observed in the SCR ratio [$F(1, 20) = 4.25$, $p = 0.01$]. Subsequent analysis indicated a significant increase in the SCR ratio from the third to fourth JVLT trials only in the sleep group ($p < 0.05$), but not awake group ($p = 0.57$). The error bars represent standard error of the mean.

When using a t-test to see whether the two groups (wake group and good sleep group) almost significantly differed before the retention interval between time point 3 and time point 4, there was a significant different between two groups [$F(1, 27) = 4.34$, $p = 0.047$].

A repeated measures ANCOVA was performed for the memory organization parameter at time point 3 as covariate in the analysis of the change in memory organization between time point 3 and 4, there was no significant difference at time point 3 and 4 [$F(1, 27) = 1.12$, $p = 0.32$]. Although no significant main effect of Group was observed [$F(1, 27) = 2.084$ $p = 0.35$], significant main effect of the Time was observed [$F(1, 27) = 18.30$ $p < 0.01$], and significant Group × Time interaction was observed [$F(1, 27) = 6.23$, $p = 0.02$].

In comparison of the index of organization with the good sleep group and the awake group, the value of SCR ratio in the third JVLT was close to the maximum (0.75) by the awake group. Therefore, it was also considered that a difference did not appear in the SCR ratio in the third JVLT and the SCR ratio in the fourth JVLT in the awake group according to the ceiling effect of subject results. Therefore, after carrying out a group division by whether the SCR ratio in the third JVLT is 0.65 or more, the awake group and the sleep group conducted same analysis again, and examined whether a difference would come out of both groups. Repeated measures ANOVA was conducted to see the effect of sleep on the SCR ratio with Group [sleepers showing the SCR ratio in the third JVLT under 0.65 ($n = 10$) vs. awake subjects showing the SCR ratio in the third JVLT under 0.65 ($n = 12$)] as between subject variable, and Time as within-subject variable. A significant Group × Time interaction was observed in the SCR ratio [$F(1, 20) = 4.25$, $p = 0.01$]. Subsequent analysis indicated a significant increase in the SCR ratio from the third to fourth JVLT trials only in the sleep group ($p < 0.05$), but not awake group ($p = 0.57$) (**Figure 8**).

DISCUSSION

In the sleep group, a significant negative correlation was observed between the changes of memory organization index wake after sleep onset. We compared memory organization between sleep and wake group, but found no significant difference between the groups. So, we needed more subanalyses. In sub analyze, sleep subjects elicited an increase in memory organization compared with awake subjects. On the other hand, sleep did not affect the number of recalled words. To our knowledge, these findings indicate that sleep may enhance memory organization.

A prominent theory proposes that three characteristic field potentials, "slow oscillations," "spindles," and "sharp" wave-ripples are involved in some forms of sleep-dependent consolidation (Lewis and Durrant, 2011). During SWS, memories newly encoded into a temporary store (i.e., the hippocampus in the declarative memory system) are repeatedly reactivated, which drives their gradual redistribution to the long-term store (i.e., the neocortex). System consolidation during SWS relies on a dialog between neocortex and hippocampus under top-down control by the neocortical slow oscillations. The depolarizing up phases of the slow oscillations drive the repeated reactivation of hippocampal memory representations together with sharp wave-ripples and thalamocortical spindles. This synchronous drive allows for the formation of spindle-ripple events where sharp wave-ripples and associated reactivated memory information become nested into succeeding troughs of a spindle (Rasch and Born, 2013).

The neural basis for memory formation has been investigated by using several modalities. In a positron emission tomography study (Fletcher et al., 1998), performance on a task to generate an organization structure in a word list was associated with activation in the left prefrontal cortex in normal subjects. Functional magnetic resonance imaging demonstrated the left inferior prefrontal cortex elicits increased activation during semantic encoding (Demb et al., 1995). Furthermore, a recent study using near-infrared spectroscopy showed activation of prefrontal cortex during a memory organization task in healthy people (Matsui et al., 2007b). These findings suggest the role for prefrontal cortex in memory performance and its organization.

Suppression of cholinergic activity during SWS alleviates tonic inhibition of hippocampal CA3 and CA1 feedback neurons, thereby it enables spontaneous reactivations of the hippocampal networks and of the memory information encoded in these networks, as well as the transfer of the reactivated information to neocortical networks (Rasch and Born, 2013).

The acetylcholine system in the hippocampus has been suggested to regulate the acquisition of new knowledge (Terry and Buccafusco, 2003). For example, cholinergic activity is low during slow-wave sleep (Gais and Born, 2004) that improves memory performance, as mentioned above. Specifically, it is assumed that the direction of cholinergic activity regulate type of sleep, which affects declarative memory. For example, Gais and Born (2004) proposed an antagonistic relationship between the acetylcholine system and memory formation, i.e., cholinergic transmissions increase during waking or REM sleep, while they are reduced during slow-wave sleep. Taken together, acetylcholine is considered a major neurochemical substance for all stages of sleep, and affects some types of cognitive abilities.

Other neurotransmitters may also play a role in the ability of sleep to enhance memory. For example, Jouvet (1972) proposed monoamines (noradrenaline, serotonin) are also involved in the regulation of non-REM sleep (Jouvet, 1972). Further, REM sleep has been reported to be regulated by monoamines, as well as by acetylcholine (Hobson et al., 1975). These observations suggest neurotransmitters affect memory performance by modulating the quality of sleep.

Results in the present study suggest nocturnal waking is disadvantageous for memory organization, suggesting the importance of the quality of sleep. Specifically, sleep selectively improved an index of memory organization but not total words recalled, a measure of learning memory itself. The reason for this discrepancy may include that the number of words in the JVLT did not pose sufficient workload. The easiness of memory tasks have been reported to make it difficult to interpret data regarding the effect of sleep (Empson and Clark, 1970). In fact, our findings indicate a ceiling effect in both groups for the total number of words recalled in the third JVLT [**Figure 3** (left) and **Figure 6** (left)]. On the other hand, the workload for memory organization may have been appropriate to assess the effect of sleep, as implicated in **Figure 3** (right) and **Figure 6** (right). It considered about the influence of the ceiling effect of a memory organization task, only the sleep subjects obtained the result that organization was promoted by sleep, to the result of having divided and examined the group again (**Figure 8**).

It is possible that the greater hike of the SCR ratio in good sleeper subjects compared to controls may have been a result of the ability of the former subjects to effectively restore semantic knowledge. Alternatively, it is also assumed that the ability to organize memory was enhanced by sleep. Recent research has shown that sleep facilitates abstraction of gist information as well as integration across multiple memories, insight into hidden solutions, and even the ability to make creative connections between distantly related ideas and concepts (Lewis and Durrant, 2011; Griessenberger et al., 2012). Our findings may also suggest these findings.

Abnormalities in the sleep structure, such as the decreased slow-wave sleep and increased nocturnal waking, have been reported in patients with depression (Tsuno et al., 2005) or schizophrenia (Zarcone et al., 1998). It is also reported that sleep-dependent memory consolidation is absent or weakened in people suffering from conditions that cause sleep disturbances. For example, consolidation of declarative memory is absent in patients with sleep apnea syndrome (Kloepfer et al., 2009). These observations suggest that adequate sleep may be effective in enhancing some types of cognitive functions, such as organizing of information, in clinical subjects.

We compared memory organization between sleep and wake group, but found no significant difference between the groups. So, we needed more subanalyses.

The difference between groups before the retention interval should be considered as a major limitation, and the fact that ceiling performance was reached for total word recall as well as for the memory organization parameter in the wake group. The absence of a significant relationship between memory organization and other sleep variables, e.g. amount of specific stages of sleep, could be due to the small sample size. We need more analyze another sleep index. In addition, the quality of sleep is much worse as in other sleep studies including young and healthy participants (Carskadon, 2005; Payne et al., 2012). This is thought that we did not set up adaptation night, so the sleep subjects would not sleep well. The sleep and the wake group would effect by circadian rhythm on learning. Further controlled study with a larger number of subjects and control procedure controlled circadian rhythm effect is warranted to investigate the role for sleep in memory and other cognitive abilities.

ACKNOWLEDGMENTS

This study was funded by grants-in-aid for Scientific Research from Japan Society for the Promotion of Science, Health and Labour Sciences Research Grants for Comprehensive Research on Disability, Health, and Welfare (H23-Seishin-Ippan-002; H24-Seishin-Ippan-002), and SENSHIN Medical Research Foundation.

REFERENCES

Achermann, P., and Borbély, A. A. (2005). "Sleep homeostasis and models of sleep regulation," in *Principles and Practice of Sleep Medicine*, 5th Edn, 377–390.

American Academy of Sleep Medicine. (2005). *The International Classification of Sleep Disorders: Diagnostic and Coding Manual*, 2nd Edn. eds P. Hauri and M. J. Sateia (Westchester: One Westbrook Corporate Center).

Carskadon, M. A. (2005). "Normal human sleep an overview," in *Principles and Practice of Sleep Medicine*, 5th Edn, 16–26.

Demb, J. B., Desmond, J. E., Wagner, A. D., Vaidya, C. J., Glover, G. H., and Gabrieli, J. D. E. (1995). Semantic encoding and retrieval in the left inferior prefrontal cortex: a functional MRI study of task difficulty and process specificity. *J. Neurosci.* 15, 5870–5878.

Empson, J. A., and Clark, P. R. (1970). Rapid eye movements and remembering. *Nature* 227, 287–288. doi:10.1038/227287a0

Fletcher, P. C., Shallice, T., and Dolan, R. J. (1998). The functional roles of prefrontal cortex in episodic memory encoding. *Brain* 121, 1239–1248. doi:10.1093/brain/121.7.1239

Fogel, S. M., Smith, C. T., and Cote, K. A. (2007). Dissociable learning-dependent changes in REM and non-REM sleep in declarative and procedural memory systems. *Behav. Brain Res.* 180, 48–61. doi:10.1016/j.bbr.2007.02.037

Gais, S., and Born, J. (2004). Low acetylcholine during slow-wave sleep is critical for declarative memory consolidation. *Proc. Natl. Acad. Sci. U.S.A.* 101, 2140–2144. doi:10.1073/pnas.0305404101

Gais, S., Mölle, M., Helms, K., and Born, J. (2002). Learning-dependent increases in sleep spindle density. *J. Neurosci.* 22, 6830–6834.

Gold, J. M. (1992). Forms of memory failure in schizophrenia. *J. Abnorm. Psychol.* 101, 487–494. doi:10.1037/0021-843X.101.3.487

Griessenberger, H., Hoedlmoser, K., Heib, D. P. J., Lechinger, J., Klimesch, W., and Schabus, M. (2012). Consolidation of temporal order in episodic memories. *Biol. Psychol.* 91, 150–155. doi:10.1016/j.biopsycho.2012.05.012

Hobson, J. A., McCarley, R. W., and Wyzinski, P. W. (1975). Sleep cycle oscillation: reciprocal discharge by two brainstem neuronal groups. *Science* 189, 55–58. doi:10.1126/science.1094539

Hori A. (2006). "Clinical sleep study manual," in *Principles and Practice of Sleep Medicine*, 5th Edn, 69–77. Japanese Society of Sleep Manual. (in Japanese)

Hsieh, S., Li, T. H., and Tsai, L. L. (2010). Impact of monetary incentives on cognitive performance and error monitoring following sleep deprivation. *Sleep* 33, 499–507.

Jouvet, M. (1972). The role of monoamines and acetylcholine-containing neurons in the regulation of the sleep-waking cycle. *Ergeb. Physiol.* 64, 166–307.

Kirimura, M. (1999). Memory organization. *A Clin. Psychiatry Lect.* 52, 272–280.

Kloepfer, C., Riemann, D., Nofzinger, E. A., Feige, B., Unterrainer, J., O'Hara, R., et al. (2009). Memory before and after sleep in patients with moderate obstructive sleep apnea. *J. Clin. Sleep Med.* 15, 540–548.

Koninck, J. D., Lorrain, D., Christ, G., Proulx, G., and Coulombe, D. (1989). Intensive language learning and increases in rapid eye movement sleep: evident of a performance factor. *Int. J. Psychophysiol.* 8, 43–47. doi:10.1016/0167-8760(89)90018-4

Lewis, P. A., and Durrant, S. J. (2011). Overlapping memory replay during sleep builds cognitive schemata. *Trends Cogn. Sci.* 15, 343–351. doi:10.1016/j.tics.2011.06.004

Matsui, M., Sumiyoshi, T., Katoh, K., and Kurachi, M. (2007a). Making for a substitute Japanese Verbal Learning Test. *Psychiatry* 49, 31–34. (in Japanese)

Matsui, M., Tanaka, K., Yonezawa, M., and Kurachi, M. (2007b). Activation of the prefrontal cortex during memory learning: near-infrared spectroscopy study. *Psychiatry Clin. Neurosci.* 61, 31–38. doi:10.1111/j.1440-1819.2007.01607.x

Matsui, M., Yuki, H., Kato, K., and Kurachi, K. (2006). Impairment of memory organization in patients with schizophrenia or schizotypal disorder. *J. Int. Neuropsychol. Soc.* 12, 750–754.

Matsuoka, K., Kim, Y., Hiro, H., Miyamoto, Y., Fujita, K., Tanaka, K., et al. (2002). Japanese version National Adult Reading Test (JART) making. *Psychiatry* 44, 503–511. (in Japanese)

Nohara, S., Suzuki, M., Kurachi, M., Yamashita, I., Matsui, M., Seto, H., et al. (2000). Neural correlates of memory organization deficits in schizophrenia: a single photon emission computed tomography study with ^{99m}Tc-ethyl-cysteinate dimer during a verbal learning task. *Schizophr. Res.* 42, 209–222. doi:10.1016/S0920-9964(99)00131-0

Payne, J., Chambers, A., and Kensinger, E. (2012). Sleep promotes lasting changes in selective memory for emotional scenes. *Front. Integr. Neurosci.* 6:108. doi:10.3389/fnint.2012.00108

Peigneux, P., Laureys, S., Delbeuck, X., and Maquet, P. (2001). Sleeping brain, learning brain. The role of sleep for memory systems. *Neuroreport* 12, A111–A124. doi:10.1097/00001756-200112210-00001

Plihal, W., and Born, J. (1997). Effects of early and late nocturnal sleep on declarative and procedural memory. *J. Cogn. Neurosci.* 9, 534–547. doi:10.1162/jocn.1997.9.4.534

Rasch, B., and Born, J. (2013). About sleep's role in memory. *Physiol. Rev.* 93, 681–766. doi:10.1152/physrev.00032.2012

Rechtschaffen, A., and Kales, A. (1968). *A Manual of Standardized Terminology, Technique and Scoring System for Sleep Stages of Human Subjects.* Los Angeles, CA: Brain Information Service/Brain Research Institute, UCLA.

Smith, C. (2001). Sleep states and memory processes in humans: procedural versus declarative memory systems. *Sleep Med. Rev.* 5, 491–506. doi:10.1053/smrv.2001.0164

Stickgold, R. (2005). Sleep-dependent memory consolidation. *Nature* 437, 1272–1278. doi:10.1038/nature04286

Stickgold, R., and Walker, M. P. (2007). Sleep-dependent memory consolidation and reconsolidation. *Sleep Med.* 8, 331–343. doi:10.1016/j.sleep.2007.03.011

Stickgold, R., and Walker, M. P. (2013). Sleep-dependent memory triage: evolving generalization through selective processing. *Nat. Neurosci.* 16, 139–145. doi:10.1038/nn.3303

Sumiyoshi, C., Matsui, M., Sumiyoshi, T., Yamashita, I., Sumiyoshi, S., and Kurachi, M. (2001). Semantic structure in schizophrenia as assessed by the category fluency test: effect of verbal intelligence and age of onset. *Psychiatry Res.* 105, 187–199. doi:10.1016/S0165-1781(01)00345-6

Sumiyoshi, C., Sumiyoshi, T., Nohara, S., Yamashita, I., Matsui, M., Kurachi, M., et al. (2005). Disorganization of semantic memory underlies alogia in schizophrenia: an analysis of verbal fluency performance in Japanese subjects. *Schizophr. Res.* 74, 91–100. doi:10.1016/j.schres.2004.05.011

Terry, A. V., and Buccafusco, J. J. (2003). The cholinergic hypothesis of age and Alzheimer's disease-related cognitive deficits: recent challenges and their implications for novel drug development. *J. Pharmacol. Exp. Ther.* 306, 821–827. doi:10.1124/jpet.102.041616

Tsuno, N., Besset, A., and Ritche, K. (2005). Sleep and depression. *J. Clin. Psychiatry* 66, 1254–1269. doi:10.4088/JCP.v66n1008

Tulving, E. C., and Fergus, I. M. (2000). *The Oxford Handbook of Memory.* Oxford: Oxford University Press.

Walker, M. P., Brakefield, T., Morgan, A., Hobson, J., Allan, H. J., and Stickgold, R. (2002). Practice with sleep makes perfect: sleep-dependent motor skill learning. *Neuron* 35, 205–211. doi:10.1016/S0896-6273(02)00746-8

Yamashita, I., Matsui, M., and Kurachi, M. (2000). Making of the word memory test to measure memory organization. *Psychiatry* 42, 1279–1283. (in Japanese)

Zarcone, V. P., Poceta, J. S., Mitler, M. M. (1998). "Sleep and schizophrenia," in *Sleep Disorders: Diagnosis and Treatment*, 2nd Edn. Humana Press. 165–188.

Permissions

All chapters in this book were first published in CDSONDCPCE, by Frontiers Media SA; hereby published with permission under the Creative Commons Attribution License or equivalent. Every chapter published in this book has been scrutinized by our experts. Their significance has been extensively debated. The topics covered herein carry significant findings which will fuel the growth of the discipline. They may even be implemented as practical applications or may be referred to as a beginning point for another development.

The contributors of this book come from diverse backgrounds, making this book a truly international effort. This book will bring forth new frontiers with its revolutionizing research information and detailed analysis of the nascent developments around the world.

We would like to thank all the contributing authors for lending their expertise to make the book truly unique. They have played a crucial role in the development of this book. Without their invaluable contributions this book wouldn't have been possible. They have made vital efforts to compile up to date information on the varied aspects of this subject to make this book a valuable addition to the collection of many professionals and students.

This book was conceptualized with the vision of imparting up-to-date information and advanced data in this field. To ensure the same, a matchless editorial board was set up. Every individual on the board went through rigorous rounds of assessment to prove their worth. After which they invested a large part of their time researching and compiling the most relevant data for our readers.

The editorial board has been involved in producing this book since its inception. They have spent rigorous hours researching and exploring the diverse topics which have resulted in the successful publishing of this book. They have passed on their knowledge of decades through this book. To expedite this challenging task, the publisher supported the team at every step. A small team of assistant editors was also appointed to further simplify the editing procedure and attain best results for the readers.

Apart from the editorial board, the designing team has also invested a significant amount of their time in understanding the subject and creating the most relevant covers. They scrutinized every image to scout for the most suitable representation of the subject and create an appropriate cover for the book.

The publishing team has been an ardent support to the editorial, designing and production team. Their endless efforts to recruit the best for this project, has resulted in the accomplishment of this book. They are a veteran in the field of academics and their pool of knowledge is as vast as their experience in printing. Their expertise and guidance has proved useful at every step. Their uncompromising quality standards have made this book an exceptional effort. Their encouragement from time to time has been an inspiration for everyone.

The publisher and the editorial board hope that this book will prove to be a valuable piece of knowledge for researchers, students, practitioners and scholars across the globe.

List of Contributors

Ishraq Siddiqui and John A. Zawadzki
Institute of Medical Science, University of Toronto, ON, Canada
Centre for Addiction and Mental Health, Campbell Family Mental Health Research Institute, Toronto, ON, Canada

Todd A. Girard
Department of Psychology, Ryerson University, Toronto, ON, Canada

George Foussias, Gary Remington and Albert H. C. Wong
Institute of Medical Science, University of Toronto, ON, Canada
Centre for Addiction and Mental Health, Campbell Family Mental Health Research Institute, Toronto, ON, Canada
Department of Psychiatry, University of Toronto, ON, Canada

Alicia Rodrigues
Centre for Addiction and Mental Health, Campbell Family Mental Health Research Institute, Toronto, ON, Canada
Collaborative Program in Neuroscience, University of Toronto, ON, Canada

Jason P. Lerch
Department of Medical Biophysics, University of Toronto, ON, Canada
Program in Neuroscience and Mental Health, the Hospital for Sick Children, Toronto, ON, Canada

Cheryl Grady
Departments of Psychology and Psychiatry, University of Toronto, ON, Canada
Rotman Research Institute at Baycrest, Toronto, ON, Canada

Mabel Rodriguez and Lucie Konrádová
Prague Psychiatric Center, Prague, Czech Republic

David Levčík, Aleš Stuchlík and Kamil Vlček
Department of Neurophysiology of Memory, Institute of Physiology, Academy of Sciences of the Czech Republic v.v.i., Prague, Czech Republic

Iveta Fajnerová
Prague Psychiatric Center, Prague, Czech Republic
Department of Neurophysiology of Memory, Institute of Physiology, Academy of Sciences of the Czech Republic v.v.i., Prague, Czech Republic
Department of Psychiatry and Medical Psychology, 3rd Faculty of Medicine, Charles University in Prague, Prague, Czech Republic

Jiří Horáček and Pavol Mikoláš
Prague Psychiatric Center, Prague, Czech Republic
Department of Psychiatry and Medical Psychology, 3rd Faculty of Medicine, Charles University in Prague, Prague, Czech Republic

Cyril Brom
Department of Software and Computer Science Education, Faculty of Mathematics and Physics, Charles University in Prague, Prague, Czech Republic

Jennifer L. Phillips and Alain Labelle
University of Ottawa Institute of Mental Health Research, Ottawa, ON, Canada

Andrée-Anne Ledoux
University of Ottawa Institute of Mental Health Research, Ottawa, ON, Canada
School of Psychology, University of Ottawa, Ottawa, ON, Canada

Andra Smith
School of Psychology, University of Ottawa, Ottawa, ON, Canada

Patrice Boyer
University of Ottawa Institute of Mental Health Research, Ottawa, ON, Canada
Université Paris Diderot–Paris 7, Paris, France

Véronique D. Bohbot
Douglas Mental Health University Institute, McGill University, Montreal, QC, Canada

Tereza Nekovarova
Department of Neurophysiology of Memory, Institute of Physiology, Academy of Sciences of the Czech Republic, Prague, Czech Republic
Ecology and Ethology Research Group, Department of Zoology, Faculty of Science, Charles University in Prague, Prague, Czech Republic

Jiri Horacek and Filip Spaniel
Prague Psychiatric Center, Prague, Czech Republic

Takashi Uehara
Department of Neuropsychiatry, Kanazawa Medical University, Ucninada-cho, Ishikawa, Japan

Tadasu Matsuoka
Department of Psychiatry, Matsuoka Hospital, Oyabe, Toyama, Japan

Tomiki Sumiyoshi
Department of Clinical Research Promotion, National Center Hospital, National Center of Neurology and Psychiatry, Tokyo, Japan

Yuko Higuchi, Tomonori Seo, Tomohiro Miyanishi and Michio Suzuki
Department of Neuropsychiatry, University of Toyama Graduate School of Medicine and Pharmaceutical Science, Toyama, Japan

Yasuhiro Kawasaki
Department of Neuropsychiatry, Kanazawa Medical University, Ishikawa, Japan

Ju-Chun Pei
Laboratory of Integrated Neuroscience and Ethology, Department of Psychology, National Taiwan University, Taipei, Taiwan

Chih-Min Liu
Department of Psychiatry, National Taiwan University Hospital, Taipei, Taiwan

Wen-Sung Lai
Laboratory of Integrated Neuroscience and Ethology, Department of Psychology, National Taiwan University, Taipei, Taiwan
Graduate Institute of Brain and Mind Sciences, National Taiwan University, Taipei, Taiwan
Neurobiology and Cognitive Science Center, National Taiwan University, Taipei, Taiwan

Lukas Rambousek, Karel Vales and Ales Stuchlik
Institute of Physiology, Academy of Sciences of the Czech Republic, Prague, Czech Republic

Tomas Palenicek
Prague Psychiatric Center, Prague, Czech Republic

Štêpán Kubík, Helena Buchtová, Karel Valeš and Aleš Stuchlík
Neurophysiology of Memory, Institute of Physiology, Academy of Sciences of the Czech Republic, Prague, Czech Republic

Thomas Enkel, Stefan M. Berger, Kai Schönig and Dusan Bartsch
Department of Molecular Biology, Central Institute of Mental Health, Medical Faculty Mannheim, University of Heidelberg, Mannheim, Germany

Björn Tews
Schaller Research Group, Division of Molecular Mechanisms of Tumor Invasion, University of Heidelberg and German Cancer Research Center, Heidelberg, Germany

Iva Prokopova, Iveta Vojtechova, Anna Zemanova and Ales Stuchlik
Department of Neurophysiology of Memory, Institute of Physiology, Academy of Sciences of the Czech Republic, Prague, Czech Republic

Tomas Petrasek
Department of Neurophysiology of Memory, Institute of Physiology, Academy of Sciences of the Czech Republic, Prague, Czech Republic
First Faculty of Medicine, Charles University in Prague, Prague, Czech Republic

Alena Sumova, Martin Sladek and Kamila Weissova
Department of Neurohumoral Regulations, Institute of Physiology, Academy of Sciences of the Czech Republic, Prague, Czech Republic

Stepan Bahnik
Department of Neurophysiology of Memory, Institute of Physiology, Academy of Sciences of the Czech Republic, Prague, Czech Republic
Social Psychology, Department of Psychology II, University of Würzburg, Würzburg, Germany

Kai Schönig, Stefan Berger and Dusan Bartsch
Department of Molecular Biology, Central Institute of Mental Health, Mannheim, Germany

Martin E. Schwab
Brain Research Institute, University of Zurich, Zurich, Switzerland
Neurosciences, Department of Biology, Swiss Federal Institute of Technology Zurich, Zurich, Switzerland

Björn Tews
Brain Research Institute, University of Zurich, Zurich, Switzerland
Neurosciences, Department of Biology, Swiss Federal Institute of Technology Zurich, Zurich, Switzerland
Division of Molecular Mechanisms of Tumor Invasion, German Cancer Research Center, Heidelberg, Germany

Malgorzata J. Wesierska and Weronika Duda
Laboratory of Neuropsychology, Department of Neurophysiology, Nencki Institute of Experimental Biology, Polish Academy of Sciences, Warsaw, Poland

Colleen A. Dockery
Laboratory of Neuropsychology, Department of Neurophysiology, Nencki Institute of Experimental Biology, Polish Academy of Sciences, Warsaw, Poland
Faculty of Life Sciences, Albstadt-Sigmaringen University of Applied Sciences, Sigmaringen, Germany

Barbora Urbanova, Ales Tomek and Hana Magerova
Department of Neurology, 2nd Faculty of Medicine, Motol University Hospital, Charles University, Prague, Czech Republic

Robert Mikulik
Department of Neurology, International Clinical Research Center, St. Anne's University Hospital, Brno, Czech Republic

Daniel Horinek
Department of Neurosurgery, 1st Faculty of Medicine, Central Military Hospital, Charles University, Prague, Czech Republic
International Clinical Research Center, St. Anne's University Hospital, Brno, Czech Republic

Kamil Vlček
Department of Neurophysiology of Memory, Institute of Physiology, Academy of Sciences of the Czech Republic, Prague, Czech Republic
International Clinical Research Center, St. Anne's University Hospital Brno, Brno, Czech Republic

Jan Laczó
International Clinical Research Center, St. Anne's University Hospital Brno, Brno, Czech Republic
Department of Neurology, 2nd Faculty of Medicine, Charles University in Prague and Motol University Hospital, Prague, Czech Republic

Rafał Marciniak, Katerina Sheardova, Daniel Hudeček and Rastislav Šumec
International Clinical Research Center, St. Anne's University Hospital Brno, Brno, Czech Republic

Pavla Čermáková
International Clinical Research Center, St. Anne's University Hospital Brno, Brno, Czech Republic
Alzheimer's Disease Research Center, Department of Neurobiology, Care Sciences and Society, Karolinska Institutet, Stockholm, Sweden

Jakub Hort
International Clinical Research Center, St. Anne's University Hospital Brno, Brno, Czech Republic
Memory Disorders Clinic, Department of Neurology, 2nd Faculty of Medicine, Charles University in Prague and University Hospital Motol, Prague, Czech Republic
Department of Neurology, 2nd Faculty of Medicine, Motol University Hospital, Charles University, Prague, Czech Republic

Kristina Holubova, Tereza Nekovarova, Ales Stuchlík and Karel Vales
Institute of Physiology, Academy of Sciences of the Czech Republic, Prague, Czech Republic

Jana Pistovcakova
Faculty of Medicine, Department of Pharmacology, Masaryk University, Brno, Czech Republic

Alexandra Sulcova
Central European Institute of Technology, Masaryk University, Brno, Czech Republic

Karel Vales and Ales Stuchlik
Institute of Physiology, Academy of Sciences of the Czech Republic, Prague, Czech Republic

Tereza Nekovarova
Institute of Physiology, Academy of Sciences of the Czech Republic, Prague, Czech Republic
Department of Zoology, Ecology and Ethology Research Group, Faculty of Natural Science, Charles University in Prague, Prague, Czech Republic

Anna Yamamotova and Richard Rokyta
Department of Normal, Pathological and Clinical Physiology, Third Faculty of Medicine, Charles University in Prague, Prague, Czech Republic

Jitka Fricova
Department of Anesthesiology and Intensive Care Medicine, Pain Management Center, First Faculty of Medicine and General University Hospital, Charles University in Prague, Prague, Czech Republic

Hana Hatalova, Dominika Radostova, Adela Pistikova, Karel Vales and Ales Stuchlik
Institute of Physiology, Academy of Sciences of the Czech Republic, Prague, Czech Republic

Ales Stuchlik
Institute of Physiology, Academy of Sciences of the Czech Republic, Prague, Czech Republic

Anna Mikulecká, Martin Šubrt, Martina Pařízková, Pavel Mareš, Aleš Stuchlík and Hana Kubová
Institute of Physiology, Academy of Sciences of the Czech Republic, Prague, Czech Republic

Ilia N. Karatsoreos
Department of Integrative Physiology and Neuroscience, Washington State University, Pullman, WA, USA

Michio Suzuki and Masayoshi Kurachi
Department of Neuropsychiatry, University of Toyama Graduate School of Medicine and Pharmaceutical Sciences, Toyama, Japan

Masashi Takeuchi
Department of Neuropsychiatry, University of Toyama Graduate School of Medicine and Pharmaceutical Sciences, Toyama, Japan
Kamiichi General Hospital, Kamiichi-machi, Japan

Yoko Ochiai, Munehito Hosokawa and Hisakazu Furuta
Sleep Disorders Center, Hokuriku National Hospital, Nanto-shi, Japan

Mie Matsui
Department of Psychology, University of Toyama Graduate School of Medicine and Pharmaceutical Sciences, Toyama, Japan

Index

A

Adult Neurogenesis, 113, 209, 211-213, 229

Allocentric Navigation, 84, 152-153, 155

Allothetic Place Avoidance Alternation Task, 128, 130, 132-134, 138

Antidepressant, 166-175, 177-187, 189, 227-229

B

Benzodiazepines, 28, 55, 175, 200, 207-208, 215, 223-225

Bipolar Disorder, 10, 43, 82-83, 113, 186, 198, 226, 228-230

C

Carousel Maze, 84-88, 112-117, 121, 123, 125-127, 190, 198-199

Central Executive Network, 36, 39-40, 44

Cerebral Microembolization, 140, 147-148

Cerebrovascular Impairment, 140

Cerebrovascular Reserve Capacity, 140, 143-145, 147-149

Chronic Pain, 158, 176-187

Circadian Clock, 114, 124-127, 226-230

Circadian Rhythmicity, 113-115, 117, 124

Clonazepam, 200-201, 207-208, 215-216, 222-224

Cognitive Deficit, 9, 11-12, 21-24, 88, 103, 114, 121, 125

Cognitive Dysfunction, 11, 26, 41-42, 46, 53, 103, 126, 129, 149, 186

Cognitive Flexibility, 24, 102-103, 125-126, 158, 161-164, 188, 197-199, 212, 227

Cognitive Impairment, 7, 23, 41, 43, 46, 51, 54, 90, 138-144, 147-152, 155-158, 162, 164-165, 189, 200, 207, 216

Cognitive Skill Learning, 128-129, 132-133, 137

Cytokines, 176, 180, 184-187

D

Default Mode Network, 36, 38-40, 43-44, 176-178, 183, 185, 187

Depressive Disorder, 167, 172-174, 179, 185-186, 199, 229

Disparate Symptoms, 36-37

Dopamine, 2, 9, 41, 43, 51-52, 55, 63, 65, 67, 90, 106-107, 110, 112, 127, 183-184, 186, 188-189, 193, 195-199, 224

E

Episodic Memory, 7, 26-27, 32-35, 82, 91, 197-199, 231, 238

Event-related Potentials, 54, 63

Extracellular Lactate Concentration, 46-47

G

Glutamate, 12, 46-47, 50-52, 67, 76, 104-105, 111, 129, 138, 166-167, 172, 174-175, 178-179, 181, 185-186

H

Hippocampal Anomalies, 26, 32, 34

Hippocampal Neurogenesis, 175, 178, 180, 187, 199, 209, 211-214, 227-228

Hypersynchrony, 91, 93, 102-103

I

Immediate-early Gene, 91-92, 94, 100, 103-104, 211

J

Japanese Verbal Learning Test, 231-233, 238

L

Locomotor Activity, 51, 65, 67, 83-87, 110, 113-114, 116-117, 121, 124-126, 128-131, 135-137, 166-169, 171-173, 190, 193-194, 196, 199, 205, 207, 229

M

Memory Acquisition, 84-87, 135-136, 138, 210, 213

Memory Organization, 231-234, 236-238

Microdialysis, 46-48, 51-52, 111

Mild Cognitive Impairment, 140, 142-143, 147-149, 151-152, 155-158, 162

Mismatch Negativity, 54-55, 57-59, 62-63, 81

Morris Water Maze, 7-8, 11-12, 23-25, 66, 69-70, 84-85, 89-90, 105, 112, 127, 153-154, 156, 189, 199-202, 205-208, 210, 227

N

Neuroactive Steroid, 166-167, 172

Neurobehavioral Function, 226-228

Neurodegenerative Diseases, 129, 135, 158, 160-165, 171

Neurogenesis, 113, 173-175, 178-180, 187, 199, 209, 211-214, 227-230

Neuromorphology, 64, 80

Neuroplasticity, 80, 174, 176, 178-179, 183, 185

Neuropsychiatric Disorder, 36

Neurotransmission, 46, 50-52, 64, 80, 102, 111, 167, 173, 175, 178

Nocturnal Waking, 231, 234-235, 237

O

Obsessive-compulsive Disorder, 84, 89, 188, 198-199, 227

P

Passive Avoidance, 113, 123, 125, 127, 200-204, 207-208, 224

Polysomnography, 233

Prefrontal Cortex, 2, 7, 10, 27, 29, 33-35, 38, 40, 43-44, 46-47, 49, 51-53, 81-82, 102-104, 106-107, 112, 128-129, 137-140, 153, 161, 177-179, 185, 188, 227, 237-238

Pregnanolone Glutamate, 166-167, 175

Psychiatric Disorder, 14, 106, 126, 176

Psychosocial Functioning, 1, 5-7

Psychotic Disorders, 9, 11, 13, 55, 230

R

Reference Memory, 7, 11-12, 15-16, 52, 87, 138, 205

Reorienting Negativity, 54-55, 57-59

Retrosplenial Cortex, 104, 139, 152-153, 156

Reward Sensitivity, 106-112, 126

Rotating Arena, 21, 85, 91-97, 101-102, 128, 130-131, 189

S

Salience Network, 36, 39-40, 43-45

Schizophrenia, 1-2, 5-13, 16-27, 29-47, 49, 51-60, 62-67, 72, 74, 76, 80-84, 89-92, 101-106, 111-116, 123, 125-127, 129-130, 137-139, 171, 173-175, 188-189, 196, 198-199, 209, 213, 226-230, 232, 237-238

Semantic Clustering Ratio, 231-232

Sensorimotor Gating, 23, 51-52, 66, 69, 81-82, 84, 123, 125, 127, 229

Serotonin, 46, 51-53, 81, 84, 89-90, 106-107, 110, 112, 166, 173-175, 179-181, 186-187, 198-199, 223-224, 230, 237

Sleep Group, 231-236

Social Behavior, 36, 83-84, 106, 125, 215-225

Spatial Behavior, 11, 22, 101

Spatial Disorientation, 152, 154-156

Spatial Learning, 11-12, 15, 20-24, 32, 88, 91, 102, 111, 121, 127, 138-139, 155, 175, 184, 201, 213

Spatial Memory, 8-11, 16-17, 23, 26-27, 31, 34, 84-86, 88-89, 91, 105, 112-113, 115, 123,, 126-127, 129-130, 135-139, 152-153, 155-157, 199-200, 202, 207-208, 210, 212-214

Spatial Navigation, 9, 11-12, 22-25, 27, 33, 85, 87-88, 92, 127, 139, 152-153, 155-157, 189, 208, 213

Synaptic Plasticity, 10, 65, 82-83, 91, 102-103, 105, 112-113, 127, 138, 178-180, 184-185, 209-210, 212-213

T

Transcranial Ultrasound, 140, 143, 147

V

Virtual Reality, 1-3, 8, 10-12, 25, 28, 155-157, 199

W

Wake Group, 231-237

Working Memory, 2, 9, 11-12, 16, 21-25, 35-36, 39, 41, 43, 45, 47, 52, 62, 81, 84-85, 89, 101, 105, 127-139, 160, 162-163, 177

www.ingramcontent.com/pod-product-compliance
Lightning Source LLC
LaVergne TN
LVHW080948210926
848485LV00004B/801

* 9 7 8 1 6 3 9 2 7 2 9 3 8 *